Textbook of Clinical Echocardiography

Textbook of Clinical Echocardiography

Second Edition

Catherine M. Otto, MD

Professor of Medicine and Director, Training Program in Cardiovascular Disease
University of Washington School of Medicine
Associate Director, Echocardiography Laboratory
Co-Director, Adult Congenital Heart Disease Clinic
University of Washington Medical Center
Seattle, Washington

W.B. SAUNDERS COMPANY
A Division of Harcourt Brace & Company
Philadelphia London Toronto Montreal Sydney Tokyo

W.B. SAUNDERS COMPANY

A Division of Harcourt Brace & Company

The Curtis Center
Independence Square West
Philadelphia, Pennsylvania 19106

Library of Congress Cataloging-in-Publication Data

Otto, Catherine M.
    Textbook of clinical echocardiography / Catherine M. Otto. — 2nd
ed.
          p.   cm.
    Includes bibliographical references and index.
    ISBN 0-7216-7669-3
    1. Echocardiography.   I. Title.
    [DNLM: 1. Echocardiography.   2. Heart Diseases—ultrasonography.
WG 141.5.E2 091t 2000]
RC683.5.U5087   2000
616.1'207543—dc21
DNLM/DLC
for Library of Congress   99-23054

TEXTBOOK OF CLINICAL ECHOCARDIOGRAPHY   ISBN 0-7216-7669-3

Printed in the United States of America

Last digit is the print number: 9   8   7   6   5   4   3   2   1

Echocardiography has become an integral part of clinical cardiology with important applications in the initial diagnosis, clinical management, and decision making for patients with a wide range of cardiovascular diseases. In addition to examinations performed in the echocardiography laboratory, echocardiographic techniques now are used in a variety of other clinical settings, including the catheterization laboratory, coronary care unit, intensive care unit, operating room, and emergency department, both for diagnosis and for monitoring the effects of therapeutic interventions. There continues to be expansion of echocardiographic applications given the detailed and precise anatomic and physiologic information that can be obtained with this technique at a relatively low cost and with minimal risk to the patient.

This textbook on general clinical echocardiography is intended to be read by individuals new to echocardiography and by those interested in updating their knowledge in this area. The text is aimed primarily at cardiology fellows on their basic echocardiography rotation but also will be of value to residents and fellows in general internal medicine, radiology, anesthesiology, and emergency medicine, as well as to cardiac sonographer students. For physicians in practice, this textbook provides a concise and practical update. A more advanced discussion of the impact of echocardiographic data in clinical medicine is available in a second book, *The Practice of Clinical Echocardiography*, CM Otto (editor), 1997, published by W.B Saunders.

After introductory chapters on practical ultrasound physics, normal tomographic transthoracic and transesophageal views, flow patterns, and indications for echocardiography, the remainder of the book is organized by disease category (for example, cardiomyopathy or valvular stenosis), emphasizing a clinical (rather than a technical) approach to echocardiographic diagnosis. In each chapter, basic principles for echocardiographic evaluation of that disease category are reviewed, the echocardiographic approach and differential diagnosis are discussed in detail, limitations and technical considerations are emphasized, and alternate diagnostic approaches are delineated. Schematic diagrams are used to illustrate basic concepts; echocardiographic images and Doppler data show typical and unusual findings in patients with each disease process. Transthoracic and transesophageal images are used throughout the text, reflecting their use in clinical practice. Tables are used frequently to summarize studies validating quantitative echocardiographic methods.

At the end of each chapter a selected list of annotated references is included. These references are suggestions for the individual who is interested in reading more about a particular subject. Additional relevant articles can be found in the suggested readings or in *The Clinical Practice of Echocardiography*. An on-line medical reference database is the best way to obtain more recent publications and to obtain a comprehensive list of all journal articles on a specific topic.

In this second edition the text of all the chapters has been revised to reflect recent advances in the field, the suggested readings have been updated, and many figures have been replaced with recent examples that more clearly illustrate the disease process. In addition, the chapter on normal anatomy and flow patterns has been expanded into two separate chapters on the normal transthoracic and the normal transesophageal examination. A recommended sequence for a complete transesophageal examination is included in this new chapter along with tables delineating the best transesophageal views for each anatomic structure.

It should be emphasized that this textbook is only a starting point or frame of reference for learning echocardiography. Appropriate training in echocardiography includes competency in the acquisition and interpretation of echocardiographic and Doppler data in real time. Additional training is needed for performance of stress and transesophageal examinations. Obviously, a textbook cannot replace the experience gained in performing studies on patients with a range of disease processes, and still photographs do not replace the need for acquisition and review of real-time data. Clearly defined guidelines for training in echocardiography have been published, as referenced in Chapter 4, that serve as guidelines for determining clinical competency in this technique. Although this textbook is not a substitute for appropriate training and experience, I hope it will enhance the learning experience of those new to the field and provide a review for those with prior training and experience.

Catherine M. Otto, MD

Acknowledgments

Special thanks go to the cardiac sonographers at the University of Washington Medical Center for acquisition of the echocardiographic figures: Caryn L. D'Jang, RDCS; Michelle C. Fujioka, RDCS; Carolyn J. Gardner, RDCS; Carol D. Kraft, RDCS; Carolyn Y. Miyake-Hull, RDCS; Scott G. Simicich, RDCS; Rebecca G. Schwaegler, RDCS; and Todd R. Zwink, RDCS. The excellent image quality is due entirely to their skill and dedication. In addition, the cardiac sonographers also contributed substantially to the text by ongoing discussions of the details of the echocardiographic examination and quantitative data analysis.

Many revisions in this second edition are the result of discussions with the Cardiology fellows during daily echocardiography interpretation sessions with special appreciation due to Robert R. Philllips, MD, and Robert B. Stewart, MD, and to my past research fellows: Ian G. Burwash, MD, Malcolm E. Legget, MD, and Brad I. Munt, MD.

Thanks are also due to the many University of Washington faculty who contributed to the preparation of this book. J. David Godwin, MD, generously provided the chest radiographs, aortogram, CT, and MRI illustrations; Dennis D. Reichenbach, MD, photographed the stenotic prosthetic valve; James H. Caldwell, MD, contributed examples of radionuclide studies; and Douglas K. Stewart, MD, provided coronary angiograms and left ventriculograms. Other individuals kindly gave permission to use previously published figures including Cornelius Rosse, MD, Daniel F. Leotta, PhD, and Gerald Basheim, MD.

Critical review of specific sections of the manuscript was provided by Gerald Basheim, MD, Carol D. Kraft, RDCS, Eric B. Larson, MD, Roy W. Martin, PhD, Donald C. Oxorn, MD, and J. Geoffrey Stevenson, MD. Their constructive comments were invaluable. The excellent anatomic illustrations of echocardiographic image planes drawn by Starr Kaplan are greatly appreciated.

A great deal of appreciation is due to Sharon A. Kemp, who bore the burden of manuscript preparation, cross-checking references, verifying figure numbers, and proofreading the galleys.

Finally, innumerable thanks are due to my family for their constant encouragement, patience, and support.

Contents

1 Principles of Echocardiographic Image Acquisition and Doppler Analysis 1

2 Transthoracic Tomographic Views, Normal Anatomy, and Flow Patterns 29

3 Transesophageal Echocardiography 59

4 Clinical Indications for Echocardiography 79

5 Echocardiographic Evaluation of Left and Right Ventricular Systolic Function 100

6 Echocardiographic Evaluation of Ventricular Diastolic Filling and Function 132

7 The Utility of Echocardiography in Patients with Ischemic Cardiac Disease 153

8 The Cardiomyopathies, Hypertensive Heart Disease, Post-Cardiac-Transplant Patient, and Pulmonary Heart Disease 183

9 Pericardial Disease: Two-Dimensional Echocardiographic and Doppler Findings . . . 213

10 Valvular Stenosis: Diagnosis, Quantitation, and Clinical Approach 229

11 Valvular Regurgitation: Diagnosis, Quantitation, and Clinical Approach 265

12 Echocardiographic Evaluation of Prosthetic Valve Dysfunction 301

13 The Role of Echocardiography in Suspected or Definite Endocarditis 329

14 Echocardiographic Evaluation of Cardiac Masses and Potential Cardiac "Source of Embolus" 351

15 Clinical Echocardiography for Diseases of the Great Vessels. 373

16 Echocardiographic Evaluation of the Adult with Congenital Heart Disease. 395

Index. 429

Color Plates 1 through 4 follow page 50

Color Plates 5 through 16 follow page 274

Color Plates 17 through 20 follow page 386

2D = two-dimensional
3D = three-dimensional
A-long = apical long-axis
A-mode = amplitude mode (amplitude versus depth)
A = late (atrial) diastolic velocity peak) or area (depends on context)
A2C = apical two-chamber
A4C = apical four-chamber
AcT = acceleration time
AF = atrial fibrillation
AMVL = anterior mitral valve leaflet
ant = anterior
Ao = aortic or aorta
AR = aortic regurgitation
AS = aortic stenosis
ASD = atrial septal defect
ASH = asymmetrical septal hypertrophy
ATVL = anterior tricuspid valve leaflet
AV = atrioventricular
AVA = aortic valve area
AVR = aortic valve replacement
BAV = balloon aortic valvuloplasty
BP = blood pressure
BS = Bjork-Shiley tilting-disk mechanical valve
BSA = body surface area
C-TGA = congenitally corrected transposition of the great arteries
C = chordae
c = propagation velocity of sound in tissue
CAD = coronary artery disease
cath = cardiac catheterization
CBV = catheter balloon valvuloplasty
Cm = specific heat of tissue
cm/s = centimeters per second
cm = centimeters
CO = cardiac output
Cont eq = continuity equation valve area
cos = cosine
CS = coronary sinus
CSA = cross-sectional area
CT = computed tomography
CW = continuous wave
Cx = circumflex coronary artery

D = diameter
D1 = first diagonal branch
D2 = second diagonal branch
DA = descending aorta
dB = decibels
dP/dt = rate of change in pressure over time
dT/dt = rate of increase in temperature
$dyne \cdot s \cdot cm^{-5}$ = units of resistance
E = early diastolic peak velocity
ECG = electrocardiogram
echo = echocardiography
ED = end-diastole
EDD = end-diastolic dimension
EDV = end-diastolic volume
EF = ejection fraction
EM-flow = volume flow rate measured by electromagnetic flowmeter
endo = endocardium
EP = electrophysiology
epi = epicardium
EPSS = E-point septal separation
ES = end-systole
ESD = end-systolic dimension
ESPVR = end-systolic pressure-volume relationship
ESV = end-systolic volume
ETT = exercise treadmill test
Δf = frequency shift
f = frequency
FL = false lumen
Fn = near field
Fo = resonance frequency
Fs = scattered frequency
FSV = forward stroke volume
Ft = transmitted frequency
fx = function
Gorlin = Gorlin formula valve area
HCM = hypertrophic cardiomyopathy
HOCM = hypertrophic obstructive cardiomyopathy
HPRF = high pulse repetition frequency
HR = heart rate
HV = hepatic vein
I = intensity of ultrasound exposure

IAS = interatrial septum
ID = indicator dilution
inf = inferior
IV = intravenous
IVC = inferior vena cava
IVCT = isovolumic contraction time
IVRT = isovolumic relaxation time
kHz = kilohertz
L = length
LA = left atrium
LAA = left atrial appendage
LAD = left anterior descending coronary artery
LAE = left atrial enlargement
LAO = left anterior oblique
lat = lateral
LCC = left coronary cusp
LLAT = left lateral
LMCA = left main coronary artery
LPA = left pulmonary artery
LSPV = left superior pulmonary vein
LV = left ventricle
LVE = left ventricular extension branch or left ventricular enlargement (depends on context)
LV-EDP = left ventricular end-diastolic pressure
LVH = left ventricular hypertrophy
LVI = left ventricular inflow
LVID = left ventricular internal dimension
LVO = left ventricular outflow
LVOT = left ventricular outflow tract
M = myxoma
M-mode = motion display (depth versus time)
MAC = mitral annular calcification
MB = moderator band
MI = myocardial infarction
MR = mitral regurgitation
MRI = magnetic resonance imaging
MS = mitral stenosis
MV = mitral valve
MVA = mitral valve area
MVL = mitral valve leaflet
MVR = mitral valve replacement
n = number of subjects
NBTE = nonbacterial thrombotic endocarditis
NCC = noncoronary cusp
OM1 = first obtuse marginal branch
OM2 = second obtuse marginal branch
ΔP = pressure gradient
P = pressure
PA = pulmonary artery
pAn = pseudoaneurysm
PAP = pulmonary artery pressure
PD = pulsed Doppler
PDA = patent ductus arteriosus or posterior descending artery (depends on context)

PE = pericardial effusion
PEP = preejection period
PET = positron-emission tomography
PISA = proximal isovelocity surface area
PLAX = parasternal long-axis
PM = papillary muscle
PMVL = posterior mitral valve leaflet
post = posterior
PR = pulmonic regurgitation
PRF = pulse repetition frequency
PRFR = peak rapid filling rate
PS = pulmonic stenosis
PSAX = parasternal short-axis
PTCA = percutaneous transluminal coronary angioplasty
PV = pulmonary vein
PVC = premature ventricular contraction
PWT = posterior wall thickness
Q = volume flow rate
Q_p = pulmonic volume flow rate
Q_s = systemic volume flow rate
r = ventricular radius or correlation coefficient (depends on context)
RA = right atrium
RAE = right atrial enlargement
RAM = random access memory
RAO = right anterior oblique
RAP = right atrial pressure
RCA = right coronary artery
RCC = right coronary cusp
Re = Reynolds number
RF = regurgitant fraction
RJ = regurgitant jet
R_o = radius of microbubble
ROA = regurgitant orifice area
RPA = right pulmonary artery
RSPV = right superior pulmonary vein
RSV = regurgitant stroke volume
RV = right ventricle
RVE = right ventricular enlargement
RVH = right ventricular hypertrophy
RVI = right ventricular inflow
RVO = right ventricular outflow
RVOT = right ventricular outflow tract
SAM = systolic anterior motion
SC = subcostal
SEE = standard error of the estimate
SPPA = spatial peak pulse average
SPTA = spatial peak temporal average
SSN = suprasternal notch
ST = septal thickness
STJ = sinotubular junction
STVL = septal tricuspid valve leaflet
SV = stroke volume or sample volume (depends on context)
SVC = superior vena cava
SWMA = segmental wall motion abnormality

$T_{1/2}$ = pressure half-time
T = thrombus
TD = thermodilution
TEE = transesophageal echocardiography
TGA = transposition of the great arteries
TGC = time gain compensation
TL = true lumen
TN = true negatives
TOF = tetralogy of Fallot
TP = true positives
TPV = time to peak velocity
TR = tricuspid regurgitation
TS = tricuspid stenosis

TSV = total stroke volume
TTE = transthoracic echocardiography
TV = tricuspid valve
v = velocity
V = volume or velocity (depends on context)
VAS = ventriculo-atrial septum
Veg = vegetation
V_{max} = maximum velocity
VSD = ventricular septal defect
VTI = velocity-time integral
WPW = Wolff-Parkinson-White syndrome
Z = acoustic impedance

Symbols	Greek Name	Used for
α	alpha	frequency
γ	gamma	viscosity
Δ	delta	difference
θ	theta	angle
λ	lambda	wavelength
μ	mu	micro-
π	pi	mathematical constant (approx. 3.14)
ρ	rho	tissue density
σ	sigma	wall stress
τ	tau	time constant of ventricular relaxation

UNITS OF MEASURE

Variable	Unit	Definition
Amplitude	dB	Decibels = a logarithmic scale describing the amplitude ("loudness") of the sound wave
Angle	degrees	Degree = $(\pi/180)$rad. Example: intercept angle
Area	cm^2	Square centimeters. A two-dimensional measurement (e.g., end-systolic area) or a calculated value (e.g., continuity equation valve area)
Frequency (f)	Hz	Hertz (cycles per second)
	kHz	Kilohertz = 1000 Hz
	MHz	Megahertz = 1,000,000 Hz
Length	cm	Centimeter (1/100 m)
	mm	Millimeter (1/1000 m or 1/10 cm)
Mass	g	Grams. Example: LV mass
Pressure	mmHg	Millimeters of mercury, 1 mmHg = 1333.2 dyne/cm^2, where dyne measures force in $cm \cdot g \cdot s^{-2}$
Resistance	$dyne \cdot s \cdot cm^{-5}$	Measure of vascular resistance
Time	s	Second
	ms	Millisecond (1/1000 s)
	μs	Microsecond

Variable	Unit	Definition
Ultrasound intensity	W/cm^2 mW/cm^2	Where watt (W) = joule per second and joule = $m^2 \cdot kg \cdot s^{-2}$ (unit of energy)
Velocity (v)	m/s cm/s	Meters per second Centimeters per second
Velocity-time integral (VTI)	cm	Integral of the Doppler velocity curve (cm/s) over time (s), in units of cm
Volume	cm^3 ml L	Cubic centimeters Milliliter, 1 ml = 1 cm^3 Liter = 1000 ml
Volume flow rate (Q)	L/min ml/s	Rate of volume flow across a valve or in cardiac output L/min = liters per minute ml/s = milliliters per second
Wall stress	$dyne/cm^2$ $kdyn/cm^2$ kPa	Units of meridional or circumferential wall stress Kilodynes per cm^2 Kilopascals where 1 kPa = 10 $kdyn/cm^2$

Principles of Echocardiographic Image Acquisition and Doppler Analysis

BASIC PRINCIPLES OF ULTRASOUND
  Ultrasound Waves
  Interaction of Ultrasound Waves with Tissues
    Reflection
    Scattering
    Refraction
    Attenuation
TRANSDUCERS
  Piezoelectric Crystal
  Types of Transducers
  Beam Shape and Focusing
  Resolution
ULTRASOUND INSTRUMENTS AND IMAGING
MODALITIES
  A-Mode/M-Mode
  2D Echocardiography
    Image Production

    Instrument Settings
    Imaging Artifacts
  3D Echocardiography
  Doppler Echocardiography
    Doppler Equation
    Spectral Analysis and Doppler Instrument
      Controls
    Continuous-Wave Doppler Ultrasound
    Pulsed Doppler Ultrasound
    Color Flow Imaging
    Doppler Artifacts
RECORDING DEVICES
EXAMINATION TECHNIQUE, EDUCATION, AND TRAINING
BIOEFFECTS AND SAFETY
  Bioeffects
  Safety
SUGGESTED READING

An understanding of the basic principles of ultrasound imaging and Doppler echocardiography is essential both during data acquisition and for correct interpretation of the ultrasound information. Although, at times, current instruments provide instantaneous images so clear and detailed that it seems as if we can "see" the heart and blood flow directly, in actuality, we always are looking at images and flow data generated by complex analyses of ultrasound waves reflected and backscattered from the patient's body. Knowledge of the strengths of this technique and, more important, its limitations is critical for correct clinical diagnosis and patient management. On the one hand, echocardiography can be used for decision making with a high degree of accuracy in a variety of clinical settings. On the other hand, if an ultrasound artifact is mistaken for an anatomic abnormality, a patient might undergo needless, expensive, and potentially risky other diagnostic tests or therapeutic interventions.

In this chapter, a brief (and necessarily simplified) overview of the basic principles of cardiac ultrasound imaging and flow analysis is presented. The reader is referred to the Suggested Reading at the end of the chapter for more information on these subjects. Since the details of image processing, artifact formation, and Doppler physics become more meaningful with experience, some readers may choose to return to this chapter after reading other sections of this book and after participating in some echocardiographic examinations.

BASIC PRINCIPLES OF ULTRASOUND

Ultrasound Waves

Sound waves are mechanical vibrations that induce alternate refractions and compressions of any physical medium through which they pass. Like other waves, sound waves are described in terms of the following (Fig. 1–1):

1. Frequency—cycles per second, or hertz (Hz)
2. Wavelength—millimeters (mm)
3. Amplitude—decibels (dB)

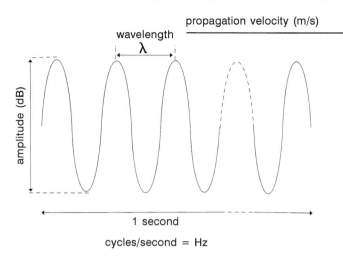

FIGURE 1–1. Schematic diagram of an ultrasound wave.

4. Velocity of propagation—which depends on each carrying medium (approximately 1540 m/s in blood)

Humans can hear sound waves with frequencies between 20 Hz and 20 kilohertz (kHz); frequencies higher than this range are termed *ultrasound.* Diagnostic medical ultrasound typically uses transducers with a frequency between 1 million and 20 million Hz or 1 and 20 megahertz (MHz).

Wavelength (λ) times frequency (*f*) equals the propagation velocity *c:*

$$c = \lambda \cdot f \qquad (1.1)$$

Since the propagation velocity in the heart is constant at 1540 m/s, the wavelength for any transducer frequency can be calculated as

$$\lambda \text{ (mm)} = 1.54/f \text{ (MHz)} \qquad (1.2)$$

as shown in Figure 1–2. Wavelength is important in diagnostic applications for at least two reasons:

1. Image resolution is no greater than 1 to 2 wavelengths (typically about 1 mm).
2. The depth of penetration of the ultrasound wave into the body is directly related to wavelength—shorter wavelengths penetrate a shorter distance than longer wavelengths.

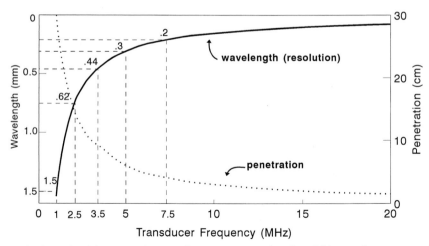

FIGURE 1–2. Graph of transducer frequency *(horizontal axis)* versus wavelength *(solid line)* and penetration *(dotted line)* of the ultrasound signal in soft tissue. Wavelength has been plotted inversely to show that resolution increases with increasing transducer frequency while penetration decreases. The specific wavelengths for transducer frequencies of 1, 2.5, 3.5, 5, and 7.5 MHz are shown.

FIGURE 1–3. Graph of the decibel scale *(horizontal axis)* showing the logarithmic relationship with the amplitude ratio *(vertical axis)*. Note that a doubling or halving of the amplitude ratio corresponds to a 6-dB change.

Thus, there is an obvious tradeoff between image resolution (shorter wavelength or higher frequency preferable) and depth penetration (longer wavelength or lower frequency preferable).

The *amplitude* (e.g., "loudness") of an ultrasound wave is described in terms of decibels. Decibels (dB) are logarithmic units based on a ratio of the measured value V of acoustic pressure to a reference value R such that

$$dB = 20 \log (V/R) \qquad (1.3)$$

Thus a ratio of 10,000 to 1 is

$$20 \times \log (10,000) = 20 \times 4 = 80 \text{ dB}$$

a ratio of 1000 to 1 is

$$20 \times \log (1000) = 20 \times 3 = 60 \text{ dB}$$

a ratio of 100 to 1 is

$$20 \times \log (100) = 20 \times 2 = 40 \text{ dB}$$

and a ratio of 2 to 1 is

$$20 \times \log (2) = 20 \times 0.3 = 6 \text{ dB}$$

A simple rule to remember is that a 6-dB change represents a doubling or halving of the signal amplitude (Fig. 1–3). The advantages of the decibel scale are that a very large range can be compressed into a smaller number of values and that low-amplitude (weak) signals can be displayed alongside very high-amplitude (strong) signals.

Interaction of Ultrasound Waves with Tissues

The interaction of ultrasound waves with the organs and tissues of the body can be described in terms of (1) reflection, (2) scattering, (3) refraction, and (4) attenuation (Fig. 1–4).

Reflection

The basis of ultrasound imaging is *reflection* of the transmitted ultrasound signal from internal structures. Ultrasound is reflected at tissue boundaries and interfaces, with the amount of ultrasound reflected dependent on the relative change in acoustic impedance between the two tissues. Acoustic impedance Z depends on

FIGURE 1–4. Diagram of the interaction between ultrasound and body tissues. Doppler analysis is based on the scattering of ultrasound in all directions from moving blood cells with a resulting change in frequency of the ultrasound received at the transducer. 2D imaging is based on reflection of ultrasound from tissue interfaces (specular reflectors). Attenuation limits the depth of ultrasound penetration. Refraction, a change in direction of the ultrasound wave, results in imaging artifacts.

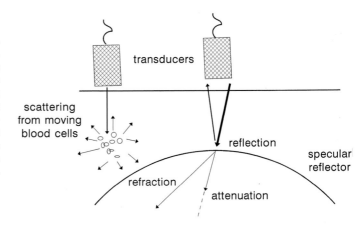

tissue density (p) and on the propagation velocity in that tissue (c):

$$Z = p \cdot c \qquad (1.4)$$

Differences in acoustic impedance largely relate to differences in tissue density, but the velocity of propagation can differ as well (e.g., bone has a propagation velocity about twice as fast as blood). Smooth tissue boundaries with a lateral dimension greater than the wavelength of the ultrasound beam act as specular, or "mirror-like," reflectors. The amount of ultrasound reflected is constant for a given interface, although the amount received back at the transducer varies with angle because (like light reflected from a mirror) the angle of incidence and reflection is equal. Optimal return of reflected ultrasound occurs at a perpendicular angle (90°). Remembering this fact is crucial for obtaining diagnostic ultrasound images. It also accounts for ultrasound "dropout" in a two-dimensional (2D) image when too little or no reflected ultrasound reaches the transducer due to a parallel alignment between the ultrasound beam and tissue interface.

Scattering

Small structures (<1 wavelength in lateral dimension) result in *scattering* of the ultrasound signal instead of reflection. Unlike a reflected beam, scattered ultrasound energy may be radiated in all directions. Only a small amount of the scattered signal reaches the receiving transducer, and the amplitude of a scattered signal is 100 to 1000 times (40–60 dB) less than the amplitude of the returned signal from a specular reflector. Scattering of ultrasound from moving blood cells is the basis of Doppler echocardiography. While some argue that the size of a single red blood cell (7–10 μm) is so much smaller (20 times) than the wavelength of ultrasound (0.2–1 mm) that it is unlikely to be an effective scatterer, most investigators consider that detectable scattering occurs due to thousands of blood cells being present in the sound beam. However, the evidence suggests that variation in hematocrit over the clinical range has little effect on the Doppler signal as used in clinical applications.

Refraction

Ultrasound waves can be *refracted*—deflected from a straight path—as they pass through a medium with a different acoustic impedance. Refraction of an ultrasound beam is analogous to refraction of light waves as they pass through a curved glass lens (e.g., prescription eyeglasses). Refraction allows enhanced image quality by using acoustic "lenses" to focus the ultrasound beam. However, refraction also occurs in unplanned ways during image formation, resulting in ultrasound artifacts, most notably the "double-image" artifact.

Attenuation

As ultrasound penetrates into the body, signal strength is progressively *attenuated* due to absorption of the ultrasound energy by conversion to heat, as well as by reflection and scattering. Overall attenuation is frequency dependent such that lower ultrasound frequencies penetrate deeper into the body than higher frequencies. The depth of penetration for adequate imaging tends to be limited to approximately 200 wavelengths. This translates roughly into a penetration depth of 30 cm for a 1-MHz transducer, 6 cm for a 5-MHz transducer, and 1.5 cm for a 20-MHz transducer, although diagnostic images at depths greater than these postulated limits can be obtained with state-of-the-art equipment.

Clinically, attenuation, as much as resolution, dictates the need for a particular transducer frequency in a specific clinical setting. For example, visualization of distal structures from the apical approach in a large adult patient requires a low-frequency transducer. From a transesophageal approach, the same structures can be imaged (at better resolution) with a higher-frequency transducer.

Attenuation also depends on acoustic impedance and on the mismatch in impedance between adjacent structures. This factor is important in transducer design so that the signal is not attenuated significantly before it leaves the transducer. It also is important during the examination. Since air has a very high acoustic impedance, any air between the transducer and the cardiac structures of interest results in substantial signal attenuation. This is avoided on transthoracic examinations by use of a water-soluble gel to form an airless contact between the transducer and the skin and on transesophageal examination by maintaining close contact between the transducer and the esophageal wall. The air-filled lungs are avoided by careful patient positioning and the use of acoustic "windows" that allow access of the ultrasound beam to the cardiac structures without intervening lung tissue. Other intrathoracic air (e.g., pneumomediastinum, residual air after cardiac surgery) results in poor ultrasound tissue penetration due to attenuation, resulting in suboptimal image quality.

TRANSDUCERS

Piezoelectric Crystal

Ultrasound transducers use a piezoelectric crystal both to generate and to receive ultrasound waves (Fig. 1–5). A piezoelectric crystal is a material (such as quartz or a titanate ceramic) with the property that an applied electric current results in alignment of polarized particles perpendicular to the face of the crystal with consequent expansion of crystal size. When an alternating electric current is applied, the crystal alternately compresses and expands, generating an ultrasound wave. The frequency that a transducer emits depends on the nature and thickness of the piezoelectric material.

Conversely, when an ultrasound wave strikes the piezoelectric crystal, an electric current is generated. Thus the crystal can serve both as a "receiver" and as a "transmitter." Basically, the ultrasound transducer transmits a brief burst of ultrasound and then switches to the "receive mode" to await the reflected ultrasound signals from the intracardiac acoustic interfaces. This cycle is repeated temporally and spatially to generate ultrasound images. Image formation is based on the *time delay* between ultrasound transmission and return of the reflected signal. Deeper structures have a longer time of flight than shallower structures, with the exact depth

calculated based on the speed of sound in blood and the time interval between the transmitted burst of ultrasound and return of the reflected signal.

The burst, or pulse, of ultrasound generated by the piezoelectric crystal is very brief, typically 1 to 6 μs, since a short pulse length results in improved axial (along the length of the beam) resolution. Damping material is used to control the ring-down time of the crystal and, hence, the pulse length. Pulse length also is determined by frequency, since a shorter time is needed for the same number of cycles at higher frequencies.

The range of frequencies contained in the pulse is described as its *frequency bandwidth*. A wider bandwidth allows better axial resolution due to the ability of the system to produce a narrow pulse. Transducer bandwidth also affects the range of frequencies that can be detected by the system with a wider bandwidth allowing better resolution of structures distant from the transducer. The stated frequency of a transducer represents the center frequency of the pulse.

Types of Transducers

The simplest type of ultrasound transducer is based on a single piezoelectric crystal (Table 1–1). Alternate pulsed transmission and reception periods allow repeated sampling along a single line, with the sampling rate limited only by the time delay needed for return of the reflected ultrasound wave from the depth of

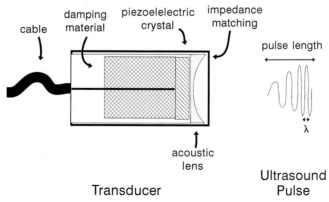

FIGURE 1–5. Schematic diagram of an ultrasound transducer. The piezoelectric crystal both produces and receives ultrasound signals, with the electric input/output transmitted to the instrument via the cable. Damping material allows a short pulse length (improved resolution). The shape of the piezoelectric crystal, an acoustic lens, or electronic focusing (with a phased-array transducer) are used to modify the beam geometry. The material of the transducer surface provides impedance matching with the skin. The ultrasound pulse length for 2D imaging is short (1–6 ms), typically consisting of two wavelengths (λ). "Ring down"—the decrease in frequency and amplitude in the pulse—depends on damping and determines bandwidth (the range of frequencies in the signal).

TABLE 1–1	**Ultrasound Transducers**

Piezoelectric Crystal Arrangements
Single (or double) crystal
Mechanical
Phased-array
Annular array

Types
Transthoracic
Transesophageal
Intravascular

Characteristics
Frequency
Focal depth
Bandwidth
Aperture ("footprint")
Power output

interest. Single nonmoving crystal transducers are used for A-mode (amplitude versus depth) or M-mode (depth versus time) cardiac recordings when a high sampling rate is desirable.

Formation of a tomographic cardiac ultrasound image is based on mechanical or electronic sweeping of the ultrasound beam across the plane of interest. This type of tomographic imaging—*sector scanning*—is used for cardiac applications, rather than a linear array of parallel ultrasound beams, to allow a faster frame rate (to show cardiac motion) and because the smaller transducer size (aperture or "footprint") fits into the narrow acoustic windows used in echocardiography. Mechanical sector scanners actually move the crystal in the transducer in either a rotational or a "wobble" fashion. Mechanical transducers have the advantage of a high signal-to-noise ratio but the disadvantages of limited Doppler capabilities and potential mechanical malfunction and now are rarely used for cardiac applications. A phased-array sector scanner consists of a series of ultrasound crystals arranged so that the beam can be electronically "steered" using combinations of the available elements. There are no moving parts prone to malfunction, and all Doppler modalities can be performed. The phased-array transducer currently is the most common type of transducer used for echocardiography.

Continuous-wave Doppler examinations use two crystals of a phased-array transducer or two separate crystals in a dedicated nonimaging transducer, with one crystal continuously transmitting and the other continuously receiving the ultrasound waves.

Beam Shape and Focusing

Beam shape and size vary predictably with distance from the transducer. However, the three-dimensional (3D) shape of the ultrasound

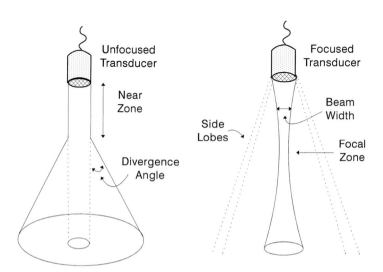

FIGURE 1–6. Schematic diagram of beam geometry for an unfocused *(left)* and focused *(right)* transducer. The length of the near zone and the divergence angle in the far field depend on transducer frequency and aperture. The focal zone of a focused transducer can be adjusted, but beam width still depends on depth. Side lobes (and grating lobes with phased-array transducers) occur with both focused and unfocused transducers and, like the central beam, are three-dimensional.

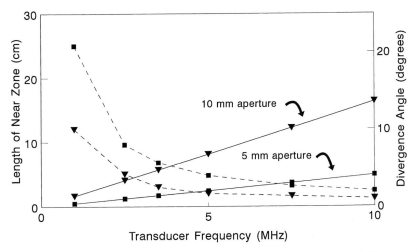

FIGURE 1–7. Graph of transducer frequency *(horizontal axis)* versus length of the near zone *(solid lines)* and divergence angle *(dashed lines)* for an unfocused 5- and 10-mm diameter aperture transducer. Equations (1.5) and (1.6) were used to generate these curves.

beam generated by a transducer is complex (Fig. 1–6) and depends on several factors, some of which can be manipulated in the design of the transducer and some of which are inherent to ultrasound physics. For an unfocused beam, the initial segment of the beam is columnar in shape (near field F_n) with a length dependent on the diameter D of the transducer face and wavelength λ:

$$F_n = D^2/4\lambda \qquad (1.5)$$

For a 3.5-MHz transducer with a 5-mm diameter aperture, this corresponds to a columnar length of 1.4 cm. Beyond this region, the ultrasound beam diverges (far field), with the angle of divergence θ determined as:

$$\sin \theta = 1.22\lambda/D \qquad (1.6)$$

This equation indicates a divergence angle of 6° beyond the near field, resulting in an ultrasound beam width of about 4.4 cm at a depth of 20 cm for this 3.5-MHz transducer. With a 10-mm diameter aperture, F_n would be 5.7 cm and beam width at 20 cm would be about 2.5 cm (Fig. 1–7).

The shape and focal depth (narrowest point) of the primary beam can be altered by making the surface of the piezoelectric crystal concave or by addition of an acoustic lens. This allows generation of a beam with optimal characteristics at the depth of most cardiac structures, but again, divergence of the beam beyond the focal zone occurs. Some transducers allow manipulation of the focal zone during the examination. Even with focusing, the ultrasound beam gen-

erated by each transducer has a lateral (azimuthal) and an elevational dimension that depends on the transducer aperture, frequency, and focusing. Beam geometry for phased-array transducers also depends on the size, spacing, and arrangement of the piezoelectric crystals in the array.

In addition to the main ultrasound beam, dispersion of ultrasound energy laterally from a single-crystal transducer results in formation of side lobes at an angle θ from the central beam where $\sin \theta = m\lambda/D$, and m is an integer describing sequential side lobes (i.e., 1, 2, 3, and so on) (Fig. 1–8). Reflected or backscattered signals from these side lobes may be received by the transducer, resulting in image or flow artifacts. With phased-array transducers, additional accessory beams termed *grating lobes* also occur as a result of constructive interference of ultrasound wave fronts (Fig. 1–9). Both the side lobes and the grating lobes affect the lateral (azimuthal) resolution of the transducer.

Resolution (Table 1–2)

Image resolution occurs for each of three dimensions: (1) *axial resolution,* that is, along the length of the ultrasound beam, (2) *lateral* or *azimuthal resolution,* that is, the resolution side to side across the 2D image, and (3) *elevational resolution,* that is, the thickness of the tomographic "slice."

Of these three, axial resolution is most precise, so quantitative measurements are made most reliably using data derived from a perpendicular alignment between the ultrasound beam

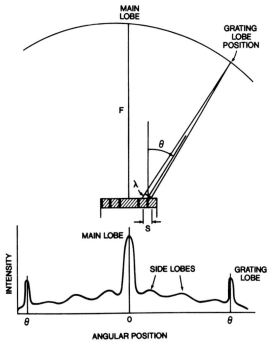

FIGURE 1–9. *(Above)* Diagram showing the position of grating lobes in phased-array transducers. The position of grating lobes is determined by the spacing between the centers of independent crystal elements in the transducer. At any point where the path length between the two crystal elements differs by one wavelength, a grating lobe is formed. The grating lobe is formed at an angle θ that depends on the wavelength λ of the crystals and spacing S between the crystal elements. *(Below)* The beam intensity plot formed at focal length F. (From Geiser EA: Chapter 25. In Skorton DJ, Schelbert AR, Wolf GL, Brundage BH (eds): Marcus Cardiac Imaging (ed 2). Philadelphia, WB Saunders, 1996, p 283.)

FIGURE 1–8. *(Above)* Diagram showing the positions at which side lobes will form. Side lobes occur at the points where the distances traversed by the ultrasound pulse from each edge of the crystal face differ by exactly one wavelength. Note that the distance from the left edge of the crystal point at point P_1 to the position of side lobe 1 is exactly one wavelength longer than the distance from point P_2 at the extreme right edge of the crystal to the position of side lobe 1. *(Below)* The beam intensity plot formed by sweeping along an arc at focal length F. (From Geiser EA: Chapter 25. In Skorton DJ, Schelbert AR, Wolf GL, Brundage BH) (eds): Marcus Cardiac Imaging (ed 2). Philadelphia, WB Saunders, 1996, p 280.)

TABLE 1–2	Determinants of Resolution in 2D Imaging

Axial Resolution
Transducer frequency
Transducer bandwidth
Pulse length

Lateral (Azimuthal) Resolution
Transducer frequency
Beam width (focusing) at each depth*
Aperture (width) of transducer
Bandwidth
Side and grating lobe levels

Elevational Resolution
Transducer frequency
Beam width in elevational plane
Side lobe levels

*Most important.

and the structure of interest (Fig. 1–10). Axial resolution depends on the transducer frequency, bandwidth, and pulse length. Since the smallest resolvable distance between two specular reflectors with conventional ultrasound is 1 wavelength, higher-frequency (shorter-wavelength) transducers have greater axial resolution. A wider bandwidth also improves resolution by allowing a shorter pulse, thus avoiding overlap between the reflected ultrasound signals from two adjacent reflectors.

FIGURE 1–10. 2D echocardiographic view of the left ventricle from a transesophageal approach at end-diastole *(above)* and end-systole *(below)*. Even with excellent image quality, as in this example, the effect of beam width can be appreciated by comparing the length of reflections from the endocardium near the transducer (point *1*) and more distal reflectors (point *2*). Note the relative "dropout" of the epicardium and endocardium when parallel to the ultrasound beam.

Lateral resolution varies with the depth of the specular reflector from the transducer, being most dependent on beam width at each depth. With a narrow beam width in the focal region, lateral resolution may approach axial resolution, and a point target will appear as a point on the 2D image. At greater depths, beam width diverges so a point target results in a reflected signal as wide as the beam width. The lack of lateral resolution at greater depths accounts for the "blurring" of the image in the far field. If the 2D image is examined carefully, progressive widening of the echo signals from similar targets along the ultrasound beam can be appreciated. Erroneous interpretations occur when the effects of beam width are not recognized. For example, beam width artifact from a strong specular reflector in the tomographic plane may appear as a linear abnormal structure. Other factors that affect lateral resolution

are transducer frequency, aperture, bandwidth, and side and grating lobe levels.

Resolution in the elevational plane is more difficult to recognize on the 2D image but is equally important in the echocardiographic examination. The thickness of the tomographic plane is variable over the 2D image, depending on transducer design and focusing, both of which affect beam width in the elevational plane at each depth. In general, cardiac ultrasound images have a "thickness" of approximately 3 to 10 mm depending on depth and the specific transducer used. The tomographic image generated by the instrument, in effect, includes reflected and backscattered signals from this entire thickness. Strong reflectors adjacent to the image plane may appear to be "in" the image plane due to elevational beam width. Even more distant strong reflectors may appear superimposed on the tomographic plane due to side lobes in the elevational plane. Examples include a calcified aortic valve appearing as a "mass" in the left atrium on apical views or a linear echo in the aortic lumen from an adjacent calcified atheroma appearing as a possible dissection flap.

ULTRASOUND INSTRUMENTS AND IMAGING MODALITIES

A-Mode/M-Mode

Historically, cardiac ultrasound began with a single-crystal transducer display of the amplitude (*A*) of reflected ultrasound versus depth on an oscilloscope screen. An A-mode display may still be shown on the 2D image screen to aid the examiner in optimal adjustment of the instrument controls. Repeated pulse transmission and receive cycles allow rapid updating of the amplitude versus depth information so that rapidly moving structures, such as the aortic or mitral valve leaflets, can be identified by their characteristic timing and pattern of motion (Fig. 1–11).

With the time dimension shown explicitly on the horizontal axis and each amplitude signal along the length of the ultrasound beam converted to a corresponding gray-scale level, a *motion (M) mode display* is produced. M-mode recordings originally were made by rolling light-sensitive paper under the brightness versus depth display. Now the M-mode data can be recorded on paper or shown on the video monitor either "scrolling" or "sweeping" across the screen at 50 to 100 mm/s. While a single-crystal transducer had to be aligned based on the M-mode output alone, 2D

FIGURE 1–11. An A-mode (along right edge) and M-mode recording of aortic root (*Ao*), left atrium (*LA*), and aortic valve motion. On the A-mode recording, the anterior and posterior aortic root (with valve closure in the center) and posterior left atrial wall are clearly identified. The rapid sampling rate of M-mode recording allows visualization of aortic valve motion. The line representing the time gain compensation curve is shown at the right of the image, superimposed on the A-mode signal.

imaging allows guidance of the M-mode beam to ensure an appropriate angle between the M line and the structures of interest.

Because only a single "line of sight" is included in an A-mode or M-mode tracing, the repetition frequency of the pulse transmission and receive phase of the transducer (the pulse repetition frequency) is limited only by the time needed for the ultrasound beam to travel to the maximum depth of interest and back to the transducer. Even a depth of 20 cm requires only 0.26 ms (given a speed of propagation of 1540 m/s), allowing a pulse frequency up to 3850 times per second. In actual practice, sampling rates of about 1800 times per second are used. This extremely high sampling rate is valuable for accurate evaluation of rapid normal intracardiac motion such as valve opening and closing. It also allows detection of high-frequency fluttering of the anterior mitral leaflet in patients with aortic regurgitation and the rapid oscillating motion of valvular vegetations. In addition, continuously moving structures, such as the ventricular endocardium, may be identified more accurately when motion versus time, as well as depth, is displayed clearly on the M-mode recording.

2D Echocardiography

Image Production

A 2D echocardiographic image is generated from the data obtained by mechanically or elec-

tronically "sweeping" the ultrasound beam across the tomographic plane. Since a finite time is needed for each scan line of data (depending on the depth of interest), the time needed to acquire all the data for one image frame is directly related to the number of scan lines. Thus there is a tradeoff between scan line density and image frame rate—the number of images per second. For cardiac applications, a high frame rate (≥30 frames per second) is desirable for accurate display of cardiac motion. This frame rate allows 33 ms per frame or 128 scan lines per 2D image at a displayed depth of 20 cm.

The reflected ultrasound signals for each scan line are received by the piezoelectric crystal and a small electric signal generated with (1) an amplitude proportional to incident angle and acoustic impedance and (2) timing proportional to distance from the transducer. This signal undergoes complex manipulation to form the final image displayed on the monitor. Typical processing includes signal amplification, time-gain compensation, filtering (to reduce noise), compression, and rectification. Envelope detection generates a bright spot for each signal along the scan line, which then undergoes analog to digital scan conversion, since the original polar coordinate data must be fit to a rectangular matrix with appropriate interpolation for missing matrix elements. This image is subject to further "postprocessing" to enhance the visual appreciation of tomographic anatomy and is displayed in "real time" (nearly simultaneous with data acquisition) on the monitor screen.

While standard ultrasound imaging is based on reflection of the fundamental transmitted frequency from tissue interfaces, *tissue harmonic imaging* instead is based on the harmonic frequency energy generated as the ultrasound signal propagates through the tissues. These harmonic frequencies result from the nonlinear effects of the interaction of ultrasound with tissue and have two properties key to generation of harmonic images. First, the strength of the harmonic signal increases with depth of propagation. Second, stronger fundamental frequencies produce stronger harmonics. Thus harmonic imaging reduces near field and side lobe artifacts and improves endocardial definition, particularly in patients with poor fundamental frequency images (Fig. 1–12). Since valves and other planar objects may appear thicker than normal with harmonic imaging, most examiners use both standard and harmonic imaging as needed throughout the examination.

FIGURE 1–12. Images obtained in an apical 4-chamber view with tissue harmonic imaging *(top)* show improved endocardial definition and reduced near field artifact compared to standard fundamental frequency images *(bottom)*.

Instrument Settings

Many of the elements in the process of image formation are features of a particular instrument that cannot be modified by the operator. Other elements can be manipulated as data are acquired ("preprocessing") or as stored data are reviewed ("postprocessing"). Incorporation of a continuous-loop digital memory to store a series (16–128) of polar images in random access memory (RAM) facilitates the evaluation of the effect of postprocessing options on the displayed image.

Standard imaging controls available in most ultrasound systems include

1. *Power output:* This control adjusts the total ultrasound energy delivered by the trans-

ducer in the transmitted bursts, thus resulting in higher-amplitude reflected signals (see "Bioeffects and Safety").

2. *Gain:* In contrast to power output, the gain control adjusts the displayed amplitude of the received signals, similar to the volume control in an audio system.

3. *Time-gain compensation (TGC):* The TGC panel allows differential adjustment of gain along the length of the ultrasound beam. Near-field gain can be set lower (since reflected signals are stronger) with a gradually increased gain over the midfield ("ramp" or "slope") and a higher gain in the far field (since reflected signals are weaker). A TGC curve is shown at the right side of Figure 1–11. On some instruments, near-field and far-field gain beyond the range of the TGC is adjusted separately.

4. *Depth:* The displayed depth affects the pulse repetition frequency and frame rate of the image, as well as allowing maximal display of the area of interest on the screen. Standard depth settings show the entire plane (from the transducer down), while "resolution" or "magnification" modes focus on a specific depth range of interest.

5. *Gray scale/dynamic range:* The number of levels of gray in the image, or *dynamic range,* can be adjusted to provide an image with marked contrast between light and dark areas or a gradation of gray levels between the lightest and darkest areas. A variation of standard gray scale is to use a color intensity for each amplitude value.

Other typical instrument controls include preprocessing and postprocessing settings that change the appearance of the displayed image. Note that image quality and resolution depend on scan-line density (as well as the factors listed in Table 1–2). Scan-line density (or frame rate or both) can be increased by using a lower depth setting or by narrowing the sector to less than the standard 60° wide image.

Imaging Artifacts (Table 1–3)

Imaging artifacts include (1) extraneous ultrasound signals that result in the appearance of "structures" that are not actually present (at least at that location), (2) failure to visualize structures that are present, and (3) an image of a structure that differs in size and/or shape from its actual appearance. Obviously, recognition of image artifacts is important for both the individual performing the study and the individual interpreting the echocardiographic data.

TABLE 1–3	Ultrasound Imaging Artifacts	
Artifact	**Mechanism**	**Example(s)**
Suboptimal image quality	Poor ultrasound tissue penetration	Body habitus (obesity, lung disease) Postcardiac surgery
Acoustic shadowing	Reflection of all the ultrasound signal by a strong specular reflector	Prosthetic valve Calcification
Reverberations	Reverberation between two strong parallel reflectors	Prosthetic valve
Beam width	Superimposition of structures within the beam profile (including side lobes) into a single tomographic image	Aortic valve "in" left atrium Atheroma "in" aortic lumen
Lateral resolution	Displayed width of a point target varies with depth	Excessive width of calcified mass or prosthetic valve
Refraction	Deviation of ultrasound signal from a straight path along the scan line	Double aortic valve or left ventricular image in short-axis view
Range ambiguity	Echo from previous pulse reaches transducer on next cycle	Second, deeper, heart image
Electronic processing	Instrument specific	Variable

The most common image "artifact" is *suboptimal image quality* due to poor ultrasound tissue penetration related to the patient's body habitus with interposition of high-impedance tissues (e.g., adipose tissue, lung, or bone) between the transducer and cardiac structures. While, strictly speaking, poor image quality is not an "artifact," a low signal-to-noise ratio makes accurate diagnosis difficult and precludes quantitative measurements. In many patients with suboptimal ultrasound penetration, image quality often is improved by use of tissue harmonic imaging. In some cases, transesophageal imaging may be needed to make an accurate diagnosis.

Acoustic shadowing (Fig. 1–13) occurs when a structure with a marked difference in acoustic impedance (e.g., prosthetic valve, calcium) blocks transmission of the ultrasound wave beyond that point. The image appears devoid of reflected signals distal to this structure, since no signal penetrates beyond the shadowing structure. The shape of the shadow (like a light shadow) follows the ultrasound path, so a small structure near the transducer casts a large shadow. When shadowing occurs, an alternate acoustic window is needed for evaluation of the area of interest. In some cases, a different transthoracic view will suffice. In other cases (e.g., prosthetic mitral valve), transesophageal imaging may be necessary.

Reverberations (Figs. 1–14 and 1–15) are multiple linear high-amplitude echo signals originating from two strong specular reflectors and resulting in a back-and-forth reflection of the ultrasound signal before it returns to the transducer. On the image, reverberations appear as relatively parallel, irregular, dense lines extending from the structure into the far field. Like acoustic shadowing, prominent reverberations limit evaluation of structures in the far field. In less dramatic cases, reverberations may

FIGURE 1–13. Example of acoustic shadowing. Transesophageal view of the left atrium and left ventricle shows shadowing *(arrow)* by mitral annular calcification.

FIGURE 1–14. Example of reverberations. Parasternal long-axis view of a mechanical aortic valve prosthesis with reverberations *(arrow)* obscuring the left atrium.

FIGURE 1–15. Reverberation artifact on transesophageal echocardiography *(top)* with the reverberation from the prominent ridge between the left atrial appendage *(large arrow)* mimicking the appearance of a mass in the left atrial appendage *(small arrow)*. M-mode *(bottom)* shows the artifact motion *(small arrow)* parallels that of the atrial ridge *(large arrow)*. With a slight change in transducer position, this artifact was no longer seen.

appear to represent abnormal structures. For example, in the parasternal long-axis view, a linear echo in the aortic root may originate as a reverberation from anterior structures (e.g., ribs) rather than representing a dissection flap.

The term *beam width artifact* is applied to two separate sources of image artifacts. First, remember that all the structures within the 3D volume of the ultrasound beam are displayed in a single tomographic plane. In the focal zone of the beam, the 3D volume is quite small and the tomographic "slice" is narrow. In the far zone, however, strong reflectors at the edge of a larger beam will be superimposed on structures in the central zone of the beam even though signal intensity falls off at the edges of the beam. In addition, strong reflectors in side lobes of the beam will be displayed in the tomographic section corresponding to the main beam. This type of beam width artifact can result in an image "showing" a calcified aortic valve in the middle of the atrium in an apical four-chamber view (Fig. 1–16).

The second type of beam width artifact is a consequence of varying lateral resolution at different imaging depths. A point target appears as a line whose length depends on the beam characteristics at that depth and the amplitude of the reflected signal. For example, the struts on a prosthetic valve can appear much longer than their actual dimension due to poor lateral resolution. Sometimes, beam width artifacts can be mistaken for abnormal structures such

FIGURE 1–16. Example of beam width artifact. Apparent "mass" in the right atrium *(arrow)* in the apical four-chamber view is beam width artifact from a calcified aortic valve.

FIGURE 1–17. Example of refraction. An overlapping double image of the aortic valve is seen in a parasternal short-axis view due to refraction of the ultrasound beam by intervening tissues. The actual *(short arrows)* and duplicate aortic valves *(long arrows)* are indicated.

as a valvular vegetation, an intracardiac mass, or an aortic dissection flap.

The appearance of a side-by-side double image results from ultrasound *refraction* as it passes through a tissue proximal to the structure of interest. This artifact often is seen in parasternal short-axis views of the aortic valve or left ventricle, where a second valve or left ventricle is "seen" medial to and partly overlapping the actual valve or left ventricle (Fig. 1–17). The explanation for this appearance is that the transmitted ultrasound beam is deviated from a straight path (the scan line) by refraction as it passes through a tissue near the transducer. When this refracted beam is reflected by the endocardium back to the transducer, the reflected signal is assumed to have originated from the scan line of the transmitted pulse (see Fig. 1–18) and thus is displayed on the image in the wrong location.

Range ambiguity occurs when echo signals from an earlier pulse cycle reach the transducer on the next "listen cycle" for that scan line, resulting in deep structures appearing closer to the transducer than their actual location. The appearance of an anatomically unexpected echo within a cardiac chamber often is due to range ambiguity, as can be demonstrated by the disappearance or a change in position of this artifact when the depth setting (and pulse-repetition frequency) is changed. Another type of range ambiguity is the appearance of an apparent second heart, deeper than the actual heart—a double image on the vertical axis. This type of range ambiguity results from echoes being re-reflected by a structure close to the transducer (such as a rib), being re-reflected by the cardiac structures and thus received at the transducer at a time *twice* normal. This artifact can be eliminated (or obscured) by decreasing the depth setting or adjusting the transducer position to a better acoustic window.

Electronic processing artifacts can be difficult to identify and vary from instrument to instrument. In addition, types of artifacts other than those listed have been described.

3D Echocardiography

While 3D echocardiography has not yet gained widespread clinical acceptance, this approach will become standard as the instrumentation is improved. There are several approaches to 3D display of echocardiographic images. One approach is to acquire images us-

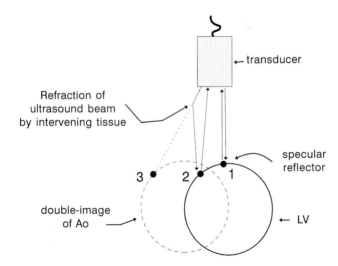

FIGURE 1–18. Schematic diagram showing the mechanism of a double-image artifact on 2D echocardiography. An ultrasound pulse reflected from point *1* of the left ventricular endocardium returns to the transducer and is shown appropriately as a bright spot in the correct position on the 2D image. Later in the scan, an ultrasound pulse is refracted by an intervening tissue so that the beam is reflected back to the transducer from point *2*. However, this reflected signal is shown along the *transmission* scan line (point *3*), since this is the presumed origin of the reflected signal.

ing a transducer that transmits and receives data simultaneously in a 3D volume. This approach has the advantage that either 3D images or 2D images in several planes can be displayed simultaneously. Currently, image quality is not ideal but is likely to improve as this technique is refined.

Another approach is to use conventional 2D imaging with a device (such as a spark-gap locator or a magnetic field locator) that identifies the 3D location of each image plane. Advantages are excellent image quality and the ability of these systems to adapt to conventional systems. However, disadvantages include nonsimultaneous 2D images from different acoustic windows and the need for 3D reconstruction of the acquired data.

Both these approaches allow display of the gray scale images in 3D from different perspectives and allow manipulation of the image data to display either 2D image planes selected after data acquisition is complete or "cutaway" 3D views to display the structures of interest. For quantitative applications, tracing of borders with reconstruction of the traced structure (such as the left ventricle) is needed.

Doppler Echocardiography

Doppler Equation

Doppler echocardiography is based on the change in frequency of the backscattered signal from small moving structures (red blood cells) intercepted by the ultrasound beam. A visual analogy is that Doppler scattering from blood is similar to scattering of light in fog, while imaging is similar to reflections from a mirror. A stationary target, if much smaller than the wavelength, will scatter ultrasound in all directions, with the frequency of the scattered signal being the same as the transmitted frequency

when observed from any direction. A moving target, however, will backscatter ultrasound to the transducer so that the frequency observed when the target is moving *toward* the transducer is higher and the frequency observed when the target is moving *away* from the transducer is lower than the original transmitted frequency (Fig. 1–19). This Doppler effect is known to all of us from audio examples of the change in sound of a car horn, siren, or train whistle as it moves toward (higher pitch) and then away (lower pitch) from the observer.

The difference in frequency between the transmitted frequency (F_T) and the scattered signal received back at the transducer (F_s) is the Doppler shift:

$$\text{Doppler shift} = (F_s - F_T) \qquad (1.7)$$

Doppler shifts are in the audible range (0–20 kHz) for intracardiac velocities using diagnostic ultrasound transducer frequencies. The relationship between the Doppler shift and blood flow velocity (v, in m/s) is expressed in the Doppler equation:

$$v = \frac{c\,(F_s - F_T)}{2\,F_T(\cos\theta)} \qquad (1.8)$$

where c is the speed of sound in blood (1540 m/s), θ is the intercept angle between the ultrasound beam and the direction of blood flow, and 2 is a factor to correct for the transit time both *to* and *from* the scattering source (Fig. 1–20).

Note that intercept angle is critically important in calculation of blood flow velocity. The cosine of an angle of 0° or 180° (parallel toward or away from the transducer) is 1, allowing this term to be ignored when the ultrasound beam is aligned parallel to the direction of blood flow. In contrast, the cosine of 90° is

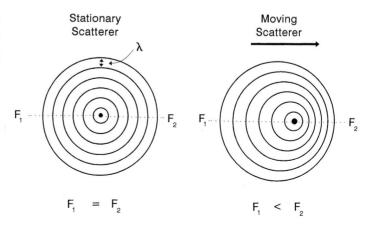

FIGURE 1–19. The Doppler effect. A stationary scatterer *(left)* scatters ultrasound symmetrically in all directions with a wavelength identical to the transmitted wavelength and with the same frequency in all directions (no Doppler shift). A moving scatterer *(right)* also scatters ultrasound symmetrically in all directions. However, the frequency will be higher when the scatterer is moving toward the transducer (F_2) than when it is moving away from the transducer (F_1) due to the movement of the scatterer resulting in waves closer together in advance of and further apart behind the moving object.

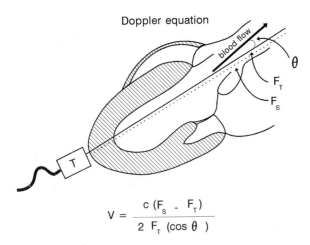

Doppler equation

$$V = \frac{c\,(F_s - F_T)}{2\,F_T\,(\cos\theta)}$$

FIGURE 1–20. The Doppler equation. The velocity V of blood flow can be calculated from the speed of sound in blood c, transducer frequency F_T, backscattered frequency F_s and the cosine of the angle θ between the ultrasound beam and direction of blood flow.

zero, indicating that no Doppler shift will be recorded if the ultrasound beam is perpendicular to blood flow.

In cardiac Doppler applications, the ultrasound beam is aligned as parallel with the direction of blood flow as possible so that the $\cos\theta$ can be assumed to be 1. Since the direction of intracardiac blood flow can be difficult to ascertain and is not predictable from the 2D image, especially with abnormal flow patterns, attempts to "correct" for intercept angle may result in significant errors in velocity calculations. Furthermore, even when blood flow direction is apparent in a 2D plane, direction in the elevational plane remains unknown. Deviation from a parallel intercept angle up to 20° results in only a 6% error in blood velocity calculation. However, a 60° intercept angle results in a 50% underestimation of flow velocity. The importance of intercept angle is particularly underlined in the setting of abnormal blood flow with high-velocity jets, such as in valvular stenosis. Note that although angle correction for the presumed direction of blood flow is used in some peripheral vascular applications, this approach is not acceptable for cardiac applications due to the likelihood that the "correction" will be erroneous.

Spectral Analysis and Doppler Instrument Controls

When the backscattered signal is received at the transducer, the difference between the transmitted and backscattered signal is determined by "comparing" the two waveforms. This is a complex process, since multiple frequencies are present in the backscattered signal. Typically, the frequency content of the signal is analyzed by a process known as a *fast Fourier transform* (FFT) that derives the component

frequencies of a complex signal. Alternate methods of frequency analysis also may be employed, such as the analog Chirp-Z method.

The display generated by this frequency analysis is termed *spectral analysis* (Fig. 1–21). By convention, this display shows time on the horizontal axis, the zero baseline in the center, and frequency shifts toward the transducer above and frequency shifts away from the transducer below the baseline. Since multiple frequencies exist at any time point, each frequency signal is displayed as a pixel on the vertical axis, with the gray (or color) scale indicat-

FIGURE 1–21. Example of a spectral Doppler display generated using a fast Fourier transform. Left ventricular inflow recorded from an apical approach is shown in the standard format. The baseline has been moved from the middle of the vertical axis to display the antegrade flow signal. Velocities toward the transducer are shown above and velocities away from the transducer below the baseline. The velocity range is determined by the Nyquist limit ($\frac{1}{2}$ PRF) with pulsed Doppler echo. Velocities are shown in shades of gray corresponding to the amplitude (decibels) of the signal.

ing the amplitude (or loudness) and the position on the vertical axis indicating the blood flow velocity (or frequency shift) component. Thus at each time point the spectral display shows (1) blood flow direction, (2) velocity (or frequency shift), and (3) signal amplitude. Each of these components is displayed at 4-ms intervals (or 250 times per second) simultaneous with data acquisition.

Pulsed and continuous-wave Doppler instrument controls typically include:

1. Power output—the electrical energy transmitted to the transducer
2. Receiver gain—the degree of amplification of returning signals
3. "Wall" or high-pass filters—elimination of low-frequency Doppler shifts due to motion of myocardium and valves (allowing only the higher frequencies to pass the filter)
4. Baseline shift—moves the zero line toward the top or bottom of the display
5. Velocity range—expands or compresses the scale (within the limits for each Doppler modality, as discussed below)
6. Postprocessing options—these often include "reject," "compression," and "dynamic range" (i.e., number of shades of gray)

In addition, pulsed Doppler controls include

7. Sample volume depth
8. Sample volume length
9. The number of sample volumes (high pulse repetition frequency Doppler echo)

The Doppler modality may be integrated with 2D imaging for each of the three major Doppler modalities: continuous-wave, pulsed, and color Doppler flow imaging. However, while color Doppler flow imaging is nearly always conjoined with 2D imaging, pulsed Doppler signal quality is optimized when the 2D image is "frozen," and continuous-wave Doppler is optimized using a dedicated, small-footprint transducer with no 2D imaging.

Continuous-Wave Doppler Ultrasound

Continuous-wave Doppler uses two ultrasound crystals—one continuously transmits and one continuously receives the ultrasound signal. The major advantage of this Doppler modality is that very high–frequency shifts (velocities) can be measured accurately since sampling is continuous. The potential disadvantage of continuous-wave Doppler is that signals from the entire length of the ultrasound beam are recorded simultaneously. However, even with overlap of flow data, a given signal often

is characteristic in timing, shape, and direction, allowing correct identification of the origin of the signal. In some cases, other methods (2D echo, color, pulsed Doppler) must be used to determine the depth of origin of the Doppler signal.

Continuous-wave Doppler optimally is performed with a dedicated, nonimaging transducer with two crystals. This type of transducer has a high signal-to-noise ratio and a small footprint, allowing it to fit into small acoustic windows (e.g., between ribs) and to be angled to obtain a parallel intercept angle between the ultrasound beam and the direction of blood flow. Use of a simultaneous imaging transducer may be helpful in some cases but signal quality may be poorer, angulation is more difficult, and the 2D image may distract the operator from optimizing the *flow* signal instead of the anatomic image (which may not coincide).

Careful technique yields a Doppler spectral signal that has a smooth contour with a well-defined edge and maximum velocity, as well as with clearly defined onset and end of flow. The audible signal is tonal and smooth. A continuous-wave Doppler velocity curve is "filled in" because lower-velocity signals proximal and distal to the point of maximum velocity also are recorded. Note that while the maximum frequency shift depends on the intercept angle between the Doppler beam and the flow of interest, amplitude (gray-scale intensity), shape, and audible quality are less dependent on intercept angle. Thus a "good quality" Doppler signal may be recorded at a nonparallel intercept angle, resulting in underestimation of flow velocity. The empirical method to ensure a parallel intercept angle is to examine the flow of interest from multiple windows with transducer angulation both in the plane of view and in the elevational plane to discover the highest-frequency shift. The highest value found is then assumed to represent a parallel intercept angle.

Pulsed Doppler Ultrasound

Pulsed Doppler echocardiography allows sampling of blood flow velocities from a specific intracardiac depth. A pulse of ultrasound is transmitted, and then, after a time interval determined by the depth of interest, the transducer briefly "samples" the backscattered signals. This transducer cycle of transmit-wait-receive is repeated at an interval termed the *pulse repetition frequency (PRF)* (Fig. 1–22). Since the "wait" interval is determined by the depth of interest—the time it takes ultrasound to travel to and from this depth—each trans-

Pulsed Doppler Ultrasound

FIGURE 1–22. With pulsed Doppler ultrasound, the transducer goes through a repetitive cycle of transmission of an ultrasound pulse at the transducer frequency (F_T), a waiting period determined by the time needed for the signal to travel to and from the depth of interest, and a receive phase when the backscattered signals are sampled. The travel-time duration determines sample volume depth. The duration of the receive phase determines sample volume.

FIGURE 1–23. Visual analogy for aliasing. The filmstrip in (**A**) shows a wheel rotating clockwise. If the frame rate of the film (or sampling rate) is halved as in (**B**), the wheel will appear to move counterclockwise when the film is played. (From Otto CM, Pearlman AS: *Echocardiography* 2:141, 1985.)

ducer cycle is longer for increasing depths. Thus the PRF also is depth dependent, being high at shallow depths and low for more distant sites.

The depth of interest in pulsed Doppler echo is called the *sample volume* because signals from a small volume of blood are sampled, with the width and height of this volume dependent on beam geometry. The length of the sample volume can be varied by adjusting the length of the transducer "receive" interval. Typically, a sample volume length of 5 mm is used to balance range resolution and signal quality, but a longer (up to 20 mm) or shorter (1–2 mm) sample volume may be useful in specific cases.

Because pulsed Doppler echo repeatedly samples the returning signal, there is a maxi-

FIGURE 1–24. The velocity of left ventricular (*LV*) outflow recorded from an apical approach exceeds the Nyquist limit so that aliasing occurs *(left)* with the appearance of the peak of the outflow curve in the reverse channel *(arrow)*. This degree of aliasing can be resolved by shifting the baseline *(right)*, in effect an electronic "cut and paste" of the spectral display.

FIGURE 1–25. In this case, LV outflow velocity exceeds 2× the Nyquist limit so that aliasing persists even after baseline shift *(left)*. The "wrapped around" peak velocity is clearly seen *(arrow)*. With high-PRF Doppler, the maximum velocity is resolved in this patient with a subaortic membrane *(right)*.

mum limit to the frequency shift (or velocity) that can be measured unambiguously. A waveform must be sampled at least twice in each cycle for accurate determination of wavelength. A visual analogy is a motion picture film of a moving wagon wheel. If the frame rate is at least twice as fast as the rotation of the wheel, the forward rotation of the wheel is "seen." If the frame rate and rotation speed are the same, the wheel will appear to stay still. Even slower frame rates result in the appearance of the wheel going backward (Fig. 1–23). This phenomenon of ambiguity in the speed and/or direction of the sampled signal is known as *signal aliasing*. In order for the frequency of an ultrasound waveform to be correctly identified, it must be sampled at least twice per wavelength. Thus the maximum detectable frequency shift (the *Nyquist limit*) is one-half the PRF.

If the velocity of interest exceeds the Nyquist limit by a small degree, signal aliasing is seen with the signal cut off at the edge of the display and the "top" of the waveform appearing in the reverse channel (Fig. 1–24). In these cases, baseline shift (in effect an electronic "cut and paste") restores the expected velocity curve and allows calculation of maximum velocity. When velocities further exceed the Nyquist limit, repeat "wraparound" of the signal occurs first into the reverse channel, then back to the forward channel, and so on. Occasionally, the shape of the waveform can be discerned (Fig. 1–25), but more often only an undifferentiated band of velocity signals can be appreciated (Fig. 1–26). Note that nonlaminar disturbed flow and aliased laminar high-velocity flow will appear (and sound) similar on spectral analysis.

Methods that can be used to resolve aliasing include (1) using continuous-wave Doppler ultrasound, (2) increasing the PRF to the maximum for that depth, (3) increasing the number of sample volumes (high-PRF Doppler), (4) using a lower-frequency transducer, or (5) shifting the baseline. Continuous-wave Doppler is the most reliable approach to resolving aliasing for very high velocities. The other approaches are useful when the aliased velocity exceeds the Nyquist limit by a modest degree (e.g., ≤ twice the Nyquist limit).

High-PRF Doppler is the deliberate use of range ambiguity to increase the maximum velocity that can be measured with pulsed Doppler echo (Fig. 1–27). When the trans-

FIGURE 1–26. Severe aliasing results in a band of frequency shifts due to multiple "wraparounds" of the velocity signal. The maximum velocity cannot be reliably identified unless continuous-wave Doppler ultrasound is used.

FIGURE 1–27. High-pulse-repetition frequency (PRF) Doppler ultrasound. High-PRF Doppler is based on the concept that with a given sample volume depth (SV_1), some ultrasound will penetrate beyond that depth. Backscattered signals from exactly twice the set depth (SV_2) will return to the transducer (T) during the receive phase of the next cycle. Thus signals from both sample volume depths are recorded simultaneously.

ducer sends out a pulse, backscattered signals from the entire length of the ultrasound beam return to the transducer. Range resolution is achieved by sampling only those signals in the short time interval corresponding to the depth of interest. However, signals from exactly twice as far away as the sample volume will reach the transducer during the "receive" phase of the next cycle. Thus signals from "harmonics" at 2×, 3×, 4×, and so on the sample volume depth, have the potential of being analyzed. Usually signal strength is low and there are few moving scatterers at these depths, so that this range ambiguity can be ig-

nored. If, instead, the sample volume is placed purposely at one-half the depth of interest, backscattered signals from this sample volume (SV_1) and a second sample volume (SV_2) twice as far away (i.e., the depth of interest) will return to the transducer during the "receive" phase (albeit one cycle later). This recording of the signal of interest at a higher PRF allows measurement of higher velocities without signal aliasing. An even higher PRF can be achieved by using additional (three or four) proximal sample volumes. Of course, the limitation of this approach is range ambiguity. The spectral analysis now includes signals from each of the sample volume depths. As with continuous-wave Doppler, the origin of the signal of interest must be determined based on ancillary data.

Color Flow Imaging

Doppler color flow imaging is based on the principles of pulsed Doppler echocardiography. However, rather than one sample volume depth along the ultrasound beam, multiple sample volumes (or multigates) are evaluated along each sampling line (Fig. 1–28). By combining data from adjacent lines, a 2D image of intracardiac flow is generated.

Along each scan line, a pulse of ultrasound is transmitted, and then the backscattered signals are received from each "gate" or sample volume along that scan line. In order to calculate accurate velocity data, several bursts along each scan line are used—typically eight—which is known as the *burst length* (Fig. 1–29). The PRF, as for conventional pulsed Doppler, is determined by the maximum depth of the Doppler signals.

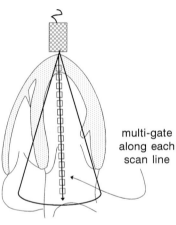

sample volume

multi-gate along each scan line

FIGURE 1–28. With pulsed Doppler, the sample volume depth is determined by the time needed for ultrasound to travel to and from the depth of interest *(left)*. With color flow imaging, multiple sample volume "gates" along each scan line are interrogated, with this process repeated for scan lines across the 2D image *(right)*.

pulsed Doppler ultrasound   color flow imaging

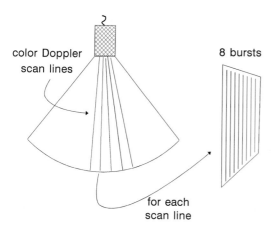

TABLE 1–4	Determinants of Color Frame Rate

Depth of sector (pulse-repetition frequency)

Sector width (number of scan lines)

Density of scan lines (number of scan lines)

Number of ultrasound bursts along each sector line (burst length)

FIGURE 1–29. Along each color Doppler scan line, several (typically eight) bursts of ultrasound are transmitted and received to allow adequate velocity resolution.

Since multiple signals are analyzed along each scan line, an audible output is not helpful and, since only a brief sample of the backscattered signal is available for analysis, an accurate spectral analysis is not possible. Instead, signals from the eight sampling lines at each position are analyzed to obtain mean velocity estimates for each sample volume along the scan line. Velocities are displayed using a color scale showing flow toward the transducer in red and flow away from the transducer in blue, with the shade of color indicating velocity up to the Nyquist limit. The option of displaying "variance" allows an additional color (usually green) to be added to indicate that the mean velocity for each of the eight bursts had excessive variability. Variance can be seen with nonlaminar disturbed flow or with laminar aliased high-velocity flow.

This process is repeated for each adjacent scan line across the image plane. Since each of these processes takes a finite amount of time depending on the speed of sound in tissue, the rapidity with which this image can be updated (the frame rate) depends on a combination of these factors (Table 1–4). During the examination, these variables may be adjusted to optimize frame rate or velocity resolution, as dictated by the specific clinical situation (Fig. 1–30).

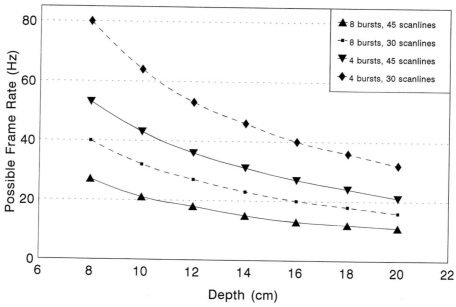

FIGURE 1–30. Graph of the maximum possible color Doppler frame rate (*y* axis) versus depth (*x* axis) for 8 or 4 bursts per scan line and 30 or 45 scan lines per frame. Note that at a depth of 16 cm, a frame rate 20 or greater can be achieved only by decreasing the burst length to 4 or narrowing the sector to 30 scan lines.

TABLE 1–5	Spectral Doppler Echo Artifacts

Artifact	Result
Nonparallel intercept angle	Underestimation of velocity
Aliasing	Inability to measure maximum velocity
Range ambiguity	Doppler signals from more than one depth along the ultrasound beam are recorded
Beam width	Overlap of Doppler signals from adjacent flows
Mirror image	Spectral display shows unidirectional flow both above and below the baseline
Electronic interference	Bandlike interference signal obscures Doppler flow
Transit-time effect	Change in the velocity of the ultrasound wave as it passes through a moving media results in slight overestimation of Doppler shifts

In addition to depth and sector scan width, color flow instrument settings typically include low-pass filter settings, gain, and power output. Most instruments provide several choices of the color "map" used to display velocity information. Velocity alone, velocity plus variance, or a power-mode display can be used. As for conventional pulsed Doppler, the zero baseline can be shifted and the PRF adjusted to vary the velocity range.

Doppler Artifacts

Spectral Doppler (Continuous Wave and Pulsed) (Table 1–5). Many Doppler artifacts are related to ultrasound physics and beam geometry, analogous to those seen with 2D imaging. Others are specific to Doppler echocardiography.

Clinically, the most important potential artifact is *velocity underestimation* due to a nonparallel intercept angle between the ultrasound beam and the direction of blood flow (Fig. 1–31). Velocity underestimation can occur with either pulsed or continuous-wave Doppler techniques and is of most concern when measuring high-velocity jets due to valve stenosis, regurgitation, or other intracardiac abnormalities. Attention to technical details with interrogation of the flow signal from multiple acoustic windows and careful angulation is needed to avoid velocity underestimation.

With pulsed Doppler echo, *signal aliasing* limits the maximum measurable velocity. If the examiner recognizes that aliasing has occurred, appropriate steps can be taken to resolve the velocity data if needed. Again the examiner needs to recognize that aliasing can be due to nonlaminar disturbed flow, as well as to high-velocity laminar flow.

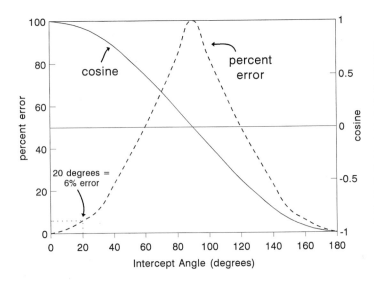

FIGURE 1–31. The importance of a parallel intercept angle between the ultrasound beam and direction of blood flow is shown. The cosine function *(solid line)* versus intercept angle *(horizontal axis)* varies from 1 at a parallel angle (0 and 180°) to 0 at a perpendicular angle (90°). The percentage error if cos θ is assumed to be 1 in the Doppler equation but, in fact, the intercept angle is *not* parallel; it varies from only 6% at a 20° angle to 50% at a 60° angle and 100% for perpendicular flows. At a perpendicular (90°) intercept angle, no blood flow velocities are recorded.

FIGURE 1–32. Doppler beam width artifact is demonstrated by the simultaneous display of superimposed aortic regurgitation *(AR)* and left ventricular *(LV)* inflow curves.

FIGURE 1–33. A mirror-image Doppler artifact with apparent weaker flow signals in the reverse channel *(arrow).*

Range ambiguity is inherent to continuous-wave Doppler but can occur with pulsed Doppler as well. With a sample volume positioned close to the transducer, strong signals from twice (or three times) the depth of the sample volume will be received in the next "receive" phase and may be misinterpreted as originating from the set sample volume depth. For example, in an apical four-chamber view, placement of a sample volume in the left ventricular apex at half the distance to the mitral annulus results in a spectral display showing the inflow signal across the mitral valve from the "second" sample volume depth. This phenomenon of range ambiguity is used constructively in the high-PRF Doppler mode.

Beam width (and side or grating lobes) affects the Doppler signal, as occurs with 2D imaging, resulting in superimposition of spatially adjacent flow signals on the spectral display. For example, left ventricular outflow and inflow may be seen on the same recording, especially with continuous-wave Doppler. Similarly, the left ventricular inflow signal may be seen superimposed on the aortic regurgitant jet (Fig. l–32).

A *mirror-image artifact* is common with spectral analysis, appearing as a symmetric signal of somewhat less intensity than the actual flow signal in the opposite direction flow channel (Fig. 1–33). Mirroring often can be reduced or eliminated by decreasing the power output or gain of the instrument. Interrogation of a flow signal from a near-perpendicular angle can result in flow signals on both sides of the baseline that must be distinguished from artifact.

Electronic interference appears as a band of signals across the spectral display that may ob-scure the flow signals. These artifacts are due to inadequate shielding of other electric instruments in the examination environment and are particularly common during studies in the intensive care unit or operating room.

The *transit time effect* is the change in propagation speed that occurs as an ultrasound wave passes through a moving medium, such as blood. This phenomenon is separate from the Doppler effect (which affects the backscattered signal) and is the basis of volume flow measurement with a transit-time flow probe. On the spectral display, the transit-time effect may result in a slight broadening of the velocity range at a given time point ("blurring" on the vertical axis), which potentially can result in slight overestimation of velocity. Some investigators argue that this should not happen, since the ultrasound signal passes through the moving blood in both directions—out (adding) and back (subtracting). In either case, this effect is insignificant clinically.

Color Doppler Flow Imaging (Table 1–6). Color flow artifacts again relate to the physics of 2D and Doppler flow image generation. *Shadowing* may be prominent distal to strong reflectors with absence of both 2D and flow data within the acoustic shadow.

Ghosting is the appearance of brief (usually one *or* two frames) large color patterns that overlay anatomic structures and do not correspond to underlying flow patterns. This artifact is caused by strong moving reflectors (such as prosthetic valve disks). Typically, this artifact is a uniform red or blue color, but it may be coded with a variance scale depending on the instrument. It is inconsistent from beat to beat.

TABLE 1–6	Color Doppler Artifacts

Artifact	Appearance
Shadowing	Absence of flow signal distal to strong reflector
Ghosting	Brief flashes of color that overlay anatomic structures and do not correlate with flow patterns
Background noise	Speckled color pattern over 2D sector due to excessive gain
Underestimation of flow signal	Loss of true flow signals due to inadequate gain
Intercept angle	Change in color (or absence at 90°) due to the angle between the flowstream and ultrasound beam across the image plane
Aliasing	"Wraparound" of color display results in a "variance" display even for laminar flow.
Electronic interference	Linear or complex color patterns across the 2D image

Color Doppler gain settings have a dramatic effect on the color flow image. Extensive gain settings result in a uniform speckled pattern across the 2D image plane due to random *background noise*. Conversely, too low a gain setting results in a smaller displayed flow area than is actually present, an effect colloquially known as "dial-a-jet." Most experienced echocardiographers recommend setting the gain level just below the level of random background noise to optimize the flow signal.

As for any Doppler technique, the *intercept angle* between the ultrasound beam and direction of blood flow *for each scan line* affects the color display in terms of both direction and velocity. Thus a uniform flow velocity traversing the image plane may appear red (toward the transducer) at one side of the sector and blue (away from the transducer) at the other edge of the sector, with a black area in the center where the flow direction is perpendicular to the ultrasound beam (Fig. 1–34).

Flow velocities that exceed the Nyquist limit at any given depth result in *signal aliasing*. Aliasing on color flow results in "wraparound" of the velocity signal, similar to that seen on a spectral display, so that an aliased velocity toward the transducer (should be red) will appear to be traveling away from the transducer (displayed in blue). Aliasing on color flow images is very common; for example, the left ventricular inflow stream appears red and then blue (due to aliasing) in the apical view (Fig. 1–35). Color aliasing can be used to advantage to quantitate flow based on the proximal isovelocity surface area method described in Chapter 11. In some cases, aliasing results in a variance display (due to an apparent range of velocities at that site),

emphasizing that a variance display does not always indicate disturbed flow.

Electronic interference on color flow displays is instrument dependent. As with other electric interference artifacts, it is most likely to occur in settings where numerous other instruments or devices are in use (e.g., operating room, intensive-care unit). Sometimes it appears as a linear multicolored band on the image along a few scan lines; sometimes more

FIGURE 1–34. Color flow in the proximal abdominal aorta showing the importance of intercept angle on the color display. Although flow in systole goes from right to left across the image plane, flow on the right side of the image appears red (since flow is directed toward the transducer) and flow on the left side of the image appears blue (since flow is directed away from the transducer). In the center, where the direction of flow is perpendicular to the ultrasound beam, no color signal (i.e., black) is seen. (See Color Plate 1, p. 50.)

FIGURE 1–35. A normal left ventricular *(LV)* inflow signal *(top)* shows aliasing from red to blue at the mitral annulus level, since the velocity exceeds the Nyquist limit of 52 cm/s. With an increase in the velocity range (to 69 cm/s) *(bottom)* aliasing no longer occurs and the *same* normal flow now appears a uniform red color. (See Color Plate 1, p. 50.)

complex patterns are seen. Caution is needed in that sometimes electronic interference results in suppression of the color flow signal. This artifact can be recognized by the absence of normal antegrade flow patterns.

RECORDING DEVICES

There are several reasons to record the echocardiographic examination, including (1) later review and/or quantitation, (2) documentation, (3) communication with the patient, referring physician, and other consultants (e.g., cardiac surgeons), (4) comparison with any future stud-

ies in that patient, and (5) clinical research. Since the entire examination may be quite lengthy, depending on the specific findings in each patient, only selected segments of the examination are recorded.

Recordings on paper can be made of M-mode, spectral Doppler, or single 2D or color flow images using a variety of page-printing devices. These recordings are of limited utility for 2D and color flow because only a single frame of information is displayed.

Video recordings are a useful method for recording data with the advantage that a large number of sequential frames can be recorded and replayed in "real time" at low cost. On videotape, the frame rate is 30 frames per second, with each frame consisting of two interlaced "fields" of information. One disadvantage of videotape is that when the tape is stopped, only one field is displayed, resulting in degradation of image quality. Other limitations of videotape are the frame rate (which is less than the achievable 2D frame rate with some ultrasound systems), image degradation in the digital-to-analog recording mode, the storage space required, and the difficulty of rapid access to different data on the same videotape. Recording video data on optical discs may obviate some of these limitations.

Digital recording and storage of echocardiographic data have the advantages of high image quality, rapid access to the data in any order, and the ability to manipulate the data in terms of image processing (such as contrast) and display formats (such as a cine-loop side-by-side display). The major limitation of digital storage is the immense amount of data contained in an echocardiographic examination (10 minutes of videotape at 30 frames per second = 18,000 image frames), which requires a combination of careful editing of the recorded data, large data storage systems, and compression of the image data (without loss of image quality). These problems have largely been resolved with current computer capacities and it is expected that most laboratories will convert to digital storage of echocardiographic examinations as cost constraints allow. Another advantage of digital storage is that selected images and cine-loops can be accessible to referring physicians using the medical center's information system.

EXAMINATION TECHNIQUE, EDUCATION, AND TRAINING

The echocardiographic examination is performed by a trained cardiac sonographer under the supervision of a qualified physician. The physician may perform all or part of the examination as well. Guidelines and recommendations for education and training in echocardiography for both sonographers and physicians have been published, as referenced in Chapter 4.

At the time of a transthoracic echocardiographic examination, the patient is positioned comfortably for each view in either a left lateral decubitus or supine position. Electrocardiographic (ECG) electrodes are attached for display of a single lead (usually lead II) on the instrument display to aid in timing cardiac events. Specially designed echocardiographic examination stretchers provide apical cutouts for optimal transducer positioning at the apex. The transducer is applied to the chest and upper abdomen using a water-soluble gel to obtain good contact without intervening air. The time needed to perform an echocardiographic examination depends on the specific clinical situation—from a few minutes in a critically ill patient to document cardiac tamponade to more than 1 hour to quantitate multiple lesions in a patient with complex valvular or congenital heart disease.

An echocardiographic examination is a technically demanding procedure, and most examiners find a significant learning curve in their ability to obtain diagnostic data. The specific examination approaches are detailed in Chapter 2 (for transthoracic) and Chapter 3 (for transesophageal) for normal anatomy and flow patterns and throughout this book for specific disease states. The examination also includes appropriate use of the echocardiographic data in patient management, as discussed in Chapter 4 and throughout the text.

BIOEFFECTS AND SAFETY

The use of ultrasound for diagnostic cardiac imaging has no known adverse biologic effects. However, ultrasound waves do have the potential to cause significant bioeffects depending on the intensity of exposure. Thus the physician and cardiac sonographer must be aware of potential bioeffects in assessing the overall safety of the procedure.

Bioeffects

Ultrasound bioeffects can be divided into three basic categories:

1. Thermal effects
2. Cavitation

3. Other (such as torque forces and microstreaming)

Thermal effects predominate with diagnostic ultrasound examinations. As the ultrasound wave passes through a tissue, heating occurs due to absorption of the mechanical energy of the sound wave. The rate of increase in temperature dT/dt depends on the absorption coefficient of the tissue for a given frequency α, the density ρ, and specific heat C_m of the tissue and the intensity I of ultrasound exposure:

$$dT/dt = 2\alpha I/\rho C_m \qquad (1.9)$$

Increases in temperature due to ultrasound exposure are offset by heat loss due to blood flow through the tissue (convective loss) and heat diffusion. More dense tissues (such as bone) heat more rapidly than less dense tissue (such as fat). However, the actual elevation in temperature for a specific tissue is difficult to predict both because of the complexity of the entire biologic system and because it is difficult to assess accurately the intensity of exposure. In addition, the actual degree of tissue heating depends on transducer frequency, focus, power output, depth, perfusion, and tissue density.

Cavitation is the creation or vibration of small gas-filled bodies by the ultrasound beam. Cavitation tends to occur only with higher-intensity exposures. Microbubbles resonate (expand and decrease in size) depending on their dimension in relation to the sound wave with a resonance frequency F_0 defined by the radius of the microbubble (R_0 in microns):

$$F_0 = 3260/R_0 \qquad (1.10)$$

Microbubbles also can be created by ultrasound by expansion of small cavitation nuclei. Cavitation has not been shown to occur with ultrasound exposure due to diagnostic ultrasound systems.

Other ultrasound bioeffects occur only with much higher exposures than occur with diagnostic ultrasound. These effects include microstreaming, torque forces, and other complex biologic effects.

Safety

The intensity I of ultrasound exposure can be expressed in several ways. The most commonly used unit of measure of intensity is power per area, where power is energy over a specific time interval:

$$\begin{aligned} I &= \text{power/area} \\ &= \text{watt/cm}^2 \end{aligned} \qquad (1.11)$$

The maximum overall intensity is then described as the highest exposure within the beam (spatial peak) averaged over the period of exposure (temporal average) and is known as the *spatial peak temporal average (SPTA) intensity.* Another common measure is the *spatial peak pulse average (SPPA),* defined as the average pulse intensity at the spatial location where the pulse intensity is maximum.

A major limitation of measuring the intensity of ultrasound exposure is that while measuring the *output* of the transducer is straightforward (e.g., in a water bath), estimating the actual tissue *exposure* is more difficult due to attenuation and other interactions with the tissue. Furthermore, tissue exposure is limited only to transmission periods and the time the ultrasound beam dwells at a specific point, both of which are considerably shorter than the total examination time. Other indices that incorporate these factors have been developed to better define the exposure levels with diagnostic ultrasound. These measures include the mechanical index (MI) and tissue thermal index (TTI) (see Suggested Reading 12 and 13).

The American Institute of Ultrasound in Medicine (AIUM) has proposed guidelines for limits *below* which ultrasound clearly has been demonstrated to be safe. These guidelines include:

1. A diagnostic exposure that produces a 1°C or less temperature elevation above normal
2. An exposure intensity less than 1 W/cm² for focused ultrasound beams

Current diagnostic ultrasound systems have outputs ranging from 10 mW/cm² (SPTA) for imaging to as high as 430 mW/cm² (SPTA) for pulsed Doppler ultrasound. There has been no evidence to date to suggest adverse effects of echocardiography at these ultrasonic outputs. Clearly, further characterization of actual tissue exposures and ongoing careful epidemiologic surveys are needed to ensure that diagnostic uses of ultrasound are safe.

While any biologic effect is likely to be small, a prudent approach is to:

1. Perform echocardiography only when indicated clinically (see Chapter 4), as part of an approved research protocol, or in appropriate teaching settings.
2. Know the power output and exposure intensity of different modalities (imaging and Doppler) of each instrument.

3. Limit the power output and exposure time as much as possible within the constraints of acquiring the necessary information.
4. Keep up to date on any new scientific findings or data relating to possible adverse effects.

SUGGESTED READING

1. Kremkau FW: Diagnostic Ultrasound: Principles and Instruments (ed 4). Philadelphia, WB Saunders, 1998.

   Basic textbook with chapters on ultrasound, transducers, imaging instruments, Doppler effect, spectral instrumentation, color-Doppler instrumentation, artifacts, and safety. Each chapter has a review section with multiple choice questions. A comprehensive examination (with answers) is included. 99 references, 590 pages.

2. Geiser EA: Echocardiography: physics and instrumentation. *In* Skorton DJ, Schelbert HR, Wolf GL, Brundage BH (eds): Marcus Cardiac Imaging: A Companion to Braunwald's Heart Disease (ed 2). Philadelphia, WB Saunders, 1996, pp 273–291.

   Advanced chapter on echocardiographic instrumentation with excellent diagrams.

3. Martin RW: Interaction of ultrasound with tissue, approaches to tissue characterization, and measurement accuracy. *In* Otto CM (ed): The Practice of Clinical Echocardiography. Philadelphia, WB Saunders, 1998, pp 113–130.

   Detailed discussion of beam patterns, ultrasound properties of tissue, scattering and measurement error. An excellent overview for the clinician. 87 references.

4. Zagebski JA: Essentials of Ultrasound Physics. St Louis, Mosby, 1996.

   Review of ultrasound physics for the beginning student. Concise text with clear schematic illustrations and tables. Topics covered include physics of diagnostic ultrasound, image storage and display, Doppler instrumentation, and bioeffects. Questions for review included with each chapter. Additional suggested readings.

5. Powis RL, Schwartz RA: Practical Doppler Ultrasound for the Clinician. Baltimore, Williams & Williams, 1991.

   Detailed but understandable book describing Doppler ultrasound techniques. An introduction to basic ultrasound principles and basic fluid dynamics also is provided.

6. Thomas JD, Rubin DN: Tissue harmonic imaging: why does it work? *J Am Soc Echocardiog* 11:803–808, 1998.

   Discussion with clear illustrations of the physical basis of tissue harmonic imaging. Contrast harmonic imaging is based on generation of harmonic frequencies by vibrating microbubbles. Tissue harmonics are generated by the nonlinear effects of ultrasound wave propagation through tissue. Instrumentation factors critical to generation of tissue harmonic images include a wide dynamic range, a narrow transmit spectrum, and a sharp receiver filter.

7. Hatle L, Angelsen B: Doppler Ultrasound in Cardiology: Physical Principles and Clinical Applications (ed 2). Philadelphia, Lea & Febiger, 1985.

   Excellent and detailed presentation on the Doppler effect, the physics of blood flow, Doppler instrumentation, and clinical applications of Doppler.

8. Stevenson JG, Otto CM: Impact of color flow Doppler physics on clinical assessment of flow abnormalities. *In* Otto CM (ed): The Practice of Clinical Echocardiography. Philadelphia, WB Saunders, 1998, pp 291–306.

   Review of the basic principles of color flow imaging, effect of instrumentation of color flow display, clinical interpretation of color flow images, and optimizing the color flow examination.

9. Harris RA, Follett DH, Halliwell M, Wells PNT: Ultimate limits in ultrasonic imaging resolution. *Ultrasound Med Biol* 17:547–558, 1991.

   Detailed review on ultrasound image resolution for readers interested in the technical details of this problem; 61 references.

10. Skorton DJ, Collins SM, Greenleaf JF, Meltzer RS, et al: Ultrasound bioeffects and regulatory issues: an introduction for the echocardiographer. *J Am Soc Echocardiogr* 1:240–251, 1988.

    Excellent review of bioeffects and safety prepared by the ASE Committee on Physics and Instrumentation.

11. Meltzer RS: Food and Drug Administration ultrasound device regulation: the output display standard, the "mechanical index" and ultrasound safety [editorial]. *J Am Soc Echocardiogr* 9:216–220, 1996.

    Brief review of ultrasound bioeffects and cavitation-related bioeffects with a discussion of the potential impact, advantages, and disadvantages of regulation of ultrasound instrument output.

12. American Institute of Ultrasound in Medicine Bioeffects Report: Bioeffects consideration for the safety of diagnostic ultrasound. *J Ultrasound Med* 7:S1–S38, 1988.

    AIUM Bioeffects Committee report of ultrasound safety and bioeffects. Detailed document with AIUM safety guidelines and discussion of thermal mechanisms, cavitation effects, epidemiologic studies, and in vivo biologic effects.

13. Frizzell LA: Conclusions regarding biological effects of ultrasound for diagnostically relevant exposures. *J Ultrasound Med* 13:69–72, 1994.

    Summary of AIUM conference held in 1992 on the Bioeffects and Safety of Diagnostic Ultrasound including definitions of the Mechanical Index (MI) and Tissue Thermal Index (TTI). Updated clinical statements are available at the AIUM web site (http:// www.aium.org).

14. Miller DL: Update on safety of diagnostic ultrasonography. *J Clin Ultrasound* 19:531–540, 1991.

    Readable review of ultrasound bioeffects; 39 references.

15. AMA Council on Scientific Affairs: Medical diagnostic ultrasound instrumentation and clinical interpretation: report of the Ultrasonography Task Force. *JAMA* 265:1155–1159, 1991.

    AMA Council on Scientific Affairs' report on diagnostic ultrasound. Review of basic principles of ultrasound with emphasis on ultrasound artifacts.

16. Barnett SB, Kossoff G, Edwards MJ: Is diagnostic ultrasound safe? Current international consensus on the thermal mechanism. *Med J Aust* 160:33–37, 1994.

    Review of the thermal effects of diagnostic ultrasound that concludes that there is no evidence of adverse effects for exposures resulting in temperatures less than 38.5°C.

17. Henderson J, Willson K, Jago JR, Whittinhgam TA: A survey of the acoustic outputs of diagnostic ultrasound equipment in current clinical use. *Ultrasound in Med Biol* 21: 699–705, 1995.

    Detailed report on the maximum acoustic power generated by 45 probes from 17 scanners using different imaging and Doppler modalities.

Transthoracic Tomographic Views, Normal Anatomy, and Flow Patterns

2

BASIC IMAGING PRINCIPLES
   Tomographic Imaging
   Nomenclature of Standard Views
   Image Orientation
   Technical Quality
   Echocardiographic Image Interpretation
TRANSTHORACIC TOMOGRAPHIC VIEWS
   Parasternal Window
      Long-Axis Views
      Right Ventricular Inflow and Outflow Views
      Short-Axis Views
   Apical Window
      Four-Chamber View
      Two-Chamber View
      Long-Axis View
      Other Apical Views
   Subcostal Window
   Suprasternal Notch Window
   Other Acoustic Windows
M-MODE RECORDINGS
   Aortic Valve and Left Atrium
   Mitral Valve
   Left Ventricle
   Other M-Mode Recordings

NORMAL INTRACARDIAC FLOW PATTERNS
   Basic Principles
      Laminar versus Disturbed Flow
      Flow-Velocity Profiles
   Clinical Quantitative Doppler Methods
      Measurement of Volume Flow
      Velocity-Pressure Relationships
      Flow Disturbances
   Normal Antegrade Intracardiac Flows
      Left Ventricular Outflow
      Right Ventricular Outflow
      Left Ventricular Inflow
      Right Ventricular Inflow
      Left Atrial Filling
      Right Atrial Filling
      Descending Aorta
   Normal Color Doppler Flow Patterns
      Impact of Color Doppler Physics on Flow Displays
      Normal Ventricular Outflow Patterns
      Normal Ventricular Inflow Patterns
      Normal Atrial Inflow Patterns
      Physiologic Valvular Regurgitation
      Technical Aspects of Color Flow Imaging
THE ECHOCARDIOGRAPHIC EXAMINATION
SUGGESTED READING

BASIC IMAGING PRINCIPLES

Tomographic Imaging

Echocardiography provides tomographic images of cardiac structures and blood flow, analogous to a thin "slice" through the heart. In contrast, angiographic techniques provide silhouette-type images; that is, structures at different distances from the imaging device are superimposed onto a single two-dimensional (2D) image. Each approach has specific advantages and disadvantages (Table 2–1). For example, a silhouette technique allows definition of the entire length of a coronary artery in a single image even though the vessel transverses numerous tomographic planes. Conversely, a single-plane right anterior oblique angiogram of the left ventricle allows assessment of regional wall motion only for those segments that form the edge of the silhouette. The lateral wall is superimposed on the opacified chamber and cannot be evaluated.

Tomographic images provide detailed anatomic data in a given image plane. However, complete evaluation of the cardiac chambers and valves requires integration of information from multiple tomographic images. Small structures that transverse numerous tomographic planes (such as the coronary arteries) are difficult to evaluate fully. Another potential problem with tomographic imaging is movement of the heart with respiration and during the cardiac cycle. Respiratory variation in cardiac location is recognized easily by its timing, but movement of the heart during the cardiac cycle is more problematic because it may not be

TABLE 2–1	Tomographic versus Silhouette Imaging	
	Tomographic	**Silhouette**
Advantages	Detailed anatomic information in a single image plane	Imaging of an entire 3D structure (such as a coronary artery)
Disadvantages	Cardiac motion Need to integrate data from multiple planes	Superimposition of structures

obvious on the 2D image. Cardiac motion relative to surrounding structures is described in three dimensions as:

1. Translation (movement of the heart as a whole in the chest)
2. Rotation (circular motion around the long axis of the left ventricle)
3. Torsion (unequal rotational motion at the apex versus the base of the left ventricle)

Even if the 2D image plane is fixed in position, the location of underlying structures may vary between systole and diastole. For example, in the apical four-chamber view, adjacent segments (which may be supplied by different coronary arteries) of the left ventricle may be seen in systole versus diastole.

Nomenclature of Standard Views (Table 2–2)

Each tomographic image is defined by its acoustic *window* (the position of the transducer) and *view* (the image plane). The standard three orthogonal echocardiographic image planes are determined by the axis of the heart itself (with the left ventricle as the major point of reference) rather than by skeletal or external body landmarks (Fig. 2–1):

1. *Long-axis plane:* Parallel to the long axis of the left ventricle and defined as an imaginary line drawn through the left ventricular apex and the center of the left ventricular base

TABLE 2–2	Transthoracic Echo Image Orientation Nomenclature

Window (Transducer Location)
Parasternal
Apical
Subcostal
Suprasternal

Image Planes
Long-axis
Short-axis
Four-chamber

2. *Short-axis plane:* Perpendicular to the long-axis view, resulting in circular cross-sectional views of the left ventricle
3. *Four-chamber plane:* Perpendicular to both long- and short-axis views, resulting in an image plane from the apex to the base intersecting the right and left ventricles and atria

Acoustic windows are transducer positions that allow ultrasound access to the cardiac structures. The bony thoracic cage and adjacent air-filled lung limit the possible acoustic windows, making patient positioning and sonographer experience critical factors in obtaining diagnostic images. Transthoracic images typically are obtained from parasternal, apical, subcostal, and suprasternal notch acoustic windows. The transducer motions used to obtain the desired view are described as follows (Figs. 2–2 and 2–3):

1. *Movement* of the transducer to a different position on the chest or in the esophagus
2. *Tilting or pointing* the transducer with a rocking motion to image different structures in the same tomographic plane
3. *Angulation* of the transducer from side to side to obtain different tomographic planes somewhat parallel to the original image plane
4. *Rotation* of the image plane at a single position to obtain intersecting tomographic planes either by manual motion of the transducer (on transthoracic imaging) or electronically (with a multiplane transesophageal transducer).

Image Orientation

Although some controversy persists regarding optimal display of echocardiographic images, most laboratories follow the American Society of Echocardiography (ASE) recommendations. The transducer position (narrowest portion of the sector scan) is shown at the top of the screen so that structures nearer to the transducer are at the top and structures farther from the transducer are at the bottom of the screen. This orientation aids in prompt recognition of ultrasound artifacts, shadowing, and re-

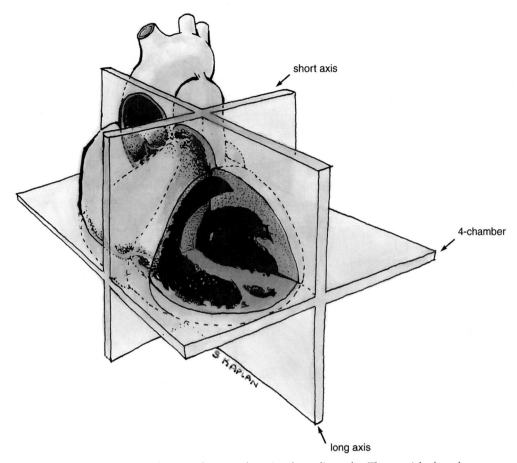

short axis

4-chamber

long axis

FIGURE 2–1. The three basic image planes used in transthoracic echocardiography. The ventricles have been cut away to show how these image planes intersect the left and right ventricles. *Dashed lines* indicate the image planes at the great vessel and atrial levels. The long-axis view extends from the left ventricular apex through the aortic valve plane. The short-axis view is perpendicular to the long-axis view resulting in a circular view of the left ventricle. The four-chamber view is perpendicular to both the long- and short-axis views and includes the left ventricular apex, right ventricle, and left and right atrium. (See Color Plate 1, p. 50.) (Courtesy Starr Kaplan, Seattle, Washington.)

verberations, since the display of the origin of the ultrasound signal is the same for all acoustic windows and image planes.

The lateral (in short-axis views) and superior (in long-axis views) cardiac structures are displayed on the right side of the screen, which is similar to the format used for other tomographic imaging techniques. Short-axis views can be thought of as the observer looking from the apex toward the cardiac base; long-axis views, as the observer looking from the left toward the right side of the heart. The four-chamber plane is displayed with lateral structures on the right side of the screen and medial structures on the left side (as for the short-axis view).

Technical Quality

Image quality is dependent on the degree of ultrasound tissue penetration, as well as on the instrument used, transducer frequency, instrument settings, and sonographer's skill. Acoustic access to the cardiac structures is determined by body habitus, specifically how the heart is positioned in the chest relative to the lungs and chest wall. Conditions that increase the separation between the transducer and the cardiac structures (e.g., adipose tissue), decrease ultrasound penetration (e.g., scar tissue), or interpose air-containing tissues between the transducer and the heart (e.g., chronic lung disease, recent cardiac surgery) lead to poor image quality. Transesophageal images tend to show better

TILT

ANGLE

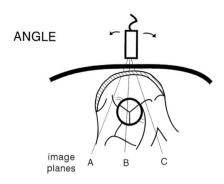

image
planes   A   B   C

ROTATE

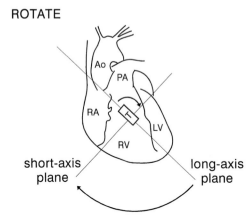

short-axis
plane   long-axis
                         plane

FIGURE 2–2. Transducer motion at a given acoustic window using the example of a left parasternal transducer position. *Tilt:* The transducer is "rocked" to provide images (*A* or *B*) in the same tomographic plane. *Angle:* Different image planes (perpendicular to the plane of the figure at lines *A, B,* and *C*) are obtained by angulation of the transducer. *Rotation:* The transducer is "twisted" with a circular motion to provide a different image plane while maintaining the same orientation between the transducer itself and the chest wall.

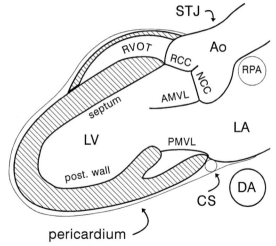

FIGURE 2–3. Schematic diagram of the parasternal long-axis view in diastole showing the aortic root *(Ao)*, sinotubular junction *(STJ)*, closed right coronary and noncoronary cusps of the aortic valve (*RCC* and *NCC*), the open anterior and posterior mitral valve leaflets (*AMVL* and *PMVL*), and the left ventricular septum and posterior wall. The medial papillary muscle has been shown for reference, although slight medial angulation is needed to visualize this structure in the long-axis view. The right ventricular outflow tract *(RVOT)* is anterior, while the coronary sinus *(CS)* in the atrioventricular groove and the descending aorta *(DA)* are seen posteriorly. The right pulmonary artery *(RPA)* lies posterior to the ascending aorta. The position of the pericardium is indicated by the thin line.

transthoracic studies, optimal patient positioning for each acoustic window brings the cardiac structures against the chest wall. In addition, respiratory variation can be used to the sonographer's advantage by having the patient suspend respiration briefly in whatever phase of the respiratory cycle that yields the best image quality. Unfortunately, even with careful attention to examination technique, echocardiographic images remain suboptimal in some patients.

Echocardiographic Image Interpretation

The physician uses the tomographic 2D echocardiographic images to build a mental three-dimensional (3D) reconstruction of the cardiac chambers and valves. To do this, an understanding of image planes and orientation and the technical aspects of image acquisition (e.g., in recognizing artifacts) is needed along with a detailed knowledge of cardiac anatomy. (A list of anatomic terminology is shown in Table 2–3.) Recording images as the tomographic plane is moved between standard image planes is important for this analysis and en-

structure definition because of greater ultrasound penetration given the shorter distance between the transducer and the cardiac structures, the use of a higher-frequency transducer, and the absence of interposed lung. On

TABLE 2–3	Terminology for Normal Echocardiographic Anatomy		
Aortic root	Sinuses of Valsalva Sinotubular junction Coronary ostia	Tricuspid valve	Anterior, septal, and posterior leaflets Chordae Commissures
Aortic valve	Right, left, and noncoronary cusps Nodules of Arantius Lambl's excrescence	Right atrium	Right atrial appendage SVC, IVC junctions Valve of IVC (Chiari network) Crista terminalis Fossa ovalis Patent foramen ovale

Mitral valve	Anterior and posterior leaflets
	Chordae (primary, secondary,
	  tertiary; basal and marginal)
	Commissures (medial and lateral)
		Left atrium	Left atrial appendage
			Superior and inferior left
			  pulmonary veins
			Superior and inferior right
			  pulmonary veins
			Ridge at junction of left atrial
			  appendage and left superior
			  pulmonary vein

Left ventricle	Wall segments (see Chapter 7) Septum, free wall Base, apex Medial and lateral papillary muscles		
Right ventricle	Inflow segment Moderator band Outflow tract (conus) Supraventricular crest Anterior, posterior, and conus papillary muscles	Pericardium	Oblique sinus Transverse sinus

SVC = Superior vena cava; IVC = inferior vena cava.

sures that abnormalities that lie outside or between our arbitrary "standard" views are not missed. In complex cases, the physician may need to perform part of the study to appreciate the 3D relationship of the different image planes. Information obtained from anatomic 2D imaging then is integrated with physiologic Doppler data and clinical information in the final echocardiographic interpretation.

TRANSTHORACIC TOMOGRAPHIC VIEWS

The normal anatomy as seen on echocardiography is described below for each tomographic view. The best views for specific cardiac structures are indicated in Table 2–4, normal changes with aging are shown in Table 2–5, and normal dimensions are shown in Table 2–6.

Parasternal Window

Long-Axis Views (Figs. 2–3 and 2–4)

With the patient in a left lateral decubitus position and the transducer in the left third or fourth intercostal space, adjacent to the sternum, a long-axis view of the heart is obtained which bisects the long axis of both aortic and mitral valves. The patient's position may need adjustment between a steep left lateral and

nearly supine position based on the images obtained in each subject. The *aortic root,* sinuses of Valsalva, sinotubular junction, and proximal 3 to 4 cm of the ascending aorta are seen in long axis. Further segments of the ascending aorta may be visualized by moving the transducer cephalad one or two interspaces. The upper limit of normal for aortic root dimensions in adults is 1.6 cm/m^2 at the annulus and 2.1 cm/m^2 at the aortic leaflet tips in systole.

In the long-axis view, the right coronary cusp of the *aortic valve* is anterior and the noncoronary cusp is posterior (the left coronary cusp is lateral to the image plane). In systole, the thin aortic leaflets open widely, assuming a parallel orientation to the aortic walls. In diastole, the leaflets are closed, with a small obtuse closure angle between the two leaflets. The leaflets appear linear from the closure line to the aortic annulus due to the hemicylindrical shape of the closed leaflets (linear along the length of the cylinder, curved along its short axis). In normal young individuals, the leaflets are so thin that only the apposed portions at the leaflets' closure line are seen. The 3D anatomy of the attachment line of the aortic leaflets to the aortic root is shaped like a crown with the three commissures attached near the tops of the sinuses of Valsalva and the midpor-

TABLE 2–4	Transthoracic Echo: Views for Specific Cardiac Structures			
Anatomic Structures	**Best Views**	**Anatomic Structures**	**Best Views**	
Aortic valve	Parasternal long-axis (PLAX) Parasternal short-axis (PSAX) Apical long-axis Anteriorly angulated apical four-chamber	Left atrium	PLAX PSAX Apical four-chamber, two-chamber, long-axis Subcostal four-chamber	
Mitral valve	PLAX PSAX-mitral valve level Apical four-chamber Apical long-axis	Right atrium	PSAX (aortic valve level) Apical four-chamber Subcostal four-chamber and short-axis	

Pulmonic valve	PSAX (aortic valve level)
	Right ventricular (RV) outflow
	Subcostal short-axis (aortic valve level)
		Aorta
		  Ascending
		
		  Arch
			High parasternal and standard parasternal long-axis
			Suprasternal notch	

Tricuspid valve	RV inflow Apical four-chamber Subcostal four-chamber and short-axis	Descending thoracic	Suprasternal notch Parasternal with angulation Apical two-chamber with modification Subcostal	
Left ventricle	PLAX PSAX Apical four-chamber, two-chamber, long-axis Subcostal four-chamber and short-axis	Interatrial septum Coronary sinus	Parasternal short-axis Subcostal four-chamber Parasternal long-axis to RV inflow view (sweep) Apical four-chamber angulated posteriorly	
Right ventricle	PLAX (RV outflow tract only) RV inflow PSAX (MV and LV levels) Apical four-chamber Subcostal four-chamber			

MV = Mitral valve; LV = left ventricle; PSAX = parasternal long axis; PLAX = parasternal short axis; RV = right ventricle.

TABLE 2–5	Echocardiographic Findings in Normal Elderly Patients
Echo Format	**Findings**
2D echo	Left and right atrial enlargement Mitral annular calcification Aortic valve fibrosis and calcification (usually without significant stenosis) Tortuosity of the aorta Prominent angle between the base of the septum and aortic root appearing as a "septal knuckle"
Doppler echo	LV inflow pattern with E < A and prolonged deceleration slope Pulmonary vein (LA inflow) pattern with increased systolic flow, reduced antegrade diastolic flow, and prominent A-wave reversal of flow

LV = Left ventricular; LA = left atrial.

tion of each leaflet attached near the base of each sinus (Fig. 2–5). This attachment line often is referred to as the aortic "annulus," although there are no distinct tissue characteristics of this attachment zone. Note that there is fibrous continuity between the aortic root and the anterior mitral leaflet. The absence of intervening myocardium between aortic and mitral valves helps identify the anatomic left ventricle in complex congenital disease.

The anterior and posterior *mitral valve* leaflets appear thin and uniform in echogenicity, with chordal attachments leading toward the medial (or posteromedial) papillary muscle seen in the long-axis view, although the papillary muscle itself is slightly medial to the long-axis plane. The anterior mitral leaflet is longer than the posterior leaflet but has a smaller annular length so that the surface areas of the two leaflets are similar (Fig. 2–6). As the mitral leaflets open in diastole, the tips separate and

TABLE 2–6	Selected Normal Echocardiographic Dimensions in Adults		
	Range	Range Indexed to BSA	Upper Limit of Normal
Aorta			
Annulus diameter (cm)	1.4–2.6	1.3 ± 0.1 cm/m²	<1.6 cm/m² (men and women)
Diameter at leaflet tips (cm)	2.2–3.6	1.7 ± 0.2 cm/m²	<2.1 cm/m² (men and women)
Ascending aorta diameter (cm)	2.1–3.4	1.5 ± 0.2 cm/m²	
Arch diameter (cm)	2.0–3.6		
Left Ventricle			
Short-axis dimension (cm)			
Diastole	3.5–6.0	2.3–3.1 cm/m²	
Systole	2.1–4.0	1.4–2.1 cm/m²	
Long-axis dimension (cm)			
Diastole	6.3–10.3	4.1–5.7 cm/m²	
Systole	4.6–8.4		
End-diastolic volume (ml)			
Men	96–157	67 ± 9 ml	
Women	59–138	61 ± 13 ml	
End-systolic volume (ml)			
Men	33–68	27 ± 5 ml	
Women	18–65	26 ± 7 ml	
Ejection fraction (%)			
Men	0.59 ± 0.06		
Women	0.58 ± 0.07		
LV-wall thickness (cm) (end-diastole)	0.6–1.1		Men ≤1.2 cm
			Women ≤1.1 cm
LV-mass (g)			
Men	<294 g	109 ± 20 g/m²	<143 g/m²
Women	<198 g	89 ± 15 g/m²	<102 g/m²
Left Atrium			
Anterior-posterior dimension (cm) (PLAX)	2.3–4.5	1.6–2.4 cm/m²	
Medial-lateral dimension (cm) (A4C)	2.5–4.5	1.6–2.4 cm/m²	
Superior-inferior dimension (cm) (A4C)	3.4–6.1	2.3–3.5 cm/m²	
Mitral Annulus			
End-diastole (cm)	2.7–0.4		
End-systole (cm)	2.9–0.3		
Right Ventricle			
Wall thickness (cm)	0.2–0.5	0.2 ± 0.05 cm/m²	
Minor dimension (cm)	2.2–4.4	1.0–2.8 cm/m²	
Length			
Diastole (cm)	5.5–9.5	3.8–5.3 cm/m²	
Systole (cm)	4.2–8.1		
Pulmonary Artery			
Annulus diameter (cm)	1.0–2.2		
Main PA (cm)	0.9–2.9		
Inferior Vena Cava Diameters			
(at RA junction) (cm)	1.2–2.3		

BSA = Body surface area; LV = left ventricle; PA = pulmonary artery; RA = right atrium.

References: Roman et al. AJC 1989 64:507; Schnittger et al. JACC 1983 2:934; Truiulzi et al. Echo 1984 1:403; Levy et al. AJC 1987 59:936; Pearlman et al. JACC 1988 12:1432; Pini et al, Circulation 1989 80:915; Erbel Dtsch Med Wschr 107:1872 (1982); Hahan et al. Z Kardiol 1982 71:445.

FIGURE 2–4. Normal parasternal long-axis 2D echo images at end-diastole *(above)* and end-systole *(below)*.

the anterior leaflet touches or comes very close to the ventricular septum. In systole, the leaflets coapt, with some overlap between the leaflets (apposition zone) and a slightly obtuse (>180°) angle relative to the mitral annulus plane. The

chordae normally remain posterior to the plane of leaflet coaptation in systole. However, some normal individuals have systolic anterior motion of the chordae, due to mild redundancy of chordal tissue that is not associated with hemodynamic abnormalities. This must be distinguished from the pathologic systolic anterior motion of the mitral leaflets seen in hypertrophic obstructive cardiomyopathy. The mitral annulus (the attachment between the mitral leaflets, left atrium, and left ventricle) is an anatomically well-defined fibrous structure with an elliptical shape. The long-axis view bisects the minor axis of the mitral annulus. (The major axis is seen in the apical four-chamber view.)

The *left atrium* is seen posterior to the aortic root with a similar anteroposterior dimension as the aortic root. The *right pulmonary artery* lies between the aortic root and superior aspect of the left atrium but may not be well seen on transthoracic images. The *coronary sinus* is seen in the atrioventricular groove posterior to the mitral annulus. Dilation of the coronary sinus due to a persistent left superior vena cava (which can be confirmed by echo-contrast injection in a left arm vein) is an occasional incidental finding of no clinical significance that can mimic a left atrial mass.

Posterior to the left atrium, the *descending thoracic aorta* is seen in cross section. A long-axis view of the descending thoracic aorta can be obtained from this window by rotating the transducer counterclockwise. Note that the oblique sinus of the pericardium lies between the left atrium and the descending thoracic

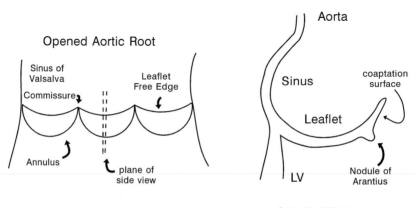

FIGURE 2–5. Schematic diagram of normal aortic valve anatomy shown in a frontal view *(left)* with the aortic root "opened" between two of the valve leaflets to demonstrate the crown-shaped "annulus." In the side view *(right)*, the commissures are near the top of each sinus so that each leaflet-sinus unit has a cuplike shape, as seen from the aortic side of the valve.

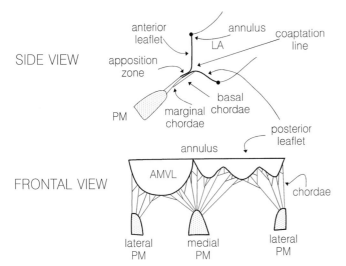

SIDE VIEW

FRONTAL VIEW

FIGURE 2–6. Schematic diagram of normal mitral valve anatomy. Definition of anatomic structures in a long-axis view *(side view)* is shown with attachments of both marginal and basal chordae. The mitral annulus has been opened *(frontal view)* between the anterior and posterior leaflets (bisecting the lateral papillary muscle) to show the relative size and shape of the two leaflets and the chordal attachments of both leaflets to both papillary muscles.

aorta so that a pericardial effusion can be seen between these two structures, while a pleural effusion will be seen only posterior to the descending thoracic aorta.

The *left ventricular* septum and posterior wall are seen at the base and midventricular level in the long-axis view, allowing assessment of wall thickness, chamber dimensions, endocardial motion, and wall thickening of these myocardial segments. From the parasternal window, the left ventricular apex is not seen—the apparent "apex" usually is an oblique image plane through the anterolateral wall.

A portion of the muscular *right ventricular outflow tract* is seen anteriorly. Unlike the symmetric prolate ellipsoid shape of the left ventricle, the right ventricle does not have an easily defined long or short axis. In effect, the right ventricle is "wrapped around" the left ventricle, with an inflow region, an apical region, and an outflow region forming a somewhat anteroposteriorly flattened U-shaped structure. Most standard image planes result in oblique tomographic sections of the right ventricle, so right ventricular size and systolic function are best evaluated from multiple views, as discussed more fully in Chapter 5.

Right Ventricular Inflow and Outflow Views

In the long-axis plane, the transducer is moved apically and then is angulated medially to obtain a view of the *right atrium, tricuspid valve,* and *right ventricle* (Fig. 2–7). In this right ventricular inflow view, the septal and anterior leaflets of the tricuspid valve are well seen. The right ventricular apex is heavily trabeculated, while the outflow tract (supracristal region) has a smoother endocardial surface. The moderator

FIGURE 2–7. Schematic *(above)* and 2D echo images *(below)* in a right ventricular inflow view showing the right ventricle *(RV)* and atrium *(RA)*, tricuspid valve *(TV)*, and ostia of the coronary sinus *(CS)* and inferior vena cava *(IVC)*.

band, a prominent muscle trabeculation that traverses the right ventricular apex obliquely and contains the right bundle branch, may be seen in both parasternal and apical views (Fig. 2–8). The papillary muscles are more difficult to identify in the right ventricle than in the left ventricle. Typically, there are two principal papillary muscles (anterior and posterior) with a smaller supracristal (or conus) papillary muscle. The moderator band attaches near the base of the anterior right ventricular papillary muscle.

The *coronary sinus* is identified as it enters the right atrium adjacent to the tricuspid annulus. By slowly scanning back to a left ventricular long-axis view, the coronary sinus can be followed along its length.

Another normal anatomic feature of the right atrium (Fig. 2–9) that may be appreciated on echocardiographic imaging is the *crista terminalis*, a muscular ridge that courses anteriorly from the superior to inferior vena cava and divides the trabeculated anterior portion of the right atrium from the posterior, smooth-walled sinus venosus segment. The right atrial appendage is rarely seen on transthoracic imaging but is a trabeculated protrusion of the right atrium extending anterior to the right atrial free wall and base of the aorta.

The *inferior vena cava* is seen entering the right atrium inferior to the coronary sinus. In some individuals, a prominent Eustachian valve is seen at the junction of the inferior vena cava and right atrium both in this view and from the subcostal window. When a more extensive fenestrated valve is present, it forms a Chiari network extending from the inferior to superior vena cava, attached to the crista terminalis posteriorly and the fossa ovalis medially, with a net-like structure that appears as mobile echos in the right atrium. Both these findings are considered normal variants of no clinical significance.

The interatrial septum is not well seen in the right ventricular inflow view, being just inferior and parallel to the image plane. However, careful angulation between the long-axis and right ventricular inflow views allows examination of the atrial septum with recognition of the thick primum septum at its junction with the central fibrous body, the thin fossa ovalis in the central portion of the atrial septum, the ridgelike limbus located superior to the fossa, and the ridge adjacent to the junction with the coronary sinus.

Moving the transducer toward the base and then angulating laterally, a long-axis view of the right ventricular outflow tract, *pulmonic valve,* and pulmonary artery is obtained. This view is particularly useful for recording flow velocities in the right ventricular outflow tract and pulmonary artery.

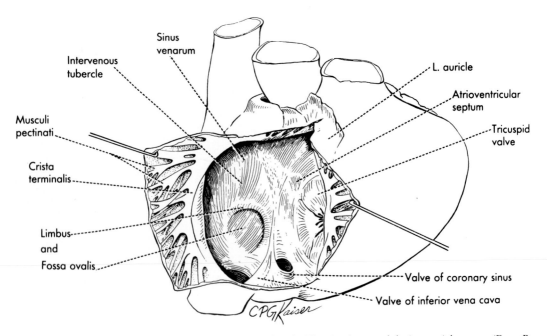

FIGURE 2–8. The interior of the right atrium seen from the right side. The view is toward the interatrial septum. (From Rosse C, Gaddum-Rosse P: Hollinshead's Textbook of Anatomy [ed 5]. Philadelphia, Lippincott-Raven, 1997, p 473.)

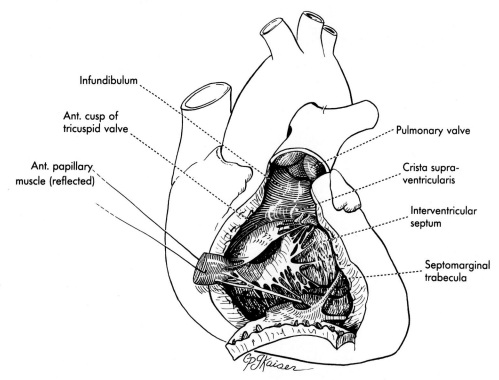

Infundibulum

Ant. cusp of
tricuspid valve

Ant. papillary
muscle (reflected)

Pulmonary valve

Crista supra-
ventricularis

Interventricular
septum

Septomarginal
trabecula

FIGURE 2–9. The interior of the right ventricle. The crista supraventricularis separates the inflow part of the ventricle from the infundibulum, or conus arteriosus. Note the great distance between the septal leaf of the tricuspid valve and the pulmonary valve. (From Rosse C, Gaddum-Rosse P: Hollinshead's Textbook of Anatomy [ed 5]. Lippincott-Raven, Philadelphia, 1997, p 473.)

Short-Axis Views

Short-axis views are obtained from the parasternal window by rotating the transducer clockwise 90° and then angulating the transducer superiorly or inferiorly to obtain specific image planes.

At the *aortic valve* level (Figs. 2–10 and 2–11), the short-axis view demonstrates all three aortic valve leaflets—right, left, and non-coronary cusps. In systole, the aortic leaflets open to a near-circular orifice. In diastole, the typical Y-shaped arrangement of the coaptation lines of the leaflets is seen. Identification of the number of aortic valve leaflets is made most accurately in systole, since a bicuspid valve may appear trileaflet in diastole due to a raphe in the position of a normal commissure. Normally, the aortic valve leaflets are thin at the base with

FIGURE 2–10. Schematic diagram of a parasternal short-axis view at the aortic valve level showing the relationship between the three cusps of the aortic valve—right coronary cusp *(RCC)*, noncoronary cusp *(NCC)*, left coronary cusp *(LCC)*—and the left atrium *(LA)*, right atrium *(RA)*, right ventricular outflow tract *(RVOT)*, and the pulmonary artery *(PA)* with right *(RPA)* and left *(LPA)* branches. The positions of the right coronary artery *(RCA)*, left main coronary artery *(LMCA)*, pulmonic valve, and tricuspid valve are shown.

FIGURE 2–11. Two-dimensional echocardiographic images at the aortic valve level in systole *(above)* and diastole *(below)*. Note the three open leaflets of the aortic valve in systole and the normal perpendicular relationship of aortic and pulmonic valves.

The close relationship between the aortic valve and other intracardiac structures is apparent in this short-axis view. In addition to the pulmonic valve and right ventricular outflow tract, which are seen anterolaterally adjacent to the left coronary cusp, portions of the tricuspid valve are seen anteriorly and slightly medially, adjacent to the right coronary cusp. The two leaflets of the tricuspid valve seen in this view are the septal and anterior leaflets.

Posteriorly, the right atrium, interatrial septum, and left atrium lie in proximity to the noncoronary cusp of the aortic valve. The left atrial appendage can be better imaged from this view by a slight lateral angulation and superior rotation of the transducer. The central location of the aortic valve illustrates how disease processes can extend from the aortic valve or root into the right ventricular outflow tract, right atrium, or left atrium. Extension of disease processes into the ventricular septum or anterior mitral leaflet also is possible, as evident in the long-axis view.

At the *mitral valve* short-axis level (Fig. 2–12), the thin anterior and posterior mitral leaflets are seen as they open nearly to the full cross-sectional area of the left ventricle in diastole and close in systole. The posterior leaflet consists of three major scallops—medial, central, and lateral—although there is considerable individual variability. The two mitral commissures—the points on the annulus where the anterior and posterior leaflets meet—are located medially and laterally. Note that this parallels the arrangement of the papillary muscles so that chordae from the medial aspects of both anterior and posterior leaflets attach to the me-

an area of thickening on the ventricular aspect in the middle of the free edge of each cusp, which serves to fill the space at the center of the closed valve. These nodules normally enlarge with age (nodules of Arantius) and can have small mobile filaments attached on the ventricular surface (Lambl's excrescences). These small but normal structures may be seen when echocardiographic images are of high quality and should not be mistaken for pathologic conditions. The origins of the left main and right coronary arteries often can be identified in this view.

The aortic and pulmonic valve planes normally lie perpendicular to each other. Thus, when the aortic valve is seen in short axis, the pulmonic valve is seen in long axis. In adults, evaluation of the leaflets of the pulmonic valve is limited; usually only one or two leaflets are seen well, and a short-axis view often is not obtainable.

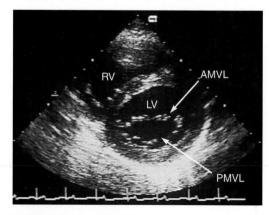

FIGURE 2–12. Short-axis 2D view at the mitral valve level showing the right ventricle *(RV)* anteriorly, the circular left ventricle *(LV)*, and the anterior *(AMVL)*, and posterior mitral valve leaflets *(PMVL)* in mid-diastole.

FIGURE 2–13. Two-dimensional echo short-axis view at the left ventricular *(LV)* papillary muscle level at end-diastole *(above)* and end-systole *(below)* showing the right ventricle *(RV)* and the medial and lateral papillary muscles. Note the circular shape of the left ventricle with symmetric wall thickening and inward endocardial motion with contraction.

dial (or posteromedial) papillary muscle and chordae from the lateral aspects of both leaflets attach to the lateral (or anterolateral) papillary muscle. Chordae branch at three levels (primary, secondary, and tertiary) between the papillary muscle tip and mitral leaflet with a progressive decrease in chordal diameter and increase in the number of chordae from approximately 12 at the papillary muscle to 120 at the mitral leaflet. Most chordae attach at the free edge of the leaflets (called *marginal chordae*), but some (called *basal chordae*) attach to the left ventricular surface of the leaflet. Occasionally, aberrant chordae to the ventricular septum or other structures are seen in an otherwise normal individual.

At the *papillary muscle* level short-axis view (Fig. 2–13), the left ventricle is seen in circular cross section. The nomenclature of left ventricular myocardial segments is discussed in Chapter 7, but basically, the ventricle is divided into

anterior (septum and free wall), lateral, posterior, and inferior (free wall and septum) segments for consistent descriptors of the location of abnormalities (Fig. 2–14).

The left ventricle typically appears circular in short axis, so that an elliptical appearance of the chamber usually is due to a nonperpendicular orientation relative to the long axis of the left ventricle. Moving the transducer superiorly with apical angulation resolves this problem. Actual distortion of the circular cross section may be seen in patients with ischemic cardiac disease, prior myocardial infarction, and aneurysm formation. The short-axis view at the papillary muscle level allows measurement of wall thickness and internal dimensions of the left ventricle in systole and diastole from either the 2D image or a 2D-guided M-mode recording. Rotating the transducer between the long- and short-axis views at this level ensures a true short-axis measurement (perpendicular to the long axis). Oblique measurements will result in overestimation of wall thickness and ventricular dimensions.

This view also allows assessment of endocardial motion and wall thickening at the midventricular level in the distribution of the left anterior descending artery (anterior septum and anterior wall), posterior descending artery (inferior septum and inferior wall), and circumflex artery (lateral and posterior walls) (see Chap. 6). Ventricular septal motion may reflect abnormalities other than coronary disease, including right ventricular volume and/or pressure overload, conduction abnormalities, and the post-cardiac-surgery state (see Fig. 5–19).

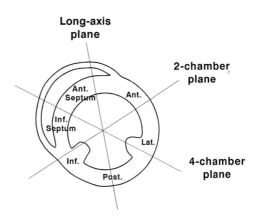

FIGURE 2–14. Relationship between the short-axis plane with left ventricular wall segments indicated, and the apical four-chamber, two-chamber, and long-axis image planes (perpendicular to the short-axis plane).

The medial and lateral papillary muscles are seen in this short-axis plane and serve as landmarks identifying the midventricular level. Rarely, one of the papillary muscles may be bifid, resulting in an appearance of three separate papillary muscles. Note that the apical segments of the left ventricular myocardium are not seen in standard parasternal views. However, in some patients, a short-axis view of the left ventricle near the apex can be obtained by moving the transducer laterally and angling medially.

Apical Window

The apical window is identified initially by palpation of the left ventricular apex with the patient in a steep left lateral decubitus position. An apical "cutout" in the examination stretcher allows optimal patient positioning and placement of the transducer on the apical impulse. Transducer position then is adjusted as needed to obtain optimal images. The relationship between the three basic apical views and the short-axis plane is shown in Figure 2–14.

Four-Chamber View (Figs. 2–15 and 2–16)

In the apical four-chamber view, the length of the *left ventricle* is seen in a plane perpendicular to both the short-axis and long-axis planes. The lateral wall, apex, and inferior septum lie in this tomographic plane. The left ventricle appears as a truncated ellipse with a longer length than width and a tapered but rounded apex. If the transducer is not positioned at the true apex, the left ventricle will appear foreshortened, with a spherical shape and little tapering of the apex. Foreshortening of the long-axis plane must be distinguished from disease processes, such as chronic aortic regurgitation, which result in increased sphericity of the ventricle. Although the right ventricle is more trabeculated than the left ventricle, prominent trabeculation also can be seen at the left ventricular apex and must be distinguished from apical thrombus. When aberrant left ventricular trabeculae transverse the ventricular chamber, a "chord" or "web" is seen on 2D echo.

Medially, the *right ventricle* is triangular in shape with a cavity about half the area of the left ventricle. The right ventricular apex is less round and more basal than the left ventricular apex. The moderator band often is seen traversing the right ventricle near the apex. The right ventricle can be further evaluated by moving the transducer medially over the right ventricular apex. Considerable individual variabil-

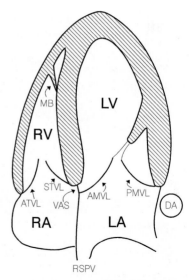

FIGURE 2–15. Schematic diagram of the apical four-chamber view showing the relationships of the left and right ventricles (*LV* and *RV*) and atria (*LA* and *RA*). In the left ventricle, the papillary muscle, chordae, and anterior and posterior mitral leaflets (*AMVL, PMVL*) are seen. The descending aorta (*DA*) is seen in partial cross section lateral to the left atrium, while the right superior pulmonary vein (*RSPV*) drains into the left atrium adjacent to the interatrial septum. In the right ventricle, the moderator band (*MB*) and the anterior and septal tricuspid valve leaflets (*ATVL* and *STVL*) are seen. Note the ventriculoatrial septum (*VAS*) separating the left ventricle from the right atrium in association with the normal, slightly more apical position of the tricuspid compared with the mitral valve annulus.

ity in the shape and wall motion of the right ventricle, particularly at the apex, is seen in normal individuals, so caution is needed in diagnosing an abnormal right ventricle from any single tomographic plane.

The four-chamber view also shows the mitral annulus in its major dimension, the anterior mitral valve leaflet (located adjacent to the septum), and the posterior mitral valve leaflet (adjacent to the lateral wall), along with chordae and attachments to the lateral papillary muscle. The mitral leaflet tips separate widely in diastole, and in systole the closure plane of the leaflets may appear "flat" (a 180° closure angle), but significant displacement of the leaflets beyond the plane of the mitral annulus is not seen unless the view is foreshortened or mitral valve disease is present.

The tricuspid annulus lies slightly (up to 1.0 cm) closer to the apex than the mitral annulus. The septal and posterior tricuspid leaflets are seen in this view with a wide diastolic opening; thin, uniformly echogenic, leaflets; and normal coaptation in systole.

FIGURE 2–16. Two-dimensional echo images in an apical four-chamber view at end-diastole *(above)* and end-systole *(below)*. Abbreviations as in Figure 2–15.

The left and right atria are distal from the apical transducer position. Although a general assessment of size and shape can be made, ultrasound resolution at this depth is poor, and detailed evaluation of atrial tumors or clots often is not possible. The interatrial septum lies parallel to the ultrasound beam in this view, so "dropout"—absence of reflected signal—from the region of the fossa ovalis is common. This should not be mistaken for an atrial septal defect.

The descending thoracic aorta may be seen lateral to the left atrium. The pulmonary veins enter the left atrium posteriorly but may be difficult to image at this depth in adults. If the transducer is angulated posteriorly from the four-chamber view, more posterior portions of the lateral and inferior septal myocardium are seen. In addition, the length of the coronary sinus comes into view in the atrioventricular groove.

Angulating the transducer anteriorly, the aortic valve and root are seen in an oblique long view. This view is sometimes referred to as the apical "five-chamber" view. More anterior portions of the septum and lateral wall are seen, especially at the base, as the transducer is angulated anteriorly. This view of the anterior mitral leaflet, left ventricular outflow tract, and aortic valve is at an angle approximately 60° to 90° from the long-axis view. In some adults, further anterior angulation of the transducer allows visualization of the pulmonary artery arising from the right ventricle. A view of the pulmonic valve from the apical window is more easily obtained in young adults and children.

Two-Chamber View (Fig. 2–17)

From the four-chamber view, the transducer is rotated counterclockwise about 60° to obtain the two-chamber view of the left ventricle, mitral valve, and left atrium. The apical two-chamber view is used for evaluation of the anterior left ventricular wall (seen to the right of

FIGURE 2–17. Apical two-chamber view showing the inferior and anterior left ventricular walls, the mitral valve, left atrium, and left atrial appendage *(LAA)*.

the screen) and the posterior wall (seen on the left). Fine adjustments in transducer position may be needed to visualize the anterior wall endocardium due to interference from adjacent lung tissue. To ensure that the proper rotation has been made for a two-chamber view, the transducer is angled posteriorly to intersect both papillary muscles symmetrically. Then the transducer is angled slightly anteriorly so that neither papillary muscle is seen in its long axis in this view. The anterior mitral leaflet is seen en face, so the apparent closure plane of the leaflet relative to the annulus can be misleading. The left atrial appendage may be visualized adjacent to the anterior wall. A long-axis view of the descending thoracic aorta can be obtained by angulating posteriorly and rotating counterclockwise from the two-chamber view.

Long-Axis View (Fig. 2–18)

Rotating the transducer another 60° from the two-chamber view (120° from the four-chamber view) yields a long-axis view similar to the parasternal long-axis view. The aortic valve, left ventricular outflow tract, and mitral valve are seen in long axis. The left ventricular walls visualized in this view are the anterior septum (on the right side of the screen) and posterior wall (on the left). Compared with the parasternal long-axis view, the left ventricular

apex now is seen, but the aortic and mitral valves are at a greater image depth (with consequent poorer image resolution).

Other Apical Views

Nonstandard short-axis views of the left ventricular apex using a higher frequency transducer (5 or 7.5 MHz) are helpful if a left ventricular apical thrombus is suspected. One useful view is obtained by sliding the transducer laterally from the left ventricular apex and then angulating medially.

Subcostal Window

With the patient supine and the legs bent at the knees (if necessary) to relax the abdominal wall musculature, subcostal images of the cardiac structures are obtained. A view of all four chambers shows the right ventricular free wall, the midsection of the interventricular septum, and the posterolateral left ventricular wall (Fig. 2–19). In this view, the interatrial septum is perpendicular to the direction of the ultrasound beam, allowing evaluation of atrial septal defects.

A subcostal short-axis view of the left ventricle allows measurements of left ventricular wall thickness and dimensions that are comparable with dimensions obtained from a parasternal short-axis view, albeit at a greater depth and through different myocardial segments. The subcostal window provides a useful alternative for qualitative and quantitative evaluation of the left ventricle when the parasternal window is inadequate.

Rotating the transducer inferiorly from the subcostal four-chamber view, a long-axis view of the inferior vena cava is obtained as it enters the right atrium. Since these 2 to 3 cm of the inferior vena cava are exposed to the negative intrapleural pressures associated with normal respiration, the size and respiratory variation of this vessel can be used to estimate right atrial pressure (see Table 5–6). The hepatic veins (particularly the central hepatic vein, which courses parallel to the ultrasound beam in this view) are helpful in assessing right atrial pressure and for recording right atrial Doppler filling patterns. The proximal abdominal aorta is imaged in long axis medial to the inferior vena cava.

Suprasternal Notch Window

With the patient supine and the neck extended, the transducer is positioned in the suprasternal notch or right supraclavicular position to obtain a view of the aortic arch in long

FIGURE 2–18. Apical long-axis view showing the left ventricle, left atrium, aorta, and aortic and mitral valves. As in the parasternal long-axis view, the posterior and anterior septal left ventricular walls are seen.

FIGURE 2–19. Schematic *(above)* and 2D echo *(below)* images from a subcostal approach showing all four cardiac chambers. The interatrial septum is perpendicular to the ultrasound beam from this window, allowing evaluation for atrial septal defects.

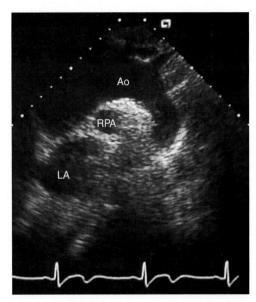

FIGURE 2–20. Schematic *(above)* and 2D echo *(below)* images of the aorta in a long-axis view from the suprasternal notch window. The ascending aortic *(Ao)* arch and descending thoracic aorta are seen with the origins of the left carotid and subclavian arteries. The right pulmonary artery *(RPA)* lies immediately inferior to the arch.

and short axis. The long-axis view (with respect to the aortic arch) shows the ascending aorta, arch, proximal descending thoracic aorta, and the origins of the right brachiocephalic and left common carotid and subclavian arteries (Fig. 2–20). The corresponding veins lie superior to the aortic arch, with the superior vena cava lying adjacent to the ascending aorta. The right pulmonary artery is seen "under" the curve of the aortic arch and can be followed to its branch point by rotating the transducer medially.

The short-axis view shows the aortic arch in cross section. The left pulmonary artery can be imaged by rotating slightly laterally. The left atrium lies inferior to the pulmonary arteries in both long- and short-axis views, so it may be possible to evaluate atrial pathology or flow disturbances from this window.

Other Acoustic Windows

In specific cases, other acoustic windows may be needed. For example, a dextropositioned heart would necessitate mirror-image acoustic windows. When a large pleural effusion is present, good-quality images may be obtained in some cases by imaging from the posterior chest wall through the effusion with the patient in a sitting position.

M-MODE RECORDINGS

Although M-mode recordings have largely been replaced by 2D imaging, M-mode recordings still have an important role in evaluation of rapid motion of cardiac structures, since the sampling rate is 1800 frames per second rather than the 30 frames per second used for 2D imaging. The rapid sampling rate also makes identification of thin moving structures, such as the left ventricular endocardium, more accurate and reproducible by showing motion as well as depth of the structure of interest. The potential disadvantage of M-mode data—a nonperpendicular orientation to the structure of interest—can be avoided by using the 2D image in two orthogonal planes to position the M-mode sampling line.

Aortic Valve and Left Atrium (Fig. 2–21)

An M-mode recording through the aortic root at the leaflet tip level shows the parallel walls of the aorta moving anteriorly in systole and posteriorly in diastole. The left atrium is posterior to the aortic root and shows filling in atrial diastole (ventricular systole) and emptying in atrial systole (ventricular diastole). Left atrial filling is largely responsible for the anterior displacement of the aortic root, so aortic root "motion" on M-mode reflects left atrium dimensions. Increased aortic root motion is seen when there is increased left atrial filling and emptying (e.g., with mitral regurgitation). Decreased aortic root motion is seen in low cardiac output states, with corresponding low volumes of atrial filling and emptying.

The aortic leaflet coaptation point is seen as a thin line in diastole. In systole, the leaflets separate rapidly and completely, forming a boxlike appearance on the M-mode recording. Fine systolic fluttering of the aortic valve leaflets may be seen in normal individuals.

Mitral Valve

An M-mode recording at the mitral valve level intercepts the anterior right ventricular wall and chamber, the interventricular septum, the anterior and posterior mitral leaflets, the posterior left ventricular wall, and the pericardium (Fig. 2–22). The coaptation point of the mitral leaflets in systole is seen as a thin line that moves slightly anteriorly during systole, paralleling the motion of the posterior wall. In early diastole, the leaflets separate widely, with the maximum early diastolic motion of the anterior leaflet termed the *E point.* Normally, there is only a small distance between the E point and the maximal posterior motion of the

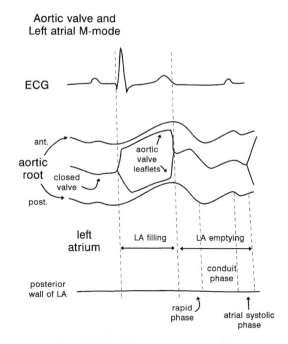

Aortic valve and Left atrial M-mode

FIGURE 2–21. Schematic *(above)* and M-mode tracing *(below)* of a normal aortic valve and left atrium. Ao = aorta; LA = left atrium.

ventricular septum—E-point septal separation (EPSS). In the absence of mitral stenosis, an increased EPSS indicates left ventricular dilation, systolic dysfunction, or aortic regurgitation.

The leaflets move together in mid-diastole (diastasis) and then separate again with atrial systole, resulting in the late-diastolic peak, the *A point.* The slope of anterior mitral leaflet closure from *A* to the closure point *(C)* is linear unless left ventricular end-diastolic pressure is elevated when a *"B bump"* or *"A-C shoulder"* may be seen on the M-mode recording of mitral valve motion. Fine fluttering of the anterior mitral leaflet is not seen in normal individuals and usually indicates aortic regurgitation.

Left Ventricle

An M-mode recording perpendicular to the long axis of and through the center of the left ventricle at the papillary muscle level provides standard measurements of systolic and diastolic wall thickness and chamber dimensions (Fig. 2–23). These measurements are limited in that they represent only a single line through the left ventricle and thus do not accurately describe the left ventricle when the disease process is asymmetric, such as with prior myocardial infarction. However, many disease processes do result in symmetric changes in the left ventricle (volume overload, hypertrophy), and the accuracy and reproducibility of these measurements make them useful in patient management. Examples of their utility include sequential evaluations of left ventricular end-systolic dimension in patients with chronic asymptomatic aortic

regurgitation or assessment of left ventricular hypertrophy in hypertensive patients.

The posterior wall endocardium is identified as the continuous line with the steepest upslope in early systole, taking care to distinguish the endocardium from reflections due to overlying mitral chordal structures. Similarly, the endocardium of the septum is identified as a continuous line with systolic inward motion. Measurements are made (using the ASE recommendations) from the leading edge of the septal endocardial echo to the leading edge of the posterior wall endocardium.

An M-mode recording at this level also may be helpful in timing the motion of the right ventricular free wall when cardiac tamponade is suspected or for detection of a small posterior pericardial effusion.

Other M-Mode Recordings

An M-mode recording through the pulmonic valve is similar to an aortic valve M-mode

FIGURE 2–22. Schematic *(above)* and M-mode tracing *(below)* of a normal mitral valve. AMVL = anterior mitral valve leaflet; PMVL = posterior mitral valve leaflet; EPSS = E-point septal separation; RV = right ventricle; LV = left ventricle.

FIGURE 2–23. Schematic *(above)* and M-mode tracing *(below)* at the left ventricular papillary muscle level. ESD = end systolic dimension; EDD = end diastolic dimension; LV = left ventricle; RV = right ventricle.

M-mode pulmonic valve

FIGURE 2–24. Patterns of pulmonic valve motion.

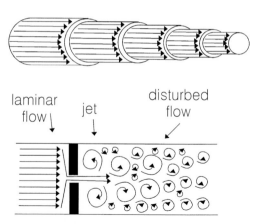

Laminar Flow

FIGURE 2–25. Laminar flow is characterized by parallel stream lines at uniform velocities with concentric layers of flow, each with a predictable and uniform direction and velocity *(above)*. Disturbed flow occurs downstream from areas of narrowing (stenotic orifice, regurgitant orifice, or intracardiac shunt) with blood flow in multiple directions and velocities *(below)*. In the orifice itself, a laminar high-velocity jet occurs.

recording except that usually only one leaflet can be recorded in adults. The slight displacement of the leaflet in diastole (after atrial contraction) is called the A wave and is increased (>7 mm) when pulmonic stenosis is present and decreased (<2 mm) when pulmonary hypertension is present. Transient midsystolic closure (or "notching") of the pulmonic valve on M-mode may be seen when pulmonary hypertension is present (Fig. 2–24).

An M-mode recording through the tricuspid valve is analogous to a mitral valve recording but rarely is useful clinically.

Use of the M-mode feature is most helpful when guided by the 2D image and used either for (1) timing of rapid cardiac motions, (2) precise measurements of cardiac dimensions, or (3) further evaluation of structures seen on 2D imaging (such as suspected vegetations) to aid in their identification.

NORMAL INTRACARDIAC FLOW PATTERNS

Basic Principles

Laminar versus Disturbed Flow (Fig. 2–25)

Normal intracardiac flow patterns are characterized by laminar flow. *Laminar flow* is defined as movement of fluid along well-defined parallel stream lines with uniform flow velocities. In three dimensions, laminar flow consists of concentric layers (or lamina) of flow, each with a predictable and uniform direction and velocity.

Steady laminar flow becomes disturbed when the dimensionless Reynolds number exceeds 2000 to 2500. The Reynolds number (Re) is directly related to blood flow velocity V, lumen diameter d, and blood density ρ and inversely related to viscosity λ:

$$\mathrm{Re} = (Vd\rho)/\lambda \qquad (2.1)$$

When blood flow patterns are disturbed, blood cells move in multiple directions at multiple velocities rather than along uniform, parallel stream lines. *Turbulence,* in fluid dynamic terms, refers to the specific situation in which the flow pattern of a particular fluid element is no longer predictable. While intracardiac flow disturbances rarely exhibit true turbulence, this term is used clinically to denote nonlaminar flow.

Flow-Velocity Profiles

The spatial distribution of velocities in cross section at a specific intracardiac location and at a specific time point in the cardiac cycle is known as the *flow-velocity profile* (Fig. 2–26). If all the parallel stream lines in a laminar flow pattern have the same velocity, then the flow-

FLOW VELOCITY PROFILES

FLAT

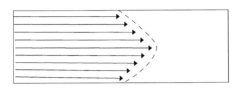

PARABOLIC

FIGURE 2–26. In a schematic longitudinal cross section of a flow stream, with the length of each arrow proportional to velocity, the difference between a flat and a parabolic flow velocity profile is shown.

velocity profile is "flat." If velocity is higher in the center of the vessel and lower at the walls of the vessel, the flow profile is "curved" (usually parabolic). While normal flow in peripheral vessels has a curved flow-velocity profile, many intracardiac flows have a relatively flat flow-velocity profile. Factors that tend to equalize the velocity distribution across the cross-sectional area of flow include tapering of the flow stream, acceleration of flow, and an inlet-type geometry. Thus the proximal aorta and pulmonary artery and the mitral and tricuspid annuli have reasonably flat flow-velocity profiles. Downstream, the spatial distribution of flow changes. For example, in the ascending aorta, the flow profile becomes skewed, with higher-velocity flow along the inside curve of the aortic arch and lower velocities along the outer curve. Many Doppler quantitative methods make assumptions about the spatial flow profile at a particular intracardiac site. In some cases, these assumptions can be verified by careful pulsed or color Doppler evaluation.

Clinical Quantitative Doppler Methods

There are three basic principles common to the clinical use of Doppler ultrasound in evaluation of cardiac disease. These will be presented briefly here and in more detail, including technical aspects and potential pitfalls, in subsequent chapters as follows: (1) measurement of volume flow in Chapter 5; (2) the relationship between velocity and pressure gradients in

Chapter 10; and (3) the concept of the 3D spatial distribution of a flow disturbance in Chapter 11.

Measurement of Volume Flow

When blood flow is laminar with a flat flow-velocity profile, it is intuitive that the instantaneous flow rate can be calculated as cross-sectional area or *CSA* (in cm^2) times flow velocity (in cm/s). Similarly, by integrating flow velocity over the duration of flow, stroke volume, *SV* (in cm^3) can be calculated as:

$$SV \text{ (cm}^3\text{)} = CSA \text{ (cm}^2\text{)} \times VTI \text{ (cm)} \quad (2.2)$$

where *VTI* is the velocity time integral (cm) of the Doppler velocity curve. This method is used clinically to measure stroke volume and cardiac output at rest or after physiologic or pharmacologic interventions, to evaluate the severity of valvular regurgitation, as a component in the equation for valve area calculations, and to quantitate the ratio of pulmonary to systemic blood flow in patients with intracardiac shunts.

Velocity-Pressure Relationships

At any area of significant narrowing in the flow stream—whether a stenotic valve, a ventricular septal defect, or a regurgitant orifice—flow velocity increases in relation to the degree of narrowing; the narrower the opening, the faster is the velocity for a given volume flow rate. In most clinical situations, the velocity in this narrow "jet" through the narrowed orifice is related quantitatively to the pressure gradient across the narrowing, as stated in the simplified Bernoulli equation:

$$\Delta P = 4v^2 \quad (2.3)$$

where ΔP is the instantaneous pressure gradient (mmHg), and v is the instantaneous velocity (m/s). This relationship between pressure gradient and velocity is important for quantitation of valve stenosis severity, noninvasive determination of pulmonary artery pressures, and evaluation of other intracardiac hemodynamics (Table 2–7) using continuous-wave Doppler ultrasound.

Flow Disturbances

Beyond an area of narrowing, disturbed flow patterns are seen. The exact location and timing of the flow disturbance allow diagnosis of valvular regurgitation, intracardiac shunts, and the anatomic level of right or left ventricular outflow obstruction. The spatial extent of the flow disturbance is helpful in evaluation of valve regurgitation. The 3D shape of the flow

TABLE 2–7	Noninvasive Hemodynamic Data Obtained by Echocardiography

Measurement	Chapter
LV systolic function	
Volume flow rate (SV, CO)	5
LV dP/dt	5
Pulmonary artery systolic pressure	5
LV diastolic function	
Filling velocities and volume flow rates	6
LV dP/dt	6
LV-EDP	6
Valve stenosis	
Pressure gradients	10
Valve areas	10
Valve regurgitation	
Regurgitant volume, fraction	11
Shunt calculations	16

LV = Left ventricular; SV = stroke volume; CO = cardiac output; dP/dt = rate of change in pressure over time; LV-EDP = left ventricular end-diastolic pressure.

TABLE 2–8	Normal Antegrade Doppler Flow Velocities

	Normal Range (m/s)
Ascending aorta	1.0–1.7
LV outflow tract	0.7–1.1
LV inflow	
E velocity	0.6–1.3 (0.72 ± 0.14)
Deceleration slope	5 ± 1.4 m/s
A velocity	0.2–0.7 (0.47 ± 0.4)
Pulmonary artery	0.5–1.3
RV inflow	
E velocity	0.3–0.7
RA filling (SVC, HV)	
Systole	0.32–0.69 (0.46 ± 0.08) m/s
Diastole	0.06–0.45 (0.27 ± 0.08) m/s
LA filling (pulmonary vein)	
Systole	0.56 ± 0.13 m/s
Diastole	0.44 ± 0.16 m/s
Atrial reversal	0.32 ± 0.07 m/s

LV = Left ventricular; E = early diastolic peak; A = late (atrial) diastolic peak; RV = right ventricular; RA = right atrial; SVC = superior vena cava; HV = hepatic vein; LA = left atrial.

References: Wilson et al. Br Heart J 53:451, 1985; Hatle and Angelsen. Doppler Ultrasound in Cardiology (ed 2). Lea & Febiger, 1985; Van Dam et al. Eur Heart J 8:1221, 1987; 9:165, 1988; Jaffe et al. AJC 68:550, 1991; Appleton et al. JACC 10:1032, 1987.

disturbance may even provide clues as to the etiology of regurgitation.

The presence, location, and extent of an intracardiac flow disturbance is evaluated with color flow imaging, which allows real-time demonstrations of the flow disturbance in each tomographic plane.

Normal Antegrade Intracardiac Flows
(Table 2–8)

Normal antegrade intracardiac flows can be evaluated with either pulsed or continuous-wave Doppler ultrasound. Accurate measurement of antegrade flow velocities is dependent on several technical factors. Most important is a parallel alignment between the ultrasound beam and the direction of blood flow. The ultrasound instrument measures Doppler frequency shifts. The displayed velocities are *calculated* with the Doppler equation based on transducer frequency, the speed of sound in blood, and the angle between the Doppler beam and flow of interest. For intracardiac flows, the 3D direction of flow is difficult to determine, particularly when flow is abnormal, and attempts to "correct" for the presumed intercept angle are likely to increase, rather than decrease, measurement error. Instead, the examiner positions the ultrasound beam as parallel as possible to the flow of interest based on

obtaining the highest calculated velocity with careful transducer positioning and angulation (Table 2–9). In the Doppler equation, cos θ = 1 (and therefore can be ignored) when flow is oriented directly away (intercept angle = 0°) or straight toward (intercept angle = 180°) the ultrasound transducer. Small deviations from a parallel intercept angle (up to 20°) result in only a small error (6%) in velocity calculations (see Fig. 1–31). While this approach generally results in accurate velocity data, the possibility of underestimation of intracardiac velocities due to a nonparallel intercept angle always must be considered in an echocardiographic examination. This potential limitation becomes significant when recording high-velocity flows in valvular stenosis, regurgitation, or intracardiac shunts.

Other technical factors pertinent to recording antegrade flow velocities include the use of an appropriate velocity scale, wall filters, and gain settings. The standard velocity format is to display flows toward the transducer above and flows away from the transducer below the zero

Color Plate 1

FIGURE 1–34. For legend, see page 24.

FIGURE 1–35. For legend, see page 25.

FIGURE 2–1. For legend, see page 31.

Color Plate 2

FIGURE 2–30. For legend, see page 55.

FIGURE 2–31. For legend, see page 55.

FIGURE 2–32. For legend, see page 56.

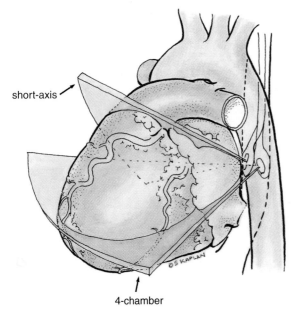

FIGURE 3–2. For legend, see page 62.

FIGURE 3–3. For legend, see page 63.

Color Plate 3

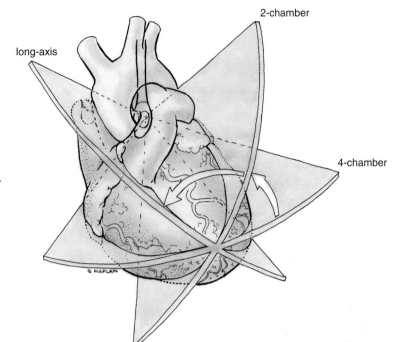

long-axis

2-chamber

4-chamber

FIGURE 3–5. For legend, see page 64.

FIGURE 3–13. For legend, see page 67.

Apical

short-axis

FIGURE 3–14. For legend, see page 68.

Color Plate 4

FIGURE 3–19. For legend, see page 71.

FIGURE 3–20. For legend, see page 72.

FIGURE 3–22. For legend, see page 74.

FIGURE 3–24. For legend, see page 75.

TABLE 2–9	Transthoracic Views for Normal Antegrade Flow Velocities
Antegrade Flow	**View**
LV outflow tract	Apical four-chamber (angulated anterior)
	Apical long-axis
Aorta (ascending)	Apical long-axis
	Suprasternal notch (SSN)
Descending aorta	
Thoracic	SSN
Proximal abdominal	Subcostal
LV inflow (mitral)	Apical four-chamber or long-axis
RV outflow tract	RV outflow
	Parasternal (aortic valve level)
	Subcostal short-axis
RV inflow (tricuspid)	RV inflow
	Apical four-chamber
LA inflow (pulmonary vein)	Apical four-chamber
RA inflow	Subcostal (central hepatic vein)
	SSN (superior vena cava)

LV = Left ventricular; RV = right ventricular; LA = left atrial; RA = right atrial; SSN = suprasternal notch.

baseline. The baseline may be shifted to maximize the flow of interest and the velocity scale adjusted so that tile velocity curve uses the entire displayed range. Wall filters are set as low as possible, without resulting in excessive noise, to allow accurate measurement of time intervals. Gain settings are adjusted to show the peak velocity and velocity curve clearly without excessive background noise. A sample volume length of 5 to 10 mm typically is used to record antegrade flow velocities because this length provides reasonable intracardiac localization with adequate signal strength.

Signal aliasing (as discussed in Chapter 1) occurs even with normal intracardiac flow velocities. Use of the baseline shift can resolve this problem in most cases. If aliasing persists, use of high pulse repetition frequency or continuous-wave Doppler is needed for unambiguous display of the maximum velocity.

With appropriate instrument setting and attention to technical details, antegrade velocities with pulsed Doppler ultrasound appear as smooth envelopes with a well-defined onset and end of flow, a well-defined maximum velocity, and a thin band of velocities at each time point. The area under the velocity curve is "clear" because the flow velocities at a specific intracardiac site are relatively uniform. Continuous-wave Doppler recordings differ in that the curve is "filled in" due to inclusion of lower velocities along the entire length of the ultrasound beam.

Left Ventricular Outflow (Fig. 2–27)

An apical or suprasternal notch window is used to obtain a parallel intercept angle between the ultrasound beam and direction of

FIGURE 2–27. Normal left ventricular outflow velocity curve recorded with pulsed Doppler from an anteriorly angulated apical four-chamber view with the sample volume (SV) positioned just proximal to the aortic valve *(above)*. The spectral display *(below)* shows a smooth velocity curve with a well-defined peak of 1.3 m/s and a clear closing click *(arrow)*.

blood flow in the left ventricular outflow tract and ascending aorta. In general, left ventricular outflow velocities are most accurately recorded from a transthoracic approach, as it is more difficult to obtain a parallel intercept angle from the transesophageal approach. In some cases, a transgastric "apical" approach may be useful but potential underestimation of velocity, due to a nonparallel intercept angle, always should be considered.

With a pulsed Doppler sample volume positioned on the left ventricular side of the aortic valve, an ejection velocity curve is recorded with a steep acceleration slope, a sharply peaked early systolic maximum velocity, and a less steep deceleration slope (Fig. 2–28). Note the narrow band of velocities at any instant in time during acceleration, reflecting the uniformity of blood flow velocity in the outflow tract during acceleration. During deceleration, the range of flow velocities at any instant is slightly wider (spectral broadening) as instability in the flow pattern during deceleration results in slight variation in flow velocities. The aortic valve closing click is seen immediately following end-ejection. Flow recordings with pulsed Doppler on the aortic side of the valve appear similar except that the aortic valve opening click is seen, instead of the closing click, and the maximum velocity is slightly higher, by 0.2 to 0.4 m/s, than the outflow tract velocity due to slight narrowing of the cross-sectional area of flow at the aortic leaflet tips.

With continuous-wave Doppler interrogation of the aortic valve, both opening and closing clicks are recorded. The area under the velocity curve is filled in with lower velocity signals because lower velocity blood flow signals that originate in the left ventricle along the length of the ultrasound beam are displayed as well (Fig. 2–28).

With a normal aortic valve, the area under the velocity curve (the velocity-time integral) reflects stroke volume, which can be calculated by multiplying by cross-sectional area. The normal antegrade maximum velocity across the valve is about 1 to 1.2 m/s and is the same whether measured by pulsed or continuous-wave Doppler methods. The normal outflow tract velocity typically is 0.8 to 1 m/s, corresponding to a velocity "step-up" across the valve or ratio of outflow tract to aortic velocity of 0.7 to 1.

The relationship between velocity and pressure gradients across *nonstenotic* valves is somewhat complex and is not fully described by the Bernoulli equation (which applies to ar-

FIGURE 2–28. Normal left ventricular outflow recorded with pulsed Doppler proximal to the aortic valve *(above)* showing an aortic closing (but not opening) click, distal to the aortic valve *(center)* showing an opening click, and with continuous-wave Doppler *(below)* showing both opening and closing clicks.

eas of narrowing). The period of acceleration corresponds to a slight pressure gradient from the left ventricle to the aorta, with the maximum pressure gradient corresponding to maximum acceleration. Left ventricular pressure falls below aortic pressure in midsystole, and at this point, deceleration of flow occurs. Thus, for the normal valve, maximum velocity occurs at the pressure crossover point (see Fig. 5–1). During deceleration, aortic pressure remains slightly higher than left ventricular pressure until flow decelerates to zero and the valve closes. At this point, left ventricular pressure continues to decline rapidly. This normal pattern of blood flow contrasts markedly with the pattern seen with a stenotic valve. With stenosis, a positive pressure gradient is present throughout the flow period, and pressure crossover corresponds to valve closure.

Right Ventricular Outflow

The right ventricular outflow tract and pulmonary artery are studied from a parasternal short-axis or right ventricular outflow tract view. In the normal individual, the right ventricular ejection curve is similar to the left ventricular ejection curve except that peak velocity is slightly lower (0.8 to 1 m/s), the ejection period is longer, and the velocity curve is more rounded, with the maximum velocity occurring in midsystole. The shapes of the right and left ventricular ejection curves appear to relate to the downstream vascular resistance. The low-resistance pulmonary vasculature results in a slower rate of acceleration of blood flow, with the maximum velocity (and pressure crossover) occurring later in the ejection cycle. When pulmonary vascular resistance is increased, the right ventricular ejection curve resembles left ventricular ejection more closely with a sharper velocity curve and earlier peak velocity.

Left Ventricular Inflow (Fig. 2–29)

Diastolic flow across the mitral valve shows two peaks: an early diastolic peak velocity (E wave) reflecting passive early diastolic filling and a late diastolic peak velocity due to atrial contraction (A wave). The normal E velocity in healthy, young individuals is about 1 m/s, with an A velocity of 0.2 to 0.4 m/s, reflecting the normal small contribution of atrial contraction to left ventricular diastolic filling. If diastole is long enough, a period of no flow, or diastasis, between the two flow curves is seen.

Even in normal individuals, the pattern of left ventricular diastolic filling varies with age, loading conditions, heart rate, and PR interval.

FIGURE 2–29. Normal left ventricular inflow velocity curve with the pulsed Doppler sample volume (SV) positioned at the mitral leaflet tips in diastole in the apical four-chamber view (above). The spectral display shows rapid early diastolic filling (E) with a small atrial (A) contribution to late diastolic filling.

With age, there is a gradual reduction in E velocity, prolongation in the rate of early diastolic deceleration, and increase in A velocity such that the ratio of E to A velocity changes from >1 in young individuals, to about 1 at ages 50 to 60, to <1 in older normal individuals.

Increased preload results in an increase in E velocity, while decreased preload has the opposite effect. When diastole is short (i.e., with a rapid heart rate), the A velocity becomes superimposed (or summated) onto the downslope of the E velocity, resulting in an apparent higher A velocity. At very high heart rates, only a single *E/A* peak may be seen. Prolongation of the PR interval has a similar effect. When atrial contraction occurs earlier in diastole, the *A* velocity is added to the downslope of the *E* velocity. These variations in the normal pattern of left ventricular diastolic filling should be recognized to avoid an inappropriate interpretation of an "abnormality."

Typically, left ventricular diastolic filling is recorded from an apical window on transthoracic studies. In addition to the physiologic variability discussed above, the peak *E* velocity and the ratio of the *E* to *A* peaks may differ depending on whether the sample volume is placed at the mitral annulus or at the mitral leaflet tips. Appropriate positioning of the sample volume depends on whether the Doppler curve is used to evaluate diastolic filling of the left ventricle (leaflet tips probably most useful) or transmitral stroke volume (mitral annular level most useful). Continuous-wave Doppler recordings show the highest velocities wherever they occur along the length of the ultrasound beam. Left ventricular diastolic filling is discussed in more detail in Chapter 5.

Right Ventricular Inflow

Right ventricular inflow can be recorded from an apical approach or from the parasternal right ventricular inflow view. The pattern of right ventricular diastolic filling is similar to left ventricular filling, although peak flow velocities are slightly lower with a normal right ventricular inflow *E* velocity of 0.3 to 0.7 m/s.

Left Atrial Filling

It is technically challenging to record left atrial filling from a transthoracic approach due to suboptimal signal strength at the depth of the pulmonary veins in many adults. However, with careful attention to technical details, this flow curve is obtainable in the right superior pulmonary vein in an apical four-chamber view in the majority of patients. From a transesophageal approach, flow in both right and left pulmonary veins can be recorded, with the clearest flow signals obtained from the left superior pulmonary vein.

Atrial contraction results in brief backflow in the pulmonary veins (a wave) followed by a biphasic filling pattern with prominent filling of the atrium (*x* descent) during ventricular systole, a second brief reversal of flow (*v* wave) following ventricular contraction, and a second atrial filling curve (*y* descent) during ventricular diastole (see Chapter 6). Abnormalities of left atrial filling can be seen in patients with mitral regurgitation (Chapter 11), constrictive pericarditis (Chapter 9), and restrictive cardiomyopathy (Chapter 8).

Right Atrial Filling

Right atrial filling can be assessed from Doppler recordings of superior vena caval flow (from a suprasternal notch approach) or central hepatic vein flow (which lies parallel to the ultrasound beam from a subcostal window). The pattern of flow again is analogous to the pulsation pattern of the neck veins seen on clinical examination, with an *a* wave, an *x* descent reflecting systolic filling, a *v* wave, and a *y* descent reflecting diastolic filling of the right atrium.

Descending Aorta

Flow patterns in the descending aorta are important in the evaluation of cardiac disorders because the downstream flow pattern depends on the presence and severity of specific cardiac lesions. Examples include aortic regurgitation, patent ductus arteriosus, and aortic coarctation. Descending thoracic aorta flow can be recorded from a suprasternal notch approach and shows antegrade flow with a systolic velocity curve, a peak velocity of about 1 m/s, and brief early diastolic flow reversal. The proximal abdominal aorta recorded from a subcostal approach shows a similar flow pattern.

Normal Color Doppler Flow Patterns

Impact of Color Doppler Physics on Flow Displays

While spectral Doppler (pulsed or continuous) is preferable for accurate measurement of specific intracardiac blood flow velocities, the overall pattern of intracardiac flow is best evaluated with color flow imaging. Unfortunately, although in theory normal laminar flow should appear as a uniform red or blue color, in fact, color flow display instrumentation results in more complex patterns.

For example, flow in the left ventricular outflow tract is a uniform red color from a parasternal long-axis view because the direction of flow is toward the transducer. The same flow is a uniform *blue* color from an apical approach because now it is directed away from the transducer (Fig. 2–30). This same phenomenon can be seen with flows in a single image plane. For example, antegrade flow in the aortic arch from a suprasternal notch view appears red (toward the transducer) in the more proximal segment and blue (away from the transducer) more distally with a small black area in the center of the image where the ultrasound

FIGURE 2–31. Color Doppler of left ventricular outflow from an apical long-axis view shows aliasing proximal to the aortic valve due to either a more parallel intercept angle between the Doppler scan line and direction of blood flow *or* a higher velocity near the septum versus adjacent to the anterior mitral valve leaflet. (See Color Plate p 2, p. 50.)

FIGURE 2–30. Flow in the left ventricular outflow tract recorded from a high parasternal position *(above)* is red (toward the transducer), while the same flow from an apical approach *(below)* is blue (away from the transducer). (See Color Plate 2, p. 50.)

beam is perpendicular to flow. Similarly, in the abdominal aorta from a subcostal approach, antegrade flow appears alternatively red and then blue as it transverses the image plane (see Fig. 1–34). In these examples, the change in color is due to a change in intercept angle between the ultrasound beam and blood flow at the left versus right edge of the sector.

Less dramatic changes in intercept angle across the 2D image also result in a complex color flow pattern for laminar normal flow. For example, evaluation of the left ventricular outflow tract in an apical long-axis view may show an apparent higher systolic velocity along the ventricular septum than along the anterior mitral leaflet (Fig. 2–31). This appearance results from a more parallel intercept angle between the Doppler beam and blood flow along the septum than adjacent to the mitral valve. The same actual velocities across the outflow tract

result in differing Doppler frequency shifts depending on this intercept angle. Since the instrument assumes that $\cos \theta = 1$ for each signal, a falsely low velocity is calculated for nonparallel intercept angles, with the resulting image showing an apparent increase in velocity across the image plane due to differing intercept angles.

In addition to intercept angle, color flow images also are affected by the phenomenon of signal aliasing. The Nyquist limit, as displayed at the top and bottom of the color scale, typically is 60 to 80 cm/s with a 2- or 3-MHz transducer at depths used for transthoracic cardiac imaging. Since normal intracardiac flow velocities often exceed this limit, signal aliasing occurs. Flow toward the transducer is displayed in red at velocities less than the Nyquist limit, but once aliasing occurs, this same flow signal is displayed in blue. Thus flow toward the transducer is red aliasing to blue, while flow away from the transducer is blue aliasing to red. In fact, multiple aliases can occur with high-velocity flows displayed sequentially as going from red to blue to red and so on. An example of normal aliasing is seen in the left ventricular inflow pattern on the apical four-chamber view, where the red flow toward the apex turns blue as it exceeds the Nyquist limit (see Fig. 1–35). While confusing at first, patterns of signal aliasing can be used to advantage in quantitation of intracardiac flows using the proximal isovelocity surface area approach discussed in Chapter 11.

Another color image pattern seen even with normal intracardiac flows is *variance,* which often is encoded as green on the color display. While the concept of variance is that a single intracardiac site exhibits multiple flow velocities and directions (such as in a regurgitant jet), from the foregoing discussions of intercept angle and aliasing, it is apparent that a normal flow pattern might meet variance criteria. For example, in a region at the aliasing limit, the instrument may sequentially measure flow toward then away from the transducer due to aliasing and then assign variance to that color pixel. Awareness that a color variance pattern can occur with normal intracardiac flows avoids erroneous interpretations.

Normal Ventricular Outflow Patterns

Color flow imaging of left ventricular outflow can be recorded from an apical approach in either an anteriorly angulated four-chamber view or a long-axis view. Flow is laminar, but aliasing typically occurs at this depth, resulting in a complex color pattern. While measurement of stroke volume proximal to the aortic valve, which *assumes* a flat flow velocity profile, has been validated, it remains controversial whether the appearance of aliasing along the ventricular septum in systole is due to a skewed flow profile or to variations in intercept angle across the color sector.

Note that while accurate measurements of antegrade velocities with pulsed or continuous-wave Doppler require a parallel intercept angle, with color flow imaging, the spatial pattern of flow is of interest rather than the absolute velocities. Thus views with nonparallel intercept angles often are helpful. For example, left ventricular outflow can be evaluated with color flow imaging in a parasternal long-axis view even though the flow direction is almost perpendicular to the ultrasound beam. As shown in Chapter 11, this view also is useful for evaluation of abnormal flows in the outflow tract, such as aortic regurgitation.

Right ventricular outflow can be visualized from a parasternal short-axis view, from the right ventricular outflow view, or from a subcostal short-axis view. Since velocities are slightly lower and the depth of interrogation is less than for left ventricular outflow, the flow pattern away from the transducer typically shows a uniform blue color.

Normal Ventricular Inflow Patterns

In the apical four-chamber view, left ventricular inflow appears as a broad flow stream extending laterally across the mitral annulus and

FIGURE 2–32. Normal pattern of left ventricular filling in mid-diastole in an apical four-chamber view shows flow toward the apex along the lateral wall simultaneously with flow away from the transducer along the septum. (See Color Plate 2, p. 50.)

lengthwise to the left ventricular apex. If the Nyquist limit is exceeded, signal aliasing occurs with a color shift at the aliasing velocity. In real time, the separate flows of early and late diastolic filling may be seen. When ultrasound penetration is optimal, diastolic flow extends from the pulmonary veins to the left ventricular apex. The normal spatial pattern of the left ventricular inflow is directed along the lateral left ventricular wall, in mid-diastole, with blue flow away from the transducer along the ventricular septum consistent with a "vortex" of flow in the left ventricle in diastole (Fig. 2–32). Interestingly, the normal counterclockwise vortex is reversed in patients after mitral valve replacement.

Right ventricular inflow patterns on color flow imaging are analogous to the patterns seen in the left ventricle, although a diastolic "vortex" is not as prominent.

Normal Atrial Inflow Patterns

Inflow into the left atrium occurs via the four pulmonary veins. On transthoracic imaging, the right superior pulmonary vein is the easiest to visualize in the apical four-chamber view. Color flow imaging showing the biphasic red inflow from this vein allows correct placement of a pulsed Doppler sample volume for recording the spectral Doppler data. All four pulmonary veins can be visualized on transesophageal echo, but again, use of color flow imaging may facilitate identification of each vein. This approach is particularly helpful with right-sided veins, which may be difficult to recognize on 2D imaging alone.

Inflow into the right atrium occurs via the superior and inferior venae cavae and the coronary sinus. Evaluation may be complicated by some degree of tricuspid regurgitation (present in 80% to 90% of normal subjects and a higher percentage of patients), which typically is directed along the interatrial septum. Flow from the inferior vena cava and coronary sinus may be seen in the right ventricular inflow view, as well as in the short-axis view at the aortic valve level and in the apical four-chamber view. Superior vena caval flow is seen from the suprasternal notch approach. In the right atrium, recognition of the several normal inflow patterns is important when an atrial septal defect is suspected. Note that 20% of normal subjects have a patent foramen ovale (demonstrable by intravenous echo contrast during a Valsalva maneuver), but color flow evidence for a patent foramen ovale is present in only about 5% of normal individuals.

Physiologic Valvular Regurgitation

With careful examination techniques, a small amount of mitral and tricuspid regurgitation is detectable in between 50% and 80% of normal people. In addition, mild pulmonic regurgitation, appearing as a narrow red "flame" in diastole, is an incidental finding (present in 70% to 80% of normal individuals). These physiologic degrees of regurgitation are characterized by a localized signal that often is seen only briefly during the cardiac cycle. Small amounts of mitral, tricuspid, and pulmonic valvular regurgitation are of no apparent clinical significance. In contrast, aortic regurgitation is rarely seen in normal subjects (5% of individuals) on color flow imaging.

Technical Aspects of Color Flow Imaging

The color flow display is dependent on each specific ultrasound instrument to some extent. However, many parameters are adjustable by the operator, so an optimal examination requires careful attention to instrument settings.

The *color flow map* usually can be varied in terms of (1) the color scale used, (2) the addition of variance to the color scale, and (3) the use of a power scale instead of a color scale. The specific color scale used is a matter of personal preference, with the diagnostic goal being to optimize the display and recognition of abnormal flow patterns.

The *velocity range* of the color flow map is determined by the Nyquist limit, and as for conventional pulsed Doppler, the range can be altered by shifting the zero baseline, changing the pulse repetition frequency, or altering the depth of the displayed image.

Color Doppler power output and *gain* are adjusted so that gain is just below the level at which random background noise appears. "Wall filters" can be varied to exclude low-velocity signals from the color flow display. In addition, many instruments allow variation in the assignment of a returning signal to 2D or Doppler display (depending on signal strength). One approach to optimizing the color flow display is to reduce the 2D gain, since the instrument does not display flow data on top of "structures" even when the 2D signal is due to excessive gain.

Perhaps the most important technical factor in color flow imaging is optimization *of frame rate*. As discussed in Chapter 1, color flow frame rate depends on sector width, depth, pulse repetition frequency, and the number of samples per sector line. The examiner optimizes frame rate by focusing on the flow of interest, narrowing the sector, and decreasing the depth as much as possible. However, use of too small a color box should be avoided as the limited field of view may lead to erroneous interpretations. When frame rate remains inadequate for timing flow abnormalities, a color M-line through the area of interest may be helpful, for example in assessment of aortic regurgitation.

THE ECHOCARDIOGRAPHIC EXAMINATION

The specific echocardiographic views and Doppler flow velocities recorded in any individual patient depend on the indication for the study, the abnormalities noted as the examination is in progress, and each laboratory's basic protocol. Chapter 4 discusses indications for echocardiography and the echocardiographic examination in detail.

SUGGESTED READING

1. Henry WL, DeMaria A, Gramiak R, et al, and the American Society of Echocardiography, Committee on Nomenclature and Standards: Report on two-dimensional echocardiography. *Circulation* 62:212–222, 1980.

   Nomenclature standards for image orientation, imaging planes, and transducer location. Clear schematic drawings.

2. American Society of Echocardiography, Doppler Standards and Nomenclature Committee: Recommendations for Terminology and Display Doppler Echocardiography. Raleigh, NC, American Society of Echocardiography, 1984, pp 1–11.

   Nomenclature standards for Doppler data plus a useful glossary of Doppler terminology.

3. Lentner C (ed): Geigy Scientific Tables, vol 5: Heart and Circulation (ed 8). Basel, Switzerland, Ciba-Geigy, 1990.

Excellent reference source summarizing normal values for cardiovascular imaging. Includes invasive and noninvasive normal data. Well referenced.

4. Netter FH: The Heart. Basel, Switzerland, Ciba, 1969.

Clear illustrations of detailed cardiac anatomy with concise accompanying text on pages 2–12. A useful introduction and review of cardiac structure.

5. Thubriker M: The Aortic Valve. Boca Raton, Fla, CRC Press, 1990.

Monograph on detailed anatomy, structure, and function of the aortic valve.

6. Roberts WC: Morphologic features of the normal and abnormal mitral valve. Am J Cardiol 51:1005–1028, 1983.

A review of anatomy and function of the mitral valve based on 1010 autopsy cases. Excellent discussion and illustrations of normal mitral valve anatomy, mitral stenosis, and mitral regurgitation. Both photographs and schematic drawings are included.

7. Schnittger I, Gordon EP, Fitzgerald PJ, Popp RL: Standardized intracardiac measurements of two-dimensional echocardiography. J Am Coll Cardiol 2:934–938, 1983.

Normal 2D echo intracardiac measurements are described in detail for 35 healthy adults.

8. Triulzi M, Gillam LD, Gentile F, et al: Normal adult cross-sectional echocardiographic values: Linear dimensions and chamber areas. Echocardiography 1:403–426, 1984.

Tabular presentation of normal echo dimensions in 72 normal adults.

9. Pearlman JD, Triulzi MO, King ME, et al: Limits of normal left ventricular dimensions in growth and development: Analysis of dimensions and variance in the two-dimensional echocardiograms of 268 normal healthy subjects. J Am Coll Cardiol 12:1432–1441, 1988.

Graphic display of normal echo dimensions in 72 adults and 196 children showing relationship of each dimension to body surface area with mean and 90% tolerance limits.

10. Roman MJ, Devereux RB, Kramer-Fox R, O'Loughlin J: Two-dimensional echocardiographic aortic root dimensions in normal children and adults. Am J Cardiol 64:507–512, 1989.

Derivation of gender-specific upper limits of normal (indexed to body size) for aortic root dimensions based on 135 adults and 52 children.

11. Benjamin EJ, Levy D, Anderson KM, et al: Determinants of Doppler indexes of left ventricular diastolic function in normal subjects (the Framingham Heart Study). Am J Cardiol 70:508–515, 1992.

Detailed study of the relationship between age and Doppler measures of left ventricular diastolic filling in the Framingham population after exclusion of subjects with hypertension, cardiac disease, or other organ system disease (n = 1485). E velocity decreased from 0.71 ± 0.14 m/s at ages 20–29 years to 0.53 ± 0.17 m/s for those ≥70 years of age. A velocity increased from 0.35 ± 0.06 to 0.64 ±0.14 m/s in the same groups. The E/A ratio was 1.03 ± 0.26 m/s at ages 60–69 years.

12. Jaffe WM, Dewhurst TA, Otto CM, Pearlman AS: Influence of Doppler sample volume location on ventricular filling velocities. Am J Cardiol 68:550–552, 1991.

Detailed study in 300 subjects showing that E velocity increases from 0.45 ± 0.15 m/s at the annulus to 0.75 ± 0.22 m/s at the leaflet tips, while A velocity increases only from 0.47 ± 0.14 to 0.64 ± 0.28 m/s. This results in differing E/A velocity ratios at the annulus (1.05 ± 0.42) versus the leaflet tips (1.36 ± 0.65).

13. Appleton CP, Hatle LK, Popp RL: Superior vena cava and hepatic vein Doppler echocardiography in healthy adults. J Am Coll Cardiol 10:1032–1039, 1987.

Normal superior vena cava and hepatic vein Doppler flows show a systolic and diastolic antegrade flow with a reduction or reversal in antegrade flow following atrial systole (A wave). Variation with respiration is prominent in normal healthy adults.

14. Basnight MA, Gonzalez MS, Kershenovich SC, Appleton CP: Pulmonary venous flow velocity: Relation to hemodynamics, mitral flow velocity and left atrial volume, and ejection fraction. J Am Soc Echocardiogr 4:547–558, 1991.

15. Klein AL, Tajik AJ: Doppler assessment of pulmonary venous flow in healthy subjects and in patients with heart disease. J Am Soc Echocardiogr 4:379–392, 1991.

16. Bartzokis T, Lee R, Yeoh TK, et al: Transesophageal echo-Doppler echocardiographic assessment of pulmonary venous flow patterns. J Am Soc Echocardiogr 4:457–464, 1991.

Each of these three references (14 to 16) provides detailed descriptions of normal pulmonary venous flow patterns and the physiologic variables that affect the flow pattern.

17. Sager KB, Nachodsky DM: Aging changes seen on echocardiography. In Otto CM, (ed): The Practice of Clinical Echocardiography. Philadelphia, WB Saunders, 1997, pp. 619–629.

Detailed review of the normal cardiac changes with aging as assessed by echocardiography including age-grouped tables of normal values for left ventricular dimensions and function and Doppler flow velocities. 47 references.

18. Stevenson JG, Otto CM: Impact of color flow Doppler physics on clinical assessment of flow abnormalities. In Otto CM (ed): The Practice of Clinical Echocardiography. Philadelphia, WB Saunders, 1997, pp. 291–306.

Discussion and examples of how the physics of color Doppler flow imaging affect assessment of both normal and disturbed flow patterns. This chapter includes a review of the basic principles of color flow imaging, the effects on instrumentation on the flow display, recognition of color flow artifacts, and methods for optimizing the color flow examination.

Transesophageal Echocardiography 3

PROCEDURE PROTOCOL AND RISKS

TOMOGRAPHIC VIEWS
  Esophageal Position
    Four-Chamber Plane
    Two-Chamber Plane
    Long-Axis Left Ventricular Plane
    Other Long-Axis Image Planes
    Short-Axis Plane
  Standard Transgastric Position
    Short-Axis Plane
    Two-Chamber Plane
  Transgastric Apical Position
    Four-Chamber Plane
    Long-Axis Plane

  Descending Thoracic Aorta

VALVE ANATOMY AND NORMAL DOPPLER FLOWS
  Left Ventricular Outflow and Aortic Valve
  Left Ventricular Inflow and Mitral Valve
  Right Ventricular Outflow and Pulmonic Valve
  Right Ventricular Inflow and Tricuspid Valve

CHAMBER ANATOMY AND ATRIAL INFLOWS
  Left Ventricle
  Left Atrium
  Right Ventricle
  Right Atrium

Transesophageal echocardiography offers the advantages of improved image quality compared to transthoracic images, particularly of posterior structures, such as the pulmonary veins, left atrium, and mitral valve. Image quality is improved both because of the decreased distance between the transducer and the structures of interest and because of the absence of intervening lung or bone tissue. A better signal-to-noise ratio and decreased image depth also allows use of higher frequency (5- and 7-MHz) transducers, which further enhances image quality.

However, transesophageal imaging is more risky than transthoracic imaging due to the insertion of the probe in the esophagus and the frequent need for conscious sedation. A transesophageal examination provides additional information but does not replace a transthoracic examination. In some situations, transthoracic imaging provides better image quality and diagnostic Doppler data. For example, anterior structures, such as a prosthetic aortic valve, may be better imaged from the transthoracic approach. For Doppler velocity measurements, the transthoracic approach offers more acoustic windows with the ability to adjust the transducer angle freely in both the transverse and elevational planes. In contrast, transducer position and angulation are constrained with the transesophageal approach by the relative positions of the esophagus and heart. The inability to align the Doppler beam parallel to the flow of interest may result in substantial velocity underestimation. In addition, it often is more difficult to obtain standard anatomic measurements from the transesophageal approach due to oblique 2D image planes. Thus, even when transesophageal imaging is necessary, data from the transthoracic examination are integrated into the final clinical interpretation.

In this chapter, the transesophageal procedure and risks are briefly outlined followed by a description of the standard views obtained from each acoustic window (transesophageal, standard transgastric, transgastric apical, and descending aorta). Sections on the transesophageal two-dimensional (2D) and Doppler evaluation of each cardiac valve and chamber are included to guide the reader to the optimal views for each anatomic structure. This chapter focuses on normal anatomy and flow patterns. Clinical indications for transesophageal imaging are discussed in Chapter 4 and pathologic images are included in subsequent chapters.

PROCEDURE PROTOCOL AND RISKS

Transesophageal echocardiography is performed by a physician skilled in both echocardiography and the endoscopy procedure, as detailed in published guidelines for physician training. Typically a cardiac sonographer assists the physician, adjusting instrument settings for optimal image quality and data acquisition. Many physicians use mild conscious sedation, in addition to local anesthesia of the pharynx, to minimize patient discomfort and improve tolerance of the procedure. When conscious sedation is used, a designated, qualified individual (usually a nurse) monitors and documents the patient's blood pressure, heart rate, respiratory rate, arterial oxygen saturation, and level of consciousness throughout the procedure. In addition, the nurse ensures patency of the airway and provides suction of oral secretions as needed (see Suggested Reading 12). The specific protocol, medications used for conscious sedation, and monitoring procedures are dictated by the operating standards of each institution.

Transesophageal echocardiography has a very low incidence of complications when performed by trained individuals with appropriate patient selection and monitoring. However, this procedure does have known risks, which must be taken into consideration in deciding whether the potential information obtained justifies use of this procedure (Table 3–1). The rate of complications serious enough to interrupt the procedure is less than 1% with a reported mortality rate of fewer than 1 in 10,000 patients. Risks are higher in patients with a history of esophageal disease, impaired respiratory status, or sleep apnea. If the preprocedure history or physical examination suggest an increased risk for conscious sedation, appropriate consultation with anesthesiology is essential. If there is a history of esophageal disease or symptoms related to impaired swallowing, a preprocedure barium swallow or gastroenterology consultation may be needed.

The risk of aspiration is minimized by having the patient fast for several hours before the procedure, use of a left lateral decubitus position during probe insertion, and having the patient continue to fast after the procedure until recovery from the local anesthesia of the pharynx. Esophageal trauma or perforation is unlikely in the absence of a history of esophageal disease or swallowing difficulty, both of which can be ascertained by clinical history. Bleeding complications are rare and usually mild, and the procedure can be safely performed with therapeutic levels of systemic anticoagulation. Initial concern that transesophageal imaging might increase the risk of endocarditis has been alleviated by several studies showing the absence of bacteremia following this procedure so that most physicians do not routinely use antibiotic prophylaxis.

TOMOGRAPHIC VIEWS

The exact views obtained on a transesophageal study vary depending on the relative positions of the heart, esophagus, and diaphragm in each patient. Even though a multiplane probe allows full rotation of the scan plane, the fixed position of the transducer in the esophagus constrains the possible image planes that can be obtained, potentially resulting in oblique image orientations compared with the three-dimensional (3D) reference system used for transthoracic images. The goal on transesophageal echocardiography is to perform a systematic and comprehensive examination, using standard short-axis, long-axis, two-chamber and four-chamber image planes whenever possible. Standard views then are supplemented with additional image planes to demonstrate the specific pathologic processes in each patient. Three-dimensional echocardiographic techniques will facilitate obtaining the optimal views as this approach becomes more usable and widely available.

A recommended sequence of images comprising a basic complete examination is shown in Table 3–2. The following sections describe views useful for evaluation of the valves and cardiac chambers that can be used to supple-

TABLE 3–1	Risks of Transesophageal Echocardiography

Risks of Esophageal Intubation
  Dental trauma
  Esophageal trauma or perforation
  Bleeding
  Aspiration
  Dislodgement of endotracheal tube, especially on
    probe withdrawal
  Displacement of nasogastric tubes

Risks of Conscious Sedation
  Hypotension
  Respiratory depression (hypoxia, respiratory arrest)
  Arrhythmias
  Bronchospasm
  Death

TABLE 3–2	**Basic Transesophageal Examination**			
Probe Position	Rotation Angle	Depth	View	Focus on:
High esophageal	0°	Include LV apex	Four-chamber	LV and RV size and function (inferior setpum and lateral wall) LA and RA size (withdraw probe to see LA appendage) Mitral and tricuspid valves (angulate anteriorly to see aortic valve)
	~60°		Two-chamber	LV size and function (inferior and anterior walls) LA and LA appendage Mitral valve
	~120°		Long-axis	LV size and function (anterior septum and posterior walls) LA and RA size Mitral and aortic valves (withdraw probe to see ascending aorta)
High esophageal	~120°	↓ depth to optimize valves	Long-axis	Mitral valve anatomy and function—2D and color Doppler (regurgitation) and antegrade mitral flow with pulsed Doppler Aortic valve anatomy and color flow
	~60°		Two-chamber	Mitral valve anatomy and function—2D and color Doppler LA appendage
	0°		Four-chamber	Mitral valve anatomy and function—2D and color Doppler Aortic valve (angulate anteriorly to "five-chamber" view) for anatomy and color flow Atrial septum
Transgastric	0°	To fit LV	Short-axis	LV wall motion, wall thickness, chamber dimensions RV size and function
Transgastric apical	0°	Increase to maximum depth	Four-chamber	Useful for antegrade aortic flow but may still be nonparallel intercept angle
Transgastric to high esophageal	0°	Decrease depth to image aorta	Short-axis descending aorta	Image aorta from the diaphragm to aortic arch

LV = Left ventricular; RV = right ventricular; LA = left atrial; RA = right atrial.

ment the basic examination as determined by the specific clinical question.

The position of the tip of the probe is described as esophageal or transgastric and is referenced to the cardiac structures seen in each view. The absolute distance of the transducer from the patient's mouth will vary depending on body size and cardiac position. There also will be variability in the exact degree of rotation, tilt, and angulation needed to obtain the best short-axis, long-axis, two-chamber, and four-chamber views. When standard views are obtained, the images correspond to the anatomy described for the equivalent transthoracic views, with the major difference being image orientation given the transesophageal transducer position.

For transesophageal echocardiograms, transducer motions will be referred to as (1) *repositioning*, defined as movement of the probe up and down in the esophagus, (2) *rotation*, defined as rotating the image plane from 0° to 180° using the multiplane control knob, (3) *turning*, defined as moving the entire transducer in a rotational fashion in the esophagus to show a mediolateral change in image plane, (4) *angulation*, defined as bending and extending the probe so that the image plane is directed superiorly or inferiorly at an angle to the original image plane, and (5) *tilt*, defined as lateral motion of the transducer tip to image different structures in the same image plane (although slight superior motion occurs as well). From the transesophageal position, most image planes are achieved using repositioning, rotation, and turning of the transducer. The use of angulation is particularly important on transgastric views. A key principle in using a multiplane probe is that the anatomic area of interest should be centered in the image before rotation to a new view to ensure that the structure of interest remains in the image plane.

Esophageal Position

Four-Chamber Plane

As the transducer is advanced into the esophagus from the mouth toward the stomach, acoustic access is limited by interposition of the air-filled trachea until the transducer passes the level of the carina. From a high

transesophageal position, with the probe located posterior to the left atrium, a standard four-chamber view usually can be obtained in the 0° position with angulation of the transducer toward the left ventricular apex (Fig. 3–1). As with transthoracic imaging, slight changes in angulation allow imaging of the coronary sinus posteriorly and the left ventricular outflow tract and aortic valve anteriorly (the "five-chamber" view) (Fig. 3–2). In the four-chamber view the lateral wall and inferior septal segments of the left ventricle are seen. Care is needed to include the full length of the ventricle in this view because in a foreshortened image the apparent apex may actually represent a more proximal segment of the anterior wall. A biplane ejection fraction can be calculated from end-diastolic and end-systolic endocardial borders traced in the four- and two-chamber transesophageal views.

When the transducer is positioned posterior to the center of the left atrium, the central portions of both the anterior and posterior leaflets of the mitral valve are well visualized in the 0° four-chamber view. Anterior angulation provides a view of the left ventricular outflow tract and anterior mitral leaflet analogous to the apical five-chamber view (Fig. 3–3). Posterior angulation provides images of more lateral seg-

FIGURE 3–1. The transesophageal four-chamber view obtained from a high transesophageal position with the multiplane probe at 0° rotation. In this view, the apparent apex may actually represent a segment of the anterior wall because of foreshortening of the long axis of the ventricle.

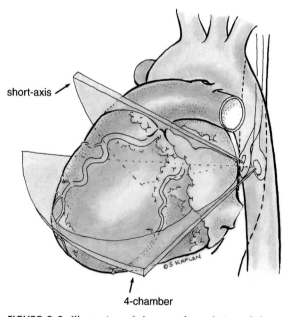

FIGURE 3–2. Illustration of the use of angulation of the transducer from a high esophageal position with the probe at 0° rotation to obtain a four-chamber view (as shown in Fig 3–1) or a short-axis view of the left atrial appendage (as shown in Fig. 3–7). (See Color Plate 2, p. 50.) (Courtesy Starr Kaplan, Seattle, Washington.)

FIGURE 3–3. Slight anterior angulation from the four-chamber view, midway between the image planes shown in Fig. 13–2, allows visualization of the aortic valve and left ventricular outflow tract *(top)*. Color flow shows normal systolic laminar flow in the outflow tract *(bottom)*. (See Color Plate 2, p. 50.)

ments of the valve leaflets with coronary sinus visualized on extreme posterior angulation.

While examining the left atrium in the four-chamber plane, it is helpful to slowly advance and withdraw the transducer to visualize the full superior and inferior extent or to slowly angulate the probe tip to provide sequential cross sections of the left atrium. Because the left atrium is in the near field of the image, careful adjustment of imaging parameters is needed to avoid misinterpretation of near-field artifacts. For this reason, identification of a small thrombus along the posterior left atrial wall is problematic.

In the standard four-chamber transesophageal image, the size, shape, and systolic function of the right ventricle can be assessed by turning the probe toward the patient's right side.

This view also provides visualization of the septal and anterior leaflets of the tricuspid valve and the right atrium. The interatrial septum is well visualized with the fossa ovalis and primum septum region clearly identifiable (Fig. 3–4).

Two-Chamber Plane

After ensuring that the left ventricular apex is in the center of the image in a four-chamber view, the image plane is slowly rotated to about 60° to obtain a two-chamber view (Fig. 3–5). Because the apex often is not exactly centered in three dimensions, the position and angulation of the transducer may need adjustment to obtain a two-chamber view that includes the full length of the left ventricle (Fig. 3–6). In this view, the inferior and anterior left ventricular walls of the left ventricle are seen allowing assessment of regional function and providing the orthogonal plane (along with the four-chamber view) for calculation of ejection fraction. With further rotation to about 90°, the left atrial appendage is visualized in a view approximately perpendicular to that obtained in the transverse plane (Fig. 3–7). The left superior pulmonary vein can be seen entering the left atrium by slightly withdrawing and turning the probe laterally. In the two-chamber view, typically only the anterior leaflet of the mitral valve is seen so that it is difficult to evaluate leaflet prolapse in this view.

FIGURE 3–4. A view of the tricuspid valve and interatrial septum is obtained by turning the transducer from the four-chamber view toward the patient's right side. The thin central region of the interatrial septum known as the fossa ovalis is between the *arrowheads*.

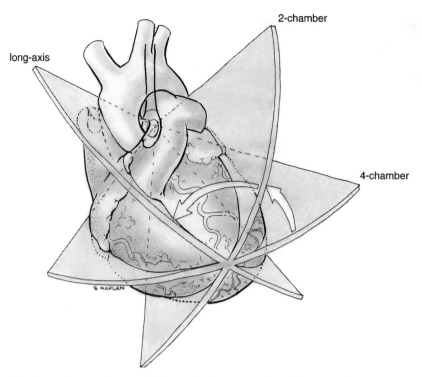

FIGURE 3–5. Rotation of the image plane starting from the four-chamber view, with the left ventricular apex centered in the image, allows a two-chamber view (see Fig. 3–6) at approximately 60° rotation and a long-axis view (see Fig. 3–8) at about 120° rotation. Slight repositioning and angulation of the transducer may be needed as the image plane is rotated to ensure inclusion of the left ventricular apex in the image. (See Color Plate 3, p. 50.) (Courtesy Starr Kaplan, Seattle, Washington.)

FIGURE 3–6. Transesophageal two-chamber view obtained from a high esophageal position with rotation of the image plane to 75° in the same patient shown in Figure 3–1*B*. LAA = left atrial appendage.

Long-Axis Left Ventricular Plane

With the transducer positioned in the high esophagus, posterior to the left atrium, further rotation of the image plane to about 120° results in a long-axis view of the left ventricle and aorta (Fig. 3–8). Again, slight adjustment of transducer position and angulation may be needed to obtain a view that includes the left ventricular apex. Similar to a transthoracic long-axis view, the proximal ascending aorta, sinuses of Valsalva, and right and noncoronary leaflets of the aortic valve are well visualized. Scanning between this view and the 90° image planes allows appreciation of the perpendicular relationship between aortic and pulmonic valve planes and the slightly more cephalad position of the pulmonic valve. The long-axis view is particularly helpful in evaluating for ascending aortic dissection, subaortic membrane, supracristal ventricular septal defect, sinus of Valsalva aneurysm, aortic valve vegetations, and abscess formation. Note that in the esophageal long-axis plane, withdrawing the transducer in the esophagus results in more cephalad images

FIGURE 3–7. *Left:* Left atrial appendage seen in the 0° image plane obtained from the four-chamber view by slight withdrawal and anterior angulation of the transducer. Note the normal trabeculation in the atrial appendage and the left main coronary artery *(arrow)* arising from the aortic root. *Right,* Orthogonal view of the atrial appendage obtained by rotation to 90°. Both these images were obtained with a 7.0 MHz transducer to optimize detection of atrial appendage thrombus.

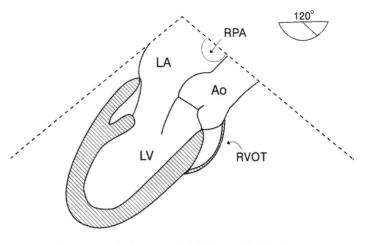

FIGURE 3–8. Schematic diagram *(top)* of the transesophageal long-axis view. This view typically is obtained at about 120° rotation, but there is considerable individual variability in the exact image plane needed to show the aorta and left ventricle in a long-axis orientation. The right pulmonary artery *(RPA)* and part of the right ventricular outflow tract *(RVOT)* may be seen in this view. Transesophageal long-axis view *(bottom)* obtained after rotation to 131° in the same patient as Figs. 3–1 and 3–6.

FIGURE 3–9. From the transesophageal long-axis view, further cephalad segments of the ascending aorta can be visualized by slight withdrawal of the transducer in the esophagus.

FIGURE 3–10. In the 90° transesophageal image plane, the right ventricular outflow tract, pulmonic valve, and pulmonary artery can be visualized with the probe turned toward the patient's left side.

of the ascending aorta with the superior limit of imaging determined by the interposed air-filled bronchus (Fig. 3–9).

The anterior and posterior mitral leaflets are seen in a long-axis orientation and the coronary sinus can be identified in cross section in the atrioventricular groove. The right pulmonary artery is visualized posterior to the aortic root at the superior aspect of the left atrium. In the long-axis view, the anterior septum and posterior wall of the left ventricle are seen. In addition, a portion of the right ventricular outflow tract is seen anterior to the aortic valve (in the far field of the image).

Other Long-Axis Image Planes

At a rotation angle of 90°, the probe can be turned from the left ventricular long-axis view toward the patient's left side to obtain a long-axis view of the pulmonic valve and right ventricular outflow tract (Fig. 3–10). In this view, the pulmonic valve is in the far field of the image and may be shadowed by the aortic valve and root if calcification is present. Portions of the right ventricle and tricuspid valve are seen, depending on the exact position of the heart relative to the esophagus in each patient.

At a 90° rotation, when the probe is turned toward the patient's right side images of the right ventricle and tricuspid valve in an inflow view are obtained. If the probe is turned further to the right, a long-axis view of the right atrium

is obtained with the superior vena cava entering from the right side of the screen and the inferior vena cava on the left (Fig. 3–11). In some individuals, a Eustachian valve at the inferior caval-atrial junction is seen.

Minor changes in the rotation angle may be needed to optimize each view. As with the left ventricular long-axis view, adjustment of transducer position (advancement and withdrawal)

FIGURE 3–11. With the probe turned toward the patient's right side, the right atrium, and superior and inferior vena cava can be visualized in the 90° transesophageal image plane. A Eustachian valve *(arrow)* often is present at the junction of the inferior vena cava with the right atrium.

allows imaging of much of the cephalad to caudal extent of the cardiac structures in each of these tomographic planes.

Short-Axis Plane

A short-axis view at the aortic valve level can be obtained by rotating the image plane to between 30° and 45° and withdrawing the probe in the esophagus to the level of the aortic valve. Visualization of aortic valve anatomy is

FIGURE 3–12. A short-axis view of the aortic valve in systole *(top)* and diastole *(bottom)* is seen in a transesophageal view at 38° rotation. The degree of rotation needed to obtain this short-axis view varies from 30° to 50°; the images themselves should be used to ensure a true short-axis image. Oblique image planes may result in artifactual distortion of the valve apparatus.

excellent, showing the three leaflets and sinuses of Valsalva (Fig. 3–12). The origin of the left main coronary artery is easily identified after minor adjustments in the depth and tilt of the image plane. The right coronary artery is more difficult to visualize and is clearly identified in only a minority of patients. The interatrial septum is well seen, with the fossa ovalis clearly defined *(arrowheads* on Fig. 3–12).

By turning the transducer laterally and angulating superiorly from the 0° esophageal position, the left atrial appendage and left superior pulmonary vein are seen (see Fig. 3–7). Prominent features include normal trabeculation of the atrial appendage and a variably prominent ridge at the junction of the anteriorly directed left superior pulmonary vein and the left atrial appendage. The laterally directed left inferior pulmonary vein is seen by advancing the transducer and angulating slightly inferiorly. The right pulmonary veins can be imaged by rotating the transducer medially and withdrawing the transducer cephalad (to see the anteriorly directed right superior pulmonary vein) or by angulating the transducer inferiorly (to see the medially directed right inferior pulmonary vein). The pulmonary veins also can be identified in the 90° image plane, turning the transducer toward the patient's right to show the right pulmonary veins and to the left for the left pulmonary veins. Again, color flow imaging often facilitates identification of the pulmonary veins based on the characteristic venous inflow patterns (Fig. 3–13).

FIGURE 3–13. The right upper *(RUPV)* and lower pulmonary veins *(RLPV)* are seen in the 90° plane with the probe turned toward the patient's right side. Color flow imaging facilitates identification of the pulmonary views as they enter the left atrium. (See Color Plate 3, p. 50.)

In many patients, the pulmonary artery can be imaged in the 0° image plane by further withdrawing the probe in the esophagus to obtain a view straight down the main pulmonary artery from the bifurcation to the valve level. In some cases, this view is limited by the position of the air-filled bronchus and some patients may find the probe uncomfortable when positioned at this level in the esophagus.

Standard Transgastric Position

Short-Axis Plane

As the transducer is passed into the stomach, slight resistance may be encountered at the gastroesophageal junction. With the probe tip in the stomach, superior angulation (flexing the scope) in the 0° image plane results in a short-axis view of the left ventricle at the papillary muscle level (Fig. 3–14). In this view, global left ventricular systolic function, left ventricular dimensions and wall thickness, and regional left ventricular function can be evaluated (Fig. 3–15).

Depending on the position of the patient's heart with respect to the diaphragm, a short-axis view at the mitral valve level may be obtainable by slight withdrawal of the transducer toward the esophagus (Fig. 3–16). The transgastric short-axis view at the mitral valve level

FIGURE 3–15. Transgastric short-axis view of the left ventricle at the papillary muscle level in diastole *(top)* and systole *(bottom)*. This view is particularly valuable for intraoperative monitoring. Regional wall motion abnormalities due to ischemia can be detected, fractional area shortening can be calculated for monitoring ventricular systolic function, and relative changes in cavity size indicate corresponding changes in intravascular volume status.

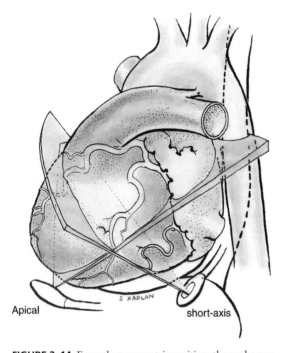

FIGURE 3–14. From the transgastric position, the probe can be positioned near the gastroesophageal junction to obtain a short-axis view of the left ventricle or can be advanced into the stomach to obtain an "apical" view. Transgastric apical images may show a foreshortened left ventricle as the true left ventricular apex often does not lie on the diaphragm. (See Color Plate 3, p. 50.) (Courtesy Starr Kaplan, Seattle, Washington.)

FIGURE 3–16. From the transgastric short-axis view of the left ventricle, slight withdrawal of the probe toward the gastroesophageal junction may allow a short-axis view of the mitral valve with definition of the anterior *(AMVL)* and posterior *(PMVL)* mitral valve leaflets. This view is particularly useful in patients with myxomatous mitral valve disease to determine the medial to lateral extent of posterior leaflet involvement.

FIGURE 3–17. From the transgastric short-axis view, 90° rotation provides a two-chamber view of the left ventricle, atrium, and atrial appendage as shown. Turning the transducer toward the patient's right side from this view provides a two-chamber view of the right atrium and right ventricle, analogous to a transthoracic right ventricular inflow view.

is helpful in precise definition of the mitral valve apparatus anatomy in patients with valve dysfunction.

Two-Chamber Plane

A two-chamber view of the left ventricle can be obtained from the transgastric position by rotating the image plane to the 90° position (Fig. 3–17). From this two-chamber view, turning the entire probe toward the patient's right side results in a view of the right atrium, tricuspid valve, and right ventricle similar to a transthoracic right ventricular inflow view. In some individuals, the right ventricular outflow tract and pulmonic valve also can be visualized.

Transgastric Apical Position

Four-Chamber Plane

From the transgastric short-axis view, the transducer is further advanced into the fundus of the stomach. In most individuals an "apical" four-chamber view can be obtained using the 0° image plane of the probe if the left ventricle lies on the diaphragm, without intervening lung.

Note that the transducer may not be on the true left ventricular apex, so this view typically is foreshortened. Anterior angulation shows the aortic valve in a view similar to the transthoracic anteriorly angulated four-chamber view, which allows Doppler interrogation of the left ventricular outflow tract and valve (Fig. 3–18).

Long-Axis Plane

From the transgastric apical four-chamber plane, rotation of the image plane to 120° results in a long-axis view of the left ventricular outflow tract, providing a more parallel intercept angle for Doppler study of outflow tract and aortic velocities. However, this view cannot be obtained in all patients, particularly if the transducer is not on the true left ventricular apex, because lung tissue is interposed between the transducer and cardiac structures as the image plane is rotated.

Descending Thoracic Aorta

From the transesophageal or transgastric position, the transducer is turned (either direction) until the image plane is directed slightly left of the patient's spine to obtain a short-axis view of the descending thoracic aorta. The aorta appears circular and shows normal systolic pulsations (Fig. 3–19). The descending thoracic aorta can be imaged in sequential short-axis views from its postgastric position to the junction with the aortic arch as the probe is

FIGURE 3–18. Transgastric apical view angulated anteriorly to include the aortic root *(top)*. This view allows recording of left ventricular outflow tract velocity with pulsed Doppler *(middle)*, and aortic jet velocity with 2D-guided continuous-wave Doppler ultrasound *(bottom)*. When a high-velocity jet is suspected, careful angulation and positioning of the transducer is needed to obtain the highest velocity signal. Because of the constraints on transducer positioning and the lack of a view equivalent to the transthoracic suprasternal notch view, the possibility of velocity underestimation should be considered.

slowly withdrawn in the esophagus. When the transducer reaches the level of the arch, turning the transducer medially, with inferior angulation, allows a long-axis view of the arch itself. The descending thoracic aorta also can be imaged in a long-axis plane by centering the aorta in the 2D sector and rotating the image plane to 90°. This long-axis view complements the short-axis view of the descending aorta in evaluation of aortic dissections, aneurysms, and atheromas and improves the differentiation of ultrasound artifacts from anatomic abnormalities. The 90° image plane also allows identification of the origin of the left subclavian artery, which is important for describing the proximal extent of dissection and for placement of an intraaortic balloon pump (see Chapter 14).

VALVE ANATOMY AND NORMAL DOPPLER FLOWS

Optimal evaluation of valve anatomy and function on transesophageal echocardiography includes the use of at least two standard orthogonal imaging planes (Table 3–3). This approach provides a reasonably complete evaluation of valve anatomy and aids recognition of ultrasound artifacts. Continuous-wave and pulsed Doppler velocities should be recorded with the ultrasound beam aligned parallel to the flow stream. However, a parallel intercept angle may be difficult to achieve given the constraints on transducer position from the transesophageal approach. As with transthoracic imaging, color Doppler is helpful for evaluation of abnormal flow patterns even at nonparallel intercept angles.

Left Ventricular Outflow and Aortic Valve

The aortic valve and left ventricular outflow tract can be imaged by anterior angulation from the 0° four-chamber view obtained with the transducer positioned posterior to the left atrium. This view is analogous to a transthoracic anteriorly angulated four-chamber view. Rotation of the image plane to about 45° provides a short-axis view of the aortic valve with clear delineation of the valve leaflets in systole and diastole. Slight withdrawal of the probe shows the sinuses of Valsalva and left main coronary artery while slight advancement provides a short-axis view of the left ventricular outflow tract. A long-axis view is obtained by rotating the image plane to about 120° (Fig. 3–20). In both the short- and long-axis views, image quality is optimized by use of a high transducer frequency and adjustment of the

FIGURE 3–19. Transesophageal 2D and color flow images of the descending thoracic aorta in short-axis *(left)* (0° rotation) and long-axis *(right)* (90° rotation) views on 2D echo *(top)* and with color flow imaging *(bottom)*. Mild atherosclerosis is present *(arrow)*. (See Color Plate 4, p. 50.)

depth to maximize the valve image. The aortic valve also can be imaged in a five-chamber view from a transesophageal position with anterior angulation from the four-chamber view at 0° rotation.

Doppler evaluation of the aortic valve on transesophageal echocardiography is problematic with color flow imaging for valvular regurgitation being the most helpful approach. With the probe positioned in the high esophagus (posterior to the left atrium), color flow imaging can be used to evaluate the flow disturbance due to aortic regurgitation in the anteriorly angulated four-chamber and long-axis views. In addition, the cross-sectional area of the aortic regurgitant jet can be evaluated starting in a short-axis view of the aortic valve and slowly advancing the probe in the esophagus to obtain a short-axis view of the outflow tract. As with transthoracic imaging, the short-axis jet area relative to outflow tract area is a reliable color flow measure of regurgitant severity.

Accurate antegrade velocity measurements across the aortic valve may not be possible because of the nonparallel intercept angle between the ultrasound beam and the direction of blood flow from the transesophageal position. In many patients, a transgastric apical view allows recording of pulsed and continuous-wave Doppler flow velocities proximal to and across the aortic valve (see Fig. 3–18). However, caution still is needed in interpretation of the

FIGURE 3–20. Long-axis images of the aortic and mitral valve with the depth adjusted to optimize evaluation of valve anatomy and motion. The 2D images *(left)* in diastole *(top)* and systole *(bottom)* show normal aortic and mitral opening and closure. The color flow images *(right)* show normal left ventricular inflow with no aortic regurgitation in diastole *(top)* and normal antegrade flow in the left ventricular outflow tract and no mitral regurgitation in systole *(bottom)*. (See Color Plate 4, p. 50.)

Doppler data obtained, since unlike a transthoracic examination, a high-velocity signal across the aortic valve cannot be studied from multiple windows with careful transducer angulation to ensure that a parallel intercept angle has been obtained. If aortic valve pathology is present, transthoracic recording of antegrade velocities is most accurate and should be performed in all cases.

Left Ventricular Inflow and Mitral Valve

The mitral valve leaflets are evaluated by slow rotation from the transesophageal four-chamber view to the long-axis view with continuous image recording. Again, adjusting the transducer frequency, image depth, and other instrument parameters are needed for optimal image quality. Adjustments in transducer angulation and position may be needed to fully evaluate pathologic findings. The subvalvular apparatus usually is well seen in these views unless there is valve calcification with shadowing of distal structures. If additional views are needed, the examiner should obtain transgastric short-axis and two-chamber views of the mitral valve. Other useful views include the transgas-

TABLE 3–3	Transesophageal Views for Cardiac Valves		
Valve	**View**	**Probe Position**	**Rotation Angle**
Aortic	Long-axis	High esophageal *or* Transgastric apical	~120°–130°
	Short-axis	High esophageal	~45°–50°
	"Five-chamber"	High esophageal *or* Transgastric apical	0° (anteriorly angulated)
Mitral	Long-axis	High esophageal Transgastric	~120°–130° 90°
	Short-axis	Transgastric (at GE junction)	May be obtained in some patients at 0° with probe flexed
	Four-chamber	High esophageal *or* Transgastric apical	0°
Pulmonic	Long-axis	Very high esophageal	0° (looking straight down PA from bifurcation)
	Outflow view	High esophageal	~90° (turn probe to left)
Tricuspid	Four-chamber	High esophageal	0°
	RV inflow (esophageal)	High esophageal	~90° (turn probe to right)
	RV inflow (transgastric)	Transgastric	~90° (turn probe to right)

PA = Pulmonary artery; RV = right ventricular.

tric apical view, although image quality may be suboptimal at the depth of the mitral valve.

The pattern of antegrade flow across the mitral valve (left ventricular diastolic filling) can be recorded with pulsed Doppler in the four-chamber or long-axis view at a parallel intercept angle (Fig. 3–21). Since the flow is directly away from the transducer, the velocity curve with the typical early diastolic peak *(E)* and late diastolic peak *(A)* velocities is shown below the baseline. Color Doppler can be used to evaluate for mitral regurgitation as the image plane is slowly rotated from the four-chamber to two-chamber to long-axis view. Alternatively, transmitral flow can be recorded from the transgastric apical approach, although signal strength is lower due to the greater depth of the mitral valve from this position. Mitral regurgitation can be evaluated with continuous-wave Doppler from the high esophageal position, using the color flow signal to align the continuous-wave Doppler beam with the vena contracta of the regurgitant jet (Fig. 3–22).

Right Ventricular Outflow and Pulmonic Valve

The right ventricular outflow tract is best imaged from a high esophageal position at 0° rotation with a long-axis view of the pulmonary artery from the valve plane to its bifur-cation. Doppler velocities can be recorded from this position at a parallel intercept angle as flow is directed straight toward the transducer (Fig. 3–23). The pulmonic valve also may be visualized in the 90° long-axis plane with the pulmonic valve seen in its perpendicular relation-

FIGURE 3–21. Left ventricular inflow recorded with pulsed Doppler with the sample volume positioned at the mitral leaflet tips from an anteriorly angulated transesophageal four-chamber view. The flow pattern is similar to a transthoracic recording of left ventricular inflow, albeit inverted as the flow is directed away from the transducer.

FIGURE 3–22. Continuous-wave Doppler recording of mitral regurgitation from a transesophageal four-chamber view. Color flow was used to identify the vena contracta of the regurgitant jet for the initial positioning of the continuous-wave Doppler beam. Transducer position and angulation then were modified as needed to obtain a clear signal with the highest flow velocity. (See Color Plate 4, p. 50.)

FIGURE 3–23. A very high transesophageal position provides a long-axis view *(left)* of the main pulmonary artery and its bifurcation into right and left pulmonary arteries. The ascending aorta is seen in short axis. This view allows recording of flow in the pulmonary artery at a parallel intercept angle because flow is directly toward the transducer *(above)*.

ship to the aortic valve in the far field of the image (see Fig. 3–10). However, velocities cannot be recorded from this approach due to a nonparallel intercept angle. In some patients, the pulmonic valve also can be imaged from the transgastric position either in the 90° image plane including the tricuspid valve or in a very anteriorly angulated apical four-chamber view.

Right Ventricular Inflow and Tricuspid Valve

The tricuspid valve is well imaged in the standard four-chamber views, both from the transesophageal position and from the transgastric apical view. Other useful views include the transesophageal right ventricular inflow view and the transgastric two-chamber view

turned to show the right heart structures. In a transgastric view obtained close to the diaphragm, the entry of the coronary sinus into the right atrium adjacent to the tricuspid valve can be seen. Further advancement of the transducer often allows a short-axis view of the tricuspid valve.

The tricuspid regurgitant jet may be recorded from either transesophageal or transgastric views; however, underestimation of velocity should be considered given the limited ability to vary transducer position to ensure a parallel intercept angle (Fig. 3–24). If high pulmonary pressures are suspected, transthoracic continuous-wave Doppler recordings or invasive measures of pulmonary pressure should be obtained.

FIGURE 3–24. Continuous-wave Doppler recording of tricuspid regurgitation from a transesophageal four-chamber view using color flow to identify the origin of the tricuspid regurgitant jet. (See Color Plate 4, p. 50.)

CHAMBER ANATOMY AND ATRIAL INFLOW

Left Ventricle

Standard views of the left ventricle are obtained from the transesophageal position in four-chamber, two-chamber, and long-axis views (Table 3–4). A standard short-axis view is obtained from the transgastric position. These views allow calculation of left ventricular volumes and ejection fraction. Comparisons with radionuclide and contrast angiography have shown that transesophageal calculation of ejection fraction is both accurate and reproducible (Fig. 3–25). End-diastolic and end-systolic volumes often are underestimated because the image plane does not include the full long axis of the ventricle. However, transesophageal echocardiography remains accurate for evaluation of relative changes in ventricular volumes based on short-axis area changes in an individual patient. Left ventricular volume status can be assessed during surgery using a combination of these views, or using a single view, such as the transgastric short-axis view for continuous monitoring.

Standard views of the left ventricle also allow evaluation of regional ventricular function for each myocardial segment with a high degree of interobserver reproducibility for grading of wall motion in standard segments. In the transgastric short-axis view, the wall segments are the same as in a transthoracic short-axis view, *except* that the entire image has been rotated approximately 180° clockwise (if standard display format is used). Compared with a transthoracic subcostal short-axis view, the image is rotated 90° clockwise (see Fig. 7–7).

Left Atrium

The location and flow patterns of the pulmonary veins are readily assessed by trans-

TABLE 3–4	Transesophageal Views for Evaluation of Cardiac Chambers		
Chamber	**View**	**Probe Position**	**Rotation Angle**
Left ventricle	Four-chamber	High esophageal	0°
	Two-chamber	High esophageal	60°
	Long-axis	High esophageal	120°
	Short-axis	Transgastric	0° with angulation of the probe tip
Left atrium	Four-chamber	High esophageal	0°, also allows assessment of all 4 pulmonary veins with medial and lateral turning and slight angulation of the transducer
	Two-chamber	High esophageal	60°
	Long-axis	High esophageal	120°
Right ventricle	Four-chamber	High esophageal	0°
	Right ventricular inflow view	High esophageal *or*	90° with probe turned toward patient's right side
		Transgastric	90° with probe turned toward patients' right side
Right atrium	Four-chamber	High esophageal	0° with posterior angulation to visualize coronary sinus
	Right atrium view	High esophageal	90° with probe turned toward patient's right side
	Low atrial view	Gastroesophageal junction	0° to visualize entry of coronary sinus into right atrium

FIGURE 3–25. Examples of endocardial border tracings at end-diastole in a transesophageal four-chamber *(top)* and two-chamber *(bottom)* for calculation of left ventricular ejection fraction, in conjunction with end-systolic border tracings.

FIGURE 3–26. Pulsed Doppler recording of normal flow in the left superior pulmonary vein shows systolic *(S)* and diastolic *(D)* inflow with a small atrial *(a)* reversal signal.

esophageal echocardiography. The flow pattern is most easily recorded in the left superior pulmonary vein where the typical systolic and diastolic antegrade flows and the reversal after atrial contraction can be appreciated (Fig. 3–26). Although flow tends to be more laminar with a narrow band on velocities on the spectral display in the left, compared to right, superior pulmonary vein, in general flow patterns are similar in all four pulmonary veins. However, exceptions do occur as, for example, when mitral regurgitation is present. In this situation, the regurgitant jet may be directed eccentrically, altering flow patterns in some, but not all, pulmonary veins.

If left atrial thrombus is suspected, the atrial appendage should be examined in at least two orthogonal views. Recognition of low flow (spontaneous contrast) and appendage thrombi are enhanced by use of a high transducer frequency (7 MHz). Care is needed to distinguish normal trabeculation from localized thrombus formation. Trabeculae tend to be more linear and are continuous with the atrial wall in more than one view. Thrombi typically protrude into the appendage, often with independent motion.

The flow pattern in the left atrial appendage can be recorded with pulsed Doppler ultrasound with the sample volume positioned in the appendage, about 1 cm from the junction with the body of the left atrium. The normal flow pattern (see Fig. 14–24) is characterized by ejection of blood from the appendage following atrial contraction at a velocity >40 cm/s. Abnormal flow patterns are seen with atrial fibrillation, atrial flutter, and other tachyarrhythmias.

The interatrial septum is well seen in the standard four-chamber view and can be evaluated in detail by centering the septum in the image and then slowly rotating the image plane with continuous recording of images. The fossa ovalis and primum septum are clearly demarcated, and the "flap valve" of a patent foramen ovale often can be identified on 2D imaging, prior to confirmation with color Doppler or an intravenous contrast injection (see Fig. 14–28).

Right Ventricle

As with transthoracic echocardiography, quantitation of right ventricular size and systolic function is difficult due to the complex geometry of this chamber. Qualitative assessment of size and function is made from the transesophageal four-chamber and apical short-axis views. In the future, 3D echocardiography may allow more precise quantitation of right ventricular geometry and function.

Right Atrium

The body of the right atrium is best imaged in the transesophageal four-chamber view. In addition, the long-axis view of the right atrium obtained with the image plane at 90° and the probe rotated toward the right with the probe tip at the left atrial level allows visualization of the atrial appendage (with normal trabeculation) and the junctions of the superior and inferior vena cava with the right atrium. Movement of the probe up in the esophagus allows evaluation of the cephalad extent of the superior vena cava, while movement toward the stomach provides additional views of the inferior vena cava.

The coronary sinus can be identified in a posteriorly angled four-chamber view. The entry of the coronary sinus into the right atrium is best seen in the 0° image plane with the trans-ducer positioned near the gastroesophageal junction and angulated superiorly (Fig. 3–27).

SUGGESTED READING

1. Porembka DT (ed): Transesophageal echocardiography and innovative echocardiographic technology. *Crit Care Clin* 12:203–497, 1996.

   This issue of Critical Care Clinics is devoted to transesophageal echocardiography. Several articles detail the techniques and pitfalls of multiplane transesophageal echocardiography. Other articles review the assessment of left ventricular systolic function, intracardiac shunts, valve repair, prosthetic valves, endocarditis, and cardiac sources of embolus.

2. Johnson SB, Sisley AC: The surgeon's use of transesophageal echocardiography. *Surg Clin North Am* 78: 311–336, 1998.

   Brief review of the basic views obtained on transesophageal echocardiography followed by a discussion of the use of transesophageal echocardiography in patients with cardiac or aortic trauma, in the critical care unit, and in patients with suspected aortic dissection. 72 references.

3. Seward JB, Khandheria BK, Edwards WD, et al: Biplanar transesophageal echocardiography: Anatomic correlations, image orientation, and clinical applications. *Mayo Clin Proc* 65:1193–1213, 1990.

   Review of biplane transesophageal views and experience in 291 patients. Useful schematic drawings, although image orientation is nonstandard.

4. Rafferty TD: Basics of Transesophageal Echocardiography. New York, Churchill Livingstone, 1995.

   Concise textbook reviewing the patient examination sequence, techniques, and procedures of transesophageal echocardiography. Clear illustrations with accompanying line drawings.

5. De Simone R, Paolella RG: Interactive atlas of transesophageal color Doppler echocardiography on CD-ROM for Windows/MAC (ed 2). New York: Springer, Heidelberg, 1997.

   Well-organized CD-ROM atlas of transesophageal echocardiographic images.

6. Oka Y, Konstadt SN: Clinical transesophageal echocardiography: A problem-oriented approach. Philadelphia, Lippincott-Raven, 1996.

   Multiauthor textbook on transesophageal echocardiography with chapters arranged by disease process in patients undergoing cardiac surgery (e.g., mitral stenosis, myxomatous mitral valve, aortic dissection) and noncardiac surgery (e.g., liver transplantation, trauma, hemodynamic monitoring).

7. Nanda NC, Domanski MJ: Atlas of transesophageal echocardiography. Baltimore, Williams & Wilkins, 1998.

   This 520-page atlas includes numerous transesophageal images with detailed figure legends. Some schematic diagrams and pathologic correlations are included. The sections on congenital heart disease are especially helpful.

FIGURE 3–27. Low transesophageal view of the right heart showing the entry of the coronary sinus *(CS)* into the right atrium. A central venous catheter *(arrow)* is present with the tip in the right atrium.

8. Daniel WG, Erbel R, Kasper W, Visser CA, Engberding R, Sutherland GR, Grube E, Hanrath P, Maisch B, Denning K, et al: Safety of transesophageal echocardiography: A multicenter survey of 10,419 examinations. *Circulation* 83:817–821, 1991.

In 10,419 transesophageal examinations performed at 15 European centers over 1 year, probe insertion was unsuccessful in only 2% of attempted studies and the procedure had to be interrupted in only 1% of cases. Reasons for interrupting the procedure included intolerance of the endoscope, pulmonary, cardiac, and bleeding complications. There was 1 death (1/10,000) due to bleeding from a lung tumor with esophageal infiltration. Since nearly all these studies were performed without conscious sedation, the additional risk associated with sedative medications must be considered. The ratio of transesophageal to transthoracic studies in this registry averaged 9% but varied from 1.4% to 23.6% between institutions.

9. Pearlman AS, Gardin JM, Martin RP, et al: Guidelines for physicians training in transesophageal echocardiography: Recommendations of the American Society of Echocardiography Committee for Physician Training in Echocardiography. *J Am Soc Echocardiogr* 5:187–194, 1992.

Recommendations for physician training in transesophageal echocardiography.

10. ACC Echocardiography Committee Position Statement: Transesophageal echocardiography. *J Am Coll Cardiol* 20:506, 1992.

Expert opinion on the clinical utility and accepted indications for transesophageal echocardiography.

11. Konstadt SM, Reich DL, Rafferty T: Validation of a test of competence in transesophageal echocardiography. *J Cardiovasc Anesth* 10:311–313, 1996.

Performance on a multiple choice question examination based on short video sequences distinguished faculty experienced in the use of transesophageal echocardiography from inexperienced operators. The need for evaluation of performance and monitoring of clinical quality is emphasized.

12. Practice guidelines for sedation and analgesia by non-anesthesiologists: A report by the American Society of Anesthesiologists Task Force on Sedation and Analgesia by Non-Anesthesiologists. *Anesthesiology* 84:459–471, 1996.

Consensus statement detailing the clinical standards for conscious sedation including patient evaluation, preprocedure preparation, monitoring (level of consciousness, ventilation, oxygenation, and hemodynamics), data recording, and availability of emergency equipment. The importance of having a staff person dedicated solely to patient monitoring and safety is emphasized, and the appropriate training of personnel is discussed.

13. Smith MD, MacPhail B, Harrison MR, Lenhoff SJ, DeMaria AN: Value and limitations of transesophageal echocardiography in determination of left ventricular volumes and ejection fraction. *J Am Coll Cardiol* 19:1213–1222, 1992.

In 36 patients undergoing left ventriculography, various transesophageal echocardiographic methods for calculation of left ventricular ejection fraction and volumes were compared with ventriculography. Ejection fraction was most accurately evaluated with the biplane Simpson's rule method (r = 0.85). However, ventricular volumes and length were consistently underestimated by transesophageal echocardiography, suggesting that foreshortening of the long axis of the ventricle occurs with transesophageal images.

14. Ryan T, Burwash I, Lu J, Otto C, Graham M, Verrier E, Spiess BD: The agreement between ventricular volumes and ejection fraction by transesophageal echocardiography or a combined radionuclear and thermodilution technique in patients after coronary artery surgery. *J Cardiothorac Vasc Anesth* 10:323–328, 1996.

Three sets of measurements of radionuclide and transesophageal echocardiographic measurement of left ventricular volumes and ejection fraction were made after coronary artery bypass grafting surgery. Ejection fraction measured by transesophageal echocardiography using Simpson's rule or the area-length method was accurate and reproducible. However, agreement for measurement of ventricular volumes was poor.

Clinical Indications for Echocardiography

4

CLINICAL DECISION ANALYSIS AS THE FRAMEWORK FOR
THE DIAGNOSTIC USE OF ECHOCARDIOGRAPHY
    Accuracy of a Diagnostic Test
    Integration of Clinical Data and Test Results
    The Threshold Approach to Clinical Decision Analysis
    Cost-Effectiveness
    Clinical Outcome
    Implications for Diagnostic Use of Echocardiography
INDICATIONS FOR ECHOCARDIOGRAPHY
    Transthoracic Echocardiography
        By Clinical Signs and Symptoms
        By Anatomic Diagnosis
        By Clinical Setting

    Stress Echocardiography
    Contrast Echocardiography
    Transesophageal Echocardiography
    Intravascular Ultrasound
    3D Echocardiography
APPROACH TO THE ECHOCARDIOGRAPHIC
EXAMINATION
    Basic Format
    Focusing the Examination
    Education and Training Guidelines
    Echocardiographic Interpretation
SUGGESTED READING

Clinical indications for echocardiographic examination are best considered within the framework of clinical decision analysis. This chapter provides a brief introduction to this approach, with suggestions for further reading indicated at the end of the chapter.

CLINICAL DECISION ANALYSIS AS THE FRAMEWORK FOR THE DIAGNOSTIC USE OF ECHOCARDIOGRAPHY

Accuracy of a Diagnostic Test

The first level of analysis in evaluating a diagnostic test is to consider its accuracy. The clinical utility of any diagnostic test, including echocardiography, depends, in large part, on the certainty with which a specific diagnosis can be confirmed or excluded based on the test results (Fig. 4–1). The *sensitivity* of a test is the degree to which it identifies all patients with the disease. *Sensitivity* is defined as the patients with a "true-positive" test result divided by all patients with the disease. The *specificity* of a test is the degree to which it identifies all patients *without* the disease. *Specificity* is defined as the patients with a "true-negative" test result divided by all patients without the disease. Sensitivity and specificity are related inversely to

each other; in general, the higher the sensitivity, the lower is the specificity and vice versa. Whether a higher sensitivity is preferable to a higher specificity depends on the specific clinical question. If the goal of the test is identification of *all* patients with the disease, a high sensitivity is preferable. If the goal is confirmation of the diagnosis in an individual patient, a high specificity is preferable. The relationship between sensitivity and specificity can be evaluated quantitatively for any given diagnostic test using receiver-operator curve (ROC) analysis (Fig. 4–2). The *accuracy* of a test is defined as the true positives plus the true negatives divided by the total number of tests performed. Accuracy indicates the percentage of patients in whom the test results are correct in identifying the presence or absence of disease.

A major limitation of applying sensitivity/specificity data to an individual patient is the problem of whether a particular patient has a "true" or a "false" test result. At first glance, it might seem that use of positive and negative predictive values would be more useful in the clinical setting. Predictive values indicate the percentage of patients with a positive test result who have the suspected disease (positive predictive value = true positives divided by all positives) and the percentage with a negative

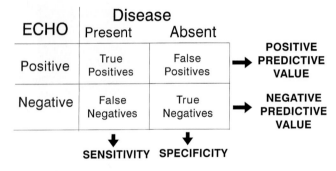

FIGURE 4–1. Sensitivity and specificity in comparison with positive and negative predictive value. Note that predictive values are dependent on the prevalence of the disease in the study population and thus cannot be extrapolated to other patient groups (*TP* = true positives; *TN* = true negatives).

test result who do not have the suspected disease (negative predictive value = true negatives divided by all negatives). However, predictive values depend on the *prevalence* of disease in a given population and therefore cannot be extrapolated to other patient groups.

The absolute number of patients with *false-positive* or *false-negative* test results depends on the prevalence of disease in the population studied as well as the sensitivity and specificity of the test. Intuitively, this is obvious comparing the use of echocardiography to "screen" healthy young subjects for endocarditis (many false-positive results due to ultrasound imaging artifacts) versus the same test in patients who have a new murmur, fever, and positive blood cultures. The finding of a valvular vegetation on echocardiography in the latter group has a much higher predictive value for a diagnosis of endocarditis than in the healthy subjects, even though the sensitivity and specificity of echocardiography for diagnosing endocarditis are the same in both groups. Again, the positive or negative predictive value of a test reflects disease prevalence as well as test accuracy.

FIGURE 4–2. Graph of sensitivity versus specificity, known as a receiver-operator curve, comparing the studies of Otto and Pearlman[9] and Oh et al.[10] In the first study a clinical decision rule was proposed for timing of valve replacement in aortic stenosis based on jet velocity breakpoints at 3 and 4 m/s. In the second study, a single breakpoint at 4.5 m/s was suggested, but the data show that a two-breakpoint approach at 3 and 4.5 m/s also would be appropriate. Patients with jet velocities between these breakpoints require calculation of aortic valve area and assessment of coexisting aortic regurgitation.

Integration of Clinical Data and Test Results

A better approach to the use of sensitivity/specificity data in patient management is to consider relevant clinical data along with the test result. The value of a diagnostic test increases when the pretest likelihood of disease is integrated with the test results to derive a posttest likelihood of disease. This approach is known as *Bayesian analysis*. For example, the pretest likelihood of severe aortic stenosis in an asymptomatic 30-year-old woman with no systolic murmur on careful auscultation is very low. An echocardiogram purporting to show severe aortic stenosis most likely is an erroneous interpretation (a false-positive test result). In this setting, the result does not increase the posttest likelihood of disease very much. In contrast, in an elderly man with a 4/6 aortic stenosis murmur and symptoms of angina, syncope, and heart failure, the diagnosis of severe valvular aortic stenosis can be made with a high level of certainty even before any test is performed. The echocardiogram serves only to confirm the diagnosis and define the severity of obstruction. In general, diagnostic tests are most helpful when the pretest likelihood of disease is intermediate so that the test result will substantially change the posttest likelihood of disease (Fig. 4–3).

The Threshold Approach to Clinical Decision Analysis

The most comprehensive approach to evaluation of a diagnostic test is *clinical decision analysis*. Clinical decision analysis incorporates several rigorous approaches to the problem of clinical prediction, with the method most applicable to a diagnostic test, such as echocardiography, being the threshold approach. The basic tenet of clinical decision analysis as applied to a diagnostic test is that the test results should have an impact on patient care by either (1) prompting a change in therapy or (2) leading to a change in the subsequent diagnostic strategy in that patient. This basic assumption is formalized in the *threshold model* of decision analysis. In this approach, two disease probability thresholds are defined for the diagnostic test: (1) a lower threshold below which the risk of the test is greater than the risk of not treating the patient, and (2) an upper threshold above which treating the patient is lower risk than performing the test. The intermediate range—where the risk of treating or not treating the patient is greater than the risk of the diagnostic test—is known as the *testing zone* (Fig. 4–4). For any *specific* indication, the testing zone for echocardiography generally is wide because of the low risk and high accuracy of this

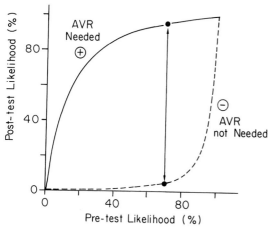

FIGURE 4–3. Bayesian analysis has been applied to the data from Otto and Pearlman.[9] The posttest likelihood (*y* axis) of need for aortic valve replacement *(AVR)* was calculated for each hypothetical pretest likelihood (*x* axis). Pretest and corresponding posttest likelihoods for the study population are indicated by the arrow. (Reprinted with permission from Otto CM, Pearlman AS: Doppler echocardiography in adults with symptomatic aortic stenosis. *Arch Intern Med* 148:2553–2560, 1988; copyright 1988, American Medical Association.)

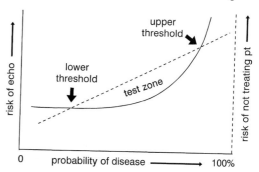

FIGURE 4–4. Diagram illustrating the threshold approach to clinical decision making. The risk of the diagnostic test—in this case, echocardiography—is shown in the solid line (left *y* axis) with the risk of *not* treating the patient for the suspected disease shown in the dashed line (right *y* axis). The probability of disease based on the clinical presentation is shown from 0 to 100% on the *x* axis. The lower threshold is the point at which the risk of not treating the patient is greater than the risk of echocardiography. The upper threshold is the point at which the risk of echocardiography (including false-negative results, delay in treatment) is greater than the risk of not treating the patient. The test zone is the pretest likelihood of disease between these two thresholds.

technique. However, both an upper and lower threshold still are definable for echocardiography. The upper threshold is reached in situations in which the diagnosis is clear, and echocardiographic examination would only delay appropriate treatment. For example, a patient with a classic presentation of an ascending aortic dissection (chest pain, wide mediastinum, peripheral pulse loss) requires prompt surgery. Any delay due to unnecessary diagnostic testing could result in additional morbidity or mortality.

It is tempting to assume that there is no lower end to the test zone for echocardiography given the absence of known adverse biologic effects of this procedure. However, the risk of the test also includes costs and, more important, the risks of additional diagnostic tests or even erroneous treatment choices resulting from a false-positive echocardiographic finding. For example, an echocardiogram is not indicated to evaluate for aortic dissection in a young patient with atypical chest pain and a normal physical examination, electrocardiogram, and chest radiograph. If a false-positive echocardiographic diagnosis leads to further evaluation with cardiac catheterization, any complications from the invasive procedure ultimately can be considered a consequence of the echocardiographic results. Thus, a lower limit to the test zone *does* exist for echocardiography and can be defined for each specific diagnostic indication by applying decision analysis techniques.

Other clinical decision analysis approaches have been applied to specific clinical problems that use echocardiographic data as a branch point in the decision analysis tree. One example is the problem of timing of valve replacement in chronic asymptomatic aortic regurgitation (see Suggested Reading 7).

Cost-Effectiveness

An additional consideration in medical practice is the cost-effectiveness of a diagnostic procedure. Note that this term includes not only the cost of the test (echocardiography compares favorably with other cardiac diagnostic tests) but also the effectiveness of the test—that is, test accuracy and its impact on patient management. This type of analysis has been applied to some echocardiographic diagnostic issues, but more widespread use of this approach is needed.

Clinical Outcome

The most important measure of the value of a diagnostic test is its impact on subsequent clinical outcome (Fig. 4–5). While the first step in evaluation of the clinical utility of a test includes various measures of diagnostic accuracy in comparison to some accepted standard, the more important assessment is whether the diagnostic test changes the subsequent diagnostic or therapeutic plan in each patient. Finally, the clinical utility of the test depends on its ability to predict prognosis; for example, survival in patients with dilated cardiomyopathy, timing of valve surgery in patients with chronic regurgitation, or the rate of hemodynamic progression in patients with valvular stenosis. Now that the accuracy and reliability of echocardiographic techniques have been well established, echocar-

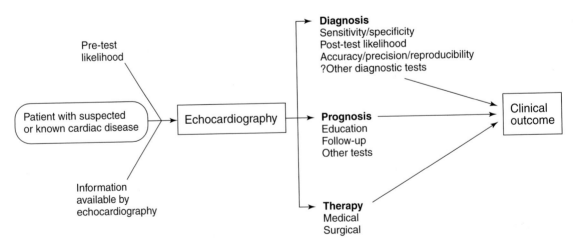

FIGURE 4–5. Flow chart illustrating the importance of the impact of the echocardiographic results on diagnosis, prognosis, and therapy. Ultimately, the effect of the echocardiographic examination on clinical outcome is the best measure of the usefulness of the test result.

diographic data are increasingly used in clinical outcome studies, as referenced in the Suggested Readings throughout this textbook.

Implications for Diagnostic Use of Echocardiography

Thus, it no longer is acceptable to consider only sensitivity and specificity in the decision whether or not to perform a diagnostic test. The echocardiogram request should indicate an appropriate clinical question (not "evaluate heart") with an estimate of the probability of the diagnosis in that patient. Next, the reliability of echocardiography for that diagnosis is considered, and most important, the likelihood that the echocardiographic results will alter patient management is formulated prior to performing the study. Often it is helpful to consider the specific branch point in the diagnostic/therapeutic plans that the echocardiographic results will be applied to in the clinical decision process.

With these considerations in mind, there are certain situations in which the use of echocardiography clearly changes patient management:

1. Making the correct anatomic diagnosis. For example, differentiating a primary valvular problem from systolic left ventricular dysfunction in a patient with heart failure symptoms.

2. Providing important prognostic data in a patient with a known anatomic diagnosis. For example, vegetation size in endocarditis or left ventricular ejection fraction in cardiomyopathy.

3. Identifying complications of a known diagnosis. For example, paravalvular abscess in endocarditis or left ventricular thrombus in cardiomyopathy.

In addition, there are numerous other settings in which echocardiography is considered to be clinically indicated. Whether all these situations meet the strict criteria of the clinical threshold model requires ongoing appraisal.

Throughout this text, the accuracy (sensitivity and specificity) of echocardiography for each specific diagnosis will be indicated, if known. The clinician then should integrate these data with the pretest likelihood of disease in each patient. Critical evaluations of the diagnostic utility of echocardiography in specific patient populations and clinical settings will be highlighted, including symptomatic adults with aortic stenosis (Chap. 10), asymptomatic chronic aortic regurgitation (Chap. 11), evaluation of chest pain in the emergency room (Chap. 7), intraoperative assessment of mitral valve repair (Chap. 11), and the diagnosis and prognosis of endocarditis (Chap. 13).

INDICATIONS FOR ECHOCARDIOGRAPHY

Transthoracic Echocardiography

By Clinical Signs and Symptoms

An echocardiogram often is requested to evaluate a specific clinical sign or symptom such as chest pain, heart failure symptoms (Fig. 4–6), a murmur, or cardiomegaly on chest radiography (Fig. 4–7). When the echocardiographer evaluates a patient with one of these indications, it is important that the differential diagnosis be considered and each possibility excluded or confirmed during the course of the examination. For example, a patient with a systolic murmur may have valvular aortic stenosis, a subaortic membrane, hypertrophic cardiomyopathy, mitral regurgitation, a ventricular septal defect, pulmonic stenosis, or tricuspid regurgitation. With two-dimensional (2D) imaging and Doppler evaluation, each of these possible diagnoses can be evaluated. If a careful examination reveals none of these abnormalities, it may be concluded that the murmur is a benign "flow" murmur (Fig. 4–8).

Similarly, in the echocardiographic examination of a patient with chest pain, even if the referring physician has made a presumptive diagnosis of coronary artery disease, the echocardiographer should be alert to any findings suggesting other causes for chest pain such as left ventricular outflow obstruction (valvular aortic stenosis or hypertrophic cardiomyopathy), aortic dissection, or pericarditis. The echocardiographic differential diagnosis for common symptoms is shown in Table 4–1 and

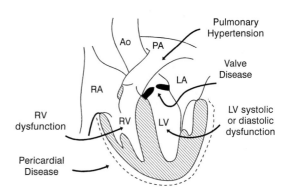

FIGURE 4–6. Diagram illustrating some of the more common causes of heart failure that should be actively excluded or confirmed during echocardiographic examination.

FIGURE 4–7. Chest radiographs demonstrating cardiomegaly due to a large pericardial effusion *(left)* and cardiomegaly due to multivalve disease with four-chamber enlargement *(right).*

for common physical signs in Table 4–2. These examples are not meant to be an exhaustive list of the possibilities but rather represent an illustration of the types of conditions the echocardiographer should consider in performing and interpreting the examination.

By Anatomic Diagnosis

In many patients referred for echocardiography, a definite or presumptive anatomic diagnosis has been made. In these patients, the echocardiographer needs to be aware of the information that can be obtained by echocardiography, the limitations of echocardiography, and alternative diagnostic approaches.

For example, in a patient with a systolic murmur known to be due to valvular aortic stenosis, the echocardiogram may be requested to evaluate the severity of obstruction, the degree of coexisting aortic regurgitation, the presence of left ventricular hypertrophy, and the

status of left ventricular systolic function, as well as to detect any associated valvular abnormalities (e.g., mitral regurgitation). Usually echocardiography provides all the needed information for clinical decision making other than coronary artery anatomy, but the echocardiographer must acknowledge that stenosis severity may have been underestimated if there was a nonparallel intercept angle between the direction of the aortic jet and the ultrasound beam. In cases where the echocardiographic re-

FIGURE 4–8. Diagram illustrating the more common etiologies for a systolic murmur. If an echocardiogram is requested for this indication, the sonographer should focus the examination toward confirmation or exclusion of each of these possibilities.

TABLE 4–1	Differential Diagnosis for the Echocardiographer: Common Symptoms
Reason for Echo	**Differential Diagnosis**
Chest pain	Coronary artery disease: acute myocardial infarction or angina Aortic dissection Pericarditis Valvular aortic stenosis Hypertrophic cardiomyopathy
Heart failure	Left ventricular systolic dysfunction (global or segmental) Valvular heart disease Left ventricular diastolic dysfunction Pericardial disease Right ventricular dysfunction
Palpitations	Left ventricular systolic dysfunction Mitral valve disease Congenital heart disease (e.g., ASD, Ebstein's anomaly) Pericarditis No structural cardiac disease

ASD = Atrial septal defect.

TABLE 4–2	Differential Diagnosis for the Echocardiographer: Common Signs
Reason for Echo	**Differential Diagnosis: Common Signs**
Cardiac murmur	
Systolic	Flow murmur (no valve abnormality)
	Aortic stenosis, subaortic obstruction, hypertrophic obstructive cardiomyopathy
	Mitral regurgitation
	Ventricular septal defect
	Pulmonic stenosis
	Tricuspid regurgitation
Diastolic	Mitral stenosis
	Aortic regurgitation
	Pulmonic regurgitation
	Tricuspid stenosis
Cardiomegaly on chest radiography	Pericardial effusion
	Dilated cardiomyopathy
	Specific chamber enlargement (e.g., left ventricle in chronic aortic regurgitation)
Systemic embolic event	Left ventricular systolic function and segmental wall motion abnormalities (aneurysms)
	Left ventricular thrombus
	Aortic valve disease
	Mitral valve disease
	Left atrial thrombus (TTE has low sensitivity)
	Patent foramen ovale

TTE = Transthoracic echocardiography.

sults appear to be discordant with the clinical impression, alternate diagnostic tests such as cardiac catheterization may be needed. Echocardiography in a patient with endocarditis is a second, more complex example. On the one hand, echocardiography can detect valvular vegetations, identify the specific valves involved, evaluate the presence and degree of valve dysfunction, and measure associated chamber enlargement. Both left and right ventricular systolic function can be qualitatively and quantitatively evaluated. In addition, abscess formation may be identified. While the potential prognostic value of measuring vegetation size remains controversial, many clinicians find this information of clinical value. On the other hand a definite diagnosis of endocarditis requires the presence of both echocardiographic and bacteriologic criteria. When echocardiographic findings are atypical, additional clinical criteria must be present to make the diagnosis. The sensitivity of echocardiography for detection of valvular vegetations varies with image quality; conversely, a healed valvular vegetation may persist after a previous episode of endocarditis. Transesophageal echocardiography is more sensitive for diagnosing valvular vegetations and should be considered if the clinical suspicion of endocarditis is moderate to high and the transthoracic study does not show typical vegetations. Transesophageal echocardiography also is much more sensitive for the diagnosis of paravalvular abscesses and for evaluation of prosthetic valve endocarditis.

In Table 4–3, the key echocardiographic findings, limitations of echocardiography, and alternate diagnostic approaches for several anatomic diagnoses are indicated. Each of these topics is covered in detail in subsequent chapters.

By Clinical Setting (Table 4–4)

The third category of indications for echocardiography is the examination requested because the patient is a member of a clinical group in whom "routine" echocardiographic studies are thought to be clinically valuable. These examinations fall into one of four categories: (1) *screening* examinations to detect cardiac abnormalities in a group of patients with a high prevalence of disease, (2) *monitoring* examinations performed as part of a therapeutic procedure, (3) *evaluation* before and after a therapeutic intervention to assess the effect of the intervention and detect possible complications, and (4) *baseline* studies performed in patients at risk for subsequent cardiac disease or progression of preexisting cardiac disease.

Screening examinations are performed in first-degree family members of patients with genetically transmitted cardiac diseases, such as

TABLE 4–3	Indications for Transthoracic Echocardiography		
Clinical Diagnosis	**Key Echo Findings**	**Limitations of Echo**	**Alternate Approaches**
Valvular Heart Disease			
Valve stenosis	Etiology of stenosis, valve anatomy Transvalvular ΔP, valve area Chamber enlargement and hypertrophy LV and RV systolic function Associated valvular regurgitation	Possible underestimation of stenosis severity Possible coexisting coronary artery disease	Cardiac cath
Valve regurgitation	Mechanism and etiology of regurgitation Severity of regurgitation Chamber enlargement LV and RV systolic function PA pressure estimate	TEE may be needed to evaluate mitral regurgitant severity and valve anatomy (especially before MV repair)	Cardiac cath
Prosthetic valve function	Evidence for stenosis Detection of regurgitation Chamber enlargement Ventricular function PA pressure estimate	Imaging prosthetic valves is limited by shadowing and reverberations TEE is needed for suspected prosthetic MR because of "masking" of the LA on TTE	Cardiac cath
Endocarditis	Detection of vegetations (TTE sensitivity 70%–85%) Presence and degree of valve dysfunction Chamber enlargement and function Detection of abscess Possible prognostic implications	TEE more sensitive for detection of vegetations (>90%) A definite diagnosis of endocarditis also depends on bacteriologic critiera TEE more sensitive for abscess detection	Blood cultures and clinical findings also are diagnostic criteria for endocarditis
Coronary Artery Disease			

Acute myocardial infarction	Segmental wall motion abnormality reflects "myocardium at risk"
	Global LV function (EF)
	Complications:
	  Acute MR vs. VSD
	  Pericarditis
	  LV thrombus, aneurysm
	  RV infarct
		Coronary artery anatomy itself not directly visualized	Coronary angio
			Radionuclide LV angio
			Cardiac cath

Angina	Global and segmental LV systolic function Exclude other causes of angina (e.g., AS, HOCM)	Resting wall motion may be normal despite significant CAD Stress echo needed to induce ischemia and wall motion abnormality	Coronary angio Stress thallium ETT

TABLE 4–3	Indications for Transthoracic Echocardiography *Continued*		
Clinical Diagnosis	**Key Echo Findings**	**Limitations of Echo**	**Alternate Approaches**
Pre-/postrevascularization	Assess wall thickening and endocardial motion at baseline Improvement in segmental function postprocedure	Viable but nonfunctioning myocardium cannot be identified	PET Thallium ETT Contrast echocardiography
End-stage ischemic disease	Overall LV systolic function (EF) PA pressures Associated MR LV thrombus RV systolic function		Coronary angio Radionuclide EF
Cardiomyopathy			
Dilated	Chamber dilation (all four) LV and RV systolic function (qualitative and EF) Coexisting atrioventricular valve regurgitation PA systolic pressure LV thrombus	No direct measure of LVEDP Accurate EF may be difficult if image quality poor	Radionuclide EF LV and RV angio
Restrictive	LV wall thickness LV systolic function Pattern of LV diastolic filling and LA filling via pulmonary veins PA systolic pressure	Diastolic dysfunction is difficult to assess Must be distinguished from constrictive pericarditis	Cardiac cath with direct, simultaneous RV and LV pressure measurement after volume loading
Hypertrophic	Pattern and extent of LV hypertrophy Dynamic LVOT obstruction (imaging and Doppler) Coexisting MR Diastolic LV dysfunction		
Hypertension	LV wall thickness and chamber dimensions LV mass LV systolic function Aortic root dilation, AR		
Pericardial Disease	Pericardial thickening Detection, size, and location of PE 2D signs of tamponade physiology Doppler signs of tamponade physiology	Diagnosis of tamponade is a hemodynamic and clinical diagnosis Constrictive pericarditis is a difficult diagnosis Not all patients with pericarditis have an effusion	Intracardiac pressure measurements for tamponade or constriction MRI or CT to detect pericardial thickening
Aortic Disease			
Aortic root dilation	Etiology of aortic dilation Accurate aortic root diameter measurements Anatomy of sinuses of Valsalva (especially) Marfan's syndrome) Associated aortic regurgitation		CT, MRI aortography

TABLE 4–3	Indications for Transthoracic Echocardiography *Continued*		
Clinical Diagnosis	**Key Echo Findings**	**Limitations of Echo**	**Alternate Approaches**
Aortic dissection	2D images of ascending aorta (PLAX, PSAX), aortic arch (SSN), descending thoracic (A2C), and proximal abdominal (SC) aorta Imaging of dissection "flap" Associated aortic regurgitation Ventricular function	TEE more sensitive (97%) and specific (100%) Cannot assess distal vascular beds	Aortography CT MRI TEE
Cardiac Masses			
LV thrombus	High sensitivity and specificity for diagnosis of LV thrombus Suspect with apical wall motion abnormality or diffuse LV systolic dysfunction	Technical artifacts can be misleading 5-Mhz transducer and angulated apical views often needed	LV thrombus may not be recognized on radionuclide or contrast angiography
LA thrombus	Low sensitivity for detection of LA thrombus, although specificity is high Suspect with LA enlargement, MV disease	TEE is needed to detect LA thrombus reliability	TEE
Cardiac tumors	Size, location, and physiologic consequences of tumor mass	Extracardiac involvement not well seen Cannot distinguish benign from malignant, or tumor from thrombus	TEE, CT, MRI (with cardiac gating)
Pulmonary Hypertension	Estimate of PA pressure Evidence of left-sided heart disease to account for increased PA pressures RV size and systolic function (cor pulmonale) Associated TR	Indirect PA pressure measurement Unable to determine pulmonary vascular resistance accurately	Cardiac cath
Congenital Heart Disease	Detection and assessment of anatomic abnormalities Quantitation of physiologic abnormalities Chamber enlargement Ventricular function	No direct intracardiac pressure measurements Complicated anatomy may be difficult to evaluate if image quality is poor (TEE helpful)	MRI with cardiac gating and realignment of images Cardiac cath

A2C = Apical two-chamber; Angio = angiography; AS = aortic stenosis; CAD = coronary artery disease; Cath = catheterization; CT = computed tomography; EF = ejection fraction; ETT = exercise treadmill test; HOCM = hypertrophic obstructive cardiomyopathy; LA = left atrial; LV = left ventricular; LVEDP = left ventricular end-diastolic pressure; LVOT = left ventricular outflow tract; MR = mitral regurgitation; MRI = magnetic resonance imaging; MV = mitral valve; ΔP = pressure gradient; PA = pulmonary artery; PE = pericardial effusion; PET = position emission tomography; PLAX = parasternal long-axis; PSAX = parasternal short-axis; RV = right ventricular; SC = subcostal; SSN = suprasternal notch; 2D = two-dimensional; TEE = transesophageal echocardiography; TR = tricuspid regurgitation; TTE = transthoracic echocardiography; VSD = ventricular septal defect.

TABLE 4–4	Other Clinical Settings in which Echocardiography Often Is Indicated

Screening Examinations

First-degree relatives of patients with genetic cardio-vascular diseases

Patients with fevers, positive blood cultures, and suspected endocarditis

Patients with cerebrovascular events for possible cardiac "source of embolus"

Patients with arrhythmia

Monitoring Studies

Intraoperative evaluation of LV function in high-risk patients

LV size and systolic function in patients with chronic valvular regurgitation

LV hypertrophy in hypertensive patients

Pre-/Postintervention Echocardiography

Possible procedural complications

Electrophysiologic studies

Endomyocardial biopsy

Effect of intervention

Revascularization (wall motion and thickening)

Pharmacologic therapy (heart failure, hypertension, HOCM)

Valve repair or commissurotomy

Baseline Studies

After valve replacement

Before chemotherapy (cardiotoxic)

LV = Left ventricular; HOCM = hypertrophic obstructive cardiomyopathy.

Marfan's syndrome or hypertrophic cardiomyopathy, to detect possible cardiac involvement in those individuals. In patients with positive blood cultures and/or a fever of unexplained etiology, an echocardiogram may be ordered to detect possible endocarditis. Similarly, in patients with cerebrovascular events that may be embolic in origin, an echocardiogram is requested to identify any potential cardiac sources of emboli. The value of echocardiography for the last two "indications" is low if the prevalence of disease in the population is low. A potential cardiac source of emboli is unlikely to be found in patients with a known noncardiac cause of the neurologic disorder. Conversely, the likelihood of identifying a potential source of embolus is high in younger patients (age <45 years) or in those with a cardiac history (e.g., left ventricular apical thrombus in a patient with prior myocardial infarction) or pertinent physical findings (e.g., mitral valve disease). Furthermore, the value of the test is directly related to the impact of the test results on the pa-tient's subsequent medical treatment. If the results of the echocardiogram will not alter therapy or the subsequent diagnostic strategy, then the echocardiogram is of little value.

Screening examinations often are requested in patients with cardiac arrhythmias to identify underlying structural abnormalities. For supraventricular arrhythmias without other evidence of underlying heart disease or a family history of a genetic disorder, the likelihood of a structural abnormality is low. Although most patients with ventricular arrhythmias will have significant structural disease, including left ventricular systolic dysfunction and/or segmental wall motion abnormalities, these diagnoses usually are known on clinical grounds or on the basis of other diagnostic tests prior to echocardiography.

The use of echocardiography as a low-yield screening examination can have a major negative impact on the diagnostic utility of this technique if only a limited number of echocardiographic studies can be performed (depending on the number of instruments, sonographers, and physicians available). In this situation, unnecessary examinations may delay or prevent diagnosis and subsequent therapy in patients with higher-priority indications for echocardiography. For example, an inpatient echocardiogram performed urgently for "source of embolus" in a patient with a low likelihood of disease may delay scheduling of an "elective" outpatient study in a patient with suspected valvular aortic stenosis. Delay in diagnosis and treatment of a patient with symptomatic severe aortic stenosis may result in an adverse medical outcome. Use of practice guidelines, as suggested by the American College of Cardiology and the American Heart Association (Suggested Reading 12) or triage of requested studies based on diagnostic yield and urgency, as suggested in Table 4–5, helps to formalize the process of prioritizing requests for echocardiographic examinations.

Monitoring examinations may be performed sequentially over brief or prolonged periods of time. Intraoperative monitoring of left ventricular size and systolic function by transesophageal echocardiography is useful in cardiac patients undergoing noncardiac surgery to optimize ventricular preload and for early identification of ischemia, thus preventing perioperative myocardial infarction. Monitoring of left ventricular size and systolic function over many years is performed in patients with chronic valvular regurgitation to determine the optimal timing of surgical intervention. In hy-

TABLE 4–5	An Example of How the Priority of Requested Echocardiographic Studies Might Be Grouped

1. High Diagnostic Yield, Emergency Indications
Hypotension—suspected pericardial tamponade
Chest pain—suspected acute aortic dissection or acute MI (nondiagnostic ECG)
Heart failure—severe, unknown etiology
Complications of acute MI
Complications of endocarditis—new murmur, heart failure, prolonged PR interval
Decompensated congenital heart disease

2. High Diagnostic Yield, Nonemergency
Cardiac murmur—stable patient with suspected significant valvular disease
Clinical diagnosis of endocarditis—stable patient with definite clinical criteria for endocarditis
Congestive heart failure—stable patient with new diagnosis of heart failure or change in clinical status
Suspected prosthetic valve dysfunction—currently stable patient with suspected valve dysfunction
Congenital heart disease—patient with new diagnosis or prior surgery
Coronary artery disease—stress echo for diagnosis or follow-up
Chronic aortic root dilation
Pulmonary heart disease or recurrent pulmonary emboli

3. High Diagnostic Yield but Can Be Scheduled Electively
Known valvular heart disease—follow-up studies for ventricular size and systolic function with no interim change
    in clinical symptoms
Preoperative assessment for elective surgery of patients with suspected cardiac dysfunction
Baseline studies after cardiac surgery or valve replacement
"Source of embolus" evaluation in patient <45 years old or in patients with suspected cardiac disease
Family history of inherited cardiac disease
Suspected cardiac mass
Hypertension

4. Moderate to low diagnostic yield
Cardiac "source of embolus" in patient >45 years of age with no evidence of cardiac disease
"Screening" examinations in arrhythmia patients, organ transplant donors or recipients, or "routine" preoperative
    patients

MI = Myocardial infarction; ECG = electrocardiogram.

pertensive patients, monitoring of left ventricular wall thickness and mass allows assessment of the effect of long-term antihypertensive therapy on end-organ damage (in this case, the left ventricle).

Preintervention and postintervention echocardiography may be used to detect possible procedural complications (e.g., pericardial effusion after electrophysiologic catheter studies or after endomyocardial biopsy). In addition, echocardiography may be used to assess the effect of the intervention by comparing preprocedure and postprocedure studies (e.g., in patients undergoing coronary revascularization procedures, percutaneous mitral balloon commissurotomy, or surgical mitral valve repair). The effects of pharmacologic therapy on a specific endpoint of interest also may be evaluated. Examples include the changes in stroke volume with vasodilator therapy in a patient with dilated cardiomyopathy or changes in the pattern of left ventricular diastolic filling after beta

blockade in a patient with hypertrophic cardiomyopathy.

Baseline echocardiographic studies serve as a reference point in patients with a high likelihood of subsequent cardiac dysfunction. In a patient with a prosthetic valve, a baseline study performed when the patient is asymptomatic and clinically stable provides the normal antegrade velocity across the valve in that individual; the degree of normal prosthetic valve regurgitation; the state of the left ventricle with respect to residual dilation, hypertrophy, or systolic dysfunction; and an estimate of postoperative pulmonary artery pressure. If the patient subsequently presents with suspected valve dysfunction, a more complete and sensitive assessment is possible by comparison with the baseline study than if no previous examination were available. Another example of the value of a baseline study is assessment of left ventricular systolic function prior to starting a potentially cardiotoxic chemotherapeutic regimen. A baseline study allows differentiation of subtle early systolic dysfunction due to chemotherapy from mild dysfunction that may be at the lower limits of the normal range.

Stress Echocardiography (Table 4–6)

In many cardiac conditions, abnormalities of cardiac function are manifested only when increased oxygen consumption results in increased cardiac demands that cannot be met by the usual compensatory changes. This basic concept has led to the widespread use of stress testing in patients with cardiovascular disease. Increased cardiac demand can be induced by exercise or with appropriate pharmacologic interventions. The risk of this approach is related to the risk of stress testing with no significant additive effect of echocardiographic imaging.

Exercise echocardiography can be performed by recording images of the left ventricle immediately before and immediately after treadmill exercise testing or by recording images during supine or upright bicycle exercise. The most common indication for exercise echocardiography is suspected or known coronary artery disease. At rest, left ventricular endocardial motion and wall thickening are normal, even if significant coronary disease is present, unless there has been prior myocardial infarction. Increased myocardial oxygen demands, such as with exercise, result in ischemia when significant stenosis of an epicardial coronary artery is present. This results sequentially in myocardial metabolic changes, decreased wall thickening and endo-

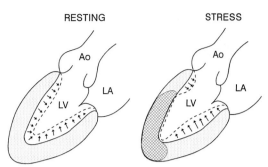

FIGURE 4–9. Diagram illustrating the concept of stress echocardiography in a patient with a 70% stenosis in the proximal third of the left anterior descending (LAD) coronary artery. At rest (left), endocardial motion and wall thickening are normal. After stress (right), either exercise or pharmacologic, the middle and apical segments of the anterior wall become ischemic, showing reduced endocardial wall motion and wall thickening. If the LAD extends around the apex, the apical segment of the posterior wall also will be affected, as shown here. The normal segment of the posterior wall shows compensatory hyperkinesis.

cardial motion, electrocardiographic changes, and angina, in that order. Echocardiographic images recorded *during* ischemia show abnormalities of wall motion, allowing detection of significant coronary artery disease (Fig. 4–9). The specific coronary arteries involved can be identified by the anatomic pattern of induced wall motion abnormalities. Exercise echocardiography, as discussed in detail in Chapter 7, has been found to be more sensitive than exercise electrocardiography (and as sensitive as thallium imaging) for detection of significant coronary artery disease. Exercise echocardiography is particularly helpful in patients with an abnormal resting electrocardiogram (such as bundle branch block or left ventricular hypertrophy). It also has been used to assess the extent of disease, to document functional improvement after revascularization, and to detect restenosis after angioplasty.

In addition to changes in segmental wall motion with exercise stress testing, parameters of global ventricular function, including ventricular volumes, ejection fraction, and the Doppler left ventricular ejection velocity curve, can be evaluated. Other Doppler parameters may be helpful in specific settings. For example, a patient with mitral stenosis will show an excessive rise in pulmonary artery systolic pressure (estimated from the tricuspid regurgitant jet) with exercise. In a patient with aortic coarctation, the increase in gradient across the coarctation with exercise can be demonstrated with Doppler recordings.

TABLE 4–6	Indications for Stress Echocardiography

Exercise Echocardiography
Coronary artery disease
   Diagnosis
   Extent of disease and vessels involved
   After revascularization
Valvular heart disease
   PA pressures in mitral stenosis patients
Congenital disease
   Aortic coarctation

Pharmacologic Stress Echo
Same indications as exercise echocardiography in patients unable to exercise due to:
   Peripheral vascular disease
   Musculoskeletal limitations
   Or as an alternate to exercise stress
Image acquisition during therapeutic pharmacologic intervention

PA = Pulmonary artery.

TABLE 4–7	Indications for Contrast Echocardiography

Standard IV Contrast (e.g., Agitated Saline Solution)
Detection of atrial septal defects and patent foramen ovale
Enhancement of TR jet signal

IV Contrast Agents with Pulmonary Transit
Enhancement of contrast between LV chamber and endocardium (improved border recognition)
Myocardial perfusion

Intracoronary Contrast (Research)
Opacification of myocardium perfused by injected vessel
Detection of myocardial ischemia

IV = Intravenous; TR = tricuspid regurgitation; LV = left ventricular.

Pharmacologic stress echocardiography replaces exercise testing when the patient is unable to exercise (e.g., peripheral vascular disease, musculoskeletal limitations). It also is an attractive alternate to exercise testing when recording of 2D and Doppler data at sequential stages of increased cardiac demand provides useful clinical data. In fact, it can be argued that pharmacologic stress testing is preferable in that the patient can be monitored carefully by echocardiography as the dose is increased, allowing termination of the "stress" as soon as a wall motion abnormality is seen. Pharmacologic stress testing most often is performed using a beta-agonists, such as dobutamine, which increases myocardial contractility, myocardial oxygen demands, and the degree of peripheral vasodilation. An alternate pharmacologic agent used in some centers is adenosine, which vasodilates normal coronary vessels, thus "stealing" blood from stenosed vessels resulting in ischemia.

Contrast Echocardiography (Table 4–7)

Intravenous injection of microbubbles formed by agitating saline solution or by using a commercially available product results in a marked increase in echogenicity of the right-sided cardiac chambers—an echocardiographic "contrast" effect (Figs. 4–10, 4–11, and 4–12). De-

FIGURE 4–10. Transesophageal view showing dense opacification of the right atrium following a peripheral venous injection of agitated saline solution, which does not pass through the pulmonary vascular bed.

FIGURE 4–11. Epicardial images of the left ventricle in an experimental model showing myocardial opacification after injection of echo contrast material directly into the aortic root, thus bypassing the pulmonary vascular bed.

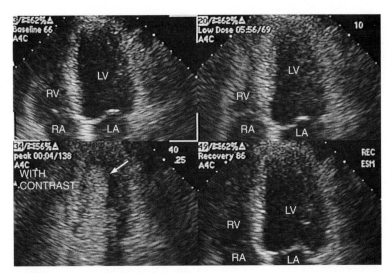

FIGURE 4–12. Example of the use of a commercially available contrast agent that passes through the pulmonary bed after an intravenous injection. In this dobutamine stress echocardiographic examination, resting images in an apical four-chamber view are shown in the upper left, images after low-dose dobutamine in the upper right, and poststress images in the lower right panel. In the lower left panel, images at peak dobutamine are recorded after intravenous injection of the contrast agent with transpulmonary passage. Note that the opacification of the left ventricular chamber enhances recognition of the endocardial border, thereby improving assessment of regional wall motion. The myocardial opacification is more difficult to appreciate given the presence of chamber opacification.

pending on the size of the microbubbles relative to the lung capillary diameter, the microbubbles are trapped in the pulmonary capillaries so that no contrast material is seen in the left side of the heart in the absence of an intracardiac right-to-left communication. Clinically, right-sided echo contrast studies are performed to document an atrial septal defect (Chap. 16) or patent foramen ovale (Chap. 14) or to increase the signal strength of the tricuspid regurgitant jet (Chap. 5) to allow a more accurate estimate of pulmonary artery pressure. Other possible uses of echo contrast include injection in a coronary artery to opacify the area of myocardium perfused by the injected vessel (Fig. 4–10) and to detect ischemia during intracoronary procedures. Commercially available contrast agents provide smaller microbubbles (4 to 10 μm in diameter) that are injected intravenously but traverse the pulmonary capillary bed. These microbubbles both provide opacification of the left ventricular chamber, which enhances endocardial definition, and ultimately, may provide a clinical method for assessing myocardial perfusion.

Transesophageal Echocardiography

The indications for transesophageal echocardiography are based on its superior image quality compared with transthoracic imaging, particularly of posterior cardiac structures (Table 4–8). Several definite indications for transesophageal echocardiography are apparent when the limitations of transthoracic imaging are considered. In Table 4–3, situations in which transesophageal echocardiography is helpful are indicated. The improved sensitivity of transesophageal versus transthoracic echocardiography for detection of paravalvular abscess in patients with endocarditis has been demonstrated convincingly (Chap. 13). Transesophageal echocardiography clearly is indicated for evaluation of prosthetic mitral valve dysfunction, since the shadows and reverberations from the prosthetic valve no longer obscure the left atrium from this approach as they do on transthoracic images (Fig. 4–13) (see also Chap. 12). Abnormalities of the posterior aspect of a prosthetic aortic valve also will be seen well with the transesophageal approach, although the anterior portion of the paravalvular region will be shadowed by the posterior aspect of the prosthetic valve.

Improved evaluation of mitral valve anatomy and the degree of mitral regurgitation are especially useful in the perioperative evaluation of patients undergoing surgical mitral valve repair (Chap. 11). In patients with congenital

TABLE 4-8	Indications for Transesophageal Echocardiography

Definite

Endocarditis with suspected paravalvular abscess

Suspected prosthetic (especially mitral) valve dysfunction

Perioperative evaluation of MV anatomy and function pre- and post-MV repair

Evaluation of posterior structures (e.g., interatrial baffle, sinus venosus ASD) in congenital heart disease

Suspected aortic dissection

Detection of left atrial thrombus (e.g., before catheter balloon mitral commissurotomy)

Probable

Search for cardiac "source of embolus" (including patent foramen ovale) in patients with an unexplained systemic embolic event

Whenever transthoracic images are non-diagnostic and echocardiography is indicated (e.g., LV function postcardiac surgery)

Suspected endocarditis when TTE nondiagnostic

MV = Mitral valve; ASD = atrial septal defect; LV = left ventricular; TTE = transthoracic echocardiography.

heart disease, transesophageal imaging improves diagnostic certainty, particularly in evaluation of posterior structures such as an interatrial baffle surgical repair or a sinus venosus atrial septal defect. The sensitivity of transesophageal echocardiography for detection of left atrial thrombus far exceeds transthoracic imaging. Finally, excellent images of the thoracic aorta, arch, and ascending aorta allow accurate diagnosis of aortic dissection by transesophageal echocardiography.

Other potential indications for transesophageal echocardiography are less firmly established. While often performed to detect a potential cardiac "source of embolus," including a patent foramen ovale, in patients with a systemic embolic event, the diagnostic utility of this test, that is, how it affects patient management, has not been critically evaluated in this patient population. Transesophageal imaging to exclude a diagnosis of endocarditis is of little utility when the pretest likelihood of disease is low. Some echocardiographers advocate the use of transesophageal imaging whenever transthoracic images are nondiagnostic. However, given that the threshold approach to clinical testing predicts a narrower test window as the risk of the test increases, it is appropriate to consider transesophageal studies somewhat more critically. The indications for a transesophageal study should be discussed with the referring physician on a case-by-case basis to determine if the information potentially obtainable justifies the slight but definite risk of the transesophageal approach.

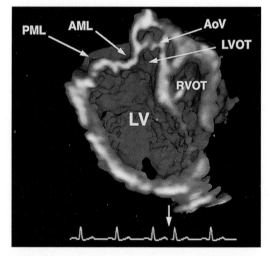

FIGURE 4-14. Voxel gray-scale 3D reconstruction of the mitral valve and left ventricle using transesophageal images in a patient with myxomatous mitral valve disease. The 3D display format allows appreciation of the relationships between the valve leaflets and annular plane. On the computer screen, these images could be viewed as full 3D images using stereoscopic glasses. (From Legget ME, Bashein G. Automatic border detection and three-dimensional reconstruction with echocardiography. *Crit Care Clin* 12: 471–496, 1996.)

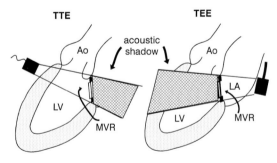

FIGURE 4-13. Diagram illustrating the problem of acoustic shadowing from a prosthetic mitral valve. On the left, with transthoracic echocardiography *(TTE),* the acoustic shadow obscures the left atrium, limiting assessment of valvular incompetence by Doppler techniques. On the right, with transesophageal echocardiography *(TEE),* the left atrium now can be evaluated for valvular incompetence. However, the acoustic shadow now obscures the left ventricular outflow tract.

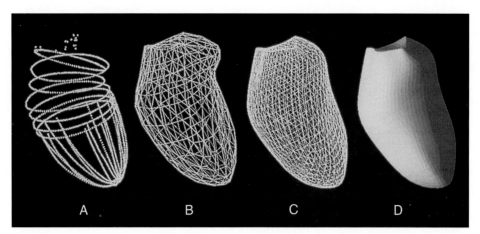

FIGURE 4–15. In vivo reconstruction of the left ventricular cavity at end-diastole. **A,** Traced borders from three acoustic windows (two short-axis views and one apical rotation) registered in 3D using a magnetic locator system with freehand transthoracic scanning. **B,** Using the piece-wise smooth subdivision method for 3D reconstruction, the second-subdivision mesh (520 faces) is fit to the traced border points. **C,** Third-subdivision fitted mesh (2080 faces). **D,** Final reconstructed surface. (See Color Plate 5, p. 274.) (From Leotta DF, Munt B, Bolson EL, Kraft C, Martin RW, Otto CM, Sheehan FS: Quantitative three-dimensional echocardiography by rapid imaging from multiple transthoracic windows: In vitro validation and initial in vivo studies. *J Am Soc Echocardiog* 10:830–839, 1997.)

Intravascular Ultrasound

Intravascular ultrasound has focused on detailed evaluation of intraarterial atherosclerotic disease. This application of ultrasound requires an "invasive" approach in the cardiac catheterization laboratory and is not addressed in this textbook. Introductory readings on this topic are included in the suggested readings.

3D Echocardiography

Three-dimensional (3D) echocardiographic techniques are likely to become more widely used as the technology becomes easier to use and is integrated into standard ultrasound systems. Voxel reconstructions are most useful for demonstrating complex intracardiac 3D relationships, particularly in cases of valvular and congenital heart disease (Fig. 4–14). Disadvantages of gray-scale voxel reconstructions are that the data are only qualitative and optimal display is dependent on the operator's choice of image plane, thus requiring considerable experience both with the 3D technique and with the anatomy of complex cardiac abnormalities.

Three-dimensional reconstructions based on tracing intracardiac borders allow highly accurate measurements of ventricular volumes and systolic function, as discussed in Chapter 5 (Figs. 4–15 and 4–16). However, this approach will remain limited to research applications until reliable methods for automatic edge detection are available.

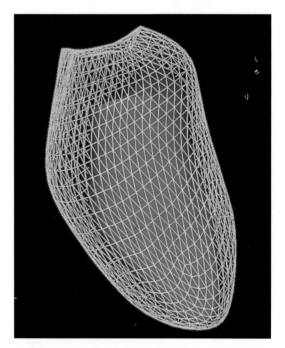

FIGURE 4–16. In vivo reconstruction of the left ventricular cavity at end-diastole (outer mesh) and end-systole (solid surface) allows accurate calculation of end-diastolic and end-systolic volumes, even when ventricular shape is distorted. (See Color Plate 5, p. 274.) (From Leotta DF, Munt B, Bolson EL, Kraft C, Martin RW, Otto CM, Sheehan FS; Quantitative three-dimensional echocardiography by rapid imaging from multiple transthoracic windows: In vitro validation and initial in vivo studies. *J Am Soc Echocardiog* 10:830–839, 1997.)

APPROACH TO THE ECHOCARDIOGRAPHIC EXAMINATION

Basic Format

The echocardiographic examination should be directed toward the specific clinical question in each individual patient. In addition, as the study is in progress, the examination should be modified to fully pursue any observed abnormalities. Most laboratories find that structuring the examination around a basic set of 2D views and Doppler recordings facilitates a directed examination while ensuring that the most important aspects of cardiac anatomy and function are examined in a systematic manner. While this "basic" examination may differ from laboratory to laboratory and may be more or less "comprehensive," it should be noted that the large number of possible imaging planes, Doppler recordings, and quantitative measurements make a truly comprehensive examination impractical in terms of examination time. An examination that includes every view and every Doppler recording without regard to the underlying pathology rarely is useful for appropriate clinical decision making, although an extensive directed examination may be needed in patients with multiple or complex cardiac lesions.

The need to focus the examination on the specific clinical question and at the same time ensure that significant abnormalities are not missed highlights the necessity for appropriate training of both the physician responsible for the examination and the sonographer performing the study, as well as for close interaction between these two individuals during the performance and interpretation of the study. Furthermore, close interaction with the referring physician is needed both before the examination is performed to clarify the differential diagnosis and clinical questions and after the examination to integrate the pretest likelihood with the echocardiographic findings and estimate the probability of any remaining diagnostic problems.

The basic echocardiographic examination should include evaluation of the following areas:

1. Left ventricle: Internal dimensions, wall thickness, segmental wall motion abnormalities, and global systolic function, with an ejection fraction estimated visually or, preferably, calculated from endocardial border tracings

2. Aortic valve and root: Aortic root dimension and appearance, aortic valve anatomy, and evidence for regurgitation or stenosis

3. Mitral valve and left atrium: Mitral valve anatomy and motion, evidence for stenosis or regurgitation, left atrial size

4. Right side of the heart: Right ventricular size and systolic function (qualitative), right atrial size, tricuspid and pulmonic valve anatomy and function, and estimate of pulmonary artery pressure

5. Pericardium: Evidence for thickening or effusion

This evaluation can be performed using the following 2D views and Doppler recordings:

1. Parasternal window
   a. 2D views
      (1) Long-axis view
      (2) Short-axis at aortic valve, mitral valve, and papillary muscle levels
      (3) Right ventricular inflow and outflow views
      (4) *Measurements* (2D or 2D-guided M-mode):
          (a) Left ventricle wall thickness and internal dimensions
          (b) Aortic root and left atrial dimensions
   b. Doppler recordings
      (1) Pulsed Doppler of pulmonary artery flow
      (2) Continuous-wave Doppler of tricuspid regurgitant jet
      (3) Color flow imaging of aortic, mitral, tricuspid and pulmonic valves
      (4) *Measurements:*
          (a) Pulmonary artery peak flow velocity
          (b) Time-to-peak velocity in pulmonary artery
2. Apical window
   a. 2D views
      (1) Apical four-chamber view with anterior and posterior angulation
      (2) Apical two-chamber view
      (3) Apical long-axis view
      (4) *Measurements:* Biplane end-systolic and end-diastolic left ventricular endocardial borders for left ventricular volumes and ejection fraction
   b. Doppler recordings
      (1) Pulsed Doppler of left ventricular inflow and outflow
      (2) Color flow imaging of mitral, aortic, and tricuspid valves
      (3) Continuous-wave Doppler of tricuspid regurgitation and of aortic and mitral antegrade flow

(4) *Measurements:*
  (a) Left ventricular inflow E and A velocities
  (b) Left ventricular outflow velocity distal to the aortic valve (continuous-wave)
  (c) Tricuspid regurgitant jet
3. Subcostal window: 2D views
  a. Subcostal four-chamber and short-axis views
  b. Inferior vena cava and abdominal aorta
4. Suprasternal notch window: Long- and short-axis 2D views of aortic arch

Starting from this basic format, a more detailed examination of the specific abnormalities in each patient and an evaluation directed toward the specific clinical question may be needed. In a patient with no abnormalities noted on this basic examination and no other specific clinical questions (e.g., suspicion of an intracardiac shunt), further evaluation may not be necessary.

Focusing the Examination

As the basic examination is in progress, the study is tailored toward the specific abnormalities noted. For example, if the aortic valve leaflets appear abnormal, attention is focused first on the precise valve anatomy—bicuspid, degenerative changes, rheumatic—and then on the function of the valve. The degree of stenosis is quantitated from the maximum aortic jet velocity (see Chap. 10), and the degree of regurgitation is evaluated with pulsed Doppler, color flow imaging, and continuous-wave Doppler techniques (see Chap. 11). Next, the left ventricular response to the pressure and/or volume load imposed by the abnormal aortic valve is assessed qualitatively (dilation, hypertrophy, overall systolic function) and quantitatively (ejection fraction, wall thickness, mass).

Another example is evaluation of a patient after myocardial infarction. In this case, attention is focused on the extent and distribution of left ventricular segmental wall motion abnormalities (see Chap. 7). If apical akinesis or dyskinesis is noted, a diligent search for an apical thrombus is indicated (see Chap. 14). If the patient has a new murmur, careful evaluation is performed to evaluate the possibility of mitral regurgitation due to papillary muscle dysfunction or the possibility of a postinfarction ventricular septal defect. Overall left ventricular systolic function is evaluated, as is right ventricular function.

Even if no obvious abnormalities are noted during the basic examination, the study may be focused toward the specific clinical question in that patient. For example, if endocarditis is suspected (see Chap. 13), more attention to valvular anatomy is needed, with careful transducer angulation and nonstandard views to optimize visualization of possible valvular vegetations. Although endocarditis cannot be excluded by echocardiography, a careful and thorough negative examination does decrease the likelihood of disease.

Close interaction between the referring physician, cardiac sonographer, and cardiologist is needed to ensure that an appropriate and complete examination is performed in each patient. Subsequent chapters detail the examination sequence and findings in each disease category.

Education and Training Guidelines

As these examples show, the sonographer must be familiar with patterns of disease in clinical cardiology, as well as with the technical aspects of performing the examination. Conversely, the physician must have expertise in the technical aspects of the examination, as well as the expected findings in each disease state, in order to guide the sonographer in optimizing data quality and to interpret the recorded data correctly. Details such as transducer frequency, gain controls, processing curves, and depth settings significantly affect 2D image quality. The appropriate choice of Doppler modality for the flow of interest—pulsed, color flow, or continuous-wave Doppler—affects the data obtained. Factors such as wall filters, gain, sample volume size, and color sector width also significantly affect data collection. Knowledge of how these factors affect data quality and knowledge of which views and approaches yield optimal data allow the physician to assess the reliability of recorded data, to suspect abnormalities that may not have been noted explicitly during the examination, to recognize imaging and flow artifacts, and to direct the sonographer in optimal data acquisition. Detailed guidelines for physician training and for education and training of cardiac sonographers have been published and should be followed.

Echocardiographic Interpretation

The interpretation session provides an opportunity for the sonographer to relay technical concerns to the physician and to direct attention to abnormalities noted during the examination. The physician can give feedback to the sonographer about the completeness and quality of data recorded and offer suggestions for future patient studies. If review suggests that additional echocardiographic recordings are needed, the patient may be asked to return for further examination.

The echocardiographic report serves at least two purposes: (1) it conveys the results of the test to the referring physician and (2) it serves as a narrative summary of the echocardiographic examination for comparison with future studies. Given the wide variety of views and flows that can be recorded, it is helpful for the report to document the structures imaged (even if normal), the flow signals recorded, the different Doppler modalities used, and the overall quality of the study. Any areas of limitation in the study are noted.

In each patient, the various echocardiographic findings then are integrated with each other in the final interpretation. For example, a report describing mitral regurgitation also would include a clear description of valve anatomy with an indication of the most likely etiology of regurgitation or the differential diagnosis if the etiology were unclear. Mitral regurgitant severity is estimated and the method(s) used to generate this estimate are indicated. In addition, the degrees of left atrial and left ventricular dilation are described, with attention to serial changes if previous studies are available. Left ventricular systolic function is quantitated, and the degree of pulmonary hypertension is estimated. All these findings fit together physiologically and thus can be reported in a logical integration of the data. For example, significant mitral regurgitation results in left ventricular and left atrial enlargement due to volume overload, while the chronically elevated left atrial pressure leads to pulmonary hypertension.

Finally, these findings are reviewed in the context of the patient's clinical presentation, potential implications of the findings are discussed with the referring physician, and additional diagnostic tests or follow-up studies are recommended as clinically indicated. If principles of clinical decision analysis are being used in patient management, the pretest and posttest likelihood of disease can be estimated. Ideally, the overall impact of the echocardiographic findings on the patient's therapy or subsequent diagnostic evaluation is reviewed with the referring physician both before and after the examination.

SUGGESTED READING

1. Sox HC Jr, Blatt MA, Higgins MC, Martin KI: Medical Decision Making. Stoneham, Mass, Butterworth Heinemann, 1988.

   A readable concise textbook summarizing the entire spectrum of medical decision making from sensitivity/specificity to cost-benefit analysis.

2. Diamond GA, Forrester JS: Analysis of probability as an aid in the clinical diagnosis of coronary-artery disease. N Engl J Med 300:1350–1358, 1979.

   Classic article on use of Bayes' theorem to determine posttest likelihood based on pretest likelihood and test results using the example of exercise electrocardiography for diagnosis of coronary artery disease.

3. Patterson RE, Horowitz SF: Importance of epidemiology and biostatistics in deciding clinical strategies for using diagnostic tests: A simplified approach using examples from coronary artery disease. J Am Coll Cardiol 13:1653–1665, 1989.

   Emphasizes integration of test results in overall patient management.

4. Wasson JH, Sox HC, Neff RK, Goldman L: Clinical prediction rules. Applications and methodological standards. N Engl J Med 313:793–799, 1985.

   Defines approach to developing and validating new clinical prediction rules. This article will be of particular value to individuals proposing new diagnostic approaches based on echocardiographic data.

5. Pauker SG, Kassirer JP: The threshold approach to clinical decision making. N Engl J Med 302:1109–1117, 1980.

   Clear and concise discussion of the concepts of decision analysis focusing on the threshold approach.

6. Pauker SG, Kassirer JP: Decision analysis. N Engl J Med 316:250–258, 1987.

   Review of decision analysis including Bayes' rule, decision trees, and outcome measures. 52 references.

7. Biem HJ, Detsky AS, Armstrong PW: Management of asymptomatic chronic aortic regurgitation with left ventricular dysfunction: A decision analysis. J Gen Intern Med 5:394–401, 1990.

   Example of the application of clinical decision methods to a clinical problem (timing of valve replacement in chronic aortic regurgitation) in which echocardiographic data (left ventricular size and systolic function) are critical to patient management.

8. Detsky AS, Naglie IG: A clinician's guide to cost-effectiveness analysis. Ann Intern Med 113:147–154, 1990.

   Outlines simplified models for cost-effectiveness analysis that should be applicable to comparisons of the use of different diagnostic tests in a specific clinical setting. Provides guidelines for setting priorities within a health care organization based on cost-effectiveness analysis.

9. Otto CM, Pearlman AS: Doppler echocardiography in adults with symptomatic aortic stenosis. Arch Intern Med 148:2553–2560, 1988.

   An example of development and validation of a clinical prediction rule for timing of valve replacement in symptomatic aortic stenosis based on Doppler echo data. Maximum aortic jet velocity (V_{max}) breakpoints are proposed at (1) >4 m/s (valve replacement indicated), (2) <3 m/s (valve replacement not needed), and (3) between 3 and 4 m/s (evaluation of valve area and coexisting aortic regurgitation needed). Simple cost analysis compares noninvasive with invasive diagnostic approach.

10. Oh JK, Taliercio CP, Holmes DR Jr, et al: Prediction of the severity of aortic stenosis by Doppler aortic valve area determination: Prospective Doppler-catheterization correlation in 100 patients. *J Am Coll Cardiol* 11:1227–1234, 1988.

Evaluation of Doppler data for diagnosis of severe aortic stenosis. Proposed single maximum aortic jet velocity breakpoint at 4.5 m/s with a sensitivity of 44% and a specificity of 93% for diagnosis of severe stenosis.

11. Popp RL: Echocardiography (2 parts). *N Engl J Med* 323:101–109, 165–172, 1990.

Review article, directed toward the general internist, summarizes major accepted indications for echocardiography. 151 references.

12. Cheitlin MD, Alpert JS, Armstrong WF, Aurigemma GP, Beller GA, Bierman FZ, et al: ACC/AHA Guidelines for the Clinical Application of Echocardiography: A Report of the American College of Cardiology/American Heart Association Task Force on Practice Guidelines (Committee on Clinical Application of Echocardiography). *J Am Coll Cardiol* 29:862–869, 1997.

Task force guidelines on indications for echocardiography divided into class I indications (general agreement that echocardiography is important), class II (divergence of opinions), and class III (not appropriate).

13. Schiller NB, Maurer G, Ritter SB, et al: Transesophageal echocardiography. *J Am Soc Echocardiogr* 2:354–357, 1989.

American Society of Echocardiography position paper on utility of transesophageal echo.

14. Fisher EA, Stahl JA, Budd JH, Goldman ME: Transesophageal echocardiography: Procedures and clinical application. *J Am Coll Cardiol* 18:1333–1348, 1991.

Review of methodology, examination technique, and indications for transesophageal echocardiography.

15. Pearlman AS, Gardin JM, Martin RP, et al: Guidelines for physicians training in transesophageal echocardiography: Recommendations of the American Society of Echocardiography Committee for Physician Training in Echocardiography. *J Am Soc Echocardiogr* 5:187–194, 1992.

Recommendations for physician training in transthoracic echocardiography.

16. ACC Echocardiography Committee Position Statement: Transesophageal echocardiography. *J Am Coll Cardiol* 20:506, 1992.

Recommendations for physician training in transthoracic echocardiography.

17. Standards and Guidelines for an Accredited Educational Program for the Diagnostic Medical Sonographer, revised 1996. Joint Review Committee on Education in Diagnostic Medical Sonography, 7108-C Alton Way/Ste 150, Englewood, CO 80112-3533; (214) 741-3533.

Standards and Guidelines for an Accredited Educational Program for the Cardiovascular Technologist, revised 1991. Joint Review Committee on Education in Cardiovascular Technology, 3525 Ellicott Mills Dr, Suite N, Ellicott City, MD 21043-4547; (410) 418-4800.

Criteria for accreditation via CAAHEP (Commission of Accreditation of Allied Health Educational Programs, 35 East Wacker Drive, Suite 1970, Chicago, IL 06601-2208) of programs offering training in diagnostic medical sonography (JRC-DMS) or in cardiovascular technology (JRC-CVT).

18. Practice Guidelines for perioperative transesophageal echocardiography. A report by the American Society of Cardiovascular Anesthesiologists Task Force on Transesophageal Echocardiography. *Anesthesiology* 84:986–1006, 1996.

These practice guidelines review and discuss the indications for perioperative transesophageal echocardiography, with classification into Category I (supported by strong evidence or expert opinion), Category II (weaker evidence and consensus opinion), or Category III (little scientific support). Training guidelines for anesthesiologists using echocardiography are proposed with a distinction between Basic Training (use of echocardiography for monitoring and screening) and Advanced Training (use of echocardiography for diagnosis and quantitation of cardiac disease).

19. Porter TR, Xie F: Myocardial contrast echocardiography: methods, analysis, and applications. *In* Otto CM (ed): The Practice of Clinical Echocardiography. Philadelphia, WB Saunders, 1997, pp 95–112.

Review of the methods for performing and analyzing contrast echocardiography plus a review of the current and potential clinical applications of this technique.108 references.

20. Clements F: Monitoring ventricular function in the OR: Impact on clinical outcome. *In* Otto CM (ed): The Practice of Clinical Echocardiography. Philadelphia, WB Saunders, 1997, pp 167–178.

This chapter focuses specifically on the use of transesophageal echocardiography by anesthesiologists for monitoring left ventricular volumes and function in the operating room.

21. MacIssac AI, Yock PG, Fitzgerald PJ: Intravascular ultrasound: histologic correlation and clinical applications. *In* Otto CM (ed): The Practice of Clinical Echocardiography. Philadelphia, WB Saunders, 1997, pp 275–290.

The correlation between intravascular ultrasound images of coronary atherosclerosis and histopathology is discussed along with an overview of the clinical applications of intravascular ultrasound. 137 references.

22. Douglas PS. Justifying echocardiography: the role of outcomes research in evaluating a diagnostic test. *J Am Soc Echo* 9:577–581, 1996.

This article strongly presents the point of view that we need to look beyond the simple issues of sensitivity and specificity or even the diagnostic accuracy of echocardiography. Instead, research should focus on the effect of the echocardiographic findings on subsequent diagnostic procedures, on the medical and/or surgical therapy of the patient and as a predictor of long-term prognosis. In addition, the issue of cost-effectiveness needs to be addressed for each clinical application of echocardiography.

Echocardiographic Evaluation of Left and Right Ventricular Systolic Function

5

BASIC PRINCIPLES
    Cardiac Cycle
    Physiology of Systolic Function
    Ventricular Volumes and Geometry
    Cardiac Output
    Response to Exercise
2D AND M-MODE EVALUATION OF LEFT VENTRICULAR SYSTOLIC FUNCTION
    M-Mode Echocardiography
        Dimensions and Fractional Shortening
        Left Ventricular Mass and Volumes
        Left Ventricular Wall Stress
        Other M-Mode Measures
    2D Echocardiography
        Qualitative Evaluation of Systolic Function
        Quantitative Evaluation of Left Ventricular Systolic Function
        Left Ventricular Mass
        Left Ventricular Wall Stress
        Other 2D Measures of Left Ventricular Systolic Function
    Limitations of 2D Evaluation of Left Ventricular Systolic Function
        Endocardial Definition
        Geometric Assumptions
        Accuracy and Reproducibility
    3D Echocardiography

DOPPLER EVALUATION OF LEFT VENTRICULAR SYSTOLIC FUNCTION
    Stroke Volume Calculation
    Sites for Stroke Volume Measurement
        Left Ventricular Outflow
        Mitral Valve
        Right Side of the Heart
        Differences in Transvalvular Volume Flow Rates
    Other Doppler Measures of Left Ventricular Systolic Function
        Acceleration Times
        dP/dt
    Limitations/Technical Considerations
    Alternate Approaches
ECHO APPROACH TO RIGHT VENTRICULAR SYSTOLIC FUNCTION
    2D/M-Mode
        Qualitative
        Quantitative
        Technical Considerations/Alternate Approaches
    Patterns of Ventricular Septal Motion
    Pulmonary Artery Pressure Estimates
        Tricuspid Regurgitant Jet plus Right Atrial Pressure
        Pulmonary Artery Velocity Curve
        Isovolumic Relaxation Time
    Limitations/Technical Considerations/Alternate Approaches
SUGGESTED READING

The degree of left ventricular systolic dysfunction is a potent predictor of clinical outcome for a wide range of cardiovascular disease, including ischemic cardiac disease, cardiomyopathies, valvular heart disease, and congenital heart disease. Echocardiography provides both qualitative and quantitative measures of systolic function. Visual estimates of global and regional function from two-dimensional (2D) echocardiographic images, quantitative ventricular volumes and ejection fractions based on endocardial border tracing, and Doppler echo-

cardiographic ejection phase indices all are valuable clinical tools.

Evaluation of ventricular systolic function is the most important application of echocardiography, so that even when evaluation of ventricular systolic function is not the focus of the examination, it plays a key role in every study. For research applications, echocardiographic measures of left ventricular systolic function provide important baseline data on disease severity. In addition, these data can serve as a sensitive and reliable surrogate endpoint for intervention trials in patients with ventricular dysfunction.

BASIC PRINCIPLES

Cardiac Cycle (Fig. 5–1)

Systole typically is defined as the segment of the cardiac cycle from mitral valve closure to aortic valve closure. The onset of systole is defined by the electrocardiogram (ECG) as ventricular depolarization (onset of the QRS complex), with the end of systole occurring after repolarization (end of T wave). In terms of ventricular pressure and volume curves over time, systole begins when left ventricular diastolic pressure exceeds left atrial pressure, resulting in closure of the mitral valve. Mitral valve closure is followed by isovolumic contraction, during which the cardiac muscle depolarizes, calcium influx and myosin-actin shortening occur, and ventricular pressure rises rapidly at a constant ventricular volume (although shape changes may occur). When ventricular pressure exceeds aortic pressure, the aortic valve opens. During ejection (aortic valve opening to closing), left ventricular volume falls rapidly as blood flows

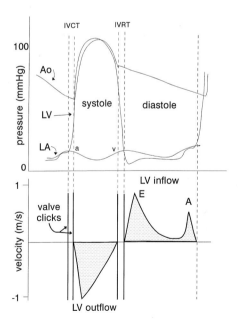

FIGURE 5–1. The cardiac cycle. Left ventricular (LV), aortic (Ao), and left atrial (LA) pressures are shown with the corresponding Doppler left ventricular outflow and inflow velocity curves. The isovolumic contraction time (IVCT) represents the time between mitral valve closure and aortic valve opening, while the isovolumic relaxation time (IVRT) represents the time between aortic valve closure and mitral valve opening.

from the left ventricle to the aorta. Left ventricular pressure exceeds aortic pressure for approximately the first half of systole, corresponding to rapid acceleration of blood flow and a small pressure difference from the ventricle to the aorta. In the normal heart, pressure crossover occurs in midsystole, so during the second half of systole, aortic pressure exceeds left ventricular pressure, resulting in continued forward blood flow but at progressively slower velocities (deceleration). Aortic valve closure occurs at the dicrotic notch of the aortic pressure tracing, immediately following end-ejection. In sum, systole includes isovolumic contraction and ventricular ejection (acceleration and deceleration phases). Ventricular volume ranges from a maximum at end-diastole (or onset of systole) to a minimum at end-systole.

Physiology of Systolic Function

Fundamentally, ventricular systolic function is best described by *contractility*: the basic ability of the myocardium to contract. However, contractility is affected by several physiologic parameters, including heart rate, coupling interval, metabolic factors, and pharmacologic agents. In addition, for a given degree of contractility, ventricular ejection performance can vary depending on *preload* (initial ventricular volume or pressure) and *afterload* (aortic resistance/impedance or end-systolic wall stress). Evaluation of contractility itself thus requires measurement of ventricular ejection performance under different loading conditions. Experimentally, contractility often is described by the slope of the end-systolic pressure-volume relationship (E_{max}). To derive this value, left ventricular pressure is graphed on the horizontal axis, with volume on the vertical axis, rather than graphing both as a function of time (Fig. 5–2). This pressure-volume "loop" then represents a single cardiac cycle, with different pressure-volume loops for the same ventricle representing different loading conditions (such as increasing or decreasing ventricular end-diastolic volume or changing afterload). E_{max} is the slope of the line that intersects the end-systolic pressure-volume point for each curve (Fig. 5–3).

The effect of preload on ventricular ejection performance is summarized by the Frank-Starling curve showing ventricular end-diastolic volume (or pressure) on the horizontal axis and stroke volume on the vertical axis (Fig. 5–4A). For a given degree of contractility, there is a curvilinear relationship between these variables such that increasing end-diastolic volume re-

Pressure-Volume Loop

FIGURE 5–2. Pressure-volume loop. Left ventricular volume is graphed on the horizontal axis, with pressure on the vertical axis. The temporal direction of pressure-volume changes is shown by the *arrows*. During diastole, volume increases with little rise in pressure. After mitral valve (MV) closure, isovolumic contraction (IVC) results in a rapid rise in pressure with no change in volume. At the onset of ejection, the aortic valve (AoV) opens with a rapid decrease in left ventricular volume during systole. Aortic valve closure is followed by isovolumic relaxation (IVR).

sults in a greater stroke volume. An increase in contractility shifts this curve up and to the left; conversely, a decrease in contractility shifts it downward and to the right.

Afterload, defined by resistance or impedance, has an inverse relationship with stroke volume such that increasing vascular resistance results in a decreased stroke volume (Fig. 5–4).

ESPVR

FIGURE 5–3. Pressure-volume loops at different loading conditions (e.g., increasing end-diastolic volumes) are used to derive a line describing end-systolic pressure-volume relationship (ESPVR), also known as elastance (E_{max}). This measure of left ventricular contractility is insensitive to changes in loading conditions.

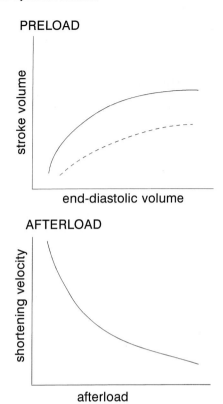

FIGURE 5–4. *(Above)* The relationship between end-diastolic volume and stroke volume is shown for a normal *(solid line)* and failing *(dashed line)* left ventricle. *(Below)* The inverse relationship between afterload and left ventricular myocardial shortening velocity is shown.

An increase in contractility shifts this curve upward and to the right; a decrease in contractility shifts it to the left.

Measurement of left ventricular systolic function independent of loading conditions is difficult using echocardiographic or other clinical approaches. It rarely is possible to construct pressure-volume loops under different loading conditions due to the problem of measuring instantaneous left ventricular volumes and the potential risk of altering loading conditions in ill patients. Thus clinical evaluation of ventricular function has focused on measurements of cardiac output, ejection fraction, and end-systolic dimension or volume, even though the load dependence of these measures is a clearly acknowledged limitation.

Ventricular Volumes and Geometry

The normal shape of the left ventricle is symmetric with two relatively equal short axes and with the long axis running from the base (mitral annulus) to the apex. In long-axis views, the apex is slightly rounded, so the apical half of the ventricle resembles a hemi-ellipse. The basal half of the ventricle is more cylindrical, so the ventricle appears circular in short-axis views. Various assumptions about left ventricular shape have been used to derive formulas for calculating ventricular volumes from M-mode or 2D images. Of course, all these formulas are simplifications to greater or lesser degrees, and there is variability among patients in the shape of the ventricle.

While ventricular volumes instantaneously throughout the cardiac cycle are of interest, usually only end-diastolic volume (EDV) and end-systolic volume (ESV) are measured in the clinical setting. Ejection fraction (EF) is:

$$EF\ (\%) = (SV/EDV) \times 100\% \qquad (5.1)$$

where stroke volume (SV) is calculated as

$$SV = EDV - ESV \qquad (5.2)$$

with cardiac output obtained by multiplying stroke volume by heart rate.

Other useful parameters of ventricular function include (1) wall stress and (2) left ventricular mass. Wall stress is the force per unit area exerted on the myocardium. Wall stress is dependent on cavity dimensions, pressure, and wall thickness. Wall stress can be described in three dimensions as circumferential, meridional (longitudinal), or radial. Typically, end-systolic calculations of circumferential and meridional wall stress are used clinically. Left ventricular mass is the total weight of the myocardium, derived by multiplying the volume of myocardium times the specific density of cardiac muscle.

Cardiac Output

The basic function of the heart is as a pump, so that measurements of cardiac output are useful in routine day-to-day patient management. *Cardiac output* is the volume of blood pumped by the heart per minute, with *stroke volume* being the amount pumped on a single beat. While cardiac output can be derived from ventricular volumes, as described above, a variety of other approaches to measurement are available, including indicator dilation methods (Fick, thermodilution), Doppler velocity data, ventricular impedance, and radionuclide methods.

Response to Exercise

Ventricular systolic function and cardiac output are dynamic, responding rapidly to the metabolic demands of the individual. Cardiac output increases from a mean of 6 L/min at rest to 18 L/min with exercise in young, healthy adults. Most of this increase in cardiac output is mediated by an increase in heart rate. With supine exercise, there is only a minimal increase in stroke volume (about 10%), whereas with upright exercise, the increase in stroke volume is approximately 20% to 35%. With exercise, end-diastolic volume is unchanged or slightly decreased, but ejection fraction increases and end-systolic volume decreases. With imaging techniques, endocardial motion and myocardial wall thickening are augmented with an appearance of "hypercontractility" during and immediately following exercise.

2D AND M-MODE EVALUATION OF LEFT VENTRICULAR SYSTOLIC FUNCTION

M-Mode Echocardiography

Dimensions and Fractional Shortening

M-mode echocardiography allows measurement of ventricular internal dimensions and wall thickness throughout the cardiac cycle. The major advantage of M-mode echocardiography is high time resolution, which facilitates recognition of the endocardial borders. Left ventricular measurements are made with the M-mode beam positioned just beyond the mitral leaflet tips (mitral chordal level), perpendicular to the long axis of the ventricle, and centered in the short-axis view. The left ventricular posterior wall endocardium is identified on the M-mode recording as the most continuous line with the steepest systolic motion. The posterior wall epicardium is identified as the echo reflection immediately anterior to the pericardium. The septal endocardium again is identified as the steepest motion in systole with a continuous reflection through the cycle. On the right ventricular side of the septum, it is important to exclude any reflections due to right ventricular trabeculations. Conversely, a dark "midseptal" stripe often is noted and should not be confused with the endocardial borders. Left ventricular wall thickness and dimensions are measured from the leading edge to leading edge of each interface of interest (American Society of Echocardiography [ASE] recommendations) for optimal measurement accuracy. For example, ventricular internal dimensions are measured from the leading edge of the septal endocardium to the leading edge of the posterior wall endocardium. Normal values for these measurements are indicated in Table 2–6.

In addition to left ventricular wall thickness and internal dimensions (LVID) at end-diastole

(d) and end-systole (s), fractional shortening can be calculated as:

$$\text{Fractional shortening (\%)} = \frac{(\text{LVID}_d - \text{LVID}_s)}{\text{LVID}_d} \times 100\% \quad (5.3)$$

Fractional shortening is a rough measurement of left ventricular systolic function, with the normal range being 25% to 45% (95% confidence limits).

A potential disadvantage of M-mode dimensions is that overestimation will occur if the beam is oblique with respect to the long or short axis of the ventricle. On the other hand, underestimation can occur if the M-line is not centered in the ventricular chamber. Both these potential errors can be avoided by using 2D imaging in both long- and short-axis planes to verify the M-mode beam orientation. With nonsymmetric disease processes (ischemic cardiac disease) or with alterations in left ventricular shape (dilated cardiomyopathy), M-mode measurements at the base may not be representative of overall left ventricular dimensions or function.

Left Ventricular Mass and Volumes

Left ventricular mass can be estimated from M-mode dimensions of septal thickness (ST), posterior wall thickness (PWT), and left ventricular internal dimensions (LVID) at end-diastole. Note that the original description of this method by Reichek and Devereux used PENN convention measurements with the endocardial echos included in wall thickness and excluded from chamber dimensions (rather than leading edge to leading edge). If ASE recommendation measurements are used, a correction factor is needed. The formula then is:

$$\text{Left ventricular mass} = 0.80 \times 1.05 \times \\ [(\text{ST} + \text{PWT} + \text{LVID})^3 - \text{LVID}^3] \quad (5.4)$$

Left Ventricular Wall Stress

Estimates of left ventricular wall stress can be calculated from M-mode data in combination with pressure data. Meridional stress σ_m is

$$\sigma_m = 0.334P \, (\text{LVID})/[\text{PWT} \times \\ (1 + \text{PWT}/\text{LVID})] \quad (5.5)$$

where P = left ventricular pressure, LVID = left ventricular internal dimensions, and PWT = posterior wall thickness. A simpler approach to

estimating wall stress is to calculate the relative wall thickness (RWT):

$$\text{RWT} = \frac{2 \times \text{PWT}}{\text{LVID}} \quad (5.6)$$

which is a useful index for evaluation of patients with left ventricular hypertrophy.

Other M-Mode Measures

Other M-mode signs of left ventricular systolic function are (1) the separation between the maximum anterior motion of the mitral leaflet and maximum posterior motion of the ventricular septum (E-point septal separation), and (2) the degree of anteroposterior motion of the aortic root (see Fig. 8–3). With normal systolic function, the anterior mitral leaflet opens to nearly fill the ventricular chamber resulting in little (0–5 mm) E-point septal separation. With systolic dysfunction, this distance is increased due to a combination of left ventricular dilation and reduced motion of the mitral valve as a result of low transmitral volume flow. Similarly, left ventricular systolic dysfunction results in reduced left atrial filling and emptying (low cardiac output), seen on M-mode as reduced anteroposterior motion of the aortic root.

Because of the limitations of M-mode echocardiography, it usually is preferable to use 2D images for measurement of left ventricular volumes and mass and for calculation of circumferential wall stress.

2D Echocardiography

Qualitative Evaluation of Systolic Function

Both global and regional ventricular function can be evaluated with 2D echocardiography on a semiquantitative scale by an experienced observer. Overall left ventricular systolic function is evaluated best from multiple tomographic planes, typically parasternal long- and short-axis views and apical four-chamber, two-chamber, and long-axis views. Attention to image acquisition is needed to obtain adequate endocardial definition. The echocardiographer then integrates the degree of endocardial motion and wall thickening from these views to classify overall systolic function as normal, mildly reduced, moderately reduced, or severely reduced. Some experienced observers can estimate ejection fraction visually from 2D images with a reasonable correlation with ejection fractions measured quantitatively by echocardiography or other techniques. Typically, ejection fraction is estimated in intervals of 5% to

10% (i.e., 20%, 30%, 40%, and so on) or an estimated ejection fraction range is reported (e.g., 20% to 30%).

Qualitative evaluation of systolic function is a simple and highly predictive index that is of great clinical utility. On the other hand, several factors can limit the usefulness of this evaluation. First, the accuracy of the estimated ejection fraction is dependent on the experience of each observer. Second, inadequate endocardial definition can result in incorrect estimates of systolic function. Third, integration of data from multiple tomographic images can be difficult when the pattern of contraction is asynchronous (with conduction defects, pacers, postoperative septal motion) or when the pattern of contraction is asymmetric (with prior myocardial infarction or with ischemia), especially when dyskinesis is present. To some extent, these limitations are minimized by an experienced observer, optimal endocardial definition, and integration of data from multiple views. However, when possible, it is preferable to avoid the limitations of estimates of systolic function by performing quantitative measurements.

Regional ventricular function also can be evaluated by imaging in multiple tomographic planes. Most often, regional function is evalu-ated qualitatively by dividing the ventricle into segments corresponding to the coronary artery anatomy and then grading wall motion on a 1 to 4 scale as normal (score = 1), hypokinetic (score = 2), akinetic (score = 3), or dyskinetic (score = 4). In some cases, hyperkinesis—that is, a compensatory increase in wall motion in regions remote from an acute myocardial infarction or the normal increase seen with exercise—also is scored. Evaluation of segmental wall motion is discussed in detail in Chapter 7.

Quantitative Evaluation of Left Ventricular Systolic Function (Table 5–1)

Quantitative evaluation of left ventricular systolic function is based on endocardial (and sometimes epicardial) border tracing at end-diastole and end-systole in one or more tomographic planes. Prerequisites for quantitative evaluation are (1) nonoblique standard image planes or image planes of known orientation relative to the long and short axis of the left ventricle, (2) adequate endocardial definition, and (3) accurate identification of the endocardial borders. In some patients, image quality is inadequate for endocardial definition. Even when image quality is adequate, endocardial borders must be traced manually by an experi-

| TABLE 5–1 | Selected Studies Validating 2D-Echocardiographic LV Volume Measurements |

First Author/ Year	Volume/Method	n	r	Regression Equation	SEE	Standard of Reference
Teicholz/74	Ejection fraction $V = [7.0/(2.4 + D)] \times D^3$	25	0.87	Echo = 0.61 angio + 0.01 ml		Biplane LV angio
Schiller/79	Modified Simpson's rule	30				Biplane angio
	Diastolic volume		0.80	Echo = 0.7 angio − 1 ml	15 ml	
	Systolic volume		0.90	Echo = 0.7 angio − 2 ml	8.5 ml	
	Ejection fraction		0.87	Echo = angio + 5	7.6%	
Folland/79	Modified Simpson's rule	35				
	Ejection fraction		0.78	Angio = 1.01 echo + 0.04	9.7%	Single-plane angio
	Ejection fraction		0.75	Radionuclide = 0.75 echo + 0.07	8.7%	Radionuclide
Parisi/79	Modified Simpson's rule	50				Single-plane angio
	Diastolic volume		0.82	Angio = 1.08 echo + 30 ml	39 ml	
	Systolic volume		0.90		29 ml	
	Ejection fraction		0.80		9%	
Gueret/80	Modified Simpson's rule	11				Cineangiography in closed-chest dogs 1 h after LAD occlusion
	Diastolic volume		0.89	Cine = 0.88 echo + 22 ml	10 ml	
	Systolic volume		0.86	Cine = 0.95 echo + 11 ml	9 ml	
	Ejection fraction		0.92	Cine = 1.13 echo − 7.5%	5%	

Table continued on following page

| TABLE 5–1 | Selected Studies Validating 2D-Echocardiographic LV Volume Measurements *Continued* | | | | | |

First Author/ Year	Volume/Method	*n*	*r*	Regression Equation	SEE	Standard of Reference
Silverman/ 80	Biplane area-length	20				Biplane angio
	Diastolic volume		0.96	Echo = 1.05 angio − 3.64		
	Systolic volume		0.91	Echo = 1.37 angio − 1.37		
	Ejection fraction		0.82	Echo = 0.87 angio + 0		
Wyatt/80	Modified Simpson's rule	21	0.98	Echo = 1.0x − 0.7 ml	6.6 ml	Directly measured fluid volume in fixed hearts
	2/3 area length		0.97	Echo = 1.0x − 8.9 ml	8.6 ml	
	Area-length (cylinder)		0.97	Echo = 1.49x − 13.4 ml	12.8 ml	
	Hemiellipsoid (bullet)		0.97	Echo = 1.25x − 11.1 ml	10.9 ml	
Starling/80	Simpson's rule	70				Single or biplane (*n* = 30) LV angio
	Diastolic volume		0.80	Echo = 0.66 angio + 42 ml	34 ml	
	Systolic volume		0.88	Echo = 0.72 angio + 18 ml	27 ml	
	Ejection fraction		0.90	Echo = 0.76 angio + 12%	7%	
Quinones/ 81	Simplified method	55				Radionuclide Angio
	Ejection fraction		0.93		6.7%	
			0.91		7.4%	
Tortoledo/ 83	Simplified method	52				Single-plane angio
	Diastolic volume		0.88	Angio = 1.07 echo − 7.3 ml	28 ml	
	Systolic volume		0.94	Angio = 1.0 echo + 1.3 ml	19 ml	
	Ejection fraction		0.92	Angio = 0.93 echo + 3.5 ml	7%	
Weiss/83	Modified Simpson's rule (15–19 "slices")	52	0.97		6.6% (mean % error)	Direct volume measurement in isolated ejecting dog hearts
Erbel/85	Simpson's rule	46				Single-plane angio
	Diastolic volume		0.91	Echo = 0.66 angio + 0.8 ml	26 ml	
	Systolic volume		0.94	Echo = 0.57 angio + 18 ml	19 ml	
	Ejection fraction		0.80	Echo = 0.61 angio + 13%	9%	
Zoghbi/90	Echo-tilt method	24				Biplane angio
	Diastolic volume		0.92	Angio = 0.80 echo + 37 ml	23 ml	
	Systolic volume		0.96	Angio = 0.97 echo − 1 ml	16 ml	
	Ejection fraction		0.82	Angio = 1.17 echo − 4	10%	
Smith/92	TEE Simpson's rule	36				Single-plane angio
	Diastolic volume		0.85	Echo = 0.75 angio + 0.2 ml	42 ml	
	Systolic volume		0.94	Echo = 0.78 angio − 3.5 ml	22 ml	
	Ejection fraction		0.85	Echo = 0.82 angio + 9.0 ml	8%	
Zile/92	Prolate ellipsoid using constant long-axis/short-axis ratio	25				LV angio in dog model
	Diastolic volume		0.96	Echo =1.0 angio − 1.8 ml		
	Systolic volume		0.95	Echo = 0.98 angio − 0.65 ml		

References: Teichholz LE et al. NEJM 291:1220–1226, 1974; Schiller NB et al. Circ 60:547–555, 1979; Folland ED et al. Circ 60:760–766, 1979; Parisi AF et al. Clin Cardiol 2:257–263, 1979; Gueret P et al. Circ 62:1308–1318, 1980; Silverman NH et al. Circ 62:548–557, 1980; Wyatt HL et al. Circ 61:1119–1125, 1980; Starling MR et al. Circ 63:1075–1084, 1981; Quinones MA et al. Circ 64:744–753, 1981; Tortoledo FA et al. Circ 67:579–584, 1983; Weiss JL et al. Circ 67:889–895, 1983; Erbel R et al. Circ 67:205–215, 1983; Zoghbi WA et al. JACC 15:610–617, 1990; Smith MD et al. JACC 19:1213–1222, 1992; Zile MR et al. JACC 20:986–993, 1992.

SEE = standard error of the estimate; angio = angiography; LAD = left anterior descending coronary artery.

enced physician or sonographer for accurate quantitation of left ventricular systolic function by echocardiography.

Since 2D-echocardiography is a tomographic technique, left ventricular volume calculations are based on geometric assumptions about the shape of the left ventricle. Obviously, accuracy in individual patients will be highest with methods that have the fewest geometric assumptions and that use data from multiple tomographic images. The greatest accuracy would be expected with three-dimensional (3D) reconstructions that use data from multiple tomographic images of known orientation and make no geometric assumptions. However, 3D methods are limited by the need for 3D localization of the image plane and the need for endocardial border tracing in multiple views. Simpler methods, based on one to three image planes, provide reasonably accurate information with less time-consuming data collection. These simpler methods are the current standard for clinical practice.

The geometric assumptions for calculating left ventricular volumes from tomographic data range from a simple ellipsoid shape to complex hemicylindrical hemi-ellipsoid shapes (Fig. 5–5). For each approach, left ventricular end-diastolic and end-systolic volumes are calculated from the corresponding tracings at that phase of the cardiac cycle. Methods that use a single dimension clearly provide only a rough approximation of left ventricular volumes but can be useful in some situations. The "cubed" method assumes that the major axis of the left ventricle is equal to twice the short-axis dimension. Then, volume *(V)* can be approximated from a single short-axis dimension *(D)* as:

$$Cubed\ formula$$
$$V = D^3 \tag{5.7}$$

The single-plane ellipsoid method uses the length *L* and 2D area *A* of a single long-axis view. Left ventricular volume is calculated assuming an ellipsoid shape as:

$$Single\ plane\ ellipsoid$$
$$V = \frac{8A^2}{3\pi L} \tag{5.8}$$

Biplane apical

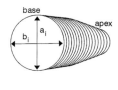

FIGURE 5–5. Examples of three formulas for left ventricular volume calculations showing the 2D echocardiographic views and measurements on the left and the geometric model on the right. For the biplane apical method, endocardial borders are traced in apical four-chamber and two-chamber views which are used to define a series of orthogonal diameters (*a* and *b*). A "Simpson's rule" assumption based on stacked disks is used to calculate volume. The single-plane ellipsoid method uses the 2D area *(A)* and length *(L)* in a single (usually apical four-chamber) view. The hemisphere-cylinder method uses a short-axis endocardial area at the midventricular level *(Am)* and a long-axis length *(L)*. For each method, both end-diastolic and end-systolic measurements are needed for calculation of end-diastolic and end-systolic volumes, respectively, and for ejection fraction determination.

Single-plane ellipsoid

Hemisphere-cylinder

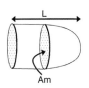

This formula also can be written as

$$V = 0.85A^2/L \qquad (5.9)$$

or

Area-length method

$$V = \left(\frac{5}{6}A^2\right)/L \qquad (5.10)$$

The biplane ellipsoid model uses a long-axis view only for length L and area A_L and incorporates an orthogonal short-axis diameter D and area A_s:

Biplane ellipsoid

$$V = \frac{\pi L}{6}\left(\frac{4A_s}{\pi D}\right)\left(\frac{4A_L}{\pi L}\right) \qquad (5.11)$$

or

$$V = \left(\frac{\pi}{6}\right)D_1 D_2 L \qquad (5.12)$$

where D_1 and D_2 are orthogonal short-axis diameters. The hemicylindrical hemi-ellipsoid model assumes that the base of the ventricle is approximated by a cylinder and the apex by an ellipsoid. Volume is calculated from a long-axis length L and the cross-sectional area A_m of an orthogonal short-axis view at the midpapillary level:

Hemisphere cylinder

$$V = (A_m)\frac{L}{2} + \frac{2}{3}(A_m)\frac{L}{2} \qquad (5.13)$$

or

"Bullet" formula
$$V = 5/6AL \qquad (5.14)$$

In the presence of regional wall motion abnormalities, all these methods will be less accurate, since if the region of abnormal wall motion is included in the dimension or area measurements, volumes will be overestimated. Apical biplane methods are more robust in this setting, using summation of a series of disks from apex to base (often called *Simpson's rule*):

Simpson's rule

$$V = \sum_{n=20}\left[\text{area} \cdot \left(\frac{L}{20}\right)\right] \qquad (5.15)$$

or a modified Simpson's rule approximation, which uses three parallel "slices" of the ventricle to obtain volume:

Modified Simpson's rule
$$V = (A_1 + A_2)h + \left(\frac{A_3 h}{2}\right) + \left(\frac{\pi h^3}{6}\right) \qquad (5.16)$$

where $h = L/3$, A_1 = mitral valve short-axis area, A_2 = papillary muscle level area, and A_3 = apex short-axis area.

For each of these formulas, end-diastolic volume is calculated from end-diastolic images and end-systolic volumes from end-systolic images. Stroke volume, then, is the difference between EDV and ESV [Eq. (5.2)], while ejection fraction (EF) is calculated with Eq. (5.1).

Other modifications and simplifications of left ventricular volume formulas have been suggested (see Table 5–1 and Suggested Reading). The ASE recommends use of biplane apical views with a modified Simpson's rule approach:

Biplane apical volume

$$V = \left(\frac{\pi}{4}\right)\sum_{i=1}^{20} a_i b_i \times \left(\frac{L}{20}\right) \qquad (5.17)$$

where the length L of the ventricle is divided into 20 disks ($i = 1$ to $i = 20$) from base to apex with a diameter of each disk determined in two apical views (a and b). The recommended alternate approach (when two views are not available) is the single-plane ellipsoid formula, Eq. (5.9). An example of the 2D images needed for left ventricular volume calculation is shown in Figure 5–6.

Left Ventricular Mass

Left ventricular mass theoretically can be determined by tracing epicardial borders to calculate the total ventricular volume (walls plus chamber), subtracting the volumes determined from endocardial border tracing, and then multiplying by the specific density of myocardium:

$$\text{LV mass} = 1.05 \text{ (total volume} - \text{chamber volume)} \qquad (5.18)$$

However, epicardial definition rarely is adequate for this approach. Instead, mean wall thickness is calculated from epicardial (A_1) and endocardial (A_2) cross-sectional areas in a short-axis view at the papillary muscle level. The short-axis radius b is calculated as:

$$b = \sqrt{\frac{A_2}{\pi}} \qquad (5.19)$$

Mean wall thickness t, then, is:

$$t = \left(\sqrt{\frac{A_1}{\pi}}\right) - b \qquad (5.20)$$

FIGURE 5–6. Examples of apical four-chamber *(left)* and two-chamber *(right)* views at end-diastole *(above)* and end-systole *(below)* showing the traced endocardial borders for calculation of ventricular volumes.

and the cross-sectional area of the myocardium (A_m) in this short-axis view is

$$A_m = A_1 - A_2 \qquad (5.21)$$

Myocardial mass is calculated from these measurements plus the left ventricular length L from the level of the short-axis plane to the base *(d)* and to the apex *(a)* such that $d + a = L$. Using a truncated ellipsoid formula,

$$\text{LV mass} = 1.05\pi\Bigg\{(b + t)^2 \bigg[2/3$$
$$(a + t) + d - \frac{d^3}{3(a + t)^2}\bigg] \qquad (5.22)$$
$$- b^2\bigg[2/3a + d - \frac{d^3}{3a^2}\bigg]\Bigg\}$$

or using an area-length formula, as

$$\text{LV mass} = 1.05\,\{[5/6A_1(a + d + t)]$$
$$- [5/2A_2(a + d)]\} \qquad (5.23)$$

FIGURE 5–7. Parasternal short-axis view at the papillary muscle level. Epicardial and endocardial borders are traced at end-diastole *(above)* for calculation of left ventricular mass, in combination with a left ventricular length measurement from an apical approach. The end-systolic short-axis image *(below)* is not used for calculaltion of ventricular mass.

The images needed for LV mass calculation are shown in Figure 5–7.

Left Ventricular Wall Stress

Both meridional and circumferential stress can be calculated from 2D echocardiographic images in combination with ventricular pressure measurements. Meridional wall stress σ_m is calculated from left ventricular peak pressure

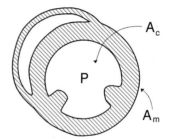

$$\sigma_m = 1.33P(A_c/A_m) \times 10^3 \text{ dynes/cm}^2$$

FIGURE 5–8. Schematic diagram of the measurements needed for calculation of meridional wall stress or σ_m. In a short-axis view at the papillary muscle level, the cavity area (A_c), and myocardial area (A_m) at end-systole are measured in combination with left ventricular pressure (P).

P, the myocardial area A_m, and cavity area A_c in a short-axis view at the papillary muscle level as (Fig. 5–8):

$$\sigma_m = 1.33P(A_c/A_m) \times 10^3 \text{ dyn/cm}^2 \quad (5.24)$$

Circumferential stress σ_c can be calculated using these variables plus ventricular length L from an apical four-chamber view as

$$\sigma_c = \left[\frac{(1.33P\sqrt{A_c})}{(\sqrt{A_m + A_c} - \sqrt{A_c})} \right] \times \\ \left[1 - \frac{(4A_c\sqrt{A_c}/\pi L^2)}{(\sqrt{A_m + A_c} + \sqrt{A_c})} \right] \text{kdyn/cm}^2 \quad (5.25)$$

Measures of wall stress are most useful in ventricular pressure or volume overall states (such as hypertension, aortic stenosis, aortic or mitral regurgitation) to evaluate left ventricular systolic function.

Other 2D Measures of Left Ventricular Systolic Function

There are several other semiquantitative 2D measures of LV systolic function. The mitral annulus moves toward the ventricular apex in systole, with the magnitude of this motion proportional to the extent of shortening in ventricular length—a useful measure of overall left ventricular systolic function. Normal subjects have motion of the mitral annulus toward the apex ≥8 mm, with a mean value of 12 ± 2 mm in both four- and two-chamber views. The sensitivity of mitral annulus motion <8 mm is 98% with a specificity of 82% for identification of an ejection fraction <50%.

In addition, the overall shape of the left ventricle provides important data. As ventricular dilation occurs, the normal elliptical shape of the apex changes to a rounded shape, and the ventricular chamber becomes spherical. The ratio of long- to short-axis dimensions (or the sphericity index) provides a semiquantitative measure of the degree of abnormality.

Limitations of 2D Evaluation of Left Ventricular Systolic Function

Endocardial Definition

Image quality remains a major potential limitation of 2D echocardiographic evaluation of left ventricular systolic function (Table 5–2). Endocardial definition is affected by the physics of ultrasound instrumentation, by anatomic factors, and by technical factors, including the skill of the sonographer. The endocardial-ventricular cavity interface is curved from any imaging window, so the endocardium appears as a thin, bright line where it is perpendicular to the ultrasound beam (axial resolution) but as a broad, "blurred" line where the beam is parallel to the endocardial-ventricular cavity interface (lateral resolution). As for other ultrasound targets, lateral resolution is depth-dependent. In addition, there may be "dropout" of signals due to attenuation, a parallel intercept angle, acoustic shadowing, or reverberations.

Anatomically, the endocardium is not a smooth surface but has numerous trabeculations that are most prominent at the left ventricular apex. The ultrasound beam is reflected from the inner edge of these trabeculations so that the "endocardium" identified by echocardiography differs from the "endocardium" identified by contrast ventriculography, in which contrast material fills these trabeculations, outlining their outer edge.

Several technical factors affect endocardial definition during image acquisition, and meticulous examination technique is needed for optimal image quality. First, acoustic access can be optimizing by (1) patient positioning so that the cardiac structures are in contact with the chest wall, (2) having the patient suspend respiration at the point in the cycle where image quality is optimal, and (3) careful adjustment of transducer position while maintaining the correct tomographic plane.

Instrument settings can dramatically affect image quality, most notably gain, and gray-scale settings, but other instrument parameters (e.g., preprocessing and postprocessing, time gain compensation curves) also may affect endocardial definition. A higher-frequency transducer is used for optimal image quality, provided penetration is adequate, and when available, the focal depth of the transducer can be adjusted to the depth of interest. In addition, newer imaging approaches, such as tissue harmonic imaging, have the potential to improve endocardial definition in many patients. The cine-loop function is used to ensure that endocardial definition is clear on freeze-frame images at end-diastole and end-systole. Finally, the individual who acquires the images should be responsible for tracing the endocardial borders. However, in some patients, even with careful attention to imaging technique, ultrasound tissue penetration is poor, precluding adequate endocardial definition.

The trained human observer remains the most accurate means for endocardial border tracing, limiting the wide application of quantitative methods because manual tracing of endocardial borders at end-diastole and end-systole in at least two views remains a tedious

---

TABLE 5–2   Optimization of 2D Echo Endocardial Definition

1. Position the patient to bring the cardiac structures in contact with the chest wall (often a steep left lateral decubitus position).

2. Have the patient suspend respiration where image quality is optimal.

3. Adjust the transducer position on the chest to improve acoustic access while maintaining the correct tomographic plane.

4. Adjust gain, gray-scale, and harmonic imaging settings to enhance identification of the endocardium.

5. Use the highest transducer frequency that provides adequate penetration.

6. Adjust the focal depth of the ultrasound beam to the depth of interest.

7. Use the cine-loop function to ensure optimal endocardial definition at end-diastole and at end-systole.

8. Have the sonographer who records the data be responsible for tracing the endocardial borders.

and time-consuming task. In many cases, identification of the endocardium requires analysis of the moving image using both the cine-loop and frame-by-frame features of the system to assist in identification of the border as the bright linear echo reflection that moves with the cardiac cycle and is spatially continuous. In the future, automatic edge-detection programs or other approaches to determination of area changes may alleviate this problem.

Geometric Assumptions

In addition to the geometric assumptions of the mathematical models themselves, quantitation of left ventricular volumes depends on accurate measurement of ventricular lengths, diameters, and cross-sectional areas. Two-dimensional echo views that foreshorten the left ventricle will result in underestimation of left ventricular length, whereas oblique short-axis views will overestimate the cross-sectional area of the chamber. Adequate apical views require a steep left lateral decubitus position with an apical cutout in the echo-stretcher mattress to obtain the true long axis of the chamber. Short-axis views should appear circular if perpendicular to the long axis of the left ventricle.

Cardiac motion during the cardiac cycle and with respiratory motion further confounds the geometric assumptions of left ventricular volume calculations. The effect of respiratory motion of the heart relative to the transducer can be avoided by measuring beats at the same phase of respiration or by having the patient briefly suspend respiration during data acquisition. It is more difficult to correct for the motion of the heart itself using a tomographic imaging procedure. Cardiac translation (movement of the heart in the chest), rotation (movement around the long axis of the heart), and torsion (unequal rotational motion of the heart) can result in images of different segments of the left ventricle during systole and diastole, even with a fixed image plane. While cardiac motion has only a limited effect on the accuracy of left ventricular volume calculations, it can have a pronounced effect on quantitative evaluation of regional ventricular function, as discussed in Chapter 7.

Accuracy and Reproducibility

Qualitative comparison of left ventricular systolic function from different studies on the same patient is facilitated by a cine-loop side-by-side format. With this approach, a single high-quality beat is captured in digital format (either the entire cardiac cycle or just the systolic phase). The study to be compared is captured similarly with the same number of frames in the cine-loop so that when the images are played side by side, heart rates are "matched" temporally. The advantage of this approach is that the same view can be examined as long as is needed for careful qualitative (or quantitative) evaluation. This approach is particularly useful for evaluation of regional ventricular function. Of course, the influence of loading conditions on left ventricular systolic function still must be considered when comparing studies performed at different time points in a patient's clinical course.

In most reported series, intraobserver variability for left ventricular volumes ranges from 5% to 10%. Interobserver variability is greater, ranging from 7% to 25% for ventricular volumes. Since ejection fraction is a calculated percentage, reproducibility is better, with variability of about 10%. These values are similar to reported variability for ventricular volumes and ejection fraction determined by contrast or radionuclide ventriculography. Note that variability between studies in an individual patient includes (1) physiologic variability (loading condition, heart rate, volume states), (2) variability in image acquisition (endocardial definition, image orientation), and (3) variability in tracing the endothelial borders. In a careful study designed to assess measurement variability for 2D echo left ventricular volumes, it was concluded that a significant change between studies is a change in ejection fraction >2%, end-diastolic volume >2%, and end-systolic volume >5% (Suggested Reading 4).

3D Echocardiography

Display of 3D echocardiographic images requires knowledge of the spatial position of each image plane or use of an ultrasound transducer that allows acquisition of a 3D data set. Most current systems use standard 2D imaging instruments in conjunction with a system that identifies the spatial location of the 2D image plane. Examples include a fixed transducer position with rotation or angulation of the image plane, a mechanical arm attached to the transducer, or a spark-gap or magnetic locater system which allows free motion of the transducer. Systems that acquire a 3D volume of ultrasound data, allowing simultaneous display of multiple tomographic images, also are under evaluation.

Three-dimensional echocardiography can be used to display the gray scale or color data in 3D space allowing improved appreciation of

TABLE 5–3	**Selected Studies Validating 3D-Echocardiograpic LV Volume Measurements**					
First Author/ Year	**Method**	*n*	*r*	**Regression Equation**	**SEE (ml)**	**Standard of Reference**
Nessly/91	Canine model	33	0.86	Echo = 0.83 RN + 4 ml	6	Radionuclide
Kuroda/91	In vitro phantom					True volume by weight
	Pull-back reconstruction		0.99	Echo = 1.1x − 10 ml	5.8	
	Rotational reconstruction		0.99	Echo = 1.0x − 7 ml	6.5	
Handschumacher/93	Ventricular phantoms		0.99	Echo = 0.96x + 2.2 ml	2.7	Direct volumes
	Gel-filled excised ventricles		0.99	Echo = 0.99x + 0.11 ml	5.9	
Gopal/93	Normal adults	15	EDV 0.92	Echo = 0.84 MRI + 22 ml	7	MRI
			ESV 0.81	Echo = 0.51 MRI + 18 ml	4	
Sapin/93	Excised porcine hearts	25	0.99	y = 1.02 Echo + 3.7 ml	7.1	Direct volumes
Sapin/94	Patients (mean age 48 yr)	35	EDV 0.97		11.0	LV angiography
			ESV 0.98		10.2	
Jiang/95	In vitro phantoms	10	0.99		3.2–6.1	Direct volumes
	Autopsy hearts with LV aneurysms	12	0.99		3.4–4.2	
	Canine LV aneurysm model	19	EDV 0.99		4.3	
			ESV 0.99		3.5	
Gopal/97	Patients with abnormal LV	30	EDV 0.90		31.8	MRI
			ESV 0.93		24.1	
Leotta/97	In vitro phantom	12	1.00	y = 1.00x − 0.6 ml		Direct volumes
	In vitro heart	5	1.00	y = 1.02x − 1.3 ml	1.3	Direct volumes
	In vivo (human)	20	0.99	3D-SV = 1.18 DOP − 17.9 ml	0.4	Doppler SV
					2.8	

References: Nessly ML et al. J Cardiothorac Vasc Anesth 5:40–45,1991; Kuroda T et al. Echocardiography 4:475–484, 1991; Handschumacher MD et al. JACC 21:743–753, 1993; Gopal AS et al. JACC 22:258–70, 1993; Sapin PM et al: JACC 22:1530, 1993; Sapin PM et al: JACC 24:1054, 1994; Jiang L et al: Circulation 91:222, 1995; Gopal AS et al: J Am Soc Echo 10:853, 1997; Leotta DF et al: J Am Soc Echo 10:830, 1997.

SEE = Standard error of the estimate; SV = stroke volume; MRI = magnetic resonance imaging; LV = left ventricle; DOP = Doppler; RN = radionuclide; EDV = end-diastolic volume; ESV = end-systolic volume.

the relationships between structures and qualitative assessment of ventricular function. Quantitative measurements using 3D echocardiography require tracing the borders of structures (such as the endocardium) in multiple image plane with 3D reconstruction of the traced borders.

Three-dimensional echocardiography provides very accurate measures of left and right ventricular volumes, ejection fraction and mass since geometric assumptions are not needed so that calculations will be accurate even with distorted ventricular geometry (Table 5–3). However, current disadvantages of 3D echocardiography include acquisition times, the need for manual border tracing, and cumbersome 3D locator systems, limiting widespread clinical utility for quantitative data analysis. Long-term, both qualitative and quantitative applications of 3D echocardiography promise to become the standard approach (see Suggested Readings 5–9).

DOPPLER EVALUATION OF LEFT VENTRICULAR SYSTOLIC FUNCTION

Stroke Volume Calculation

Doppler echocardiographic evaluation of left ventricular systolic function usually is based on calculation of stroke volume and cardiac output. Using Doppler and 2D echo data, stroke volume (SV) is calculated as cross-sectional area (CSA) of flow times the velocity-time integral (VTI) of flow through that region:

$$SV = CSA \times VTI \qquad (5.26)$$

Conceptually, the left ventricle ejects a volume of blood into the cylindrical aorta on each beat (Fig. 5–9). The base of this cylinder is the systolic cross-sectional area of the outflow tract, while its height is the distance the average blood cell traveled during ejection for that beat. This distance is expressed as the integral of the Doppler systolic velocity-time curve, since velocity is the first derivative of distance. Alternatively, this distance also can be thought of as mean velocity (cm/s) multiplied by ejection duration(s). Again, since the volume of a cylinder is base times height, stroke volume is cross-sectional area multiplied by the velocity-time integral.

This approach to stroke volume calculation depends on several basic assumptions (Table 5–4). First, the cross-sectional area must be measured accurately. Typically, diameter is measured and 2D area calculated as $\pi(D/2)^2$

TABLE 5–4	Assumptions for Accurate Volume Flow Measurement by Doppler Echo

- Accurate cross-sectional flow area measurement
- Laminar flow
- Spatially "flat" flow velocity profile
- Parallel intercept angle between Doppler beam and direction of blood flow
- Velocity and diameter measurements are made at the same anatomic site

based on the assumption of a circular geometry. Deviations from a circular geometry or changes in cross-sectional area during the flow period will result in inaccuracies unless appropriate corrections are included in the calculations. Of note, small errors in 2D diameter measurements become large errors in cross-sectional area calculations because of the quadratic relationship between these variables. Using a transducer orientation and instrument settings that maximize image quality, performing measurements based on axial (rather than lateral) resolution, performing diameter measurements in two orthogonal planes (when possible), and averaging several beats can help minimize this source of error.

Second, the pattern of flow is assumed to be laminar, and (in most clinical applications) the spatial flow profile across the flowstream is assumed to be relatively flat. These assumptions ensure that the velocity curve represents the spatial (as well as temporal) average flow in that region. The validity of the assumption of laminar flow in the great vessels and across normal cardiac valves is demonstrated by the narrow band of velocities and smooth spectral signal seen on pulsed Doppler echo recordings. A flat flow profile also is a reasonable assumption at the inlet to the great vessels and across the valve planes due to the effects of geometric convergence and acceleration. A flat flow velocity profile can be confirmed by moving the sample volume across the flowstream in two orthogonal views to demonstrate uniform velocities at the center and the edges of the flowstream.

Third, the Doppler signal is assumed to have been recorded at a parallel intercept angle to flow, resulting in an accurate velocity measurement (based on a $\cos \theta = 1$ in the Doppler equation). In practical terms, the sonographer aligns the Doppler beam in the presumed direction of flow and then carefully moves the ultra-

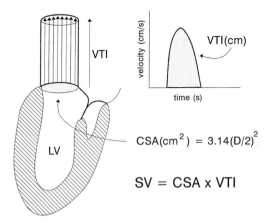

FIGURE 5–9. Doppler stroke volume calculation. The cross-sectional area (CSA) of flow is calculated as a circle based on a 2D echo diameter *(D)* measurement. The length of the cylinder of blood ejected through this cross-sectional area on a single beat is the velocity-time integral (VTI) of the Doppler curve. Stroke volume (SV) then is calculated as CSA × VTI.

sound beam across the image plane and in the elevational plane to obtain the highest-velocity signal, indicating the most parallel alignment with flow. Note that the optimal window for Doppler interrogation is when the ultrasound beam and flowstream are parallel, while the optimal window for diameter measurement is when the ultrasound beam and tissue-blood interfaces are perpendicular.

Fourth, it is crucial that the diameter and velocity measurements be made *at the same anatomic site* since the cross-sectional area and flow velocity curves must be temporally and spatially congruent for accurate volume flow rate calculations. As the cross-sectional area of flow narrows or expands, flow velocity will increase or decrease correspondingly so that conjoining information from two different anatomic sites will result in erroneous stroke volume data. Similarly, dynamic changes in stroke volume occur with changes in heart rate, loading conditions, exercise, etc. so that measurements made at disparate times cannot be combined. In clinical practice, diameter and velocity recordings are made in close sequence and are repeated if there is any question of an interval physiologic change.

Sites for Stroke Volume Measurement

Stroke volume can be measured by this approach at any intracardiac site where both cross-sectional area and the flow velocity integral can be recorded given the assumptions of laminar flow and a flat flow profile.

Left Ventricular Outflow (Fig. 5–10)

Left ventricular stroke volume can be measured in the aorta either at the aortic valve leaflet tips or in the ascending aorta. While some would argue which anatomic level (ascending aorta or leaflet tips) should be used, measurements at each of these levels can be accurate provided that diameter and flow velocity are measured at the same anatomic site. Ascending aortic diameter is measured from a parasternal long-axis view, and the flow velocity curve is recorded from either an apical or a suprasternal notch window. If continuous-wave Doppler ultrasound is used, the highest velocities along the path of the beam will be recorded, so the narrowest segment of the aorta (the sinotubular junction) should be used for diameter measurements. Alternatively, a circular orifice area can be calculated from an M-mode diameter of aortic leaflet opening, and pulsed Doppler can be used to record the flow velocity in the aortic orifice itself. Note that if aortic valve disease is

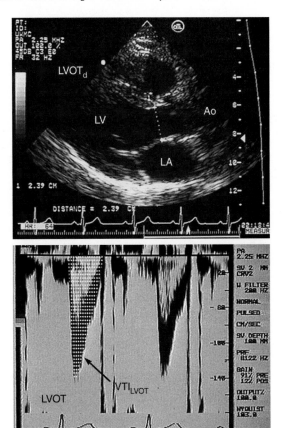

FIGURE 5–10. Examples of left ventricular outflow tract diameter measurement for a parasternal long-axis view *(above)* and the pulsed Doppler left ventricular outflow just proximal to the aortic valve from an apical approach *(below)* for stroke volume calculation.

present, stroke volume measurement in the ascending aorta will be inaccurate due to nonlaminar flow distal to the valve.

Measurement of stroke volume in the left ventricular outflow tract, at the aortic annulus just proximal to the valve leaflets, offers the advantages that (1) flow remains laminar proximal to a stenosis (allowing transaortic stroke volume calculations in patients with aortic valve disease) and (2) the needed data can be recorded in nearly all patients. Left ventricular outflow tract diameter is measured in a parasternal long-axis view parallel and immediately adjacent to the aortic valve, in midsystole, from the septal endocardium to the leading edge of the anterior mitral leaflet. Pulsed Doppler is used from an apical approach to record the velocity curve, using the closing click of the aortic valve to ensure that the sample volume is located at the annulus (the same site as the diameter measurement). The small region of flow convergence proximal to the narrowed aortic valve is avoided by moving the sample volume slightly apically until a narrow spectral width is seen at the velocity peak.

Mitral Valve (Fig. 5–11)

Transmitral stroke volume can be calculated by one of two basic approaches. Given the complex motion of the mitral leaflets in diastole, the first approach uses a "mean" mitral orifice area derived from the maximal 2D opening of the mitral valve in early diastole multiplied by the ratio of the mean degree of leaflet separation throughout diastole. Mean leaflet separation is calculated as the average M-mode leaflet separation (six measurements) divided by the maximum opening:

$$\text{Maximum orifice} \times (\text{Mean/Max}) = \text{Average mitral valve orifice} \quad (5.27)$$

Transmitral flow then is recorded with pulsed Doppler at the leaflet tips. Although accurate, this approach is tedious to perform in the clinical setting.

The alternate approach to transmitral stroke volume determination postulates that the mitral annulus is the limiting cross-sectional flow area, with the leaflets moving passively in response to the flowstream. This approach multiplies cross-sectional annulus area by the velocity-time integral of flow recorded at the mitral annulus level. The mitral annulus is assumed to be circular, using a parasternal long-axis diameter, or, more accurately, elliptical, using an apical four-chamber view for the major axis of the ellipse and the long-axis view for the minor axis.

Right Side of the Heart (Fig. 5–12)

In the right side of the heart, stroke volume can be calculated by analogous methods in the pulmonary artery or across the tricuspid valve. In adult patients, use of the pulmonary artery site may be limited by poor image quality resulting in unobtainable or inaccurate pulmonary artery diameter measurements. How-

FIGURE 5–11. *(Above)* Example of mitral annulus diameter measurement *(arrow)* in an apical four-chamber view with the sample volume (SV) positioned at the mitral annulus. *(Below)* The pulsed Doppler left ventricular inflow signal is recorded for transmitral stroke volume calculation.

FIGURE 5–12. Examples of pulmonary artery diameter measurement in a parasternal right ventricular outflow view *(above)* and pulsed Doppler pulmonary artery flow recorded from a parasternal approach *(below)* for transpulmonic stroke volume calculation.

ever, from a transesophageal echocardiography approach, pulmonary artery flow and diameter often can be measured.

Differences in Transvalvular Volume Flow Rates

In a normal heart, stroke volume across each of the four valves will be equal, and measurement at more than one site only serves as an internal accuracy check. However, in the presence of valvular regurgitation or an intracardiac shunt, calculation of stroke volume at two intracardiac sites allows quantitation of the degree of regurgitation or pulmonic-to-systemic shunt ratio, as detailed in Chapters 11 and 16.

Other Doppler Measures of Left Ventricular Systolic Function

Acceleration Times

In addition to stroke volume calculations, the shape of the Doppler ejection curve may provide information about ventricular function. When systolic function is normal, the isovolumic contraction period is short, and the rate of pressure rise in early systole is rapid. These features are reflected in the Doppler velocity curve, which shows a short isovolumic contraction time, a rapid acceleration of blood in early systole, and a short time interval from the onset of flow to maximum velocity. With impaired left ventricular systolic function, the isovolumic contraction time (also known as the *preejection period*) becomes progressively longer, the rate of acceleration diminishes, and the time to maximum velocity increases, with all these changes mirrored in the Doppler velocity curve (Fig. 5–13). In addition to measuring these variables at rest, some centers have found evaluation of aortic ejection curves with exercise useful in detection of left ventricular systolic dysfunction.

dP/dt

When mitral regurgitation is present, the continuous-wave Doppler velocity curve indicates the instantaneous pressure difference between the left ventricle and the left atrium in systole, assuming a constant intercept angle between the mitral regurgitant jet and the ultrasound beam. Given the rapid rate of rise of left ventricular pressure with normal systolic function (and the low left atrial pressure), mitral regurgitation typically shows a rapid rise to maximum velocity as per the Bernoulli equation. If the rate of rise in ventricular pressure is reduced due to left ventricular systolic dysfunction, the rate of increase in velocity of the mitral regur-

FIGURE 5–13. In a patient with severely reduced left ventricular systolic function, the left ventricular outflow velocity *(above)* shows a delayed time to peak and low peak velocity (compare with Fig. 5–10). The mitral regurgitant jet *(below)* is a low velocity with a depressed rate of velocity rise in early systole.

gitant jet also is reduced. For example, in patients with premature ventricular beats, the altered contractility of the premature beat will be evidenced by a marked difference in the rate of velocity increase of the mitral regurgitant jet. The slope of the mitral regurgitant jet can be quantitated as the rate of change in pressure over time (*dP/dt*) by measuring the time interval between the mitral regurgitant jet velocity at 1 and at 3 m/s (Fig. 5–14). At each velocity, the corresponding pressure gradient is $4v^2$ per the Bernoulli equation. Then,

$$dP/dt = \frac{[4(3)^2] - [4(1)^2]}{\text{Time interval}} = \frac{32 \text{ mmHg}}{\text{Time interval}} \qquad (5.28)$$

Thus a longer time interval indicates a depressed *dP/dt*, and vice versa. Of course, the

FIGURE 5–14. Left ventricular *dP/dt* can be calculated from the mitral regurgitant jet. Continuous-wave Doppler mitral regurgitation curves are consistent with normal *(above)* and severely reduced *(below)* left ventricular systolic function.

calculation of *dP/dt* can be performed only when a recordable mitral regurgitant jet is present and assumes a constant (and parallel) intercept angle between the mitral regurgitant jet and the ultrasound beam throughout the cardiac cycle.

Limitations/Technical Considerations

The major limitation of Doppler evaluation of left ventricular systolic function in adults is accurate diameter measurement for cross-sectional area calculations. While the Doppler velocity curves can be recorded consistently with little interobserver measurement variability (2% to 5%), the variability of 2D diameter measurements is significantly greater (8% to 12%). Again, measurement variability includes (1) technical differences in *recording* the data (such as intercept angle, image quality, tomographic plane), (2) variability in *measuring* the

recorded data, and (3) *physiologic* variability occurring between the time of repeat data recording. For Doppler velocity data, the major source of measurement variability is data recording, given the critical importance of obtaining a parallel intercept angle between the ultrasound beam and the flow of interest. For 2D diameters, the major source of variability is measuring the 2D images, particularly when image quality is suboptimal or when lateral resolution limits accurate border recognition. Despite these potential limitations, Doppler measurement of stroke volume has been well validated in a variety of clinical and research settings (Table 5–5).

Measurement of *dP/dt* is limited by the need for enough mitral regurgitation to generate a Doppler signal with a well-defined velocity curve. Changes during ejection in the intercept angle between the ultrasound beam and the regurgitant jet will result in an erroneous measurement, since the assumption that cos $\theta = 1$ in the Doppler equation will not be valid.

Alternate Approaches

Thermodilution cardiac outputs, measured with an indwelling right-sided heart catheter, are the standard approach to evaluation of cardiac output both in the catheterization laboratory and in the coronary care unit. Thermodilution outputs offer the advantages that measurements can be repeated frequently by the nurse caring for the patient and pulmonary artery pressures can be monitored continuously as well. Disadvantages of this approach are that it is invasive (risks, discomfort) and it provides only a volumetric flow rate, without direct visualization of ventricular function. Stroke volume can be maintained despite a low ejection fraction due to compensatory left ventricular dilation. For example, the same stroke volume of 60 ml may result from an ejection fraction of 20% with a left ventricular end-diastolic volume of 300 ml or from a normal ejection fraction (60%) with a smaller left ventricular end-diastolic volume (100 ml).

Available alternate approaches to measurement of left ventricular volumes and ejection fraction are contrast angiography in the cardiac catheterization laboratory (Fig. 5–15) and radionuclide ventriculography (Fig. 5–16). Both computed tomography and magnetic resonance imaging are capable of left ventricular volume calculation, although they may not be available routinely. The choice of imaging technique in an individual patient will depend on what other clinical questions are present (e.g.,

TABLE 5–5	Selected Studies Validating Doppler Volume Flow Measurement					

First Author/ Year	Volume Flow Site/Method	n	r	Regression Equation	SEE	Standard of Reference
Huntsman/83	Ascending aorta	100	0.94	DOP = 0.95x + 0.38	0.58 L/min	TD-CO
Fisher/83	Mitral leaflets	52	0.97	DOP = 0.98x + 0.02	0.23 L/min	Roller pump
Meijboom/83	Mitral leaflets	26	0.99	DOP = 0.97x + 0.07	0.13 L/min	EM flow
	RVOT	26	0.99	DOP = 0.96x + 0.11	0.16 L/min	Roller pump
Lewis/84	Mitral annulus	35	0.96	TD = 0.91x + 5.1	5.9 ml	TD-SV
	LVOT	39	0.95	TD = 0.91x + 7.8	6.4 ml	TD-SV
Stewart/85	Mitral leaflets	29	0.97	DOP = 0.98x + 0.3	0.3 L/min	Roller pump
	Aortic annulus	33	0.98	DOP = 1.06x + 0.2	0.3 L/min	Roller pump
	Pulmonary annulus	30	0.93	DOP = 0.89x + 0.4	0.5 L/min	Roller pump
Bouchard/87	Aortic leaflets	41	0.95	DOP = 0.97x + 1.7	7 ml	TD-SV
Dittmann/87	Mitral annulus	40	0.86	DOP = 0.88 + 1.75	0.80 L/min	TD-CO
	LVOT (M-mode)	40	0.93	DOP = 0.94x + 0.44	0.59 L/min	TD-CO
DeZuttere/88	Mitral orifice (instantaneous)	30	0.91	DOP = 0.92x + 0.35	0.53 L/min	TD-CO
Holt/88	Mitral leaflets	48	0.93	DOP = 1.1x − 0.45	0.36 L/min	TD-CO
Otto/88	LVOT (proximal to stenotic aortic valve)	52	0.91	DOP = 1.0x + 0.03	0.25 L/min	EM-flow and timed collection
Burwash/93	LVOT (proximal to aortic stenosis)	75	0.86	CO = 0.92 DOP + 0.26	0.50 L/min	Transit-time flow probe

Data from Huntsman et al. Circ 67:593–601, 1983; Fisher et al. Circ 67:872–877, 1983; Meijboom et al. Circ 68:437–445, 1983; Lewis et al. Circ 70:425–431, 1984; Stewart et al. JACC 6:653–662, 1985; Bouchard et al. JACC 9:75–83, 1987; Dittman et al. JACC 10:818–823, 1987; DeZuttere et al. JACC 11:343–350, 1988; Holt et al. AJC 62:131–135, 1988; Otto et al. Circ 78:435–441, 1988; Burwash et al. Am J Physiol 265 (Heart Circ Physiol 34):1734, 1993.

SEE = Standard error of the estimate; TD = thermodilution; CO = cardiac output; DOP = Doppler; RVOT = right ventricular outflow tract; LVOT = left ventricular outflow tract; SV = stroke volume; EM-flow = volume flow rate measured by electromagnetic flowmeter.

FIGURE 5–15. Left ventricular angiography is an alternate approach to evaluation of left ventricular systolic function, which is performed most often in patients undergoing cardiac catheterization for other indications, such as coronary artery disease. End-diastolic *(left)* and end-systolic *(right)* frames are shown.

Regions of Interest

End Diastolic   End Systolic

Time-Activity Curve

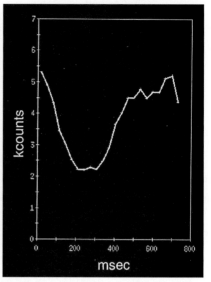

FIGURE 5–16. A radionuclide ventriculogram. Standard view radionuclide ventriculographic images at end-diastole (dias) and end-systole (syst) in a patient with normal cardiac chamber size and global function of both ventricles. The region of interest (ROI) and background region (BKG) for measurement of counts and calculation of ejection fraction is shown. The time-activity curve in kilo-counts per milliseconds is graphed. (Courtesy of James H. Caldwell, MD.)

possible valvular disease) as well as availability and cost.

ECHO APPROACH TO RIGHT VENTRICULAR SYSTOLIC FUNCTION

2D/M-Mode

Qualitative

The right ventricle is evaluated qualitatively by 2D imaging from several different windows: parasternal long- and short-axis, right ventricular inflow, apical four-chamber, and subcostal four-chamber views (Fig. 5–17). In each view, the area of the right ventricular chamber (relative to the left ventricular chamber), the shape of the right ventricular cavity, right ventricular wall thickness, the degree of motion of the right ventricular free wall, and the pattern of ventricular septal motion are evaluated.

The *normal shape* of the right ventricle is complex in three dimensions, with the inflow segment located medial to the left ventricle, the body and apex located anterior to the left ventricle, and the right ventricular outflow tract located superior to the left ventricle and aortic valve. There is no simple geometric shape that approximates the right ventricular chamber; rather, it is "wrapped around" the left ventricle in a U-shaped fashion. Since echocardiographic long- and short-axis views are oriented with respect to the left ventricle, the right ventricle may appear abnormal in some individuals due to the position of the right ventricle relative to the image plane. This occurs most often in parasternal views, where the right ventricle may be imaged in an oblique orientation. Both subcostal and apical four-chamber windows tend to offer more consistent views of the right ventricle, with the right ventricle appearing somewhat triangular in shape with a broad base and narrow apex. The right ventricular apex is slightly closer to the base than the left ventricular apex (by about one third of the left ventricular length) in normal individuals.

With right ventricular dilation, the right ventricular outflow tract may be enlarged in the parasternal long-axis view. On apical and subcostal views, the right ventricular chamber will be larger and the right ventricular apex is either closer to or encompasses the left ventricular apex. The degree of right ventricular dilation is described as mild (enlarged but a

2D area <left ventricular area), moderate (right ventricular = left ventricular area), or severe (right ventricular >left ventricular area) using the combination of multiple image planes in this overall assessment. Right ventricular dilation is the normal response of the ventricle to volume overload, and its presence mandates a careful search for etiology, such as an atrial septal defect, tricuspid regurgitation, or pulmonic regurgitation. Long-standing pressure overload of the right ventricle also can lead to dilation.

Right ventricular hypertrophy is manifested as increased thickness of the right ventricular free wall as seen on 2D images or by M-mode, with a wall thickness >0.5 cm being abnormal in adults. The presence of right ventricular hypertrophy suggests right ventricular pressure overload and should prompt a search for evidence of elevated pulmonary pressures or pul-

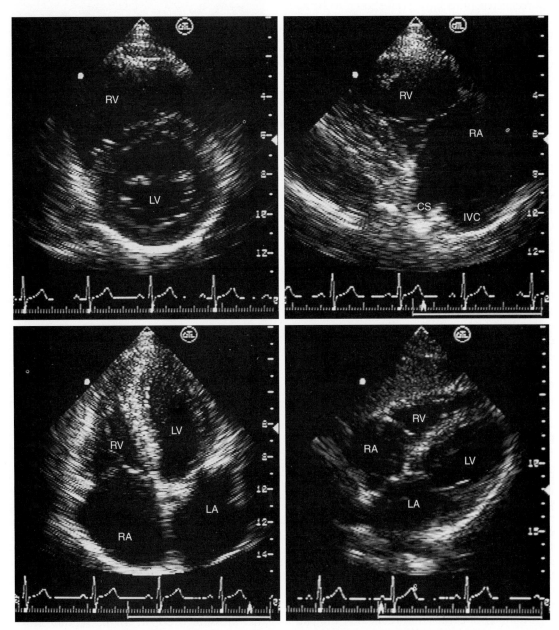

FIGURE 5–17. Evaluation of right ventricular size and systolic function is based on multiple image planes including parasternal short-axis *(above, left)*, right ventricular inflow *(above, right)*, apical four-chamber *(below, left)*, and subcostal four-chamber *(below, right)* views. CS = coronary sinus; IVC = inferior vena cava.

monic valve stenosis. Increased thickness of the right ventricular free wall also may be seen in some infiltrative cardiomyopathies or in hypertrophic cardiomyopathy.

Quantitative

Quantitative evaluation of right ventricular systolic function by 2D/M-mode echo is difficult. Standard geometric formulas for volume calculations have only limited applicability given the shape of the right ventricle, and while 3D reconstructions have been shown to be accurate, the need for tedious endocardial border tracing and extensive data analysis has restricted its use to the research setting. In most cases, qualitative evaluation is sufficient for clinical decision making.

Technical Considerations/Alternate Approaches

Evaluation of right ventricular systolic function may be limited by poor ultrasound tissue penetration in some individuals. With careful patient positioning and a search from multiple windows, the right ventricle usually can be visualized, but endocardial definition may be suboptimal. If clinically indicated, transesophageal echo offers superior images of the right ventricle both in the high esophageal four-chamber view and from a transgastric approach.

Right ventricular contrast angiography can be performed at catheterization, but there is wide variability in the appearance of the normal right ventricle. Radionuclide ventriculography can be used to derive a right ventricular ejection fraction. The right ventricle also can be imaged on computed tomography or magnetic resonance imaging scanning, and cine-views may be helpful, when available, for evaluation of systolic function.

Patterns of Ventricular Septal Motion

The interventricular septum functions as part of the left ventricle in the normal heart. During diastole, the left ventricle is circular in a short-axis view, with the normal septal curvature convex toward the right ventricle and concave toward the left ventricle. With the onset of systole, the septal myocardium thickens, and the septal endocardium moves toward the center of the left ventricle such that at end-systole the short-axis image shows a circular left ventricular chamber.

A number of cardiac disorders alter the pattern of ventricular septal motion, the most prominent being right ventricular pressure and volume overload. The basic principle underly-

FIGURE 5–18. Abnormal septal motion on M-mode in a patient after cardiac bypass surgery. In systole, the septum moves anteriorly but thickens normally. (For septal motion with right ventricular volume overload, see Fig. 16–17.)

ing the pattern of septal motion with right ventricular dilation or hypertrophy is that the septum moves toward the center of mass of the entire heart. Normally, the center of cardiac mass coincides with the center of the left ventricle. When right and left ventricular masses are equal, septal motion will be "flat" (on M-mode) or minimal (on 2D echo). When right ventricular mass exceeds left ventricular mass, the septum moves "paradoxically" anterior in systole (on M-mode) and flattens or reverses its curvature in diastole (on 2D echo) (Fig. 5–18).

On 2D echocardiography, pressure overload of the right ventricle (increased mass due to increased wall thickness with a nondilated chamber) results in a leftward shift of septal motion throughout the cardiac cycle with the maximum reversed curvature at end-systole. With predominant right ventricular volume overload, the maximum reversed curvature is seen in mid-diastole with normalization of curvature in systole (see Suggested Reading 22).

With increased right ventricular mass due to volume overload, the additional factor of increased right ventricular filling and emptying accentuates the diastolic reverse motion of the septum (due to rapid right ventricular diastolic filling), resulting in a D shape of the left ventricular chamber in early diastole, with the reversed curvature of the septum persisting throughout diastole. Anterior motion with systole may appear less prominent than with isolated pressure overload as the septum moves from its abnormal diastolic position back toward the center of the heart, resulting in a more convex curve relative to the right ventricular chamber. Often, the observation of abnormal septal motion during the examination is the first clue of right ventricular pressure and/or volume overload.

Other abnormalities that affect the pattern of ventricular septal motion are summarized in Figure 5–19. Conduction defects affect the pattern of motion by altering the sequence of right and left ventricular contraction. Valvular disease can affect the timing of right ventricular versus left ventricular diastolic filling, particularly in early diastole. Pericardial tamponade or constriction results in a fixed total cardiac volume so that respiratory changes in right ventricular filling result in respiratory shifts in the pattern of septal motion.

An abnormal pattern of septal motion may be appreciated on 2D imaging; however,

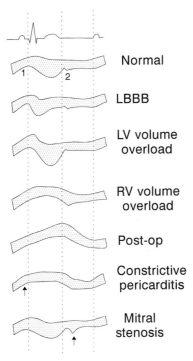

FIGURE 5–19. Schematic diagram of different patterns of septal motion on M-mode echocardiography. The normal pattern is characterized by systolic brief anterior motion *(1)* followed by posterior motion and myocardial thickening. In diastole, a small diastolic dip *(2)* following mitral valve opening may be seen. Left bundle branch block (LBBB) is characterized by systolic rapid downward septal motion. Left ventricular (LV) volume overload results in exaggerated septal (and posterior wall) motion. Right ventricular (RV) volume overload results in paradoxical anterior motion of the septum in systole. A similar pattern is seen in patients after cardiac surgery (Post-op). Constrictive pericarditis is characterized by anterior motion of the septum with atrial filling (before the QRS), while mitral stenosis typically shows a prominent early diastolic dip.

M-mode echo offers more detailed time resolution for studying the pattern of motion. Abnormal septal motion rarely is diagnostic in and of itself, but it may raise a diagnostic possibility that had not been considered previously or may support a suspected diagnosis. For example, a pattern of paradoxical septal motion in association with right ventricular and right atrial enlargement suggests the possibility of an atrial septal defect. This possibility then can be specifically excluded (or confirmed) during the echocardiographic examination. Another example is the patient with a pericardial effusion; in this situation a changing pattern of septal motion with respiration supports a diagnosis of tamponade physiology.

Pulmonary Artery Pressure Estimates

Clinically, one of the most important quantitative parameters of right ventricular systolic function is an estimate of pulmonary artery pressures. Pulmonary hypertension often occurs in response to chronic left-sided heart diseases, such as mitral stenosis, mitral regurgitation, cardiomyopathy, and ischemic cardiac disease. Knowledge of the degree of pulmonary pressure elevation is critical in patient management (Tables 5–6 and 5–7).

Tricuspid Regurgitant Jet plus Right Atrial Pressure

The most reliable method for estimating pulmonary artery pressures noninvasively is based on measurement of the velocity in the tricuspid regurgitant jet. This velocity V_{TR} reflects the right ventricular (RV) to right atrial (RA) pressure difference ΔP, as stated in the Bernoulli equation (Fig. 5–20):

$$\Delta P_{RV-RA} = 4(V_{TR})^2 \qquad (5.29)$$

When added to an estimate of right atrial pressure, right ventricular systolic pressure (RVP) is obtained:

$$RVP = \Delta P_{RV-RA} + RAP \qquad (5.30)$$

In the absence of pulmonic stenosis (which is rare in adults), right ventricular systolic pressure equals pulmonary artery systolic pressure, so that

$$PAP_{systolic} = 4(V_{TR})^2 + RAP \qquad (5.31)$$

as diagrammed in Figure 5–21.

This method has been shown to be highly accurate compared with invasive measurements of pulmonary artery pressure over a wide range of values. Of course, the reliability of this approach is dependent on obtaining a parallel in-

TABLE 5–6	Doppler Echo Methods for Pulmonary Artery Pressure Estimation

Method	Advantages	Potential Limitations
$4(V_{TR})^2 + RAP$	Accurate Measurable in a high percentage of patients overall (90%)	Nonparallel intercept angle between jet and ultrasound beam Misidentification of jet signal Right atrial pressure estimate (not available in ventilated patients) Presence of pulmonic stenosis Inadequate signal in patients with chronic lung disease
TPV in pulmonary artery	Readily measured in nearly all patients, including patients with chronic lung disease Estimates *mean* pulmonary artery pressure	Skewed flow profile in pulmonary artery Measurement variability
RV-IVRT	Alternate approach	Difficulty in recording tricuspid and pulmonic valve closure in adults Measurement variability

V_{TR} = Velocity of tricuspid regurgitation; RAP = right atrial pressure; TPV = time to peak velocity; RV-IVRT = right ventricular isovolumic relaxation time.

TABLE 5–7	Selected Studies Validating Noninvasive Pulmonary Artery Pressure Measurement

First Author/ Year	Method	n	r	Regression Equation	SEE
Kitabatake/83	Time to peak flow (RVOT)	33	−0.88	Log (mean PAP) = 0.0068 (AcT) + 2.1 mmHg	—
Stevenson/84	IVRT (Burstin method, in sedated patients)	95	0.97	Doppler mean PAP = 0.97 (cath) + 1.7 mmHg	6.4 mmHg
Isobe/86	PEP/AcT	45	0.89	PEP/AcT = 0.023 mean PAP + 0.48 mmHg	—
Stevenson/89	TR-jet Time to peak flow (PA)	50	0.96 0.63		6.9 mmHg 16.4 mmHg
	IVRT Pulmonic regurgitation		0.97 0.96		5.4 mmHg 4.5 mmHg
Yock/84	TR-jet	62	0.95	Doppler RV-RA ΔP = 1.03 ΔP + 0.71 mmHg	7 mmHg
Berger/85	TR-jet	69	0.97	Systolic PAP = 1.23 (Doppler ΔP) − 0.09 mmHg	4.9 mmHg
Currie/85	TR-jet	127	0.96	Doppler RV-RA ΔP = 0.88 ΔP + 2.2 mmHg	7 mmHg
Lee/89	Pulmonic regurgitation	29	0.94	Diastolic PAP (echo) = 0.95 (cath) − 1 mmHg	Mean difference: 3.3 ± 2.2 mmHg

References: Kitabatake A et al. Circ 68:302–309, 1983; Stevenson JG et al. JACC 4:1021–1027, 1984; Isobe M et al. AJC 57:316–332, 1986; Stevenson JG et al. JASE 2:157–171, 1989; Yock PG, Popp RL. Circ 70:657–662, 1984; Berger M et al. JACC 6:359–365, 1985; Currie PJ et al. JACC 6:750–756, 1985; Lee RT et al: AJC 64:1366–1370, 1989.

RVOT = Right ventricular outflow tract; PAP = pulmonary artery pressure; AcT = acceleration time; cath = cardiac catheterization; PEP = preejection period; PA = pulmonary artery; TR = tricuspid regurgitation; IVRT = isovolumic relaxation time; RV-RA = right ventricle to right atrium; ΔP = pressure gradient.

FIGURE 5–20. Relationship between the velocity in the tricuspid regurgitant (TR) jet and the right ventricular–right atrial (RV-RA) pressure difference as calculated with the simplified Bernoulli relationship.

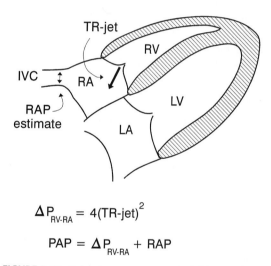

$$\Delta P_{RV-RA} = 4(TR\text{-jet})^2$$

$$PAP = \Delta P_{RV-RA} + RAP$$

FIGURE 5–21. Pulmonary artery pressure (PAP) can be calculated noninvasively based on the velocity in the tricuspid regurgitant (TR) jet and the respiratory variation in inferior vena cava (IVC) size as an estimate of right atrial pressure (RAP).

FIGURE 5–22. Tricuspid regurgitant jet in a patient with normal pulmonary pressures and a maximum jet velocity of 2.7 m/s.

tercept angle between the tricuspid regurgitant jet and the ultrasound beam. Most often the apical or right ventricular inflow view yields the highest-velocity signal given careful angulation of the ultrasound beam in three dimensions. Occasionally, the highest-velocity tricuspid regurgitant jet is recorded from a subcostal approach. Although this method requires the presence of tricuspid regurgitation, this rarely is a limitation, since about 90% of normal indi-

viduals and patients have some degree of tricuspid regurgitation (Fig. 5–22).

The same concept can be applied to the pulmonic regurgitant velocity curve. The end-diastolic pulmonic regurgitant velocity reflects the pulmonary artery to right ventricular end-diastolic pressure gradient per the Bernoulli equation. When added to an estimate of right atrial pressure, this provides a noninvasive estimate of diastolic pulmonary artery pressure.

Right atrial pressure is best estimated from evaluation of the inferior vena cava during respiration (Fig. 5–23). From a subcostal window,

FIGURE 5–23. Subcostal view of the junction between the inferior vena cava *(IVC)* and the right atrium *(RA)* during normal expiration *(above)* and inspiration *(below)*.

TABLE 5–8	Estimation of Right Atrial Pressure		

Inferior Vena Cava	Change with Respiration or "Sniff"	Estimated Right Atrial Pressure
Small (<1.5 cm)	Collapse	0–5 mmHg
Normal (1.5–2.5 cm)	Decrease by >50%	5–10 mmHg
Normal	Decrease by <50%	10–15 mmHg
Dilated (>2.5 cm)	Decrease <50%	15–20 mmHg
Dilated with dilated hepatic veins	No change	>20 mmHg

An alternate approach to estimation of right atrial pressure is clinical examination of the degree of jugular venous distension. However, while this approach is reliable in distinguishing changes (increases or decreases) over time in filling pressures in an individual patient, it is less accurate in determining the absolute right atrial pressure.

Pulmonary Artery Velocity Curve

Another approach to estimating pulmonary pressure is based on the shape of the pulmonary artery Doppler velocity curve. Comparison of the normal left ventricular and right ventricular ejection curves reveals that left ventricular ejection shows very rapid acceleration with a short time from flow onset to maximum velocity, whereas right ventricular ejection shows a slower acceleration, a longer time from onset of flow to peak flow, and a more "rounded" velocity curve (see Figs. 5–10 and 5–12). As pulmonary vascular resistance increases, the shape of the right ventricular ejection curve more closely approximates the left ventricular ejection curve, suggesting that the shapes of these velocity curves are related to the downstream resistance or impedance. A logarithmic relationship between the time from onset of flow to peak velocity and mean pulmonary artery pressure has been described, as shown in Table 5–6 and Figure 5–24.

The time to peak velocity estimates of pulmonary artery pressure are not as reliable as tricuspid regurgitant jet estimates for two reasons. First, this method depends on measurement of a relatively short time interval, so measurement error is high and reproducibility is

this segment of the inferior vena cava is imaged during quiet respiration (see also Chapter 6, section on right atrial pressure). If the inferior vena cava diameter is normal (1.2 to 2.3 cm) and the segment adjacent to the right atrium collapses by at least 50% with respiration, then right atrial pressure is equal to normal intrathoracic pressures (i.e., 5 to 10 mmHg). Failure to collapse with respiration and/or dilation of the inferior vena cava and hepatic veins is associated with higher right atrial pressures (Table 5–8). When no response is noted with normal respiration, the patient is asked to "sniff". This generates a sudden decrease in intrathoracic pressure, resulting in a change in inferior vena cava diameter.

FIGURE 5–24. Graph of the relationship between mean pulmonary artery pressure and the pulmonary artery acceleration time or time to peak velocity (TPV).

low. Second, the spatial flow velocity profile in the pulmonary artery is skewed, with higher acceleration and velocity along the inner edge of the curvature. Even when the sample volume appears positioned in the center of the vessel in a 2D image plane, it may be near the inner wall in the elevational plane, since this curvature is 3D. Thus the shape of the pulmonary artery velocity curve is most helpful when it is normal. An apparent short time to peak velocity can be due to measurement variability or to the nonuniform spatial flow velocity distribution in the vessel.

Isovolumic Relaxation Time

Pulmonary hypertension is associated with prolongation of the right ventricular isovolumic relaxation time (IVRT). This time can be measured as the interval between pulmonic valve closure and tricuspid valve opening, recorded either with M-mode echocardiography (showing leaflet closure) or Doppler echo (showing the valve "clicks"). Nomograms relating the right ventricular IVRT to the degree of pulmonary hypertension have been shown to be accurate in pediatric populations. In adults, this approach is rarely used because of the difficulty in recording pulmonic valve closure given suboptimal acoustic access in many patients. In addition, as with the time to peak velocity in the pulmonary artery velocity curve, the IVRT is a short interval that is subject to considerable measurement variability.

Limitations/Technical Considerations/ Alternate Approaches

Determination of pulmonary artery systolic pressure derived from the continuous-wave Doppler tricuspid regurgitant jet velocity is only as accurate as the primary data. Underestimation of tricuspid regurgitant jet velocity due to a nonparallel intercept angle between the jet and the ultrasound beam results in underestimation of pulmonary artery pressures. Overestimation of pulmonary artery pressures can occur if the mitral regurgitant jet is mistaken for tricuspid regurgitation. Although both signals occur in systole and are directed away from the left ventricular apex, the duration of tricuspid regurgitation is slightly longer than mitral regurgitation (when right and left ventricular systolic function are normal) due to a slightly longer right ventricular systolic ejection period (Fig. 5–25). The shapes of the velocity curves tend to differ as well, with tricuspid regurgitation having a slower upstroke and a peak later in systole, although the shapes of both velocity curves are affected by changes in ventricular function or atrial pressure. Note that the velocity of mitral regurgitation always is high, since it reflects the systolic left ventricular (approximately 100 mmHg) to left atrial (approximately 10 mmHg) pressure difference. With normal pulmonary artery pressures, tricuspid regurgitant jet velocity is 2 to 2.5 m/s. With pulmonary hypertension, pulmonary pressure may approach systemic pressures, with

FIGURE 5–25. Comparison of the flow duration typically shows that tricuspid regurgitation *(above)* is slightly longer than mitral regurgitation *(below).*

a corresponding tricuspid regurgitant jet velocity in the range of 5 m/s.

It is important conceptually to keep separate the grading of regurgitant *severity*—which is a measure of the *volume* of reverse flow across the valve—and regurgitant jet *velocity*—which reflects the instantaneous *pressure gradient* across the valve.

The tricuspid regurgitant jet can be used to estimate pulmonary artery pressure when right ventricular and pulmonary artery systolic pressures are equal, specifically in the absence of

pulmonic stenosis. When pulmonic stenosis is present, pulmonary pressures can be estimated by subtracting the right ventricle to pulmonary artery pressure difference derived from the pulmonic stenotic jet velocity (V_{PS}) from the estimated right ventricular systolic pressure:

$$PAP = [4(V_{TR})^2 + RAP] - [4(V_{PS})^2] \quad (5.32)$$

The estimate of right atrial pressure from the appearance of the inferior vena cava also can affect the accuracy of Doppler echo pulmonary artery pressure estimates. The importance of this source of error is greatest at intermediate tricuspid regurgitant jet velocities: a tricuspid regurgitant jet velocity of 2.5 m/s with a right atrial pressure of 5 mmHg indicates a pulmonary artery pressure of only 30 mmHg (normal to mildly elevated), but if right atrial pressure is 20 mmHg, then pulmonary artery pressure is 45 mmHg (mild to moderate pulmonary hypertension). At the extreme (i.e., a tricuspid regurgitant jet of 5 m/s), pulmonary hypertension clearly is severe regardless of the right atrial pressure estimate.

If images of the inferior vena cava are suboptimal, or if the degree of change with respiration is equivocal, it is appropriate to report the range of possible pulmonary artery pressures or to indicate that the right ventricle to right atrial pressure gradient should be added to a clinical estimate of right atrial pressure. Evaluation of respiratory variation in inferior vena cava diameter can be confounded by respiratory motion in the position of the inferior vena cava such that the center of the vessel moves in and out of the image plane. Of course, evaluation of inferior vena cava size and respiratory variation is not helpful in patients supported by positive-pressure ventilation, since intrathoracic pressures are abnormal.

The time to peak velocity in the pulmonary artery can appear short when the Doppler sample volume is positioned along the inner curve of the pulmonary artery. Conversely, impaired right ventricular systolic function may result in an apparently normal time to peak velocity even in the presence of pulmonary hypertension.

The alternative to noninvasive Doppler echo estimate of pulmonary artery pressures is direct measurement in the coronary care unit or cardiac catheterization laboratory with a pulmonary artery (Swan-Ganz) catheter. This approach has the advantages of precision, a high degree of accuracy (assuming appropriate transducer calibration and balancing), and the ability to continuously record measurements over a period of several days. Disadvantages are its costs, potential complications of line placement, and the difficulty of performing repeat measures over longer time intervals.

SUGGESTED READING

2D Echocardiographic Ventricular Volumes and Ejection Fraction

1. American Society of Echocardiography Committee on Standards, Subcommittee on Quantitation of Two-Dimensional Echocardiograms: Recommendations for quantitation of the left ventricle by two-dimensional echocardiography. *J Am Soc Echocardiogr* 2:361–367, 1989.

    Clear description of methods for quantitation of left ventricular systolic function by 2D echocardiography as recommended by the American Society of Echocardiography. Technical details of image acquisition, diagrams illustrating quantitative techniques, and tables of normal values are included.

2. Folland ED, Parisi AF, Moynihan PF, et al: Assessment of left ventricular ejection fraction and volumes by real-time, two-dimensional echocardiography. A comparison of cineangiographic and radionuclide techniques. *Circulation* 60:760–766, 1979.

    Key paper comparing five different algorithms for determining left ventricular volumes by 2D echocardiography in comparison with both radionuclide ventriculography and contrast angiography.

3. Smith MD, MacPhail B, Harrison MR, et al: Value and limitations of transesophageal echocardiography in determination of left ventricular volumes and ejection fraction. *J Am Coll Cardiol* 19:1213–1222, 1992.

    Calculation of left ventricular volumes using a modified Simpson's rule can be made from transesophageal images using short-axis views at the mitral valve, papillary muscle, and apical levels plus left ventricular length measured in the four-chamber view. Underestimation of left ventricular length on transesophageal echocardiographic images results in smaller calculated left ventricular volumes than angiographic measurements.

4. Gordon EP, Schnittger I, Fitzgerald PJ, et al: Reproducibility of left ventricular volumes by two-dimensional echocardiography. *J Am Coll Cardiol* 2: 506–513, 1983.

    Repeat recordings and measurement of left ventricular volumes by 2D echocardiography showed 95% confidence limits for individual subjects' measurements of ±15% for end-diastolic volume, ±25% for end-systolic volume, and ±10% for ejection fraction.

3D Echocardiography

5. Leotta DF, Munt B, Bolson EL, Kraft C, Martin RW, Otto CM, Sheehan FS: Quantitative three-dimensional echocardiography by rapid imaging from multiple transthoracic windows: in vitro validation and initial in vivo studies. *J Am Soc Echocardiogr* 10:830–839, 1997.

    Three-dimensional image acquisition using a magnetic field system allowed continuous image acquisition with free scanning from multiple acoustic windows. Interactive 3D border tracing and reconstruction using the piecewise smooth subdivision model provided accurate volumes for in vitro phantoms (with distorted shapes) and in vitro hearts. This 3D technique also provided accurate stroke volume measurement in human subjects with image acquisition times <90 seconds.

6. Jiang L, Vazquez-de-Prada JA, Handschumacher MD, et al: Quantitative three-dimensional reconstruction of aneurysmal left ventricles: in vitro and in vivo validation. *Circulation* 91:222–230, 1995.

    Using an external spark-gap locator system to identify the 3D orientation of the scan plane, 3D reconstructions of aneurysmal ventricles were performed in vitro and in vivo. Calculated volumes and mass by 3D echocardiography correlated closely with direct measurements for the in vitro hearts. In vivo data were compared to actual instantaneous ventricular volumes using an intracavitary balloon attached to an external column. In vivo 3D volumes and ejection fraction correlated closely with the actual measurements, despite the presence of distorted ventricular geometry.

7. Gopal AS, Schnellbaecher MJ, Shen Z, et al: Freehand three-dimensional echocardiography for determination of left ventricular volume and mass in patients with abnormal ventricles: comparison with magnetic resonance imaging. *J Am Soc Echocardiogr* 10:853–861, 1997.

    Freehand scanning using a "line of intersection" display allows 3D determination of left ventricular volumes and mass. Using this approach in 30 patients with abnormal ventricular geometry, 3D volumes were more accurate than 2D volumes when compared to volumes obtained by magnetic resonance imaging. The elimination of geometric assumptions with 3D echocardiography is especially important when ventricular shape is altered by disease.

8. Gopal AS, King DL: Three-dimensional echocardiography: approaches and applications. *In* Otto CM (ed): The Practice of Clinical Echocardiography. Philadelphia, WB Saunders, 1997. pp. 131–166.

    This chapter reviews the basic principles of the acquisition, display, and clinical applications of 3D echocardiography. Image acquisition using acoustic or electromagnetic spatial locator systems are contrasted with images acquired by rotational scanning. The use of surface-rendered volume displays versus wire-frame models is discussed. Quantitative applications of 3D echocardiography include measurement of left ventricular volumes, ejection fraction, and mass. Right ventricular, left and right atrial, and pericardial fluid volume calculations also can be performed. 202 references.

Other 2D Measures of Systolic Function

9. Collins M, Hsieh A, Ohazama CJ, Ota T, Stetten G, Donovan CL, Kisslo J, Ryan T: Assessment of regional wall motion abnormalities with real-time 3-dimensional echocardiography. *J Am Soc Echocardiogr* 12:7–14, 1999.

    Real-time volumetric imaging allows recording of a 3-dimensional pyramidal shaped volumetric data set that contains the entire left ventricle. This allows display of simultaneous tomographic planes for evaluation of the extent and location of regional wall motion abnormalities from a single cardiac cycle.

10. Gorsan J III, Romand JA, Mandarino WA, et al: Assessment of left ventricular performance by on-line pressure-area relations using echocardiographic automated border detection. *J Am Coll Cardiol* 23: 242–252, 1994.

Echocardiographic images of the left ventricle were analyzed using automated border detection to derive ventricular areas from short-axis images throughout the cardiac cycle. Using directly measured ventricular pressure, pressure-area loops were generated and used to calculate stroke area, stroke force, end-systolic elastance, and preload recruitable stroke force.

11. Simonson JS, Schiller NB: Descent of the base of the left ventricle: An echocardiographic index of left ventricular function. J Am Soc Echocardiogr 2:25–35, 1989.

The motion of the mitral annulus toward the ventricular apex in systole (lengthwise ventricular shortening) provides a simple method for quantitation of left ventricular systolic function. Average motion in normal individuals was 12 ± 2 mm, with motion <8 mm sensitive (98%) and specific (82%) for diagnosis of an ejection fraction of less than 50%.

12. Aurigemma GP, Douglas PS, Gaasch WH: Quantitative evaluation of left ventricular structure, wall stress and systolic function. *In* Otto CM (ed): The Practice of Clinical Echocardiography. Philadelphia, WB Saunders, 1997. pp. 1–24.

2D echocardiography allows sophisticated evaluation of left ventricular geometry and systolic function. This chapter provides a detailed and critical discussion of approaches to measurement of wall stress and systolic performance. The calculation of circumferential as well as meridional stress is described. 143 references.

Doppler Evaluation of Systolic Function

13. Chen C, Rodriguez L, Guerrero JL, et al: Noninvasive estimation of the instantaneous first derivative of left ventricular pressure using continuous-wave Doppler echocardiography. *Circulation* 83:2101–2110, 1991.

The rate of ventricular pressure rise in early systole (dP/dt) can be calculated from the mitral regurgitant jet velocity curve. Both dP/dt$_{max}$ and −dP/dt$_{max}$ can be determined accurately and reliably.

14. Chung N, Nishimura RA, Holmes DR Jr, Tajik AJ: Measurement of left ventricular dP/dt by simultaneous Doppler echocardiography and cardiac catheterization. J Am Soc Echocardiogr 5:147–152, 1992.

Doppler measurement of left ventricular dP/dt from the mitral regurgitant velocity curve was most accurate using the time interval from 1 to 3 m/s on the velocity curve.

15. Bouchard A, Blumlein S, Schiller NB, et al: Measurement of left ventricular stroke volume using continuous-wave Doppler echocardiography of the ascending aorta and M-mode echocardiography of the aortic valve. J Am Coll Cardiol 9:75–83, 1987.

Description of stroke volume measurement based on a continuous-wave Doppler recording of ascending aortic flow and an M-mode tracing of the aortic valve (assuming a circular systolic orifice).

16. Lewis JF, Kuo LC, Nelson JG, et al: Pulsed Doppler echocardiographic determination of stroke volume and cardiac output: clinical validation of two new methods using the apical window. *Circulation* 70:425–431, 1984.

Description of left ventricular outflow tract and mitral annulus methods for stroke volume calculation. Validation in 39 patients versus thermodilution cardiac output and application of Doppler stroke volume measurement at two intracardiac sites to calculation of regurgitant volume is described. Interobserver variability for stroke volume or cardiac output (mean percentage error ± 1 SD) was 16.4% ± 13% for the mitral annulus method and 6.8% ± 5% for the left ventricular outflow method.

17. Otto CM, Pearlman AS, Gardner CL, et al: Experimental validation of Doppler echocardiographic measurement of volume flow through the stenotic aortic valve. *Circulation* 78:435–441, 1988.

Validation of left ventricular outflow tract method for measurement of stroke volume proximal to a stenotic aortic valve. Repeat measurement of left ventricular outflow tract diameter showed a mean coefficient of variation of 2%.

18. Sjoberg BJ, Ask P, Loyd D, et al: Subaortic flow profiles in aortic valve disease: a two-dimensional color Doppler study. *J Am Soc Echocardiogr* 7:276–285, 1994.

Using time-corrected quantitative color Doppler echocardiography, the spatial flow velocity profile proximal to the aortic valve was examined. In 10 patients with aortic stenosis, the flow profile was fairly flat; however, deviations from a flat flow profile were observed in five healthy control subjects.

Right Ventricular Systolic Function

19. Jiang L, Siu SC, Handschumacher MD, et al: Three-dimensional echocardiography: in vivo validation for right ventricular volume and function. *Circulation* 89:2342–2350, 1994.

Echocardiographic three-dimensional reconstructions of the right ventricle (using epicardial image acquisition with a spark-gap locater system) were performed during 20 hemodynamic states in five dogs. Both end-diastolic (r = 0.99, y = 1x − 3.4, SEE = 1.8 ml) and end-systolic (r = 0.98, y = 1x + 2, SEE = 2.5 ml) echocardiographic volumes correlated well with actual volumes measured using an intracavity balloon connected to an external calibrated column.

20. Louie EK, Rich S, Levitsky S, Brundage BH: Doppler echocardiographic demonstration of the differential effects of right ventricular pressure and volume overload on left ventricular geometry and filling. J Am Coll Cardiol 19:84–90, 1992.

Right ventricular pressure overload results in a leftward septal shift on 2D echocardiography that is maximal at end-systole and in early diastole. In contrast, right ventricular volume overload results in the maximal leftward septal shift at end-diastole with a rela-

tively normal septal contour at end-systole and early diastole. Recognition of these differing patterns of septal motion focuses the examination on the relevant differential diagnosis.

Noninvasive Pulmonary Pressures

21. Yock PG, Popp RL: Noninvasive estimation of right ventricular systolic pressure by Doppler ultrasound in patients with tricuspid regurgitation. *Circulation* 70:657–662, 1984.

    Description and validation of calculating the right ventricular to right atrial maximum systolic pressure difference from the maximum tricuspid regurgitant jet velocity using the simplified Bernoulli equation. While the Doppler and invasive pressure gradient correlated well (r = 0.95), clinical estimates of right atrial pressure from the degree of jugular venous distension correlated only modestly with measured right atrial pressure (r = 0.80).

22. Currie PJ, Seward JB, Chart K-L, et al: Continuous-wave Doppler determination of right ventricular pressure: a simultaneous Doppler-catheterization study in 127 patients. J Am Coll Cardiol 6:750–756, 1985.

    Further validation of the use of tricuspid regurgitant jet velocity to estimate right ventricular systolic pressure in a larger series of patients. An adequate tricuspid regurgitant jet velocity signal was obtained in 111 of 127 (87%) of patients. The average coefficient of variation for measurement of maximum velocity was 2% (range 0 to 18%).

23. Kitabatake A, Inoue M, Asao M, et al: Noninvasive evaluation of pulmonary hypertension by a pulsed Doppler technique. *Circulation* 58:302–309, 1983.

    Estimation of pulmonary artery mean pressure from the shape of the right ventricular outflow tract velocity curve; specifically, the time interval from onset of flow to maximum velocity is described (see Fig. 5–24).

24. Stevenson JG: Comparison of several noninvasive methods for estimation of pulmonary artery pressure. *J Am Soc Echocardiogr* 2:157–171, 1989.

    In a pediatric population, noninvasive methods for estimation of pulmonary artery pressure were compared. Both the Burstin method (pulmonic valve closure to tricuspid opening) and the tricuspid regurgitant jet method were highly accurate (r = 0.97 and 0.96, respectively) and could be recorded in nearly all subjects (82% to 89%). The right ventricular output tract time to peak velocity (TPV) correlated better (r = 0.94) with directly measured pulmonary artery pressure than did TPV from the pulmonary artery velocity curve (r = 0.63).

25. Lee RT, Lord CP, Plappert T, St John Sutton M: Prospective Doppler echocardiographic evaluation of pulmonary artery diastolic pressure in the medical intensive care unit. *Am J Cardiol* 64:1366–1370, 1989.

    Estimation of pulmonary artery diastolic pressure from the pulmonic regurgitant velocity curve was possible in 17 of 29 (59%) of intensive care unit patients. The pulmonary artery to right ventricular diastolic pressure difference was calculated at $4V^2$, where V is the end-diastolic pulmonic regurgitant jet velocity, and then added to a clinical estimate of right atrial pressure. Correlation with invasively measured pulmonary artery pressure was excellent (r = 0.94, mean absolute difference = 3.3 mmHg).

Echocardiographic Evaluation of Ventricular Diastolic Filling and Function

6

BASIC PRINCIPLES
  Phases of Diastole
  Parameters of Diastolic Function
    Ventricular Relaxation
    Ventricular Compliance
    Ventricular Diastolic Pressures
    Ventricular Diastolic Filling (Volume) Curves
    Atrial Pressures and Filling Curves
  Normal Respiratory Changes
  Clinical Etiologies of Diastolic Dysfunction
ECHOCARDIOGRAPHIC APPROACH TO LEFT
VENTRICULAR DIASTOLIC FUNCTION
  2D/M-Mode Evaluation
  Doppler Evaluation of Left Ventricular Filling
    Description of Left Ventricular Filling by Doppler Echo
    Quantitative Ventricular Filling Velocity and Time Interval Measurements
    Volumetric Flow Rates
  Doppler Data Recording
  Factors That Affect Doppler Left Ventricular Filling
    Normal Variations
    Physiologic Factors
    Left Ventricular Relaxation
    Left Ventricular Compliance

RIGHT VENTRICULAR DIASTOLIC FUNCTION
  Right Ventricular Filling
  Doppler Data Recording
  Physiologic Factors That Affect Right Ventricular Filling
LEFT ATRIAL FILLING
  Doppler Assessment
  Doppler Data Recording
  Physiologic Factors That Affect Left Atrial Filling
RIGHT ATRIAL FILLING
  Doppler Assessment
    Right Atrial Filling Curves
    Right Atrial Pressure
  Doppler Data Recording
  Limitations
CLINICAL UTILITY
  Left Ventricular Hypertrophy
  Cardiomyopathy
  Pericardial Disease
  Ischemic Cardiac Disease
  Noninvasive Estimates of Left Ventricular Diastolic Pressure
ALTERNATE APPROACHES TO EVALUATION OF
DIASTOLIC DYSFUNCTION
SUGGESTED READING

There has been increasing recognition that *diastolic* ventricular function often plays a key role in the clinical manifestations of disease in patients with a wide range of cardiac disorders. For example, many patients with clinical heart failure have normal systolic function with predominant diastolic dysfunction. Diastolic dysfunction may be an early sign of cardiac diseases (as in hypertension), often antedating clinical or echocardiographic evidence of systolic dysfunction. In addition, the degree of diastolic dysfunction may explain the difference in clinical symptoms between patients with similar degrees of systolic dysfunction.

Echocardiographic techniques allow evaluation of right and left ventricular diastolic filling patterns and right and left atrial filling patterns.

The relationship between these noninvasive measures and ventricular diastolic function and the utility of these measures in patient evaluation are discussed in this chapter.

BASIC PRINCIPLES

Phases of Diastole

Although several different definitions of diastole have been proposed, the most widely accepted clinical definition is the interval from aortic valve closure (end-systole) to mitral valve closure (end-diastole) (Fig. 6–1). The isovolumic contraction period, from mitral valve closure to aortic valve opening, typically is considered to be part of systole.

FIGURE 6–1. The relationship between left ventricular *(LV)*, left atrial *(LA)*, and aortic *(Ao)* pressures and M-mode tracings of the aortic and mitral valve is shown. The isovolumic relaxation time *(IVRT)* is the interval from aortic valve closure to mitral valve opening. During this interval, left ventricular pressure declines rapidly. A rapid rise in left ventricular pressure occurs during the isovolumic contraction time *(IVCT)*, the interval between mitral valve closure and aortic valve opening.

Diastole can be divided into four phases: (1) isovolumic relaxation, (2) the early rapid diastolic filling phase, (3) diastasis, and (4) late diastolic filling due to atrial contraction. During the isovolumic relaxation interval, left ventricular pressure falls rapidly following aortic valve closure. At the point where left ventricular pressure falls below left atrial pressure, the mitral valve opens, ending the isovolumic relaxation period. With mitral valve opening, blood flows from the left atrium to the left ventricle, with the rate and time course of flow being determined by several factors, including the pressure difference along the flow path, ventricular relaxation, and the relative compliances of the two chambers. Maximal opening of the mitral leaflets typically occurs rapidly, within 100 ± 10 ms of valve opening, in normal individuals.

As the ventricle fills, pressures between the atrium and ventricle equalize, resulting in a period of *diastasis,* during which there is little movement of blood between the chambers and the mitral leaflets remain in a semiopen position. The duration of diastasis is heart rate–

dependent, being longer at slow heart rates and entirely absent at faster heart rates. With atrial contraction, left atrial pressure again exceeds left ventricular pressure, resulting in mitral leaflet opening and a second pulse of left ventricular filling. In normal individuals, the atrial contribution to ventricular filling typically is small, comprising only about 20% of total ventricular filling (Fig. 6–2).

The phases of diastole for the right ventricle are analogous to those described for the left ventricle, with the difference that the total duration of diastole is slightly shorter in normal individuals due to a slightly longer right ventricular systolic ejection period.

Parameters of Diastolic Function

There are several physiologic parameters that can be used to describe different aspects of diastolic function, but there is no single measure of overall diastolic function. The most clinically relevant parameters identified to date include ventricular relaxation, myocardial compliance, and chamber compliance. Additional parameters of interest include elastic recoil of the ventricle and the effect of pericardial constraint, but the importance of these factors in

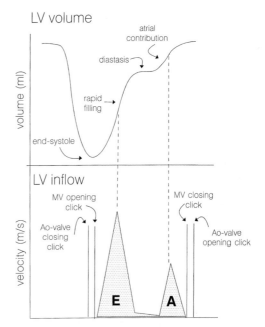

FIGURE 6–2. The relationship between left ventricular volume and the diastolic left ventricular Doppler filling pattern is shown. Early rapid filling coincides with the *E* velocity, followed by diastasis, with little or no flow from left atrium to left ventricle, and atrial contraction, which coincides with the late diastolic *A* velocity. The Doppler velocity curve, in effect, is the first derivative of the left ventricular volume curve.

normal diastolic ventricular function remains controversial.

Ventricular Relaxation

Left ventricular relaxation, occurring during isovolumic relaxation and the early diastolic filling period, is an active process involving utilization of energy by the myocardium. Factors affecting isovolumic relaxation include internal loading forces (cardiac fiber), external loading conditions (wall stress, arterial impedance), inactivation of myocardial contraction (metabolic, neurohumoral, and pharmacologic), and nonuniformity in the spatial and temporal patterns of these factors. Abnormal relaxation results in prolongation of the isovolumic relaxation time, a slower rate of decline in ventricular pressure, and a consequent reduction in the early peak filling rate (due to a smaller pressure difference between the atrium and the ventricle when the atrioventricular valve opens). Measures of left ventricular relaxation include the isovolumic relaxation time (IVRT), the maximum rate of pressure decline *(−dP/dt)*, and the time constant of relaxation (tau or τ). There are several different mathematical ap-

proaches to calculation of tau, but basically it reflects the rate of pressure decline from the point of maximum $-dP/dt$ to mitral valve opening. While peak rapid filling rate is affected by ventricular relaxation, it is only an indirect measure of this physiologic parameter, since several other factors also affect peak filling (Fig. 6–3).

Ventricular Compliance

Compliance is the ratio of change in volume to change in pressure *(dV/dP)*. Stiffness is the inverse of compliance: the ratio of change in pressure to change in volume *(dP/dV)*. Conceptually, compliance can be divided into myocardial (the characteristics of the isolated myocardium) and chamber (the characteristics of the entire chamber) components. Chamber compliance is influenced by ventricular size and shape, as well as by the characteristics of the myocardium. Extrinsic factors also may affect measurement of compliance, including the pericardium, right ventricular volume, and pleural pressure. Evaluation of ventricular compliance is based on diastolic passive pressure-volume curves showing the degree to which pressure and volume change in relation to each other over the physiologic range of pressures and volumes (Fig. 6–4).

Ventricular Diastolic Pressures

Clinically, evaluation of diastolic pressures alone often is used in patient management. Measurement of left ventricular end-diastolic pressure (LV-EDP) (or its surrogate, pulmonary artery wedge pressure) is the most commonly available measure of diastolic "function," although its limitations as a descriptor of diastole are well recognized.

Ventricular Diastolic Filling (Volume) Curves

Another clinically available measure related to diastolic function is the time course of ventricular filling: the ventricular diastolic filling curve. Experimentally, filling curves can be measured on a beat-to-beat basis from implanted sonocrystal-derived ventricular dimensions or from impedance catheter data. Clinically, filling curves can be generated for an individual cardiac cycle from frame-by-frame measurements of ventricular volumes using angiographic, computed tomography, magnetic resonance, or echocardiographic images or from high-temporal-resolution radionuclide studies. Doppler echocardiography offers the ability to measure left ventricular diastolic filling, noninvasively, on a beat-to-beat basis.

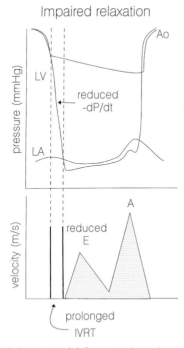

FIGURE 6–3. Impaired left ventricular relaxation is described by a reduced *−dP/dt*, and a prolonged time constant of relaxation. The Doppler velocity curve shows a prolonged IVRT, reduced *E* velocity (corresponding to a low left atrial–left ventricular gradient at mitral valve opening), and an increased *A* velocity.

Decreased compliance

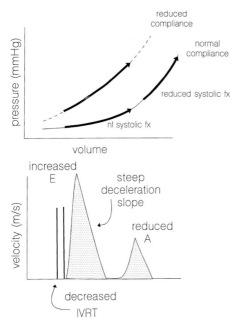

FIGURE 6–4. Reduced diastolic compliance is described by a steeper passive pressure-volume relationship of the left ventricle. As left ventricular volume increases in diastole, pressure rises rapidly, resulting in an initial high left atrial–left ventricular pressure gradient with a rapid decrease in the filling gradient during diastole. The Doppler velocity curve shows a decreased IVRT, steep deceleration slope, and reduced *A* velocity. Note that even with normal compliance, reduced systolic function results in a rightward shift along the normal pressure-volume relationship, resulting in a similar pattern of diastolic filling.

Unfortunately, while ventricular *diastolic function* is one of the major factors affecting the pattern of *diastolic filling,* these two concepts are not identical. Several physiologic parameters other than diastolic function affect diastolic filling. Given no change in diastolic function (i.e., relaxation, compliance, etc.), the peak early diastolic filling rate will be affected by (1) changes in the pressure difference between the ventricle and the atrium (the opening pressure) due to changes in preload (e.g., increased with volume loading, decreased with volume depletion), (2) a change in transmitral volume flow rate (e.g., increased with coexisting mitral regurgitation), or (3) a change in atrial pressure (e.g., elevated left ventricular end-diastolic pressure or a *v* wave due to mitral regurgitation).

Late diastolic filling is affected by cardiac rhythm, atrial contractile function, ventricular end-diastolic pressure, heart rate, and the timing of atrial contraction (PR interval), as well as

by ventricular diastolic function. In addition, it is obvious that the utility of ventricular diastolic filling patterns for assessing diastolic function is valid only in the absence of obstruction at the atrioventricular valve level (i.e., mitral stenosis). The importance of considering the influence of these factors on the pattern of diastolic filling as assessed by Doppler echocardiography is discussed in more detail in the following sections.

Atrial Pressures and Filling Curves

Another somewhat indirect approach to evaluation of ventricular diastolic function is measurement of atrial filling patterns and pressures. This approach is conceptually sound given that elevations in ventricular diastolic pressures will be reflected in elevated pressures in the atrium. Atrial filling patterns obviously are closely linked with diastolic ventricular function, especially in early diastole, when the atrioventricular valve is open, since the atrium serves as a "conduit" for flow from the venous circulation to the ventricle (Fig. 6–5).

Right atrial pressures normally are quite low (0 to 5 mmHg), with only small increases in

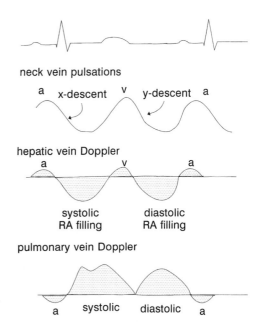

FIGURE 6–5. Schematic diagram of right atrial (hepatic vein) and left atrial (pulmonary vein) filling patterns and the close correspondence with the pattern of jugular venous pulsations. Pulmonary and hepatic vein patterns appear "opposite" in direction, since the direction of flow in the hepatic vein using a transthoracic subcostal view is away from the transducer (into the right atrium), while the direction of flow from a transthoracic apical view of the pulmonary vein is toward the transducer (into the left atrium).

pressure following atrial (*a* wave) and ventricular (*v* wave) contraction. Right atrial filling is characterized by: (1) a small reversal of flow following atrial contraction (*a* wave), (2) a systolic phase (which is effectively "diastole" for the atrium) when blood flows from the superior and inferior vena cava into the atrium, (3) a small reversal of flow at end-systole (*v* wave), and (4) a diastolic filling phase when the atrium serves as a conduit for flow from the systemic venous return to the right ventricle. These filling phases are reflected in the patterns of jugular venous pulsation familiar to the clinician: the *a* wave following atrial contraction, the *x* descent corresponding to atrial systolic filling, the *v* wave with ventricular contraction, and the *y* descent corresponding to atrial diastolic filling. Disease processes affect the jugular venous pulsations and the Doppler pattern of right atrial filling in similar ways.

Left atrial filling from the pulmonary veins also is characterized by (1) a small reversal of flow following atrial contraction (*a* wave), (2) a systolic filling phase, (3) a blunting of flow or brief reversal at end-systole, and (4) a diastolic filling phase. In normal individuals, the systolic and diastolic filling phases are approximately equal in volume. Normal left atrial pressure is low (5 to 10 mmHg), corresponding to the normal left ventricular end-diastolic pressure, with slight increases in pressure following atrial (*a* wave) and ventricular (*v* wave) contraction.

Normal Respiratory Changes

The patterns of right and left ventricular diastolic filling show normal respiratory variation. With inspiration, negative intrapleural pressure results in an increase in systemic venous return into the thorax and, thus, into the right atrium. This increased right atrial volume and pressure results in a transient increase in right ventricular diastolic filling volumes and velocities, with a normal magnitude of increase of up to 20% compared with end-expiratory values.

Left atrium filling does *not* increase with inspiration, since pulmonary venous return is entirely intrathoracic and thus not affected significantly by respiratory changes in intrathoracic pressure. In fact, left atrial and, consequently, left ventricular diastolic filling is slightly higher at end-expiration than during inspiration. The mechanism of the observation remains controversial. Some postulate a delay in transit of the increased right ventricular filling to the left side of the heart. Others suggest a decrease in left atrial filling during inspiration due to an increased volume (or "pooling") in the pulmonary venous bed. Less likely, in normal individuals, is impaired left ventricular diastolic filling due to an increase in right ventricular diastolic volume within a fixed-volume pericardium. This last mechanism may become important in patients with pericardial disease (constriction, tamponade) and may partly account for the exaggerated respiratory changes in right ventricular and left ventricular diastolic filling seen in these conditions.

Clinical Etiologies of Diastolic Dysfunction

While diastolic dysfunction can be seen with a wide range of cardiac disorders, there are three basic mechanisms of disease that lead to diastolic dysfunction. First, diseases that affect the ventricular myocardium with preserved contractile (systolic) function present with "isolated" diastolic dysfunction. Examples include left ventricular hypertrophy due to hypertension, hypertrophic cardiomyopathy, ischemic disease without prior myocardial infarction, and restrictive cardiomyopathy. Second, pericardial disease (tamponade, constriction) results in impaired cardiac filling due to extrinsic compression of the heart. Third, diastolic dysfunction often accompanies systolic dysfunction of the left ventricle (e.g., in dilated cardiomyopathy or end-stage ischemic disease).

ECHOCARDIOGRAPHIC APPROACH TO LEFT VENTRICULAR DIASTOLIC FUNCTION

2D/M-Mode Evaluation

Evaluation of ventricular chamber dimensions and wall thickness is an integral part of the echocardiographic evaluation of diastolic function. In a patient with clinical heart failure, the findings of increased wall thickness with a nondilated chamber and normal systolic function suggest that diastolic dysfunction may be the etiology of "heart failure." Of course, this finding is neither sensitive nor specific for the diagnosis of diastolic dysfunction. Diastolic dysfunction can be present concurrently with systolic dysfunction (e.g., in dilated cardiomyopathy) and may be absent despite ventricular hypertrophy in some situations, such as physiologic hypertrophy in an athlete. On M-mode echocardiography, early studies suggested that the degree and rate of motion of the posterior left ventricular wall might provide a useful measure of diastolic function. In practical terms, the magnitude of these changes is too small to be measured reliably. Other findings on two-dimensional (2D) or M-mode echocardiography that raise the question of diastolic dysfunction include pericardial thickening (as in constrictive pericarditis), the pattern of ventricular septal motion with respiration (especially with tamponade physiology), and dilation of the inferior vena cava and hepatic veins (consistent with elevated right atrial pressures). Tissue characterization of the myocardium using ultrasound techniques may prove to be useful in evaluation of patients with suspected diastolic dysfunction, but further studies are needed. Thus direct evaluation of ventricular diastolic function by 2D or M-mode techniques is limited. Instead, attention has focused on the utility of Doppler echocardiography for evaluation of diastolic function.

Doppler Evaluation of Left Ventricular Filling (Table 6–1)

Description of Left Ventricular Filling by Doppler Echo

Doppler recordings of left ventricular diastolic filling velocities correspond closely with ventricular filling parameters measured by other techniques. The normal Doppler ventricular inflow pattern is characterized by a brief time interval between aortic valve closure and the onset of ventricular filling (the isovolumic

TABLE 6–1	Doppler Measures of Left Ventricular Diastolic Filling

Velocities
E velocity
A velocity
E/A ratio

Intervals
Isovolumic relaxation time (IVRT)
Rapid filling period
Diastasis
Atrial filling period

Acceleration/Deceleration
Time from mitral valve opening to E velocity
Maximal acceleration
Early diastolic deceleration slope (or half-time)

Filling Rates/Volumes
Peak rapid filling rate
Peak atrial filling rate
Stroke volume
Fractional filling rates (first third)

Color M-Mode Doppler
Propagation velocity

Doppler Tissue Imaging Wall Motion Velocity

relaxation time). Immediately following mitral valve opening, there is rapid acceleration of blood flow from the left atrium to the ventricle with an early peak filling velocity of 0.6 to 0.8 m/s occurring 90 to 110 ms after the onset of flow in young, healthy individuals. This early maximum filling velocity (E velocity) occurs simultaneously with the maximum pressure gradient between the atrium and ventricle. After this maximum velocity, flow decelerates rapidly (i.e., with a steep slope) in normal individuals with a normal deceleration slope of 4.3 to 6.7 m/s². Early diastolic filling is followed by a variable period of minimal flow (diastasis), depending on the total duration of diastole. With atrial contraction, left atrial pressure again exceeds ventricular pressure, resulting in a second velocity peak (late diastolic or atrial velocity), which typically ranges from 0.19 to 0.35 m/s in young, normal individuals (Fig. 6–6).

Quantitative Ventricular Filling Velocity and Time Interval Measurements

Quantitative measurements that can be made from the Doppler velocity curve include (Fig. 6–7):

1. *Maximum velocities:* The E velocity, the A velocity, and their ratio (E/A ratio).
2. *Velocity-time integrals:* Total, early diastolic, atrial contribution, first third or half of diastole, and their ratios.
3. *Time intervals:* The isovolumic relaxation time, the total duration of diastole, the rapid filling period, the length of diastasis, and the atrial filling period.
4. *Measures of acceleration and deceleration:* The time from onset of flow to the E velocity, the maximum rate of rise in velocity, and the slope of early diastolic deceleration.

Instead of deceleration slope, some centers measure the deceleration *pressure half-time*, as is used in evaluation of mitral stenosis. The *half-time* is defined as the time interval from the maximum E velocity to the point where the maximum pressure gradient has fallen to half its initial value (see Chap. 10). When assessing diastolic dysfunction (which presumes the absence of mitral stenosis), use of the deceleration time is preferable, since the half-time depends on both this slope and the maximum E velocity.

Volumetric Flow Rates

In order to convert the Doppler ventricular inflow *velocity curve* to a *volume curve*, the cross-sectional area of flow must be taken into account. As described in Chapter 2, volumetric

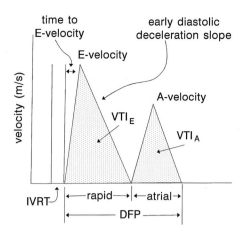

FIGURE 6–7. Schematic diagram of quantitative measurements that can be made from the Doppler left ventricular filling curve.

FIGURE 6–6. Normal pattern of left ventricular diastolic filling recorded with pulsed Doppler in an apical four-chamber view. The sample volume is positioned at the mitral leaflet tips. In this normal young individual, the E velocity is high and the A velocity is low.

flow rates can be calculated as the product of velocity and cross-sectional area in regions where flow is laminar with a spatially symmetric flow pattern. Thus the instantaneous volume flow rate across the mitral valve can be calculated as instantaneous velocity times the flow cross-sectional area (CSA). Similarly, transmitral stroke volume (SV) can be determined from the integral of the flow velocity curve (VTI) over the diastolic filling period:

$$SV_{transmitral} = VTI \times CSA$$

The standard approach to determining the cross-sectional area of flow across the mitral valve is to calculate the cross-sectional area of flow at the mitral annulus level. Motion of the mitral leaflets is a passive process, with the degree of motion reflecting flow across the valve (in the absence of mitral stenosis). Although there is some tapering of the flow area from the annulus to the leaflet tips, the more rigid mitral annulus is a preferable site for flow measurement rather than the flexible, mobile leaflets. Although the shape of the mitral annulus is complex in three dimensions, area often is calculated as an ellipse, based on diameter measurements in apical four-chamber and parasternal long-axis views. The even simpler assumption of a circular geometry, using the four-chamber view diameter, also is a reasonable approximation in most clinical situations (Fig. 6–8).

Combining Doppler left ventricular inflow velocity data with the cross-sectional area of the mitral annulus, additional filling parameters that can be calculated include:

1. *Peak filling rates*: Peak rapid filling rate, atrial peak filling rate, and their ratio
2. *Stroke volume*
3. *Fractional filling rates*: For example, first third filling fraction or the ratio of early to late filling

For each of these parameters, the filling rate is calculated by multiplying the appropriate velocity or velocity-time integral by cross-sectional area. For example, peak rapid filling rate (PRFR) is:

$$PRFR \ (ml/s) = E \ velocity \ (cm/s) \times CSA \ (cm^2)$$

Of course, volume flow measurements are accurate only when velocities and diameters are measured at the same anatomic location, for example, at the annulus level.

FIGURE 6–8. Calculation of volumetric flow rates across the mitral annulus.

FIGURE 6–9. Transesophageal recording of left ventricular filling. Flow is directed away from the transducer from this approach.

Doppler Data Recording

Left ventricular inflow can be recorded in nearly all patients from an apical approach in either a four- or two-chamber view (Table 6–2). This window allows parallel alignment between the ultrasound beam and the direction of left ventricular filling. On transesophageal echocardiography, left ventricular inflow can be recorded from a high esophageal position, taking care to align the Doppler beam parallel to the inflow stream (Fig. 6–9). In some patients, a

TABLE 6–2	Selected Normal Parameters of Diastolic Function
Time Intervals	
IVRT	63 ± 11 ms
Derived Measures	
Tau	33 ± 6 ms
$-dP/dt$	2048 ± 335 mmHg/s
Filling Rates	
Peak filling rate	288 ± 66 ml/s
Peak filling rate normalized to LV-EDV	2.9 ± 1 s^{-1}
Atrial filling rate	229 ± 83 ml/s
Ratio of early to atrial velocity integral	1.71 ± 0.43
Velocities	
E/A ratio	1.32 ± 0.42
Deceleration slope	5 ± 1.4 m/s^2

References: Tebbe et al: Clin Cardiol 3:19, 1980; Shapiro and McKenna: Br Heart J 51:637, 1984; Pearson et al: Am Heart J 113:1417, 1987; Snider R et al: Am J Cardiol 56:921, 1985.

IVRT = Isovolumic relaxation time; dP/dt = rate of change in pressure over time; LV-EDV = left ventricular end-diastolic volume.

transgastric apical view also may allow recording of left ventricular inflow, although caution is needed to avoid foreshortening of the ventricle and a nonparallel intercept angle (with resultant underestimation of velocities) from this window.

Inflow velocities can be recorded with pulsed or continuous-wave Doppler modalities. With continuous-wave ultrasound, signals from the entire length of the ultrasound beam are recorded so that the maximal velocities—wherever they occur in relation to the mitral leaflet tips and annulus—are recorded. This lack of range resolution may lead to errors in calculation of volumetric flow rates in some individuals, since the site of cross-sectional area measurement may not correspond to the site of maximal velocity.

With pulsed Doppler ultrasound, the sample volume depth can be placed at the mitral annulus level or can be moved slowly along the length of the ultrasound beam to identify the site of maximal velocity, usually at the mitral leaflet tip level. The normal increase in velocities seen between the annulus and leaflet tips is consistent with some tapering of the flow-stream area, although there is marked individual variation. If volumetric flow rates will be calculated using the annulus diameter, velocities should be recorded at the annulus level. Conversely, many of the studies using velocity, time interval, or deceleration slope data to describe left ventricular filling patterns are based on maximal inflow velocities at the leaflet tips (without calculation of volumetric flow rates). Since even the pattern of inflow (e.g., E/A ratio), not just the absolute velocities, can vary between the annulus and leaflet tips, this inconsistency in methodology has led to a dilemma for the clinician echocardiographer. One approach is to record left ventricular inflow both at the annulus and leaflet tips in each patient so that volumetric flow rates can be calculated if indicated. Alternatively, if volumetric flow rates are not needed, recording left ventricular inflow at the leaflet tips may be adequate for patient management.

Optimal recordings of left ventricular inflow velocities are dependent on careful patient positioning and transducer angulation both to obtain a parallel intercept angle between the direction of flow and the ultrasound beam and to enhance the signal-to-noise ratio. Typically, with pulsed Doppler, a sample volume size of 5 mm is used with the velocity range adjusted to maximize the display of the velocity of interest. Wall filters are reduced (as allowed by signal quality) so that the velocities approach the baseline, allowing accurate time interval measurements. While normal left ventricular filling shows slight respiratory variation, care is needed to ensure that apparent velocity changes are not simply due to respiratory changes in the intercept angle between the ultrasound beam (which is held still) and the inflow stream (which moves with the heart during respiration).

Color Doppler flow imaging of left ventricular filling provides a spatial display of the flow pattern but is less useful for evaluation of left ventricular diastolic function. The normal pattern seen with color Doppler imaging is laminar inflow rapidly filling the ventricular chamber from base to apex, with flow predominantly along the posterior lateral wall. Inflow is associated with flow within the ventricle away from the transducer along the anteroseptal walls (often referred to as a *vortex*) in mid-diastole. Situations in which the normal color inflow pattern are disturbed include left ventricular systolic dysfunction (with lower velocity "puffs" of inflow and an abnormal apical flow pattern) and prosthetic mitral valves (with inflow along the anteromedial wall instead of the posterolateral wall).

Newer approaches to evaluation of diastolic function include color Doppler M-mode and Doppler tissue imaging techniques. Color Doppler M-mode recordings of left ventricular inflow from an apical approach can be used to measure the propagation velocity as blood moves from the annulus to the apex. The flow propagation velocity is decreased with restrictive ventricular filling and increased with constrictive pericarditis (see Suggested Reading 28). Doppler tissue imaging allows evaluation of regional wall motion in diastole with the pattern of diastolic wall velocities corresponding to the E and A filling velocities (see Suggested Reading 29).

TABLE 6–3	Diastolic Filling Diastolic Function: Factors That May Affect the Doppler Left Ventricular Filling Pattern

Technical
Sample volume location
Doppler modality
Intercept angle

Normal Variations
Respiration
Heart rate
Age
PR interval

Physiologic
Preload (LA pressure)
Volume flow rate (MR)
Left ventricular systolic function (LV-ESV)
Atrial contractile function
Diastolic "function"
Relaxation
Compliance/stiffness

LA = Left atrial; MR = mitral regurgitation; LV-ESV = left ventricular end-systolic volume.

Factors That Affect Doppler Left Ventricular Filling (Table 6–3)

Normal Variations

As previously discussed, there may be normal slight variation (<20%) in ventricular inflow velocities with respiration. In addition, the pattern of left ventricular inflow is affected by heart rate and the timing of atrial versus ventricular contraction. At higher heart rates, diastole is shorter—particularly the period of diastasis—so that the A velocity more closely succeeds the E velocity. When overlap of these two velocity curves occurs, the A velocity, in ef-

FIGURE 6–10. Schematic diagram showing the overlap or "summation" of A velocity with E velocity that occurs with higher heart rates.

fect, is "added" to the *E*-velocity curve, resulting in a higher *A* velocity and lower *E/A* ratio (Fig. 6–10). Similarly, a longer PR interval results in an *A* velocity earlier in diastole that may become superimposed on the *E*-velocity curve. At very high heart rates (short diastolic filling periods), the *E*- and *A*-velocity curves become merged into a single *E/A* velocity. Evaluation of a patient with complete heart block but intact atrial contraction often demonstrates this

nicely, with the location of the *A* velocity relative to the *E* velocity affecting its magnitude accordingly (Fig. 6–11).

Diastolic left ventricular inflow patterns also are affected by patient age (Table 6–4). In children and young adults, the majority of ventricular filling occurs in early diastole, with a prominent *E* velocity and only a small contribution to ventricular filling due to atrial contraction (20% of total left ventricular volume). With age, the *E*

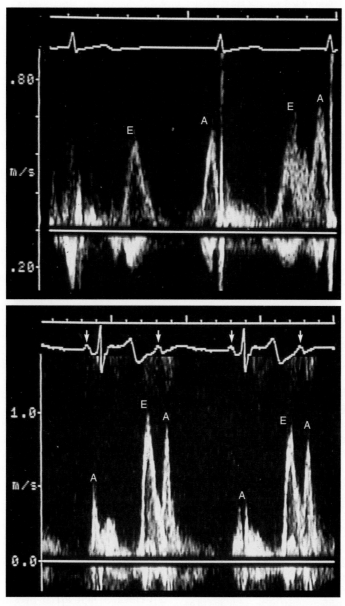

FIGURE 6–11. Left ventricular filling in a patient with an atrial arrhythmia *(top)* showing the effect of a shorter diastolic interval on the *E/A* pattern and in a patient with second-degree heart block showing two *a* waves for each diastole *(bottom)*.

TABLE 6–4	Effect of Aging on Parameters of Left Ventricular Diastolic Filling in Normal Subjects		
	Mean (95% CI)		
	Age 21–49 y*	Age >50 y*	Age >70 y†
E- velocity (m/s)	0.72 (0.44–1.00)	0.62 (0.34–0.90)	0.44 (0.25–0.76)
A- velocity (m/s)	0.40 (0.20–0.60)	0.59 (0.31–0.87)	59 (0.38–0.84)
E/A ratio	1.9 (0.7–3.1)	1.1 (0.5–1.7)	0.8 (0.5–1.2)
Deceleration time (ms)	179 (139–219)	210 (138–282)	140 (90–230)
IVRT (ms)	76 (54–98)	90 (56–124)	

CI = Confidence interval, IVRT = isovolumic relaxation time.

*Data from Cohen GI, Pietrolungo JF, Thomas JD, Klein AL: A practical guide to assessment of ventricular diastolic function using Doppler echocardiography. *J Am Coll Cardiol* 27:1753–1760, 1996. Normal reference values were derived from 61 subjects age 21 to 49 years and 56 subjects over age 50 years.

†Data from Sagie A, Benjamin EJ, Galdersisi M, et al: Reference values for Doppler indexes of left ventricular diastolic filling in the elderly. *J Am Soc Echocardiogr* 6:570–576, 1993.

References values were derived from 114 healthy elderly subjects in the Framingham Heart Study.

velocity diminishes, and the atrial contribution becomes more prominent, with equalization of *E* and *A* velocities at approximately age 60 years and reversal of the *E/A* ratio after that age in normal individuals. Early diastolic deceleration time also is progressively prolonged with age (Fig. 6–12). Presumably the mechanism of the changes in left ventricular filling patterns with age is a gradual reduction in the rate of early diastolic relaxation.

Physiologic Factors

Several physiologic variables other than left ventricular diastolic function also affect the pattern of left ventricular diastolic filling. While it is clear that Doppler velocity recordings accurately represent left ventricular filling patterns, it should be emphasized again that left ventricular *filling* is not equivalent to left ventricular *diastolic function*.

Left atrial pressure, *preload*, dramatically affects the pattern of left ventricular filling (Fig. 6–13). Increased preload results in an increase in the *E* velocity, a shortened IVRT, and steeper deceleration slope of early diastolic filling. As the left ventricle fills rapidly in early diastole, left ventricular diastolic pressure rises, so atrial contraction results in only a small pressure gradient between the left atrium and the left ventricle and a small *A* velocity. Examples of elevated preload include volume infusion or an elevated left atrial pressure due to elevation of left ventricular end-diastolic pressure.

Mitral regurgitation also results in an increase in *E* velocity both via the mechanism of an elevated left atrial pressure and because of the increased volume flow rate across the mitral valve. Again, the *A* velocity tends to be reduced (Fig. 6–14).

FIGURE 6–12. Schematic diagram showing the changes in left ventricular *(top)* and left atrial inflow and pulmonary venous flow *(bottom)* patterns that occur with age. The typical pattern seen in younger (age <50 years) subjects *(solid lines)* is compared with middle-aged *(dotted lines)* and older (age >70 years) subjects *(dashed lines)*.

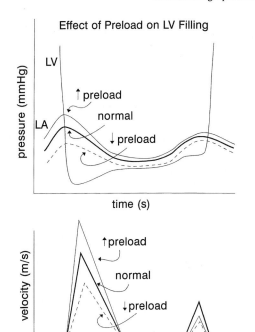

FIGURE 6–13. Effect of preload on left ventricular filling pattern. With increased preload, an increased pressure gradient from the left atrium to the left ventricle at the time of mitral valve opening results in a higher E velocity. The A velocity remains the same or is reduced if a high end-diastolic pressure results in a smaller left atrial to left ventricular pressure gradient following atrial contraction. The opposition changes occur with decreased preload.

Situations with a reduced left atrial pressure have a reduced E velocity due to a smaller gradient between the left atrium and left ventricle at mitral valve opening. Thus hypovolemia or use of a venodilator (such as nitroglycerin) results in a decrease in the E velocity. Reduced preload is unlikely to affect atrial contraction, so the A-velocity peak is either unaffected or enhanced if left ventricular diastolic pressure remains low at the time of atrial contraction.

Left ventricular systolic function affects the pattern of diastolic filling in that, for a given diastolic pressure-volume curve, an increased end-systolic volume results in a shift to a steeper portion of the pressure-volume curve. Diastolic filling then occurs with a greater increase in pressure for a given increase in volume. This results in an increased E velocity and reduced A velocity, similar to the pattern seen with decreased compliance due to a shift to a different diastolic pressure-volume curve (see Fig. 6–4).

Atrial contractile function, although not always recognized clinically, can affect the pattern of left ventricular diastolic filling. This is obvious in the case of atrial fibrillation, when no atrial contribution to ventricular filling is seen (Fig. 6–15), or with atrial flutter, when small "flutter" waves in the inflow velocity pattern may be noted, but is less obvious in sinus rhythm with ineffective atrial contraction, which may result in a small A velocity.

Despite the potential influence of all these factors on the pattern of left ventricular diastolic filling, the Doppler velocity data still can provide useful information on diastolic dysfunction if carefully interpreted. The two parameters of diastolic function that are most readily evaluated with Doppler velocity data are ventricular relaxation and ventricular compliance.

FIGURE 6–14. Left ventricular inflow in a patient with severe mitral regurgitation showing a high E velocity due to increased volume flow across the mitral valve and an increased left atrial pressure.

FIGURE 6–15. Left ventricular inflow in a patient with atrial fibrillation shows a single velocity peak and no A velocity.

FIGURE 6–16. Left ventricular inflow in a patient with amyloidosis showing a pattern consistent with impaired relaxation.

Left Ventricular Relaxation

Impaired ventricular relaxation results in the classic pattern of diastolic dysfunction with impaired early diastolic filling and an increased atrial contribution to total left ventricular filling (Fig. 6–16). Impaired relaxation is associated with a reduced *E* velocity, a lengthened IVRT, a prolonged early diastolic deceleration time, and an *E/A* ratio <1 (see Fig. 6–3).

Left Ventricular Compliance

Abnormal ventricular compliance results in rapid early diastolic filling following mitral valve opening with a short IVRT and rapid acceleration time. As the ventricle fills, left ventricular diastolic pressure rises rapidly, so a high *E* velocity is followed by a steep deceleration slope. The atrial contribution to filling is relatively small, since LV-EDP is elevated with only a small left atrial to ventricular pressure gradient following atrial contraction (see Fig. 6–4).

In the clinical setting, evaluation of diastolic ventricular function is complicated by the coexistence of more than one of the factors that affect diastolic filling. For example, patients with reduced compliance also may have an elevated preload. Thus an elderly patient with reduced compliance may have a pattern of left ventricular filling similar to a younger patient with normal diastolic function (a pattern referred to as *pseudonormalization*). A patient with impaired relaxation may have coexisting mitral regurgitation. As these examples illustrate, sorting out the relative contribution of diastolic dysfunction from other physiologic parameters can be difficult in an individual patient. Furthermore, the factors that affect diastolic filling are not independent. A change in one physiologic parameter (such as left atrial pressure) may affect other parameters (such as atrial compliance and left ventricular contractility). The interdependence of these physiologic parameters complicates not only our ability to evaluate individual patients but also our understanding of the physiology of diastolic filling. Elegant in vitro studies by Thomas and colleagues provide insight into the interdependence of these relationships (see Suggested Reading 5).

RIGHT VENTRICULAR DIASTOLIC FUNCTION

Right Ventricular Filling

The pattern of right ventricular diastolic filling is similar to left ventricular diastolic filling except that maximal velocities are lower (because the tricuspid annulus is larger) and the diastolic filling period is slightly shorter. Although few studies have addressed right ventricular diastolic filling, the same measurements described for left ventricular diastolic filling are applicable.

Doppler Data Recording

On transthoracic echocardiography, right ventricular inflow can be recorded from the parasternal right ventricular inflow view or from the apical four-chamber view (Fig. 6–17). Either pulsed or continuous-wave ultrasound can be used with the same technical considerations as apply to recording left ventricular inflow velocities. Again, evaluation of respiratory

FIGURE 6–17. Doppler right ventricular inflow shows an *E* velocity and *A* velocity similar to left ventricular inflow.

variation on inflow velocities is complicated by the respiratory motion of the heart, so care must be taken to ensure a parallel intercept angle between the ultrasound beam and inflow stream throughout the respiratory cycle. This can be accomplished in most patients by using a window where 2D echo shows little respiratory variation in the image plane itself or in the Doppler beam orientation relative to the 2D image.

Physiologic Factors That Affect Right Ventricular Filling

Right ventricular filling appears to be affected by all the same physiologic parameters that affect left ventricular filling, although less attention has been directed toward right ventricular inflow patterns. Again, the major differences between right ventricular and left ventricular filling are (1) timing, (2) reciprocal respiratory variation (as described earlier), and (3) absolute velocities, which are lower for right ventricular inflow because the tricuspid annulus is larger than the mitral annulus.

LEFT ATRIAL FILLING

Doppler Assessment

Left atrial filling is evaluated by Doppler recordings of pulmonary vein flow either from a transesophageal or a transthoracic approach. Again, the Doppler pattern of velocities parallels the normal filling curves, with inflow into the left atrium occurring in two phases, systolic and diastolic. In addition, there is flow deceleration following ventricular contraction and a

small reversal of flow after atrial contraction (Fig. 6–18). On transesophageal recordings, the systolic inflow pattern is biphasic in most patients, with an early systolic peak related to atrial relaxation and a second late systolic peak related to displacement of the mitral annulus toward the left ventricular apex. Respiratory variation in flow may be seen in left-heart filling patterns (atrial and ventricular) but is less prominent than the variation seen in right-heart filling *and* is directionally opposite: left-heart filling diminishes slightly with inspiration. Both the pulmonary veins and the left atrium are intrathoracic in their entirety, so negative intrathoracic pressure does not result in a pressure gradient between them. Instead, atrial filling may diminish during inspiration as blood "pools" briefly in the expanded pulmonary veins, which then empty during expiration.

Doppler Data Recording

From a transesophageal approach, left atrial inflow patterns can be easily recorded in each of the four pulmonary veins in the transverse plane. Careful positioning and angulation are needed to ensure that the pulsed Doppler sample volume is located in the pulmonary vein itself rather than in the adjacent left atrium. A sample volume size of 5 mm typically is used with wall filters lowered to show the low-velocity components associated with atrial and ventricular contraction. The flow pattern varies somewhat with distance from the pulmonary vein orifice. A distance of 0.5 to 1 cm from the orifice provides optimal signal strength with the most consistent inflow pattern.

The left superior pulmonary vein is most easily visualized adjacent to the left atrial appendage, directed somewhat anteriorly. The left inferior pulmonary vein can be visualized by advancing the transducer a short distance to see the inflow pattern from this horizontally directed vein. The right pulmonary veins can be imaged by turning the transducer medially to identify the superior right pulmonary vein (again anteriorly directed) and advancing the probe slightly to image the horizontally positioned right inferior pulmonary vein (Fig. 6–19).

From a transthoracic approach, recording pulmonary venous flow patterns is more challenging. Most echocardiographers use the apical four-chamber view, which allows a parallel alignment between the right superior pulmonary vein flowstream and the ultrasound beam. Signal strength may be a limiting factor at this depth of interrogation (typically about 14 cm), so careful attention to sample volume

FIGURE 6–18. Normal pattern of left atrial inflow recorded in the right superior pulmonary vein from a transthoracic apical four-chamber view. Note the systolic *(S)* and diastolic *(D)* filling phases with a slight flow reversal following atrial contraction *(A)*.

FIGURE 6–19. Normal pattern of left atrial inflow recorded in the left superior pulmonary vein from a transesophageal approach.

TABLE 6–5	Factors That Affect Left Atrial Filling Patterns

Systolic Atrial Filling
Age
Left atrial size
Left atrial pressure
Atrial contractile function

Diastolic Atrial Filling
Gradient from pulmonary veins to left ventricle
Left ventricular diastolic relaxation
Left atrial compliance
Left ventricular compliance

Reversal Following Atrial Contraction
Atrial contraction function
Left atrial compliance
Left ventricular compliance
Cardiac rhythm

position, wall filters, and gain settings is needed to optimize the velocity data. Sample volume positioning may be facilitated by the use of color flow imaging to identify the flowstream from the pulmonary vein into the left atrium. Again, the sample volume should be positioned *in* the pulmonary vein within 0.5 to 1 cm of the orifice. Of note, the biphasic pattern of systolic inflow and atrial reversal may be more difficult to demonstrate on transthoracic compared with transesophageal imaging due to a lower signal-to-noise ratio. In addition, the flow pattern in the left upper pulmonary vein (on trans-esophageal echocardiography) shows a more laminar flow pattern than the right upper pulmonary vein (on transesophageal or transtho-racic echocardiography). Alternate transtho-racic windows that may allow recording of pulmonary vein flow in some individuals include subcostal and parasternal short-axis views at the aortic valve level or suprasternal notch views of the left atrium and pulmonary veins. However, intercept angle tends to be sub-optimal from these windows.

Physiologic Factors That Affect Left Atrial Filling (Table 6–5)

Left atrial filling is affected by many of the same variables that affect left ventricular dias-tolic filling. Higher heart rates result in merging of the systolic and diastolic phases of left atrial filling, while lower heart rates result in clearer separation between them. Changes in left atrial inflow with aging have been described, includ-ing a reduction in the diastolic filling phase, a compensatory increase in the systolic filling phase, and a more prominent atrial reversal in subjects older than age 50 (see Fig. 6–12).

Since, during diastole, the flowstream is con-tinuous from the pulmonary veins to the left ventricle, the diastolic flow pattern is affected mostly by the pressure gradient from the pul-monary veins to the left ventricle, left ventricu-lar relaxation, and left atrial and left ventricu-lar compliance.

The systolic phase of atrial filling is most af-fected by left atrial size, pressure, compliance, and atrial contractile function.

Atrial reversal is dependent on left atrial contraction/relaxation, left atrial and left ven-tricular compliance, and cardiac rhythm. In-creases in preload will augment the diastolic filling phase by augmenting the pressure gradi-ent along this flowstream.

With impaired left ventricular relaxation, the pulmonary venous pattern is expected to show a prominent atrial reversal and blunting of the diastolic filling phase corresponding to the low E/A ratio seen on the left ventricular in-flow pattern.

With reduced left ventricular compliance, the pulmonary venous flow pattern is expected to show prominent diastolic inflow. Atrial re-versal is prominent as well, since a high left ventricular diastolic pressure reduces late dias-tolic left ventricular filling so that atrial con-traction results in reversal of flow in the pul-monary veins.

Note that these pulmonary venous flow pat-terns allow differentiation of a high E/A ratio with normal diastolic function (normal pul-monary venous flow pattern) from a high E/A ratio due to "pseudonormalization" with re-duced ventricular compliance (pulmonary ve-nous flow pattern with prominent diastolic phase and atrial flow reversal). For example, a left ventricular filling pattern characterized by a high E and low A velocity in association with a normal pulmonary vein flow pattern is consistent with normal left ventricular diastolic function. Conversely, the same left ventricular filling pattern in association with a pulmonary venous flow pattern showing an increased atrial reversal and decreased ratio of systolic to diastolic antegrade flow suggests impaired ventricular compliance.

RIGHT ATRIAL FILLING

Doppler Assessment

Right Atrial Filling Curves

Doppler velocity curves of right atrial filling can be recorded in the superior vena cava (from a suprasternal notch approach) or the central hepatic vein (from a subcostal approach), since these central veins empty directly into the right atrium without intervening venous valves. The pattern of right atrial filling recorded by Doppler parallels the jugular venous pressure curves seen clinically (Fig. 6–20). However, the Doppler data represent a more reliable approach, since evaluation of jugular venous patterns is difficult in some patients due to body habitus and interpretation is subjective (with no recorded data).

Again, right atrial filling patterns show respiratory variation in normal individuals with augmentation of right atrial inflow during inspiration, as is seen in the right ventricular inflow pattern. A plausible explanation for these observations is that the negative intrathoracic pressure with voluntary inspiration (but not with mechanical ventilation) results in an extrathoracic to intrathoracic pressure gradient

FIGURE 6–20. Normal pattern of right atrial inflow recorded in the central hepatic vein from a subcostal approach. Again, systolic *(S)* and diastolic *(D)* antegrade filling with slight flow reversal following atrial *(A)* contraction is seen.

from the great veins into the right atrium, leading to increased blood flow into the right side of the heart.

Right Atrial Pressure

Right atrial pressure can be estimated by echocardiographic evaluation (from the subcostal window) of the inferior vena cava as it enters the right atrium (see Table 5–8). First, the *size* of the inferior vena cava reflects the intraluminal volume, resulting in dilation with elevated right atrial pressures and a reduction in size with low atrial pressures. Second, the segment of the thin-wall vessel immediately adjacent to the atrium responds to the changes in right atrial pressure and volume that are seen with the normal changes in intrathoracic pressure with spontaneous respiration. As the right atrium fills more rapidly during inspiration, the inferior vena cava partially "collapses" due to flow from the inferior vena cava into the right atrium when inferior vena cava and right atrial pressures are low. Thus a low right atrial pressure (0 to 5 mmHg) is present when the inferior vena cava is small (<1.5 cm diameter) with respiratory "collapse" to >50% of the original diameter. Right atrial pressure is normal (5 to 10 mmHg) when the inferior vena cava size is normal (1.5 to 2.5 cm diameter) with <50% collapse of the proximal segment with normal respiration (or a "sniff"). When inferior vena cava size is normal but respiratory collapse is <50%, estimated right atrial pressure is 10 to 15 mmHg. Elevated right atrial pressure (15 to 20 mmHg) is manifested by inferior vena cava dilation with little respiratory variation. More severe elevations in right atrial pressure (>20 mmHg) tend to be associated with dilation of the hepatic veins as well. The validity of this approach to right atrial pressure estimation has been well established, with reported sensitivities and specificities of 87% and 82%, respectively, for detection of elevated right atrial pressures (>10 mmHg). Of course, this approach is not valid in patients supported by mechanical ventilation, since the changes in intrathoracic pressure are not physiologic in this situation.

Doppler Data Recording

Right atrial filling is most often evaluated from the subcostal window. After the long-axis view of the inferior vena cava is obtained, the transducer is rotated and angulated to visualize the central hepatic vein, which tends to be directed toward the transducer in this view, allowing a parallel intercept angle between the pulsed Doppler beam and hepatic vein flow.

Hepatic vein flow is assumed to be representative of inferior vena caval flow, since both enter into the right atrium without intervening venous valves. Direct study of inferior vena caval flow is limited by a nearly perpendicular intercept angle.

Right atrial inflow also can be recorded in the superior vena cava from the suprasternal notch window. From the standard aortic arch view, the transducer is angulated toward the patient's right to visualize the superior vena cava adjacent and slightly anterior to the ascending aorta. The pulsed Doppler sample volume is positioned in the superior vena cava, with adjustment of transducer angle and sample volume depth to obtain a well-defined velocity curve. As for other inflow patterns, wall filters are minimized (as allowed by signal-to-noise ratio) to demonstrate the low-velocity flows associated with atrial filling.

Limitations

From both the superior vena cava and hepatic vein recordings it is important to distinguish respiratory variation in the Doppler curves due to (1) respiratory variation in the angle between the ultrasound beam and blood flow direction from (2) true variations in atrial filling volumes. The hepatic vein is small, so several positions often need to be tried to find one that maintains the sample volume in the hepatic vein throughout the respiratory cycle.

The physiologic factors that affect left atrial filling also affect right atrial filling, although (as for ventricular filling) less attention has been focused on physiologic parameters affecting the right side of the heart. Respiratory variation in right atrial filling typically is much more prominent than the respiratory variation seen in left atrial filling.

CLINICAL UTILITY

The four major disease categories that affect left ventricular diastolic function are secondary hypertrophy, cardiomyopathies, ischemic cardiac diseases, and pericardial disease. These categories include examples of diastolic dysfunction per se, including (1) abnormal relaxation, (2) reduced compliance, and (3) pericardial restraint, as well as the confounding effects of other physiologic variables on the pattern of left ventricular filling.

Left Ventricular Hypertrophy

The "classic" pattern of left ventricular diastolic dysfunction is seen with left ventricular hypertrophy due to hypertension or to valvular aortic stenosis. The predominant abnormality is impaired relaxation, resulting in a pattern of reduced early diastolic filling and an enhanced atrial contribution to filling. The Doppler velocity curve typically shows a prolonged IVRT, reduced acceleration to a reduced E velocity, prolonged early diastolic deceleration slope, an increased A velocity, and an E/A ratio <1. When left ventricular systolic dysfunction supervenes, the elevated LV-EDP and elevated left atrial pressure may result in "pseudonormalization" of this pattern with an enhanced E velocity (related to a higher mitral valve opening gradient) and reduced A velocity (due to the elevated left ventricular end-diastolic pressure). Coexisting mitral regurgitation also can lead to a "paradoxical" higher E velocity despite impaired ventricular relaxation.

Cardiomyopathy

Patients with hypertrophic cardiomyopathy often have a pattern of left ventricular diastolic filling consistent with impaired relaxation. Some studies have suggested that Doppler evaluation of left ventricular diastolic filling can be used to assess the effects of medical therapy (e.g., beta blockers or calcium channel blockers) on diastolic function in this disease.

A variety of diastolic filling patterns can be seen in patients with dilated cardiomyopathy (see Chapter 8). Preliminary evidence suggests that differences in diastolic function may explain differences in clinical symptoms between patients with similar degrees of systolic dysfunction. When systolic dysfunction is present, the elevated end-systolic volume results in a shift along the pressure-volume curve to a steeper segment. This means that for a given diastolic pressure-volume relationship, compliance is reduced at higher left ventricular volumes (see Fig. 6–4). Thus the expected pattern of diastolic filling in dilated cardiomyopathy is that of reduced compliance: a high E velocity, rapid deceleration slope, low A velocity, and an E/A ratio >1. Keeping in mind that E velocity and E/A ratio usually decrease with age, the finding of a "normal" left ventricular filling pattern in a patient older than 50 years should raise the question of abnormal ventricular compliance.

In cardiac amyloidosis, a specific example of restrictive cardiomyopathy, the patterns of left ventricular diastolic filling and the change in these patterns during the disease course are particularly instructive. With amyloid infiltration of the myocardium, the first change is impaired relaxation, resulting in the classic pattern of diastolic dysfunction with a reduced E velocity and increased A velocity. As the disease progresses, compliance also becomes abnormal, resulting in a shift from $E/A <1$ to an $E/A >1$, with all the other findings of reduced compliance. This "pseudonormalized" pattern can be distinguished from normal (if the patient is seen at only one point in the disease course) by the pattern of pulmonary venous inflow, which shows a diastolic component greater than the systolic component with an enhanced atrial reversal. To some extent, this description oversimplifies the changes seen in amyloid heart disease, since concurrent changes in left ventricular systolic function, the degree of mitral regurgitation, and left atrial filling pressures also occur, all of which affect the pattern of left ventricular diastolic filling. However, it does serve as a useful framework for understanding the complex changes that occur with diastolic dysfunction.

Pericardial Disease

With both pericardial tamponade and pericardial constriction, cardiac filling is impaired by pericardial "restraint." In the case of tamponade physiology, filling is impaired in both early and late diastole, with an accentuation of the normal variation seen in right and left ventricular filling with respiration. With constrictive pericarditis, early diastolic filling tends to be normal, with marked impairment of filling late in diastole when the heart has expanded to the maximum allowed by the fibrotic pericardial encasement. Both these conditions are discussed in more detail in Chapter 9.

Ischemic Cardiac Disease

In patients with coronary artery disease and no prior myocardial infarction, induction of ischemia results in diastolic dysfunction prior to systolic dysfunction (see Chapter 7). Diastolic filling curves with ischemia induced by balloon inflation during percutaneous transluminal angioplasty show rapid onset of a reduced E velocity, with resolution of these changes as ischemia is relieved. In acute myocardial infarction, a pattern of delayed relaxation is seen acutely. At follow-up, one of several patterns of left ventricular filling may be observed. (1) With successful reperfusion and little myocardial damage, left ventricular diastolic filling returns to normal. (2) With an infarction but preserved left ventricular systolic function, the pattern of impaired relaxation often persists. (3) With a large infarction and significant left ventricular systolic dysfunction, the "pseudo-normalized" pattern of a high E velocity and low A velocity due to a combination of reduced compliance, a high LV-EDP, and a shift along the diastolic pressure volume curve (increased end-systolic volume) can be seen. Thus an apparent "normal" pattern of left ventricular filling late after myocardial infarction may be due to normal left ventricular diastolic and systolic function or to impaired diastolic and systolic function. As for cardiomyopathy patients, these two groups can be distinguished by a higher E/A ratio, shorter IVRT, and steeper deceleration slope than normal and by the pattern of pulmonary venous flow.

Noninvasive Estimates of Left Ventricular Diastolic Pressure

Accurate noninvasive assessment of left atrial pressure (which usually is equivalent to LV-EDP) has been an elusive goal, but several promising approaches to this problem have been proposed. One approach is to use the end-diastolic velocity of the aortic regurgitant velocity curve, recorded with continuous-wave Doppler, to calculate the end-diastolic pressure gradient between the aorta and left ventricle using the Bernoulli equation. Diastolic blood pressure then is subtracted from this pressure gradient to obtain LV-EDP. For example, if the end-diastolic aortic regurgitant velocity is 3.9 m/s, then the aortic to left ventricular gradient is $4(3.9)^2$ or 61 mmHg. With a diastolic blood pressure of 72 mmHg, LV-EDP would be $(72 -61) = 11$ mmHg. While conceptually sound, this approach is limited by (1) the need for a recordable aortic regurgitant jet, (2) dependence on an accurate cuff diastolic blood pressure measurement, and (3) derivation of a small number (LV-EDP) from two larger numbers, so small errors in either measured variable lead to large errors in the calculated result.

Another proposed approach is based on the pattern of pulmonary venous inflow. The ratio of flow in systole relative to total flow is inversely related to the LV-EDP. The higher the LV-EDP, the lower is the contribution of systolic filling to total pulmonary venous flow (i.e., "blunting" of the systolic flow signal). Using velocity-time integrals (VTI), a ratio of the systolic VTI to total left atrial-filling VTI that is greater than 55% is predictive of a left atrial pressure greater than or equal to 15 mmHg with a sensitivity of 91% and a specificity of 87% (see Suggested Reading 15).

A more complicated approach is based on the pattern of left ventricular diastolic filling.

The variables most closely correlated with LV-EDP are the IVRT, deceleration rate of early left ventricular filling, and the atrial filling fraction. Regression equations incorporating these measures plus the pulmonary venous systolic fraction have been proposed (see Suggested Readings 16 and 17). Further evaluation of these methods is needed to verify their accuracy in the clinical setting.

ALTERNATE APPROACHES TO EVALUATION OF DIASTOLIC DYSFUNCTION

Despite the numerous potential shortcomings of Doppler echocardiographic evaluation of diastolic filling, it has great promise as a repeatable, noninvasive, widely available method for evaluation of diastolic function. Techniques used in the research laboratory (time constant of relaxation, pressure-volume curves, etc.) rarely are applicable to clinical patient management. The other available clinical modalities for evaluation of diastolic function include

1. Direct intracardiac pressure measurements
2. Contrast angiographic filling curves based on frame-by-frame volume calculations
3. Radionuclide high-resolution time-activity curves

SUGGESTED READING

Reviews

1. Smith, MD: Left ventricular diastolic function: Clinical utility of Doppler echocardiography. *In* Otto CM (ed): The Practice of Clinical Echocardiography. Philadelphia, WB Saunders, 1997, pp 49–74.
   Advanced discussion of the principles and applications of Doppler evaluation of diastolic function in clinical practice. Includes tables of normal values, case examples, literature review, and 147 references.

2. Bonow RO, Udelson JE: Left ventricular diastolic dysfunction as a cause of congestive heart failure: Mechanisms and management. *Ann Intern Med* 117:502–510, 1992.
   Review of mechanisms of diastolic dysfunction and the effects of physiologic changes (heart rate, loading conditions) and aging on diastolic filling. The diagnosis and management of heart failure due to diastolic dysfunction are also reviewed. 85 references.

3. Nishimura RA, Tajik AJ: Evaluation of diastolic filling the left ventricle in health and disease: Doppler echocardiography is the clinician's Rosetta stone. *J Am Coll Cardiol* 30:8–18, 1997.
   Review emphasizing the Doppler evaluation of diastolic function with examples of venous inflow patterns, as well as ventricular inflow patterns, in normal and abnormal subjects. 93 references.

4. Cohen GI, Pietrolungo JF, Thomas JD, Klein AL: A practical guide to assessment of ventricular diastolic function using Doppler echocardiography. *J Am Coll Cardiol* 27:1753–1760, 1996.
   An excellent and concise review of standard Doppler measurements, patterns of diastolic function, and future directions in Doppler assessment of diastolic function. 77 references.

Physiologic Principles and Measurement of Ventricular Filling

5. Thomas JD, Weyman AE: Echocardiographic Doppler evaluation of left ventricular diastolic function: Physics and physiology. *Circulation* 84:977–990, 1991.
   Detailed mathematical approach to left ventricular diastolic filling with clear diagrams showing the effects of changes in specific parameters on the pattern of diastolic filling.

6. Spirito P, Maron BJ, Bonow RO: Noninvasive assessment of left ventricular diastolic function: Comparative analysis of Doppler echocardiographic and radionuclide angiographic techniques. *J Am Coll Cardiol* 7:518–526, 1986.
   Comparison of Doppler and radionuclide angiographic evaluation of diastolic filling in 12 normal subjects and 25 patients with cardiac disease. Good correlations were noted between Doppler and radionuclide measures of the ratio of early to late diastolic filling (r = 0.76), the time interval from end-systole to end of early rapid filling (r = 0.83), and the slope of the early flow velocity peak versus peak filling rate (r = 0.79).

7. Rokey R, Kuo LC, Zoghbi WA, et al: Determination of parameters of left ventricular diastolic filling with pulsed Doppler echocardiography: Comparison with cineangiography. *Circulation* 71:543-550, 1985.
   Comparison of Doppler and cineangiographic measures of left ventricular diastolic filling in 30 patients showed that the Doppler curve resembles the first derivative of the angiographic volume curve. Doppler and angiographic peak filling rate (r = 0.87) and normalized peak filling rate (r = 0. 83) correlated well.

8. Nishimura RA, Schwartz RS, Tajik AJ, Holmes DR: Noninvasive measurement of rate of left ventricular relaxation by Doppler echocardiography: Validation with simultaneous cardiac catheterization. *Circulation* 88:146–155, 1993.
   The time constant of left ventricular relaxation (tau) can be calculated from the Doppler mitral regurgitant velocity signal using a semilogarithmic method with a zero asymptote, after conversion of velocities to pressures, using the Bernoulli equation. However, this approach requires knowledge of left atrial pressure and has only limited accuracy for detection of changes in tau in an individual patient.

9. Chen C, Rodriguez L, Lethor JP, et al: Continuous wave Doppler echocardiography for non-invasive assessment of left ventricular dP/dt and relaxation time constant from mitral regurgitant spectra in patients. *J Am Coll Cardiol* 23:970–976, 1994.
   In 12 patients with mitral regurgitation, Doppler-derived measures correlated well with invasive data for

maximum +dP/dt *(r = 0.91), maximum −dP/dt (r = 0.89), and tau (r = 0.93).*

10. Berk MR, Xie G, Kwan OL, et al: Reduction of left ventricular preload by lower body negative pressure alters Doppler transmitral filling patterns. *J Am Coll Cardiol* 16:1387–1392, 1990.

    To avoid confounding effects of pharmacologic intervention, preload was reduced by lower body negative pressure. Decreased preload resulted in a reduced E velocity, no change in A velocity, a reduced E/A ratio, and a reduction in mean acceleration and deceleration with a corresponding prolongation of the pressure half-time.

11. Stoddard MF, Pearson AC, Kern MJ, et al: Influence of alteration in preload on the pattern of left ventricular diastolic filling as assessed by Doppler echocardiography in humans. *Circulation* 79:1226–1236, 1989.

    Preload reduction with nitroglycerin in 50 patients resulted in a reduced left ventricular end-diastolic pressure, peak early filling velocity, and E/A ratio. Relaxation and chamber stiffness were unchanged. The importance of preload in the Doppler patterns of left ventricular diastolic filling is emphasized.

12. Thomas JD, Choong CYP, Flachskampf FA, Weyman AE: Analysis of the early transmitral Doppler velocity curve: Effect of primary physiologic changes and compensatory preload adjustment. *J Am Coll Cardiol* 16:644–655, 1990.

    Elegant description of early diastolic filling with mathematical explanations (for the mathematically inclined) and clear diagrams showing the effects of changes in each parameter (for the rest of us).

13. Harrison MR, Clifton GD, Pennell AT, DeMaria AN: Effect of heart rate on left ventricular diastolic transmitral flow velocity patterns assessed by Doppler echocardiography in normal subjects. *Am J Cardiol* 67:622–627, 1991.

    In 20 adult volunteers, heart rate was varied by transesophageal atrial pacing. Although E velocity was unchanged, A velocity increased from 0.37 ± 0.06 m/s at a heart rate of 70 bpm to 0.50 ± 0.07 m/s at a heart rate of 88 bpm (P<0.003), demonstrating the significant effects of minor changes in heart rate on left ventricular filling.

Evaluation of Atrial Filling Parameters

14. Castello R, Pearson AC, Lenzen P, Labovitz AJ: Evaluation of pulmonary venous flow by transesophageal echocardiography in subjects with a normal heart: Comparison with transthoracic echocardiography. *J Am Coll Cardiol* 18:65–71, 1991.

    Pulmonary venous flow consists of four phases: two antegrade flows in systole (due to atrial relaxation and ventricular contraction), antegrade flow in diastole, and flow reversal during atrial contraction. Flows are more clearly demonstrated on TEE, particularly in the left superior pulmonary vein at a depth of 0.5 to 1 cm from entry into the left atrium.

15. Kuecherer HF, Muhiudeen IA, Kusumoto FM, et al: Estimation of mean left atrial pressure from transesophageal pulsed Doppler echocardiography of pulmonary venous flow. *Circulation* 82:1127–1139, 1990.

    In 47 patients undergoing cardiovascular surgery, the systolic fraction of pulmonary venous inflow correlated with mean left atrial pressure (r = −0.88). A systolic fraction <55% had a sensitivity of 91% and a specificity of 87% for detection of a left atrial pressure ≥15 mmHg.

16. Mulvagh S, Quinones MA, Kleiman NS, et al: Estimation of left ventricular end-diastolic pressure from Doppler transmitral flow velocity in cardiac patients independent of systolic performance. *J Am Coll Cardiol* 20:112–119, 1992.

    A combined approach to estimates of left ventricular end-diastolic pressure (LV-EDP) is proposed: LV-EDP = 46 − (0.22IVRT) − (0.10AFF) − (0.03DT) − (2 + E/A) + (0.05MAR) where IVRT = isovolumic relaxation time, in ms, AFF = atrial filling fraction, DT = deceleration time, E/A = E to A velocity ratio, and MAR = time from end of mitral flow to R wave. In the test group, this equation was 90% sensitive and specific for detection of an LV-EDP > 15 mmHg.

17. Pozzoli M, Capamolla S, Pinna G, et al: Doppler echocardiography reliably predicts pulmonary artery wedge pressure in patients with chronic heart failure with and without mitral regurgitation. *J Am Coll Cardiol* 27:883–893, 1996.

    Simultaneous right heart catheterization and Doppler studies were performed in 231 patients with chronic heart failure. Pulmonary wedge pressure correlated most closely with the deceleration rate of early mitral filling and the systolic fraction of pulmonary venous flow. Regression equations for noninvasive calculation of pulmonary wedge pressure are proposed.

18. Marino P, Prioli AM, Destro G, et al: The left atrial volume curve can be assessed from pulmonary vein and mitral valve velocity tracings. *Am Heart J* 127:886–898, 1994.

    A novel approach to derivation of the left atrial volume curve from the instantaneous transmitral volume flow rate (annular area × mitral velocity) and the right upper pulmonary vein flow curve is described. Left atrial volumes by 2D echocardiography correlated well with Doppler derived volume (r − 0.95, SEE − 11.9 ml).

19. Hofmann T, Keck A, van Ingen G, et al: Simultaneous measurement of pulmonary venous flow by intravascular catheter Doppler velocimetry and transesophageal Doppler echocardiography: Relation to left atrial pressure and left atrial and ventricular function. *J Am Coll Cardiol* 26:239–49, 1995.

    In 32 patients undergoing open heart surgery, simultaneous measurement of left atrial pressure, pulmonary venous flow velocity by Doppler catheter, and transesophageal recording of pulmonary venous flow demonstrate close agreement between Doppler catheter and velocity data. Left atrium pressure correlated with the ratio of systolic to diastolic peak velocity, the systolic velocity-time integral, the time to maximal flow velocity, and the ratio of systolic to diastolic flow duration.

20. Nishimura RA, Appleton CP, Redfield MM, et al: Noninvasive Doppler echocardiographic evaluation of left ventricular filling pressures in patients with cardiomy-

opathies: A simultaneous Doppler echocardiographic and cardiac catheterization study. *J Am Coll Cardiol* 28:1226–1233, 1996.

In patients with systolic left ventricular dysfunction, left atrial pressure correlated directly with the E/A ratio, and inversely with the early diastolic deceleration time. In contrast, correlation was poor in patients with hypertrophic cardiomyopathy due to multiple other factors affecting diastolic filling in these patients.

21. Kircher BJ, Himelman RB, Schiller NB: Noninvasive estimation of right atrial pressure from the inspiratory collapse of the inferior vena cava. *Am J Cardiol* 66:493–496, 1990.

The inferior vena cava size and respiratory motion are related to right atrial pressure such that a 50% respiratory collapse in inferior vena cava diameter has a sensitivity of 87% and specificity of 82% for detection of a right atrial pressure <10 mmHg.

Clinical Outcome Studies

22. Vanoverschelde JLJ, Essamri G, Michel X, et al: Hemodynamic and volume correlates of left ventricular diastolic relaxation and filling in patients with aortic stenosis. *J Am Coll Cardiol* 20:813–821, 1992.

Doppler measures of left ventricular diastolic filling were used, in conjunction with invasive measures of right and left heart pressures, to evaluate the parameters of diastolic function in 17 patients with isolated severe aortic stenosis. Patients with normal systolic function had evidence of impaired relaxation with an increased atrial contribution to diastolic filling (reduced E- velocity, increased A- velocity). In contrast, those with systolic dysfunction had rapid early diastolic filling with a reduced atrial contribution. These distinct filling patterns were largely attributable to differences in left atrial pressure.

23. Appleton CP, Hatle LK, Popp RL: Demonstration of restrictive ventricular physiology by Doppler echocardiography. *J Am Coll Cardiol* 11:757–768, 1988.

In 14 patients with a clinical diagnosis of restrictive cardiomyopathy, the pattern of left ventricular diastolic filling was characterized by a shortened deceleration time and a reduced A velocity. The venous inflow pattern (superior vena cava, hepatic vein) showed reduced systolic inflow and a prominent atrial reversal.

24. Poulsen SH, Jensen SE, Botzsche O, Egstrup K: Evaluation and prognostic significance of left ventricular diastolic function assessed by Doppler echocardiography in the early phase of a first acute myocardial infarction. *Eur Heart J* 18:1882–1889, 1997.

*In 65 patients with acute myocardial infarction, on univariate analysis both ejection fraction and parameters of diastolic function were predictors of the development of congestive heart failure. However, on multi-*variate analysis only the Doppler mitral early diastolic deceleration slope was a significant independent predictor of heart failure in the first week after myocardial infarction.*

25. Johannessen K-A, Cerqueira MD, Stratton JR: Influence of myocardial infarction size on radionuclide and Doppler echocardiographic measurements of diastolic function. *Am J Cardiol* 65:692–697, 1990.

In 83 patients studied 8 to 12 weeks after acute myocardial infarction, infarct size measured by thallium-201 tomography was inversely correlated with peak A velocity and directly correlated with peak E velocity, deceleration slope, and E/A ratio.

26. Xie GY, Berk MR, Smith MD, DeMaria AN: Relation of Doppler transmitral flow patterns to functional status in congestive heart failure. *Am Heart J* 131:766–771, 1996.

In a series of 60 consecutive patients with congestive heart failure and an ejection fraction <40%, a restrictive pattern of left ventricular diastolic filling was predictive of more severe clinical symptoms and impaired exercise tolerance.

27. Pinamonti B, Zecchin M, Di Leanarda A, et al: Persistence of restrictive left ventricular filling pattern in dilated cardiomyopathy: An ominous prognostic sign. *J Am Coll Cardiol* 29:604–612, 1997.

In 110 patients with dilated cardiomyopathy, a restrictive pattern of ventricular filling at baseline, with persistence of this pattern at a 3-month follow-up study, was predictive of high mortality and cardiac transplantation rates.

New Approaches

28. Takatsuji H, Mikami T, Urasawa K, et al: A new approach for evaluation of left ventricular diastolic function: Spatial and temporal analysis of left ventricular filling flow propagation by color M-mode Doppler echocardiography. *J Am Coll Cardiol* 27:365–371, 1996.

Propagation velocity on a color M-mode of left ventricular filling from an apical approach was defined as the distance/time ratio between the mitral orifice and the point where velocity decreased to 70% of its initial value. Compared to micromanometer pressure data, propagation velocity correlated with the time constant of relaxation (tau) and with peak −dP/dt in a series of 40 patients.

29. Derumeauz G, Ovize M, Loufoua F, et al: Doppler tissue imaging quantitates regional wall motion during myocardial ischemia and reperfusion. *Circulation* 97:1970–1977, 1998.

Color Doppler tissue imaging allowed assessment of both regional systolic and diastolic function during myocardial ischemia and after reperfusion.

The Utility of Echocardiography in Patients With Ischemic Cardiac Disease

7

BASIC PRINCIPLES
  Relationship Between Coronary Artery Anatomy and
    Segmental Wall Motion
  Echocardiographic Views for Evaluation of Left
    Ventricular Wall Motion
    Transthoracic Imaging
    Transesophageal Imaging
  Sequence of Events in Ischemia
  Evaluation of Global and Regional Ventricular
    Function in Coronary Artery Disease
MYOCARDIAL ISCHEMIA
  Basic Principles
  Stress Echocardiography
    Exercise Echocardiography
    Dobutamine Stress Echocardiography
    Other Stress Modalities
  Limitations/Technical Aspects
  Alternate Approaches
    Exercise Electrocardiography
    Doppler Stress Echocardiography
    Direct Echocardiographic Imaging of the
      Coronary Arteries
    Radionuclide Techniques/Positron Emission
      Tomography
    Coronary Angiography

Clinical Utility
  Diagnosis of Coronary Artery Disease
  Extent and Location of Ischemic Areas
  Prognostic Implications
MYOCARDIAL INFARCTION
  Basic Principles
  Echocardiographic Imaging
  Limitations/Alternate Approaches
  Clinical Utility
    Diagnosis of Acute Myocardial Infarction in the
      Emergency Department
    Evaluation of Interventional Therapy for Acute
      Myocardial Infarction
    Complications of Myocardial Infarction
END-STAGE ISCHEMIC CARDIAC DISEASE
  Differentiation from Other Causes of Left Ventricular
    Systolic Dysfunction
  Echocardiographic Approach
  Limitations/Alternate Approaches
SUGGESTED READING

Given the high prevalence of coronary artery disease, evaluation of patients with suspected or documented ischemic disease is one of the most common indications for echocardiography. Echocardiographic evaluation focuses on the functional outcome of coronary artery disease—specifically systolic wall thickening and endocardial motion—rather than on direct imaging of the coronary arteries. While the proximal left main and right coronary arteries often can be identified, even on transthoracic images, tomographic imaging techniques currently do not provide the detailed knowledge of distal vessel anatomy or the location and severity of coronary artery narrowings that is needed for patient management. Coronary angiography remains the procedure of choice for direct assessment of coronary artery anatomy.

However, echocardiography offers detailed functional assessment of segmental and global left ventricular systolic function both at rest and after interventions to induce ischemia (Table 7–1). In many cases, this functional assessment provides critical data for patient management. For example, stress echocardiography is a reliable approach for the initial diagnosis of coronary artery disease, especially in patients with a nondiagnostic stress electrocardiogram (ECG). Another example is the use of echocardiography in the emergency department for early diagnosis of acute myocardial infarction in patients with an equivocal electrocardiogram. In addition, the central role of echocardiography in evaluation for complications of acute myocardial infarction has long been recognized. Finally, echocardiography often pro-

TABLE 7–1	Echocardiography for Coronary Artery Disease

Myocardial Ischemia
Diagnosis of coronary artery disease
Severity of disease (number of vessels involved, extent of myocardium at risk)
Overall LV systolic function
Diastolic LV function

Acute Myocardial Infarction
Detection of wall motion abnormalities
Evaluation of recurrent chest pain after myocardial infarction
Assessment of the response to reperfusion therapy

Complications of Acute Myocardial Infarction
LV systolic dysfunction
LV thrombus
Aneurysm formation
Acute mitral regurgitation
Ventricular septal defect
LV rupture
Pericardial effusion

End-Stage Ischemic Disease
LV and RV systolic dysfunction
Associated mitral regurgitation
Pulmonary artery pressures
LV thrombus

LV = Left ventricular; RV = right ventricular.

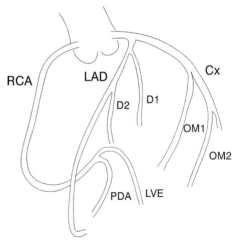

FIGURE 7–1. Schematic drawing of coronary artery anatomy showing the left anterior descending (LAD) artery with diagonal (D1 and D2) branches, the circumflex artery (Cx) with obtuse marginal branches (OM1 and OM2), and the right coronary artery (RCA) giving rise to the posterior descending artery (PDA) and left ventricular extension (LVE) branch.

FIGURE 7–2. Normal left coronary artery in a right anterior oblique (RAO) projection showing the left anterior descending (LAD) and circumflex (Cx) coronary arteries.

vides important prognostic data in patients with coronary artery disease.

BASIC PRINCIPLES

Relationship Between Coronary Artery Anatomy and Segmental Wall Motion

While coronary anatomy varies to some degree from patient to patient, the overall pattern of coronary artery branching is relatively uniform (Fig. 7–1). The left main coronary artery arises from the superior aspect of the left coronary sinus of Valsalva and divides into (1) the left anterior descending artery, which extends via the interventricular groove down the anterior wall to (and sometimes around) the left ventricular apex, and (2) the circumflex artery, which continues laterally in the atrioventricular groove. The right coronary artery arises from the superior aspect of the right coronary sinus of Valsalva and extends inferomedially following the atrioventricular groove. Approximately 80% of patients have a *right-dominant* coronary circulation; the right coronary gives rise to the posterior descending artery, which lies in the inferior interventricular groove supplying both the inferior aspect of the ventricular sep-

tum and the inferior free wall (Figs. 7–2 and 7–3). In about 20% of patients, the coronary circulation is *left dominant;* the circumflex artery gives rise to the posterior descending artery.

The posterior left ventricular wall may be supplied by extension branches from the right coronary artery or by obtuse marginal branches of the circumflex arteries. The lateral wall is supplied by obtuse marginal branches of the circumflex artery. The left anterior descending artery supplies the anterior portion of the interventricular septum via septal perforating branches and the anterior wall via diagonal branches. There is marked individual variability in the blood supply to the left ventricular apex. In some cases, the left anterior descending artery extends around the apex to supply the apical segment of the inferior wall. In other cases, the posterior descending artery extends around the apex to supply the apical segment of the anterior wall. More commonly, the blood supply to the apex arises from both the left an-

terior descending and the posterior descending coronary arteries.

Segmental wall motion abnormalities seen by echocardiography correspond closely with the coronary artery blood supply to the myocardium. Several different schemes for reporting the location of wall motion abnormalities on echocardiography have been proposed. These approaches differ mainly in the number of segments into which the left ventricle is divided; all are similar in the use of nomenclature that corresponds both to coronary anatomy and to the application of these terms for other cardiac imaging modalities.

From base to apex, the left ventricle typically is divided into three segments—basal, midventricular, and apical—to correspond to proximal, middle, and apical lesions of the coronary arteries. In a short-axis view, both at the basal (mitral valve) and mid–left ventricular (or papillary muscle) levels, the ventricle is divided clockwise, beginning with the interventricular groove, into the anterior wall, the lateral wall, the posterior wall, and the inferior wall (Fig. 7–4). The ventricular septum is divided into at least two segments (inferior and anterior), since it receives blood flow from both the posterior

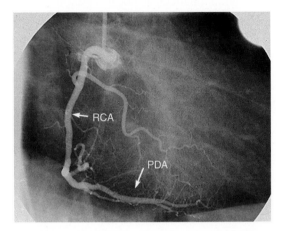

FIGURE 7–3. Normal right coronary anatomy with the posterior descending artery (PDA) seen in a right anterior oblique (RAO) projection.

Echo Views for Wall Motion

FIGURE 7–4. Echocardiographic views for wall motion evaluation. In the short-axis view, at the base and midventricular levels, the left ventricle is divided into anterior septum *(1, 7)* and free wall *(2, 8)*, lateral *(3, 9)*, posterior *(4, 10)*, inferior free wall *(5, 11)*, and inferior septal *(6, 12)* segments. These same wall segments are seen in apical views as indicated, plus the anterior *(13)*, inferior *(15)*, and posterolateral *(14)* apical segments are seen.

descending and the left anterior descending arteries. The apical region often is divided into only three or four segments (instead of five to eight segments at the base) because of the normal tapering of the ventricle toward the apex. Depending on the exact scheme used, this results in between 15 and 20 myocardial segments. While a more elaborate segmental system may be needed for research purposes, for routine patient evaluation a 15-segment scheme provides sufficient detail for clinical correlation between coronary anatomy and echocardiographic findings. The location of wall motion abnormalities can be reported descriptively, using a series of drawings showing different echocardiographic views, using a target diagram with the apex in the center and the base around the circumference (Fig. 7–5), or using more quantitative display formats.

The segmental wall motion abnormalities seen with ischemia or infarction correspond to the coronary anatomy as follows:

1. Left anterior descending artery disease results in wall motion abnormalities of the anterior septum, anterior free wall, and anterior left ventricular apex. Depending on the degree to which diagonal branches supply the lateral wall, abnormalities may be seen for these segments as well. If the left anterior descending artery extends around the apex, apical segments of the inferior and posterolateral walls may be affected. The location of the lesion along the length of the coronary artery obviously affects the pattern of wall motion. A lesion in the distal third of the vessel affects only

the apex, a lesion in the midsegment of the vessel affects the midventricular and apical segments, while a proximal lesion affects the entire wall including the basal segments.

2. Circumflex artery disease affects wall motion of the lateral and posterior left ventricular walls. Again, the extent of segmental wall motion is related to the exact coronary anatomy in an individual patient. Echocardiography is particularly helpful in patients with circumflex disease because this myocardial region often is "silent" electrocardiographically and is not well seen on a single-plane right anterior–oblique left ventricular angiogram.

3. Posterior descending artery disease results in abnormal wall motion in the inferior septum, inferior free wall, and posterior left ventricular segments. If the posterior descending artery is a short vessel, the apex will not be affected, while extensive wall motion abnormalities of the apex may be seen if the posterior descending artery extends to supply the ventricular apex.

Other patterns of abnormal wall motion are seen with lesions of the branches of the three major coronary arteries. For example, isolated disease in a diagonal branch of the left anterior descending artery results in a discrete wall motion abnormality in the portion of the anterolateral wall supplied by that vessel. Proximal right coronary artery disease can result in ischemia or infarction of the right ventricular free wall.

Collateral vessels and previous bypass surgery also affect the pattern of wall motion. If a myocardial segment has a balanced oxygen demand/supply ratio, wall motion will be normal whether blood flow is supplied antegrade by the native vessel, by collateral vessels, or by a bypass graft.

Echocardiographic Views for Evaluation of Left Ventricular Wall Motion

Transthoracic Imaging

Regional systolic function for each segment of the left ventricle can be assessed on transthoracic imaging by combining data from multiple image planes. In the parasternal long-axis view, the basal and midventricular segments of the anterior septum and posterior left ventricular walls are seen. In the parasternal short-axis view, circumferential images of the left ventricle at the base and midventricular levels are obtained. Note that if the transducer is angulated toward the apex from a fixed parasternal position, progressively more apical segments of the

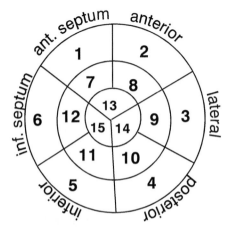

FIGURE 7–5. "Target" diagram for reporting left ventricular segmental wall motion with the apex in the center of the circle and the base around the circumference. Segment numbers correspond to those shown in Figure 7–4.

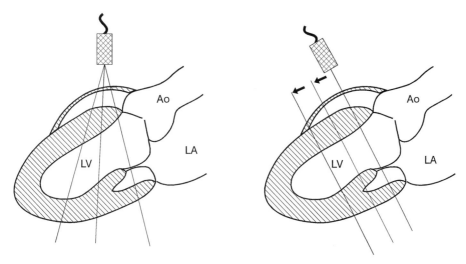

FIGURE 7–6. Angulation of the transducer from a fixed parasternal position results in short-axis views that intersect similar segments of the septum but progressively more apical segments of the posterior wall. By moving the transducer apically, more parallel image planes can be obtained.

posterior wall are imaged while the *same* segment of the septum is included in the ultrasound image plane. A more parallel alignment between image planes may be obtained by moving the transducer apically to obtain short-axis midventricular and (sometimes) apical views of the left ventricle (Fig. 7–6). In either case, evaluation of wall motion from other windows is helpful for avoiding misdiagnosis related to an oblique image plane. Of note, the apical segments rarely are adequately visualized from the parasternal window.

From the apical window, evaluation of left ventricular wall motion is performed in four-chamber, two-chamber, and long-axis views. Detailed evaluation of the extent of abnormal myocardium is possible by slow rotation of the image plane between the standard views. In the four-chamber view, the inferior septum and lateral wall are seen. Anterior angulation to include the aortic valve allows visualization of portions of the anterior septum. In the two-chamber view, the anterior and inferior free walls are seen. Endocardial and epicardial definition of the anterior wall may be difficult due to attenuation by adjacent overlying lung tissue. This problem can be alleviated by careful patient positioning and imaging during held respiration. In the apical long-axis view, the anterior septum and posterior wall are seen (analogous to the parasternal long-axis view).

Note that while these three apical image planes are approximately 60° to each other, there is some individual variation in their exact relationship. In addition, variation in coronary anatomy between individuals results in variable patterns of abnormal wall motion. Care is needed in positioning the transducer at the apex to avoid foreshortening of the ventricle from this approach. Integration of data from parasternal and apical approaches, taking into account image quality in each view, allows assessment of each myocardial segment in at least two views.

Finally, evaluation from a subcostal approach may be helpful. In the subcostal four-chamber view, the inferior septum and lateral wall are imaged. In the subcostal short-axis view, the inferior and posterior walls are nearest the transducer and the anterior and lateral walls most distal (Fig. 7–7).

Transesophageal Imaging

When transthoracic images are inadequate or in certain monitoring situations (e.g., intraoperative monitoring of left ventricular function), regional left ventricular function can be evaluated from a transesophageal approach. From the high left atrial position, a four-chamber view of the left ventricle is obtained (in the 0° plane of the transesophageal echocardiographic probe) showing the inferior septum and lateral wall. Rotating the image plane to approximately 60° provides a two-chamber view with visualization of the anterior and inferior walls, while further rotation to about 120° results in a long-axis view with imaging of the anterior septum and posterior wall. Again, the exact degree of rotation to obtain these views varies slightly from patient to patient. In

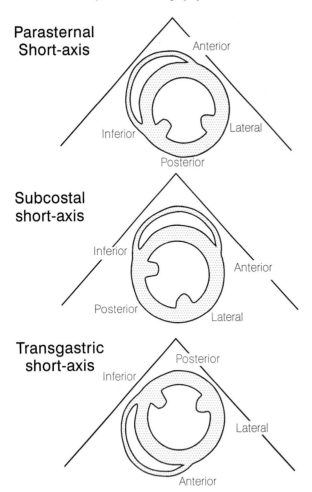

Parasternal Short-axis

Subcostal short-axis

Transgastric short-axis

FIGURE 7–7. The wall segments seen in the short-axis view from transthoracic parasternal and subcostal, and transesophageal transgastric approach are shown. Correct identification of wall segments is facilitated by noting the position of the septum and the papillary muscles.

addition, transducer position and angulation may require adjustment as the image plane is rotated using anatomic landmarks to ensure optimal images with inclusion of the apical segments. Even with optimal technique, these views may be foreshortened; that is, the apparent apex represents an oblique plane through the anterolateral wall, while the true left ventricular apex is not seen.

From the transgastric position the transverse image plane provides short-axis views of the left ventricle at the base (mitral valve) and midventricular (papillary muscle) level. Rotation of the image plane at this position provides a two-chamber view, although the apex may be foreshortened. Further advancement of the probe may allow acquisition of an "apical" four-chamber view (in the 0° plane) by flexing the probe tip. However, the ventricle may be foreshortened and the true apex missed if the left ventricular apex does not lie on the diaphragm without intervening lung tissue in a position accessible from the transgastric approach.

Transesophageal imaging of left ventricular wall motion is indicated:

1. For intraoperative assessment of global and segmental left ventricular function.
2. In critically ill patients when transthoracic views are inadequate.

Sequence of Events in Ischemia

Irreversible myocardial damage (e.g., infarction) results in wall motion abnormalities that are present at rest. With an acute infarction, wall thickness is normal, but systolic wall thickening and endocardial motion are reduced or absent. An old myocardial infarction is characterized by thinning and increased echogenicity of the affected segments due to scarring and fibrosis, in addition to abnormal motion and absent wall thickening.

In contrast, ischemia is a reversible imbalance in the myocardial oxygen demand/supply ratio. Even with substantial coronary artery narrowing, blood flow is adequate for myocar-

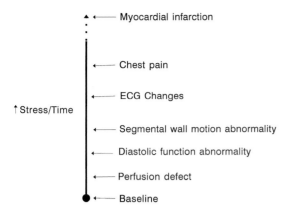

FIGURE 7–8. Schematic diagram of the sequence of events in myocardial ischemia.

dial oxygen demands at rest. However, when the narrowing exceeds approximately 70% of the luminal cross-sectional area, blood flow becomes inadequate to meet increased myocardial oxygen demands with exercise, pharmacologic interventions, or mental stress, resulting in ischemia. When oxygen demand returns to baseline, blood flow again is adequate, ischemia resolves, and wall motion returns to normal. Thus, wall motion *at rest* is normal in patients with coronary artery disease if there has been no prior myocardial infarction.

The sequence of changes as a region of myocardium becomes ischemic is as follows (Fig. 7–8). The first detectable changes associated with heterogeneity of flow to the left ventricle are biochemical followed by a significant perfusion defect (detectable by radionuclide techniques). Next, regional myocardial dysfunction, characterized by both abnormal diastolic relaxation and compliance and impaired systolic wall thickening and endocardial motion, occurs in rapid succession (within a few cardiac cycles). Ischemic ST-segment depression on electrocardiography and clinical angina are relatively late manifestations of ischemia and are not seen consistently. Echocardiography, by detecting abnormal regional wall motion, provides a useful noninvasive method for evaluating ischemia that should be more sensitive than electrocardiography given this sequence of events. Echocardiography differs from radionuclide techniques in that the functional consequences of ischemia, rather than the pattern of myocardial perfusion, are assessed.

Evaluation of Global and Regional Ventricular Function in Coronary Artery Disease

Global left ventricular systolic function can be evaluated either qualitatively or quantitatively in patients with coronary artery disease using the approaches described in Chapter 5. Since the pattern of left ventricular dysfunction typically is *not* uniform, it is important that qualitative evaluation be based on multiple tomographic views. If quantitative methods are applied, approaches that incorporate endocardial borders from at least two tomographic planes are most appropriate. In patients with coronary artery disease, the left ventricular ejection fraction is essential clinical data because it is a crucial variable in clinical decision making concerning surgical intervention.

Segmental (or regional) left ventricular systolic function most often is evaluated using a semiquantitative scoring system. The endocardial motion for each defined myocardial segment is described as normal, hypokinetic, akinetic, or dyskinetic, with a score from 1 to 4 corresponding to these descriptive terms. Hyperkinesis also may be scored (Table 7–2). Some clinicians prefer to subclassify the degree of hypokinesis as mild, moderate, or severe, but such a subclassification often has significant in-

TABLE 7–2	Qualitative Scale for Assessment of Segmental Wall Motion on Echocardiography	

Score*	Wall Motion	Definition
1	Normal	Normal endocardial inward motion and wall thickening in systole
2	Hypokinesis	Reduced endocardial motion and wall thickening in systole
3	Akinesis	Absence of inward endocardial motion or wall thickening in systole
4	Dyskinesis	Outward motion or "bulging" of the segment in systole, usually associated with thin, scarred myocardium

*A score of 0 may be used for hyperkinesis, defined as increased endocardial inward motion and wall thickening in systole.

terobserver and intraobserver variability. An overall wall motion score index can be derived by dividing the sum of scores for each segment by the number of segments evaluated:

$$\text{Wall motion score index} = \text{Sum of individual segment scores/} \text{Number of segments visualized}$$

Several more quantitative approaches to echocardiographic segmental wall motion have been proposed. Most of these represent modifications of angiographic techniques, such as the centerline method for quantitative wall motion analysis. Limitations of the application of these approaches to echocardiographic images include:

1. The need to identify and manually trace the endocardium at end-diastole and end-systole. Accurate automatic edge-detection algorithms minimize this problem.
2. The need to evaluate wall motion in multiple tomographic views.
3. The need for knowledge of the degree of variability of normal wall motion for each view.
4. The effects of translation, rotation, and torsion of the left ventricle during the cardiac cycle. This potentially could result in imaging different regions of myocardium in systole versus diastole for a given tomographic plane.
5. The question of whether wall thickening or endocardial motion is a more appropriate method for describing regional ventricular function.

As automated edge-detection programs become faster and are validated for echocardiographic data, quantitative analysis of segmental function will become more feasible in the clinical setting. Approaches that incorporate three-dimensional (3D) reconstruction of the left ventricle also appear promising.

MYOCARDIAL ISCHEMIA

Basic Principles

Since echocardiographic wall motion at rest is normal in a patient with significant coronary artery disease and no prior myocardial infarction, imaging *during ischemia* is needed for diagnosis. Inducing ischemia during echocardiographic imaging is referred to as *stress echocardiography*. Ischemia can be induced by increasing myocardial oxygen demand either with exercise or by pharmacologic interventions (Table 7–3).

Stress Echocardiography

Exercise Echocardiography

Exercise echocardiography typically is performed using standard exercise-test protocols. Supine or upright bicycle exercise protocols have the advantage that echocardiographic imaging can be performed during exercise at each progressive level of exertion, including maximal exercise. Treadmill exercise protocols have the advantage that a higher total workload can be achieved but the disadvantage that imaging can only be performed after exercise. Wall motion abnormalities that resolve very rapidly after exercise may be missed.

Resting images are acquired in digital format for standard views of the left ventricle. Stan-

TABLE 7–3	Stress Echocardiography		
Type of Stress	**Advantages**	**Disadvantages**	
Treadmill exercise	Widely available High workload	Imaging post-ETT only	
Upright bicycle	Imaging during exercise	Imaging may be technically difficult Lower workload	
Supine bicycle	Imaging during exercise	Lower work load Supine position affects exercise physiology	
Dobutamine	Continuous imaging Does not require physically active patient	Potential adverse effects of dobutamine Level of stress achieved	
Dipyridamole	Continuous imaging Does not require physically active patient	Potential adverse effects of dipyridamole Induction of relative flow inequality rather than ischemia per se	

ETT = Exercise treadmill test.

FIGURE 7–9. Flowchart of an exercise echocardiography protocol.

dard exercise protocols are used with monitoring of the 12-lead ECG, blood pressure, and symptoms by a qualified physician during and following the exercise protocol. The risks of exercise echocardiography are the risks of the exercise test itself.

Either during maximal exercise (supine or sitting bicycle) or immediately after exercise (treadmill), image acquisition is repeated. A repetitive cine-loop acquisition cycle is helpful because respiratory motion limits the examiner's ability to select a good quality beat quickly in real time. Typically, four or more sequential cycles are recorded digitally, and the examiner subsequently chooses the best image for comparison with the baseline views (Fig. 7–9). Next, the rest and exercise cine-loop digital images are displayed side by side so that endocardial motion and wall thickening for each myocardial region can be compared. A systematic approach, comparing each segment in turn, is needed for detection of subtle abnormalities (Fig. 7–10).

Interpretation of an exercise stress echocardiogram includes incorporation of data on the maximum workload achieved (exercise duration), the heart rate and blood pressure response to exercise, the presence of arrhythmias, and clinical symptoms, as well as evaluation of the echocardiographic images.

Dobutamine Stress Echocardiography

Pharmacologic stress testing with intravenous dobutamine is based on the increased heart rate and contractility induced by this potent beta agonist. Typically, infusions are started at a low dose (5 μg/kg/min) and increased incrementally every 3 to 5 minutes with a calibrated infusion pump until the maximum dose (30 to 40 μg/kg min) or an endpoint has been

reached. Atropine is added, if needed, to achieve an appropriate increase in heart rate with a typical goal of 85% of the patient's maximum predicted heart rate. In order to minimize the likelihood of significant adverse effects and to optimize the quality of the data obtained, a dobutamine stress echocardiography examination requires a well-defined study protocol performed in the appropriate clinical setting.

Patient monitoring during dobutamine stress echocardiography includes periodic blood pressure measurement (usually every 2 to 3 minutes), continuous ECG rhythm monitoring, and careful observation for clinical symptoms or signs. Appropriate equipment, medications, and trained personnel should be immediately available in the event of an adverse effect, including a cardiac defibrillator, emergency cardiac medications, intravenous esmolol (a beta blocker that counteracts the effects of dobutamine), and a qualified physician.

After an intravenous line for administration of the dobutamine has been placed, the patient is positioned in a left lateral decubitus position on an echo-stretcher with an apical cutout to allow optimal image acquisition throughout the study protocol. Initially, the intravenous line is filled only with saline solution while resting data are obtained. At baseline, after 3 minutes at each dosage level, and during recovery, data collection includes recording of heart rate, blood pressure, symptoms, a 12-lead ECG, and echocardiographic images (Fig. 7–11). Standard views include parasternal short-axis images at the base and papillary muscle levels and apical four-chamber, two-chamber, and long-axis images. Digital image acquisition in a cine-loop format facilitates interpretation of the study. Some centers also record Doppler left ventricular filling and ejection velocities at each stage of the stress protocol.

Endpoints for stopping the test are (1) reaching the maximum protocol dose, (2) patient discomfort, (3) a definite wall motion abnormality on echocardiography involving two or more adjacent segments, (4) ST-segment elevation on ECG, (5) reaching 85% of maximum predicted heart rate for age, (6) a systolic blood pressure >200 or <100 mmHg *or* a diastolic blood pressure >120 mmHg, or (7) significant ventricular arrhythmias.

Although complications are uncommon when appropriate precautions are observed, reported adverse effects include anxiety, tremulousness, palpitations, arrhythmias, paresthesias, and chest pain. Note that since the purpose of the test is to induce ischemia, many

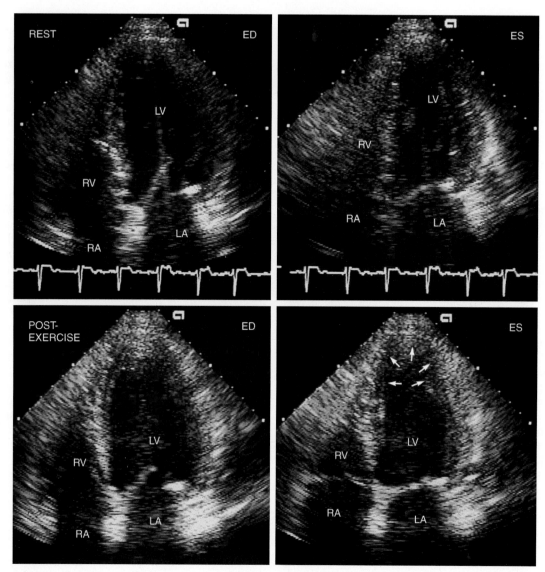

FIGURE 7–10. Frames from an abnormal exercise echo study showing the development of apical akinesis *(arrows)* with exercise. End-diastolic (ED) images are shown on the left, end-systolic (ES) on the right, with rest images on the top and exercise images on the bottom. The patient was found to have a severe proximal left anterior descending artery stenosis on coronary angiography.

patients will have either echocardiographic changes or ECG evidence of ischemia and may experience angina. However, the frequency of angina may be less than with standard ECG stress testing because the protocol can be stopped as soon as wall motion abnormalities are seen (which often is before angina occurs). Hypotension occurs in up to 10% of patients because of peripheral β_2-receptor-mediated vasodilation but, unlike hypotension with exercise testing, is *not* associated with severe coronary disease or a worse prognosis. Contraindications to dobutamine stress echocardiography

are unstable angina, uncontrolled hypertension, or sensitivity to dobutamine or sulfites.

The echocardiographic images are interpreted after reformatting the digital images so that each quadrant of the screen shows a single view at rest (upper left), low-dose (upper right), maximal dose (lower left), and recovery phase (lower right). For each myocardial segment, wall motion is compared on these images in a systematic fashion. Since wall thickening and endocardial motion normally increase with dobutamine, an abnormal test is defined as the observation of hypokinesis or akinesis in a re-

Typical Dobutamine Stress Echo Protocol

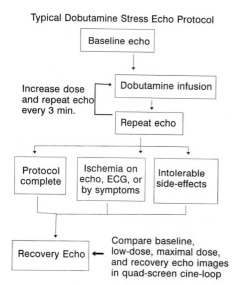

FIGURE 7–11. Flowchart of dobutamine stress echo protocol.

gion that had normal wall motion at rest (Figs. 7–12 and 7-13).

In addition to detection of ischemic myocardium, dobutamine stress echocardiography has been proposed as a method to evaluate for myocardial viability in regions that are "stunned" or "hibernating." For example, after treatment of myocardial infarction with thrombolytic therapy, the extent of residual viable myocardium in the area at risk may be unclear early after the event because of myocardial "stunning." Alternatively, a patient with chronic coronary artery disease may have hypokinesis or akinesis at baseline due to "hibernating" myocardium, which may recover with revascularization. In both these settings, echocardiographic imaging during low-dose (5 to 10 μg/kg/min) dobutamine infusion has been reported to show improved wall thickening and endocardial motion in viable segments of the myocardium. Of course, at higher dobutamine doses, worsening of regional function may occur due to induction of ischemia. This pattern of initial improvement at low dose, with subsequent worsening of myocardial function at higher dobutamine doses, is referred to as a biphasic response.

Other Stress Modalities

Dipyridamole has been proposed for echocardiographic stress testing by some investigators based on the differential pattern of coronary blood flow induced by this agent: increased blood flow in normal coronary arteries with a *relative* decrease in blood flow in diseased vessels. Overall success with this approach has been higher with perfusion imaging (e.g., thallium) because the difference in blood flow between regions supplied by normal versus abnormal coronary arteries can be seen on the

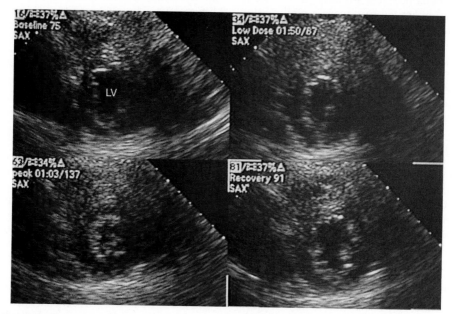

FIGURE 7–12. Normal dobutamine stress echocardiography showing the parasternal short-axis view at end-systole at baseline *(upper left)*, low-dose (5 μg/kg/min) dobutamine *(upper right)*, high-dose (40 μg/kg/min) dobutamine *(lower left)*, and recovery images *(lower right)*. Note the baseline heart rate of 75 bpm, and the heart rate of 137 bpm at peak dose dobutamine. There is a marked decrease in end-systolic cavity area from baseline to peak dose images.

FIGURE 7–13. Example of an abnormal dobutamine stress echocardiographic study. *Top,* Baseline images; *Bottom,* Peak dose images (40 μg/kg/min dobutamine plus 0.5 mg atropine); *Left,* End-diastolic images; *Right,* End-systolic images. The apical segment of the septum became dyskinetic at peak dobutamine dose *(arrows)*, indicating significant coronary artery disease. In this case, angiography showed severe stenosis in the proximal left anterior descending artery.

radionuclide images. Results with echocardiographic imaging have been less consistent, since actual ischemia (not just a relative difference in blood flow) is needed to discern a wall motion abnormality.

Whichever method of inducing ischemia is used, diagnosis of coronary disease is based on comparison of resting and stress echocardiographic images. Preferably, this is performed using digital image acquisition with cine-loop formatting of a single (good-quality) beat in each tomographic view. Side-by-side display of rest and stress images allows reliable detection of new wall motion abnormalities. Typical views for echocardiographic stress testing are a parasternal short-axis view at the papillary muscle level, an apical long-axis view, an apical two-chamber view, and an apical four-chamber view. Other views may be helpful in individual patients depending on image quality and the area of myocardium involved.

Limitations/Technical Aspects

Stress echocardiography has a high sensitivity and specificity for diagnosis of significant coronary artery disease (Tables 7–4 and 7–5). In addition, it allows reliable definition of the anatomic location and extent of ischemic myocardium. However, stress echocardiography does have both technical and physiologic limitations.

The most important potential technical limitation of stress echocardiography is image quality, specifically endocardial definition. Assessment of endocardial wall motion and wall thickening requires adequate delineation of the endocardium for each myocardial segment. Careful attention to patient positioning, transducer orientation, and image processing parameters can improve image quality, but definition of certain segments, particularly the anterior wall, may be difficult in some individuals due to adjacent lung tissue.

Exercise and postexercise imaging can be limited by respiratory interference due to a rapid respiratory rate. Digital acquisition in cine-loop format of several cycles, followed by selection of the best images, is necessary for correct interpretation. The possible effects of translation and rotation, both between systole and diastole and between baseline and stress, should be considered in comparisons of wall motion. Given these potential limitations, the interpretation of a stress echocardiographic

| TABLE 7–4 | Selected Studies on the Diagnostic Accuracy of Exercise Echocardiography Compared with Coronary Angiography* |

First Author/Year	N	Percentage with Documented CAD	Sensitivity (%)	Specificity (%)
Limacher/1984	73	—	91	88
Armstrong/1987	123	82	87	86
Ryan/1988	64	47	78	100
Sawada/1989	57 (women)	49	86	86
Crouse/1991	228	77	97	64
Marwick/1992	179	64	84	86
Quinones/1992	112	77	74	88

*In all studies, significant coronary artery disease was defined as a ≥50% stenosis in an epicardial vessel.
ETT = Exercise treadmill testing; CAD = coronary artery disease.
Data from Limacher et al: Circ 67:1211–1218, 1984; Armstrong et al: JACC 10:531–538, 1987; Ryan et al: 11:993–999, 1988; Sawada et al: 14:1440–1447, 1989; Crouse et al: AJC 67:1213–1218, 1991; Marwick et al: JACC 19:74–81, 1992; Quinones et al: Circ 85:1026–1031, 1992.

study includes a description of image quality as an indicator of the reliability of these results. Suboptimal images should be interpreted with caution. Some centers use contrast agents that opacify the left ventricle after intravenous administration to enhance detection of regional wall motion abnormalities when endocardial definition is suboptimal with fundamental or harmonic frequency imaging.

Potential physiologic limitations are related to the fact that abnormal wall motion occurs only *during* ischemia. First, if the "stress" used does *not* induce ischemia, no wall motion abnormality will be seen even if significant coronary disease is present. For example, a patient with limited exercise duration due to hip pain may not achieve a level of exertion that results in ischemia. Similarly, a pharmacologic "stress"

| TABLE 7–5 | Selected Studies on Diagnostic Accuracy of Dobutamine Stress Echocardiography Compared with Coronary Angiography |

First Author/Year	Source of Subjects	N	Percentage with Documented CAD	Percentage Stenosis Considered Significant	Sensitivity (%)	Specificity (%)
Berthe/1986	Post-AMI	30	100	50	85	88
Cohen/1991	Chest pain	70	27	70	86	95
Sawada/1991	Coronary angio	103	44	50	89	85
Mazeika/1992	Coronary angio	50	26	70	78	93
Martin/1992	Coronary angio	40	35	50	76	60
Segar/1992	Coronary angio	85	—	50	95	82
Marcovitz/1992	Coronary angio	141	21	50	96	66
Marwick/1993	Coronary angio	217	65	50	72	83

References: Berthe et al: AJC 58:1167–1172, 1986; Cohen et al: AJC 67:1311–1318, 1991; Sawada et al: Circ 83:1602–1614, 1991; Mazeika et al: JACC 19:1203–1211, 1992; Martin et al: AIM 116:190–196, 1992; Segar et al: JACC 19:1197–1202, 1992; Marcovitz et al: AJC 69:1269–1273, 1992; Marwick et al: JACC 22:159–167, 1993.
CAD = Coronary artery disease; AMI = acute myocardial infarction; Angio = angiography.

that does not induce ischemia will not induce a wall motion abnormality. Second, the duration of ischemia is important. If ischemia has resolved by the time imaging is performed, the wall motion abnormality will not be detected. This is of particular concern with treadmill exercise, since echocardiographic imaging is performed after exertion, although this possible limitation may be offset by the higher maximum workload achieved prior to the recovery period compared with bicycle exercise protocols.

Stress echocardiography in patients with abnormal global or regional function at rest is more difficult to interpret than in subjects with normal resting left ventricular systolic function. The presence of a segmental motion abnormality at rest implies that coronary artery disease, with prior myocardial infarction, is present. With stress imaging, new wall motion abnormalities in regions remote from the site of resting abnormal wall motion indicate additional areas of ischemia. Evaluation of areas adjacent to the resting wall motion abnormality may be problematic due to a potential tethering effect by the abnormal region.

In patients with global systolic dysfunction at rest—which may be due to end-stage ischemic disease, cardiomyopathy, or chronic valvular disease—stress echocardiography is much less specific for the diagnosis of coronary disease. Differentiation of end-stage ischemic disease from a primary cardiomyopathy is discussed under the section on myocardial infarction below. Stress echocardiography also may be helpful in some patients with cardiomyopathy or valvular disease, depending on the specific clinical question.

Alternate Approaches

Exercise Electrocardiography

Exercise ECG remains a standard test for evaluation of patients with suspected or known coronary artery disease. Even though it has a lower sensitivity and specificity for diagnosis of coronary disease compared with imaging techniques, it continues to provide important prognostic data at a low cost in many patients. Imaging techniques most often are needed in subgroups with high false-positive (e.g., women with chest pain) or false-negative rates and in patients with an abnormal resting ECG that obscures exercise-induced ischemic changes.

Doppler Stress Echocardiography

Doppler stress echocardiography has been proposed as an approach that can be used in-stead of, or in addition to, evaluation of segmental wall motion. Left ventricular ejection parameters derived from the aortic outflow Doppler velocity curve, including maximum velocity, the velocity-time integral, and the maximum and mean acceleration rates, can be recorded at rest and with stress. The actual changes in an individual patient can be compared with the expected changes for these variables.

Left ventricular diastolic filling is abnormal during ischemia and may be assessed from the Doppler left ventricular inflow curve. Several studies have found that *during* ischemia (e.g., with balloon inflation during percutaneous transluminal angioplasty), the early diastolic filling velocity is reduced, the isovolumic relaxation period is prolonged, and the E/A ratio falls. These findings are consistent with an acute abnormality in diastolic relaxation. Other studies have found seemingly contradictory results, for example, an increase in the E velocity and E/A ratio with exercise-induced ischemia. Confounding variables that affect the pattern of diastolic filling, most importantly left atrial pressure and heart rate, most likely account for these discrepant results. Another possible explanation is rapid temporal changes in diastolic function during and after ischemia so that the pattern of left ventricular filling varies depending on the time interval between onset of ischemia and the Doppler recording. This possibility is supported by several studies showing that the pattern of left ventricular filling later returns to baseline. Of course, it is simplest to compare changes in an individual patient with his or her own baseline Doppler findings. When comparing patients with each other, other variables that affect diastolic filling, such as age, coexisting mitral regurgitation, PR interval, and ventricular systolic function, further hamper the clinical application of these data.

Direct Echocardiographic Imaging of the Coronary Arteries

The origins of the right and left coronary arteries often can be identified on transthoracic imaging (Fig. 7–14). On transesophageal imaging, the proximal left coronary can be followed to its bifurcation into left anterior descending and circumflex arteries (Figs. 7–15 and 7–16), and often these branches can be imaged for a portion of their length, as can the right coronary artery (see Suggested Reading 40). However, clinical decision making usually requires detailed knowledge of the entire extent of the coronary anatomy. Tomographic imaging is a

FIGURE 7–14. Right coronary artery (RCA) seen on a transthoracic parasternal short-axis view.

FIGURE 7–16. Doppler recording of coronary artery blood flow in the left main coronary artery from a transesophageal approach showing predominant diastolic flow.

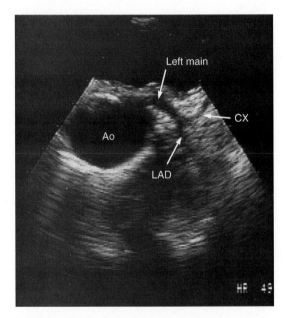

FIGURE 7–15. Left main coronary artery on transesophageal imaging showing its bifurcation into left anterior descending (LAD) and circumflex (Cx) arteries.

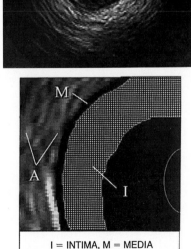

I = INTIMA, M = MEDIA
A = ADVENTITIA

FIGURE 7–17. Intravascular ultrasound scan of mild coronary disease illustrating the typical three-layered appearance generated by the acoustic difference between the layers of the artery: intima, media, and adventitia. (From MacIsaac AI, Yock PG, Fitzgerald PJ: Intravascular ultrasound: Histologic correlation and clinical applications. In Otto CM [ed]: The Clinical Practice of Echocardiography. Philadelphia, WB Saunders, 1997, p. 278.)

suboptimal method for evaluation of the relatively small coronary vessels that move with the epicardial surface of the heart.

Intravascular ultrasound techniques, in which an imaging transducer is mounted on an intracoronary catheter, provide detailed cross-sectional views of proximal coronary arteries (Fig. 7–17). This application of ultrasound imaging is not covered in this book; suggested readings are indicated at the end of Chapter 4.

Radionuclide Techniques/Positron Emission Tomography

Radionuclide perfusion imaging techniques with thallium or sestamibi immediately after exercise and at rest after redistribution are well-validated techniques for evaluation of coronary artery disease patients (Fig. 7–18). These techniques also can be performed using dipyridamole to induce heterogeneity in blood flow or with dobutamine to induce ischemia. Compared with stress echocardiography, radionuclide techniques have the advantage that image quality is less dependent on each patient's body habitus, although attenuation due to breast tissue may be a problem in women. Disadvantages of radionuclide techniques include a higher cost, it is less easily performed at the bedside, and it uses ionizing radiation (albeit a

FIGURE 7–18. Exercise stress dual-isotope radionuclide study; resting images were acquired with 201-thallium and exercise images with Tc-Sestamibi. Three views are shown. At the top the vertical long-axis (VLA) images from the septum to lateral wall are shown with the stress images on the top and the rest images on the bottom. In the middle, horizontal long-axis (HLA) images are shown from posterior to anterior. At the bottom, short-axis (SA) images from apex to base are displayed. On the exercise images, there is an inferior wall perfusion defect starting in the apical slice on the short-axis view and extending to the midcavity and basal slices. On the rest images, there is complete redistribution consistent with ischemia without prior infarction in the inferior wall. (See Color Plate 6, p. 274.) (Courtesy of James H. Caldwell, Jr., MD.)

low dose). Technical factors are important with both techniques, and data quality at a particular institution depends in part on experience.

Positron emission tomography (PET) combines physiologic and anatomic data and theoretically allows assessment of myocardial metabolism and perfusion. This technique is not widely available clinically, although research applications are considerable.

Coronary Angiography

Coronary angiography remains the standard of reference for evaluation of coronary artery disease. Cinefluoroscopic films of coronary anatomy in multiple views allow detailed assessment of both proximal and distal coronary anatomy.

Clinical Utility

Diagnosis of Coronary Artery Disease

Stress echocardiography is used for the diagnosis of significant coronary artery disease. The accuracy of stress echocardiography is highly dependent on image quality, specifically endocardial definition, with most investigators reporting success rates for obtaining diagnostic images after treadmill exercise of 85% to 100%. The success rate for image acquisition and the quality of the images obtained tend to be greater with supine exercise (in which the patient can be positioned optimally) and with pharmacologic stress (which has the added advantage of little increase in respiratory interference).

Compared with coronary angiography, with significant disease defined as 50% narrowing of an epicardial coronary artery, exercise echocardiography has an overall sensitivity of 74% to 97% and a specificity of 64% to 100% for diagnosing the presence of coronary artery disease (see Table 7–4). Sensitivity is highest for multivessel disease (>90%) and lowest for single-vessel disease (60% to 80%) in these studies. In comparison, exercise electrocardiography had a much lower sensitivity at 51% to 63% and specificity at 62% to 74%, while exercise thallium-201 perfusion imaging tended to have an accuracy similar to echocardiography, with a sensitivity of 61% to 94% and a specificity of 81%.

Extent and Location of Ischemic Areas

When image quality is adequate, stress echocardiography also allows accurate evaluation of the location and extent of the area of ischemic myocardium. By integrating data from multiple views, a reasonable estimate of the lo-

cation of significant coronary lesions can be made. Echocardiographic estimates of which and how many coronary arteries are affected correlate well with angiographic findings.

Prognostic Implications

The relationship between stress echocardiographic results and clinical outcome has been evaluated in several studies. Exercise echocardiography in patients after myocardial infarction predicts subsequent cardiac events with a positive predictive value of 63% to 80% and a negative predictive value of 78% to 95%. In patients with suspected coronary artery disease, the presence of an inducible wall motion abnormality predicts cardiac events (myocardial infarction, revascularization, death) over the subsequent 12 months with a sensitivity of 45% (positive predictive value of only 34%) but a specificity of 86% (negative predictive value of 91%). In patients undergoing noncardiac vascular surgery, dobutamine stress echocardiography is 100% sensitive and 69% specific for prediction of perioperative unstable angina, myocardial infarction, or death. However, the perioperative cardiac event rate is low, so a positive dobutamine stress echocardiogram has a predictive value of only 19%. Thus, this test is most helpful when results are *normal,* indicating a low likelihood of a perioperative event (negative predictive value of 100%). Further studies on the relationship between stress echocardiography and clinical outcome are needed.

MYOCARDIAL INFARCTION

Basic Principles

Myocardial infarction is irreversible injury to the myocardium due to prolonged ischemia, usually secondary to acute thrombotic occlusion of an epicardial coronary artery at the site of an atherosclerotic plaque. Initially, the affected myocardium becomes akinetic, with normal wall thickness. Over time (4 to 6 weeks), the involved myocardial segments show thinning of the wall and increased echogenicity. A transmural infarction (>50% of wall thickness pathologically, Q waves on ECG clinically) results in a definite area of akinesis and wall thinning. A nontransmural infarction (<50% wall thickness pathologically, no Q waves on ECG) may result in a lesser degree of wall thinning and in hypokinesis rather than akinesis.

Since ischemic myocardium also is akinetic in a patient with chest pain, echocardiography cannot distinguish acute infarction from ongoing ischemia. Furthermore, with prolonged ischemia or with successful reperfusion therapy for acute myocardial infarction, a phenomenon called *stunned myocardium* may be seen, where the wall motion abnormality persists for 24 to 72 hours even though irreversible damage has not occurred. Some investigators also propose that prolonged persistence of wall motion abnormalities that can be reversed by reperfusion can occur—termed *hibernating myocardium.* Echocardiographic imaging cannot distinguish between these conditions since it shows the regional myocardial function at the time imaging is performed. The converse of this principle also should be kept in mind. Normal wall motion implies that there is no ischemia *at the time* the images were acquired. Thus normal wall

motion *between* episodes of chest pain does not exclude a diagnosis of unstable angina.

Echocardiographic Imaging

The myocardial segments affected and the echocardiographic views for assessment of myocardial infarction are the same as described for myocardial ischemia.

An occlusion of the left anterior descending artery results in akinesis of the anterior septum, anterior free wall, and apex (Fig. 7–19). Imaging in parasternal long- and short-axis views and in apical views demonstrates these segmental wall motion abnormalities. In the acute setting (Fig. 7–20), the unaffected walls may be hyperkinetic. Overall left ventricular systolic function typically is moderately depressed with

FIGURE 7–19. Old anterior myocardial infarction with thinning and increased echogenicity of the distal septum *(arrows)* seen in the parasternal long-axis view *(left top)* and short-axis views at the mid–left ventricular level *(right top).* With this mid–left anterior descending artery occlusion, the basal septum *(left bottom)* is normal.

FIGURE 7–21. M-mode recording of an old anterior myocardial infarction with thinning and increased echogenicity of the septum *(above)*. The left ventricular outflow velocity curve shows a reduced antegrade velocity consistent with a reduced stroke volume.

FIGURE 7–20. Acute anterior myocardial infarction seen in an apical four-chamber view in diastole *(top)* and systole *(bottom)*. The apical septum is akinetic *(arrows)*, although the myocardium is not yet thinned and scarred.

an average ejection fraction of 41% ± 11% after an unreperfused anterior myocardial infarction due to a proximal left anterior descending artery occlusion (Fig. 7–21).

Occlusion of the posterior descending artery results in an inferior myocardial infarction with akinesis of the inferior septum, the inferior free wall, and (to a variable extent) the posterior wall (Fig. 7–22). Parasternal and apical views again are used. The subcostal approach may be particularly helpful in patients with poor image quality from parasternal and apical windows. Typically, overall left ventricular systolic func-

tion is only mildly depressed, with an average postinfarction ejection fraction of 53% ± 10% after an unreperfused inferior infarction. With inferior infarction, the echocardiographer also should evaluate for possible concurrent right ventricular infarction.

Occlusion of the circumflex artery, resulting in a lateral myocardial infarction, is less common and often is electrocardiographically "silent." Akinesis of the lateral and posterior walls is seen, with a mild to moderately depressed ejection fraction depending on the extent of myocardium supplied by the circumflex artery in that individual.

Note that these "classic" patterns of wall motion abnormalities will vary with individual variation in coronary anatomy and the location of the occlusion along the length of the coronary artery. Also, these patterns will be altered by the use of reperfusion therapy.

FIGURE 7–22. Mitral regurgitation due to papillary muscle dysfunction after inferior myocardial infarction. (See Color Plate 6, p. 274.)

In acute myocardial infarction, diastolic function, as well as systolic function, is abnormal. Acutely, early diastolic relaxation is impaired, with a reduced E velocity on the left ventricular inflow curve. With successful reperfusion, this pattern of diastolic filling tends to normalize over the subsequent 1 to 2 weeks. With large infarctions that are not reperfused, the E velocity also increases after infarction; however, in this situation, this change in inflow velocity reflects an increased left ventricular end-diastolic pressure rather than "normalization" of the left ventricular filling pattern. In patients with moderate to severely reduced systolic function, the E/A ratio correlates positively with left ventricular end-diastolic and left atrial pressures (i.e., a higher E/A ratio indicates a higher left ventricular end-diastolic pressure) due to the overriding effect of left atrial pressure on the early diastolic filling velocity. It is most helpful to interpret patterns of left ventricular diastolic filling in an individual patient over time with side-by-side comparisons of the echocardiographic findings and integration with other clinical data. Comparisons between patients are limited by the numerous other factors that affect the pattern of left ventricular inflow (see Chap. 6).

Limitations/Alternate Approaches

As for other applications of echocardiography, image quality can be a limiting factor in patients with poor ultrasound tissue penetra-tion. However, with optimal patient positioning, an experienced sonographer, and a state-of-the-art instrument, diagnostic images can be obtained in nearly all patients.

The standard approach to the diagnosis of acute myocardial infarction includes two of the following three findings: (1) a typical clinical presentation, (2) diagnostic ECG changes, and (3) a consistent pattern of elevation in serum cardiac enzyme levels. When typical findings of acute myocardial infarction are present, the diagnosis rarely is in doubt. Unfortunately, many patients have an atypical clinical presentation, and ECG changes may be nondiagnostic. In these equivocal cases or when a rapid diagnosis is needed for clinical management, prompt echocardiographic imaging may be helpful.

Radionuclide imaging for acute myocardial infarction is based on the principle of detection of areas of hypoperfusion. The finding of a normal radionuclide perfusion pattern in patients presenting with chest pain has a high specificity for the absence of acute myocardial infarction. Sensitivity for acute infarction is lower since an old infarction cannot be distinguished from an acute infarction with this approach.

Coronary angiography, of course, remains the standard of reference for identification of an occluded coronary artery. Concurrent left ventriculography can identify wall motion abnormalities using a right anterior oblique view, showing the anterior wall, apex, and inferior wall in silhouette (Fig. 7–23), and a left anterior oblique view to evaluate the lateral wall (which is superimposed on the ventricular chamber in the right anterior oblique view).

Clinical Utility

Diagnosis of Acute Myocardial Infarction in the Emergency Department

In a patient presenting to the emergency department with chest pain, echocardiographic assessment of global and segmental wall motion can be helpful in clinical decision making. The presence of a segmental wall motion abnormality indicates that coronary artery disease is present—either an acute infarction, ischemia, or an old infarction. Associated hyperkinesis of uninvolved segments suggests an acute event. Some physicians use contrast echocardiography to evaluate myocardial perfusion in the emergency department, but this approach largely is limited to research centers.

Normal wall motion *during pain* is consistent with a very low likelihood of acute myocardial infarction, so it may be possible to triage the patient to a noncoronary care unit bed depending on the clinical setting. Normal wall motion once pain has resolved is less diagnostic, since unstable angina may be present with wall motion abnormalities seen only *during* episodes of ischemia.

Global left ventricular systolic dysfunction also is an important prognostic sign, indicating significant cardiac disease and the need for further evaluation.

Some clinical centers now use exercise echocardiography in the early evaluation of patients presenting with chest pain to allow triage to further inpatient versus outpatient evaluation. Patients with a diagnostic ECG, previous history of coronary disease, or unstable hemodynamics receive prompt standard treatment. In the remainder, after exclusion of myocardial infarction by serial enzyme level measurement, stress testing is performed to identify those with coronary artery disease. Other centers use radionu-clide imaging techniques in the chest pain evaluation unit (see Suggested Readings 20 and 21).

Evaluation of Interventional Therapy for Acute Myocardial Infarction

In a patient with a history suggestive of acute myocardial infarction but a nondiagnostic ECG, a definite segmental wall motion abnormality on echocardiography may significantly alter decisions regarding reperfusion therapy or may prompt emergency coronary angiography, depending on the specific clinical situation.

In a patient with a definite myocardial infarction by clinical and ECG criteria, echocardiography allows assessment of the location and extent of "myocardium at risk." Once reperfusion therapy has been initiated, echocardiography can be used to assess its effects, although the several-day time lag between successful reperfusion and normalization of wall motion ("stunned" myocardium) makes this evaluation most meaningful before hospital discharge or at outpatient follow-up. However, echocardiography can be helpful in identification of recurrent ischemia in patients with recurrent chest pain by identification of wall motion abnormalities in regions that previously were normal.

At long-term follow-up after myocardial infarction, echocardiography allows assessment of global ventricular function and long-term ventricular dilation due to "infarct expansion."

Complications of Myocardial Infarction

Echocardiography is the procedure of choice for initial evaluation of the post–myocardial infarction patient with a new systolic murmur. Most commonly, the etiology of the murmur is *mitral regurgitation* due to either papillary muscle dysfunction, abnormal wall motion of the segment underlying a papillary muscle, or papillary muscle rupture. The presence and severity of mitral regurgitation are evaluated using Doppler techniques (see Chap. 11), and the etiology is inferred from two-dimensional (2D) imaging. Partial or complete rupture of the papillary muscle is a catastrophic complication that can be recognized as a flail leaflet with an attached mass (the papillary muscle head) that prolapses into the left atrium in systole (Fig. 7–24). Transesophageal imaging is indicated when this diagnosis is suspected unless the diagnosis is clear on transthoracic images.

Another cause of a new systolic murmur after myocardial infarction is a *ventricular septal*

FIGURE 7–23. Left ventricular angiography with diastolic *(top)* and systolic *(bottom)* frames showing an akinetic apex *(between arrows)* due to myocardial infarction.

FIGURE 7–24. On a transesophageal image in a two-chamber orientation, papillary muscle (PM) rupture is seen with an abrupt discontinuity in the anterolateral papillary muscle. In systole, the papillary muscle head prolapsed into the left atrium in association with severe mitral regurgitation. The patient underwent emergency mitral valve repair. MV = mitral valve.

defect due to necrosis and rupture of a focal area of the interventricular septum (Figs. 7–25 and 7–26). Identification of the rupture site may be difficult with 2D imaging, especially since this complication tends to occur with *small* infarcts so that the wall motion abnormality may be subtle. Evaluation with Doppler ultrasound establishes the diagnosis, with a high-velocity left-to-right systolic jet recorded with continuous-wave Doppler ultrasound and systolic turbulence on the right ventricular side of the septum recorded with conventional pulsed Doppler or color flow imaging.

When *ventricular rupture* occurs in the free wall of the left ventricle (instead of in the septum), mortality is extremely high due to extravasation of blood into the pericardial space and acute pericardial tamponade. However, some patients have a temporary respite due to containment of the rupture by pericardial adhesions or by thrombosis at the rupture site. In these patients, echocardiography may establish the diagnosis, prompting emergency surgery (Fig. 7–27). Echocardiographic clues of ventricular rupture (in the appropriate clinical setting) include a diffuse or localized pericardial effusion and a discrete segmental wall motion abnormality. Occasionally, the site of rupture can be visualized on 2D imaging, and rarely, flow

FIGURE 7–25. Color flow image showing left-to-right flow across an apical ventricular septal defect (VSD) after myocardial infarction *(above)*. Continuous-wave Doppler *(below)* shows high-velocity left-to-right flow in systole with lower-velocity left-to-right flow in diastole across the defect. (See Color Plate 7, p. 274.)

from the ventricle into the pericardial space can be demonstrated with Doppler techniques.

A chronic, contained ventricular rupture is called a *pseudoaneurysm.* A left ventricular pseudoaneurysm has a wall composed of pericardium (no myocardial fibers). Characteristic features are a narrow "neck" at the site of rupture with an abrupt transition from normal myocardium to the aneurysm, and a ratio of the diameter at the "neck" to the maximum diameter of the aneurysm of <0.5 (Fig. 7–28). Typically, the pseudoaneurysm is partially filled with thrombus. Often, flow in and out of the pseudoaneurysm is seen, and clinically, a corresponding apical murmur may be appreciated on auscultation. While long-term survival has

FIGURE 7–26. Postmyocardial infarction ventricular septal defect seen on left ventriculography in a left anterior oblique image plane. There is rapid appearance of contrast in the right ventricle after injection into the left ventricle.

been described occasionally in patients with a pseudoaneurysm, correct echocardiographic diagnosis is essential. Surgical repair usually is recommended given a high likelihood of spontaneous rupture.

A *pericardial effusion* also can be seen after myocardial infarction as a nonspecific response to transmural infarction. This effusion may be asymptomatic or may be associated with clinical symptoms (chest pain) and signs (ECG changes) of acute pericarditis. While usually benign, tamponade physiology can occur.

Another complication of acute myocardial infarction for which echocardiography is the diagnostic procedure of choice is *right ventricular infarction*. Clinical diagnosis requires a high level of suspicion. Other clinical tests, such as ST-segment elevation in right-sided ECG leads, are not as sensitive or specific as echocardiography. Right ventricular infarction most often is associated with an inferior left ventricular infarct. Echocardiographic findings include right ventricular hypokinesis or akinesis with variable degrees of right ventricular dilation. This diagnosis significantly changes the clinical management of these patients (i.e., low cardiac output is treated with volume infusions rather than with afterload reduction or inotropic agents).

Longer-term complications of acute myocardial infarction include aneurysm formation, left ventricular thrombi, and the sequelae of the irreversible decrease in left ventricular systolic function. A *left ventricular aneurysm* is defined echocardiographically as a dyskinetic region with a diastolic contour abnormality (Fig. 7–29). Apical aneurysms are most common,

FIGURE 7–27. Transgastric short-axis image showing acute left ventricular rupture after myocardial infarction. There in an abrupt discontinuity in the left ventricular wall *(arrows)* with flow in and out of a thrombus lined section of the pericardium. Rapid diagnosis allowed surgical intervention in this patient.

but inferobasal aneurysms also may be seen. Note that a "true" left ventricular aneurysm, unlike a "false" or pseudoaneurysm, is lined by (thinned) myocardium. There is a smooth transition from normal myocardium to the thinned area with an obtuse angle between the aneurysm and body of the left ventricle. The ratio of the diameter of the junction between the aneurysm and the remainder of the left ventri-

FIGURE 7–28. Apical long-axis view showing a chronic basal aneurysm filled with thrombus with a narrow neck *(left)* consistent with a pseudoaneurysm (pAn). Angiography (oriented to match the apical long-axis view) shows a similar appearance *(right)*.

FIGURE 7–29. Apical dilation and systolic dyskinesis *(above left)* consistent with an apical aneurysm. The pattern of left ventricular inflow *(above right)* shows a prominent E velocity consistent with an elevated left ventricular end-diastolic pressure. The mitral regurgitant velocity curve in this patient *(below right)* shows a reduced dP/dt.

cle to the maximum aneurysm diameter is >0.5 (see Fig. 9–16).

Left ventricular thrombi form in regions of stasis of blood flow, such as in an apical aneurysm or overlying an area of akinesis in other regions of the left ventricle. Evidence of severely reduced overall ventricular function, an aneurysm, an akinetic area, and the appearance of a spontaneous contrast effect in the left ventricle all increase the likelihood of left ventricular thrombus formation. Only rarely (as in hypereosinophilic syndrome) do ventricular thrombi occur in the absence of an underlying wall motion abnormality.

A thrombus is identified as an area of increased echogenicity within the ventricular chamber, distinct from the endocardium. Often, the thrombus protrudes into the chamber with a convex contour, but laminated thrombus with a concave contour following the endocardial curve also can be seen. Care is needed to distinguish a thrombus from prominent apical trabeculation with a false tendon or "web" traversing the apex of the left ventricular chamber.

Diagnosis of apical thrombi is enhanced by using a 5-MHz transducer (improved near-field resolution), sliding the transducer laterally from the apical window and then angulating medially and superiorly to obtain a short-axis view of the apex. These procedures allow clear definition of the apical endocardium in most individuals. However, if images are suboptimal, appropriate interpretation should indicate that a thrombus "cannot be excluded," especially if the patient is at high risk of left ventricular thrombus formation. Note that transesophageal imaging is rarely helpful for this diagnosis because the apex often cannot be visualized and is in the far field of the image plane.

END-STAGE ISCHEMIC CARDIAC DISEASE

Differentiation from Other Causes of Left Ventricular Systolic Dysfunction (Table 7–6)

The diagnosis of coronary artery disease is clear in patients with definite segmental wall motion abnormalities that correspond to the distribution of coronary blood flow. In end-stage ischemic disease, repeated transmural and subendocardial infarctions result in a diffuse pattern of abnormal wall thickening and endocardial motion. Thus, when global systolic dysfunction is present, it may be difficult to differentiate between end-stage ischemic disease and systolic dysfunction due to long-standing valvular disease or a dilated cardiomyopathy (Fig. 7–30).

Echocardiographic Approach

Several features of the echocardiographic examination help in this differentiation. The segmental pattern of left ventricular wall motion is examined carefully in each tomographic plane. While patients with a dilated cardiomyopathy may have a somewhat asymmetric pattern of wall motion with relative preservation at the ventricular base, definite areas of akinesis or wall thinning suggest ischemic disease. The degree of reduction in overall ventricular function (ejection fraction) is important in patient management but does not assist in determining the etiology of disease.

Right ventricular size and systolic function are normal in patients with ischemic disease unless there has been a previous right ventricular infarction. Dilated cardiomyopathy occasionally affects the two ventricles in differing degrees but most often results in a symmetric pattern of right and left ventricular dilation and reduced systolic function.

TABLE 7–6	Differentiation of Left Ventricular Systolic Dysfunction Due to End-Stage Ischemic Disease from Dilated Cardiomyopathy or Chronic Valvular Disease		
Findings	**End-Stage Ischemic Disease**	**Dilated Cardiomyopathy**	**Chronic Valvular Disease**
Left ventricular ejection fraction	Moderate to severely depressed	Moderate to severely depressed	Moderate to severely depressed
Segmental wall motion abnormalities	May be present	Absent	Absent
Right ventricular systolic function	Normal	Decreased	Variable
Pulmonary artery pressures	Elevated	Elevated	Elevated
Mitral regurgitation	Moderate	Moderate	Moderate to severe
Aortic regurgitation	Not significant	Not significant	Moderate to severe

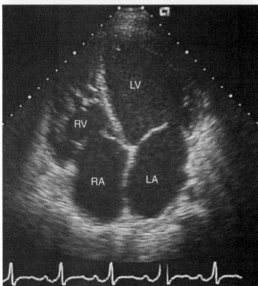

FIGURE 7–30. End-stage ischemic heart disease *(above)* and a dilated cardiomyopathy *(below)* often appear similar on 2D echocardiography. Note that the patient with ischemic disease has normal right ventricular size and systolic function.

Mitral valve regurgitation typically accompanies both dilated cardiomyopathy and end-stage ischemic disease due to one of several mechanisms, including mitral annular dilation, reduced papillary muscle systolic function, or malalignment of the papillary muscles. Left ventricular dilation and systolic dysfunction *due to* chronic mitral regurgitation, in contrast to mitral regurgitation due to ventricular dilation and dysfunction, usually are associated with anatomic abnormalities of the mitral leaflets themselves (e.g., myxomatous or rheumatic disease).

Pulmonary artery pressures are elevated to variable degrees in patients with left ventricular dysfunction of any etiology, due to chronic elevation in left ventricular end-diastolic pressure. Pulmonary pressures can be estimated from the tricuspid regurgitant jet velocity or from the pulmonary artery systolic velocity curve as described in Chapter 5.

Mild degrees of tricuspid valve regurgitation are common in ischemic disease, but moderate or severe regurgitation usually is a response to chronic pulmonary hypertension or chronic right ventricular dilation and systolic dysfunction.

Note that aortic regurgitation is *not* a consequence of left ventricular dilation or systolic dysfunction. Left ventricular dilation typically does not result in an increase in the diameter of the aortic annulus or adjacent outflow tract. The finding of moderate or severe aortic regurgitation implies primary valvular disease or aortic root dilation.

Left ventricular thrombi may be present with severe left ventricular dysfunction of any etiology. The observation of reduced systolic function should prompt a search for apical thrombi, but this finding does not help in the differential diagnosis.

Limitations/Alternate Approaches

If a diagnosis of end-stage ischemic disease versus a primary cardiomyopathy would alter patient management, coronary angiography may be needed for a definitive diagnosis, to document the exact site and severity of coronary lesions, and to assess the distal vessel anatomy.

SUGGESTED READING

General

1. Armstrong VF, Pellikka PA, Ryan T, et al: Stress echocardiography: Recommendations for performance and interpretation of stress echocardiography. *J Am Soc Echocardiogr* 11:97–104, 1998.
    This position paper from the American Society of Echocardiography summarizes the optimal methods of performing pharmacologic and stress echocardiography. Details include the imaging technique, required equipment, personnel, and analysis techniques. Contraindications, accuracy, and prognostic implications also are summarized.

Exercise Echocardiography

2. Marcovitz PA: Exercise echocardiography: Stress testing in the initial diagnosis of coronary artery disease and in patients with prior revascularization or myocardial infarction. *In* Otto CM (ed): The Practice of Clini-

cal Echocardiography. Philadelphia, WB Saunders, 1997, pp. 217–236.

The clinical application of exercise echocardiography is discussed in detail including necessary equipment and personnel, interpretation of stress images, a comparison of treadmill versus bicycle exercise testing, and the relative advantages and disadvantages of exercise echocardiography compared to other diagnostic approaches. Topics include the utility of exercise echocardiography for detection of coronary artery disease, and evaluation after revascularization or acute myocardial infarction. The value of exercise echocardiography for detection of coronary artery disease in women (sensitivity 86% to 88%, specificity 84% to 86%) is emphasized. 84 references.

3. Olmos LI, Dakik J, Gordon R, Dunn JK, Verani MS, Quinones MA, Zoghbi WA: Long-term prognostic value of exercise echocardiography compared with exercise ^{201}Tl, ECG, and clinical variables in patients evaluated for coronary artery disease. *Circulation* 98: 2679–2686, 1998.

In 225 patients undergoing exercise echocardiographic and nuclear stress tests, cardiac events at a mean follow-up of 3.7 years were predicted by induction of ischemia on echocardiography (odds ratio 4.1, 95% confidence interval 1.32 to 12.79) or a perfusion defect on [201]thallium (odds ratio 4.93, 95% confidence interval 1.72 to 14.08). The authors conclude that echocardiographic and radionuclide stress studies provide comparable prognostic data.

4. Marwick TH, Mehta R, Arheart K, Lauer MS: Use of exercise echocardiography for prognostic evaluation of patients with known or suspected coronary artery disease. *J Am Coll Cardiol* 30:83–90, 1997.

In 463 patients undergoing exercise echocardiography, ischemia was defined as an exercise-induced new or worsened wall motion abnormality on 2D echocardiography. Multivariate predictors of cardiac events or revascularization at 44 ± 11 months were the percent age-predicted maximal heart rate and ischemia (relative risk 5.06, 95% confidence interval [CI] 3.09 to 8.29, P < .001). Echocardiographic data provided incremental predictive value compared to clinical and exercise data alone.

5. Heupler S, Mehta R, Lobo A, et al: Prognostic implications of exercise echocardiography in women with known or suspected coronary artery disease. *J Am Coll Cardiol* 30:414–420, 1997.

In 508 women undergoing stress echocardiography, there was no evidence of ischemia in 81%, 13% had an new or worsened wall motion abnormality with exercise, and 6% had evidence of old myocardial infarction. At follow-up (41 ± 10 months), 7% had cardiac events including 17 cardiac deaths and 19 patients with myocardial infarction or revascularization for progressive symptoms. Independent predictors of outcome were known coronary artery disease and echocardiographic ischemia (odd ratio 4.3, 95% CI 2.1 to 8.7, P < .0001).

6. Kafka HF, Leach AJ, Fitzgibbon GM: Exercise echocardiography after coronary artery bypass surgery: Correlation with coronary angiography. *J Am Coll Cardiol* 25:1019–1023, 1994.

A total of 213 exercise echocardiographic studies were performed in 182 patients 2 weeks to 21 years after coronary artery bypass grafting for suspected recurrent ischemia. Compared to coronary angiography, exercise echocardiography had a positive predictive value of 71% for vascular compromise in one vascular territory and 98% for ischemic involving more than one coronary artery distribution. False-negative results were most likely with ischemia isolated to the posterolateral region of the left ventricle.

Dobutamine Stress Echocardiography

7. Marwick TH: Stress echocardiography with non-exercise techniques: Principles, protocols, interpretation, and clinical applications. *In* Otto CM (ed): The Practice of Clinical Echocardiography. Philadelphia, WB Saunders, 1997, pp. 237–266.

Concise summary of the principles, technical aspects, and clinical utility of pharmacologic stress echocardiography. Comprehensive tables summarize clinical studies evaluating the sensitivity and specificity of dobutamine stress, vasodilator stress, and atrial pacing stress echocardiography. 150 references.

8. Picano E, Mathias W Jr, Pingitore A, et al: Safety and tolerability of dobutamine-atropine stress echocardiography: A prospective, multicenter study. *Lancet* 344: 1190–1192, 1994.

In 2949 dobutamine-atropine stress echocardiographic studies performed at 24 experienced centers, there were 14 serious complications (1/240 tests) including 5 significant ventricular arrhythmias, 2 myocardial infarctions, 1 prolonged myocardial ischemia, and 5 cases of atropine-induced hallucinations. Minor complications occurred in 12% of cases and often precluded a diagnostic examination.

9. Mertes H, Sawada SG, Ryan T, et al: Symptoms, adverse effects, and complications associated with dobutamine stress echocardiography: Experience in 1118 patients. *Circulation* 88:15–19, 1993.

Complications of dobutamine stress echocardiography that required termination of the test protocol included noncardiac symptoms (nausea, anxiety, headache, tremor, urgency) in 3%, and angina pectoris in 19.3% (which was relieved by sublingual nitroglycerin or a short-acting beta blocker in all cases). Arrhythmias included premature ventricular contractions in 15%, premature atrial contractions in 8%, and nonsustained ventricular tachycardia in 40 (3.5%) patients. There were no deaths, myocardial infarctions, or episodes of sustained ventricular tachycardia.

10. Geleijnse ML, Fioretti PM, Roelandt JR: Methodology, feasibility, safety and diagnostic accuracy of dobutamine stress echocardiography. *J Am Coll Cardiol* 30:595–606, 1997.

This review summarizes the data from 2246 patients having dobutamine stress echocardiography at 28 different centers. The risk of ventricular fibrillation or myocardial infarction was ~1/2000 and there were no reported deaths. Dobutamine stress echocardiography was nondiagnostic in about 5% due to poor image quality and in 10% due to submaximal stress. In the remainder, the overall sensitivity was 80% with a specificity of 84% for detection of coronary artery disease.

Sensitivity was higher for three-vessel (92%) compared to two-vessel (86%) or one-vessel (74%) disease and was lowest for circumflex artery disease.

11. Poldermans D, Arnese M, Fioretti PM, et al: Improved cardiac risk stratification in major vascular surgery with dobutamine-atropine stress echocardiography. *J Am Coll Cardiol* 26:648–653, 1995.

    Dobutamine atropine stress echocardiography allows cardiac risk stratification in patients undergoing major vascular surgery. Stress testing is low yield in the one-third of patients with no clinical risk factors (angina, diabetes, Q- waves on ECG, symptomatic ventricular tachyarrhythmias, age >70 years) as the cardiac event rate is only 1% in this group. A resting wall motion abnormality on echocardiography is associated with an increased risk of perioperative events. In addition, inducible ischemia on dobutamine stress echocardiography has a 38% positive predictive value and a 100% negative predictive value for perioperative death, myocardial infarction, or angina. Risk can be further stratified based on the heart rate at which ischemia occurred; those with ischemia at a maximum heart rate ≤70% of age predicted are at higher risk (53% event rate) compared to those with ischemia at a heart rate >70% predicted (21% event rate).

12. Poldermans D, Arnese M, Fioretti PM, et al: Sustained prognostic value of dobutamine stress echocardiography for late cardiac events after major noncardiac vascular surgery. *Circulation* 95:53–58, 1997.

    The risk of cardiac events after major noncardiac vascular surgery (mean follow-up 19 ± 11 months) is increased in those with extensive (risk 6.5 times higher) or limited inducible ischemia (risk 2.9 times higher) on preoperative dobutamine stress echocardiography compared to those with no wall motion abnormalities. Risk also is increased (3.8 times) in those with a resting wall motion abnormality on echocardiography. See accompanying editorial by Bach and Eagle on pages 8 to 10 in the same issue of Circulation).

13. Bates JR, Sawada SG, Segar DS, et al: Evaluation using dobutamine stress echocardiography in patients with insulin-dependent diabetes mellitus before kidney and/or pancreas transplantation. *Am J Cardiol* 77: 175–179, 1996.

    An abnormal dobutamine stress echocardiographic study was associated with a cardiac event rate of 45% compared to an event rate of only 6% in those with a normal study (mean follow-up 1.1 ± 0.7 years).

Myocardial Infarction

14. Foster E, Cooper SG: Echocardiography in the coronary care unit: Management of acute myocardial infarction, detection of complications, and prognostic implications. *In* Otto CM (ed): The Practice of Clinical Echocardiography. Philadelphia, WB Saunders, 1997, pp. 195–216.

    This chapter summarizes the pathophysiologic correlates of the echocardiographic findings in acute myocardial infarction, the role of echocardiography in patient management, and the utility of echocardiography for detecting complications of acute myocardial infarction. 194 references.

15. Pearlman AS, Otto CM: Role of echocardiography in evaluating patients presenting to the emergency room with acute chest pain: Diagnosis and patient triage. *In* Otto CM (ed): The Practice of Clinical Echocardiography. Philadelphia, WB Saunders, 1997, pp. 179–194.

    Review of the potential utility of echocardiography for triage, risk stratification, and detection of other causes of chest pain in patients with suspected myocardial infarction. Clinical trials, practical aspects of data collection, and potential research applications are discussed. 79 references

16. Mohler ER 3rd, Ryan T, Segar DS, et al: Clinical utility of troponin T levels and echocardiography in the emergency department. *Am Heart J* 135:253–260. 1998.

    The combination of cardiac troponin T levels and a new wall motion abnormality on echocardiography performed in the emergency department had a positive predictive value of 84% and a negative predictive value of 90% for adverse cardiac events in 100 patients admitted for chest discomfort.

17. Fleishmann KE, Goldman L, Robiolio PA, et al: Echocardiographic correlates of survival in patients with chest pain. *J Am Coll Cardiol* 23:1390–1396, 1994.

    In 513 presenting to the emergency department with chest pain, 92% were admitted to the hospital, 48% had ischemic changes on ECG, 46% had a history of coronary artery disease, and 21% suffered an acute myocardial infarction. At 28$^1/_2$-month follow-up 20% had died (57% cardiovascular) with echocardiographic predictors of overall mortality, and death from cardiovascular causes being severe left ventricular systolic dysfunction and moderate or severe mitral regurgitation (even when adjusted for clinical and ECG variables).

18. Otto CM, Stratton JR, Maynard C, et al: Echocardiographic evaluation of segmental wall motion early and late after thrombolytic therapy in acute myocardial infarction: The Western Washington Tissue Plasminogen Activator Emergency Room Trial. *Am J Cardiol* 65: 132–138, 1990.

    Concordance between infarct location by echocardiography and angiography was 81% (versus 76% for ECG) in 92 patients with acute myocardial infarction. Improvement in wall motion between the acute presentation and 3-month follow-up was seen only in subjects with reperfusion within 2 hours of symptom onset.

19. Gibler WV, Runyon JR, Levy RC, et al: A rapid diagnostic and treatment center for patients with chest pain in the emergency department. *Ann Emerg Med* 25:1–8, 1995.

    A protocol for rapid diagnosis in patients presenting to the emergency department with possible cardiac ischemia, no history of coronary artery disease, a nondiagnostic ECG, and stable hemodynamic is proposed. Serial testing for creatine kinase isoenzyme MB subunit (CK-MB) levels is performed with continuous ECG monitoring for 9 hours, followed by echocardiography and stress testing if the CK-MB level is not elevated. This approach allowed discharge home of 82% of patients with normal test results. Of those admitted after the 9-hour period, 34% had an acute myocardial infarction, unstable angina, or stable angina.

20. Kontos MC, Arrowood JA, Paulsen WH, Nixon JV: Early echocardiography can predict cardiac events in emergency department patients with chest pain. *Ann Emerg Med* 31:550–557, 1998.

Echocardiography performed within 4 hours of presentation for chest pain in 260 patients had a higher sensitivity (91%) than ECG (40%) for prediction of cardiac events (myocardial infarction or revascularization). Specificity of echocardiography (75%) was lower than ECG (94%), most likely related to the definition of an abnormal echocardiogram as a regional wall motion abnormality or an ejection fraction <40%.

21. Heller GV, Stowers SA, Hendel RC, et al: Clinical value of acute rest technetium-99m tetrofosmin tomographic myocardial perfusion imaging in patients with acute chest pain and nondiagnostic electrocardiogram. *J Am Coll Cardiol* 31:1011–1017, 1998.

In 357 patients with chest pain, Tc-99m tetrofosmin SPECT imaging was performed within 6 hours of symptoms. An abnormal resting perfusion study had a sensitivity of 90% and a specificity of 60% for detection of acute myocardial infarction. The negative predictive value of a normal perfusion scan was 99%, indicating that a normal study is associated with a very low cardiac event rate. The cost implications of using SPECT imaging in the emergency department are discussed.

Myocardial Viability

22. Lualdi JC, Douglas PS: Echocardiography for the assessment of myocardial viability. *J Am Soc Echocardiogr* 10:772–781, 1997.

Excellent review on the use of low-dose dobutamine stress echocardiography for assessment of myocardial viability. Other methods for assessing viability also are discussed.

23. Cigarroa CG, deFilippi CR, Brickner E, et al: Dobutamine stress echocardiography identifies hibernating myocardium and predicts recovery of left ventricular function after coronary revascularization. *Circulation* 88:430–436, 1993.

In 25 patients with multivessel coronary artery disease and depressed ventricular function, dobutamine stress echocardiography was performed preoperatively and after revascularization. After revascularization, ventricular function improved in 9 of 11 patients with contractile reserve (defined as improvement in wall thickening in two adjacent segments or greater than a 20% improvement in the regional wall thickening score) but in only 2 of 14 patients without contractile reserve.

24. Smart SC, Sawada S, Ryan T, et al: Low-dose dobutamine echocardiography detects reversible dysfunction after thrombolytic therapy of acute myocardial infarction. *Circulation* 88:405–415, 1993.

In 51 patients with dobutamine echocardiographic studies performed within 7 days and again 4 weeks after myocardial infarction, dobutamine-responsive wall motion had a specificity of 90% and a sensitivity of 86% for reversible myocardial dysfunction.

25. Arnese M, Corvel JH, Salustri A, et al: Prediction of improvement of regional left ventricular function after surgical revascularization: A comparison of low dose dobutamine echocardiography with 201 Tl singlephoton emission computed tomography. *Circulation* 91:2748–2752, 1995.

The sensitivity of wall motion with low-dose dobutamine for prediction of recovery of function after revascularization was 74% compared to 89% for 201-thallium poststress reinjection scintigraphy. However, the specificity of low dose dobutamine was 95% compared to 48% for 201-thallium SPECT imaging suggesting that the nuclear technique overestimates the probability of postoperative recovery.

26. Baer RM, Voth E, Deutsch HJ, et al: Assessment of viable myocardium by dobutamine transesophageal echocardiography and comparison with fluorine-18 fluorodeoxyglucose positron emission tomography. *J Am Coll Cardiol* 24:343–353, 1994.

Dobutamine stress echocardiography had a positive predictive value of 81% and a negative predictive value of 97% for assessment of myocardial viability, as defined by F-18 fluorodeoxyglucose uptake.

27. Meza JF, Kates MA, Barbee W, et al: Combination of dobutamine and myocardial contrast echocardiography to differentiate postischemic from infarcted myocardium. *J Am Coll Cardiol* 29:974–984, 1997.

The combination of contrast and dobutamine echocardiography increased the sensitivity (88%) for detection of myocardial viability in a canine model, but specificity was low (61%) even with a combined approach.

28. Qureshi U, Nagueh SF, Afridi I, et al: Dobutamine echocardiography and quantitative rest-redistribution 201Tl tomography in myocardial hibernation: Relation of contractile reserve to 201Tl uptake and comparative prediction of recovery of function. *Circulation* 95: 626–635, 1997.

In patients with stable coronary disease and resting regional dysfunction, a biphasic response on dobutamine echocardiography had only a 74% sensitivity, but an 89% specificity for recovery after revascularization. Qualitative thallium assessment had a high sensitivity (98%) with low specificity (27%), while quantitative thallium uptake had a 90% sensitivity and 56% specificity for recovery of myocardial function after revascularization.

Complications of Acute Myocardial Infarction

29. Come PC, Riley MF, Weintraub R, et al: Echocardiographic detection of complete and partial papillary muscle rupture during acute myocardial infarction. *Am J Cardiol* 56:787–789, 1985.

Mechanism and echocardiographic diagnosis of postmyocardial infarction mitral regurgitation are discussed.

30. Raitt MH, Kraft CD, Gardner CJ, et al: Subacute ventricular free wall rupture complicating myocardial infarction. *Am Heart J* 126:946–955, 1993.

Review of the literature and four case reports of left ventricular rupture after myocardial infarction emphasizing that this diagnosis may be made by echocardiography and can be successfully treated surgically. 73 references.

31. Kishon Y, Iqbal A, Oh JK, et al: Evolution of echocardiographic modalities in detection of post-myocardial infarction ventricular septal defect and papillary muscle rupture: Study of 62 patients. *Am Heart J* 126: 667–675, 1993.

   In 40 patients with a postmyocardial ventricular septal defect, 2D transthoracic echocardiography was diagnostic in only 68% but 95% were detected using Doppler plus 2D imaging. In 22 patients with papillary muscle rupture, the site of rupture was visualized in only 45%, but 100% had severe mitral regurgitation on Doppler examination.

32. Oliva PB, Hammill SC, Edwards WD: Cardiac rupture, a clinically predictable complication of acute myocardial infarction: Report of 70 cases with clinicopathologic correlations. *J Am Coll Cardiol* 22:720–726, 1993.

   Cardiac rupture should be suspected after myocardial infarction in the setting of pericarditis, repetitive emesis, restlessness and agitation, or if there is a deviation from the expected pattern of T-wave evolution on ECG. Prompt echocardiography can establish the diagnosis of cardiac rupture, allowing rapid intervention.

33. Visser CA, Kan G, Meltzer RS, et al: Incidence, timing, and prognostic value of left ventricular aneurysm formation after myocardial infarction: A prospective, serial echocardiographic study in 158 patients. *Am J Cardiol* 57:729–732, 1986.

   Left ventricular aneurysm formation was seen within 3 months in 22% of patients with nonreperfused myocardial infarctions—29 of 90 (32%) anterior and 6 of 68 (9%) posterior infarctions.

34. Asinger RW, Mikell FL, Elsperger J, Hodges M: Incidence of left ventricular thrombosis after acute transmural myocardial infarction. *N Engl J Med* 305:297–302, 1981.

   In the prethrombolytic era, the incidence of apical thrombus detectable by 2D echocardiography was 0 of 35 inferior infarctions and 12 of 35 (34%) anterior infarctions. Thrombi occurred only in areas of akinesis or dyskinesis.

35. Kinch JW, Ryan TJ: Right ventricular infarction. *N Engl J Med* 330:1211–1217, 1994.

   A concise and well-written review of the clinical presentation, diagnosis, and management of right ventricular infarction. The echocardiographic approach is emphasized and compared with ECG and hemodynamic and radionuclide findings. 78 references.

Clinical Outcome after Myocardial Infarction

36. Krivokapich J, Child JS, Gerber RS, et al: Prognostic usefulness of positive or negative exercise stress echocardiography for predicting coronary events in ensuing twelve months. *Am J Cardiol* 71:646–651, 1993.

   In 360 patients with suspected coronary artery disease (60% of whom had resting wall motion abnormalities on echocardiography), an inducible wall motion abnormality on exercise echocardiography predicted cardiac events (myocardial infarction, revascularization, or death) over 12 months of follow-up with a sensitivity of 45% and a specificity of 86%. Patients unable to reach an appropriate stress level had a high rate of cardiac events even when the echocardiogram was nondiagnostic (17 of 27 patients).

37. St. John Sutton M, Pfeifer MA, Happert T, et al: Quantitative two-dimensional echocardiographic measurements are major predictors of adverse cardiovascular events after acute myocardial infarction. *Circulation* 89:68–75, 1994.

   In 512 patients with echocardiograms 11 days and 1 year after myocardial infarction, baseline left ventricular end-systolic area and percent change in area were strong predictors of cardiac death and cardiac events. Patients treated with captopril had smaller left ventricular areas at 1 year with a greater percent change in cavity area in the captopril group and a lower rate of adverse outcomes (risk reduction 35%). These data suggest that left ventricular enlargement and function after myocardial infarction are predictors of outcome and that prevention of left ventricular enlargement, as assessed by echocardiography, improves clinical outcome.

38. Greco CA, Salustri A, Seccareccia F, et al: Prognostic value of dobutamine echocardiography early after uncomplicated acute myocardial infarction: A comparison with exercise electrocardiography. *J Am Coll Cardiol* 29:261–267, 1997.

   An abnormal predischarge dobutamine stress echocardiographic study after myocardial infarction was associated with a relative risk of 5.5 (95% CI 1.14 to 23.16) for cardiac death and myocardial infarction at follow-up (mean 17 ± 13 months). Dobutamine stress echocardiography was an independent predictor of outcome on multivariate analysis when other clinical and exercise variables were included in the analysis.

39. Sicari R, Picano E, Landi P, et al: Prognostic value of dobutamine-atropine stress echocardiography early after acute myocardial infarction. *J Am Coll Cardiol* 29:254–260, 1997.

   Dobutamine atropine stress echocardiography was performed an average of 12 days after myocardial infarction in 778 patients. Evidence of myocardial viability in regions with abnormal resting wall motion was associated with unstable angina over a follow-up interval of 9 ± 7 months, whereas inducible ischemia was predictive of cardiac-related death.

Direct Visualization of Coronary Anatomy

40. Petrovic O, Eisner GB, Wilensky RL, et al: Transthoracic echocardiography detection of coronary atherosclerosis. *Am J Cardiol* 77:569–574, 1996.

   A modified short-axis view using a broad-band (3- to 5-MHz) transducer can be used to identify the left main and proximal left anterior descending artery and the proximal right coronary artery on transthoracic imaging. Analysis of segmental regions of the coronary and wall thickness measurements allowed detection of coronary atherosclerosis. Improvements in image quality may allow improved direct evaluation of coronary anatomy using ultrasound techniques.

The Cardiomyopathies, Hypertensive Heart Disease, Post-Cardiac-Transplant Patient, and Pulmonary Heart Disease

8

DILATED CARDIOMYOPATHY
  Basic Principles
  Echocardiographic Approach
  Limitations/Technical Considerations
  Clinical Utility
  Alternate Approaches
HYPERTROPHIC CARDIOMYOPATHY
  Basic Principles
  Echocardiographic Approach
    Left Ventricular Asymmetric Hypertrophy
    Left Ventricular Diastolic Function
    Dynamic Outflow Tract Obstruction
    Mitral Valve Abnormalities
  Limitations/Technical Considerations
  Clinical Utility
    Diagnosis and Screening
    Evaluation of Medical Therapy
    Surgical Therapy
  Alternate Approaches
RESTRICTIVE CARDIOMYOPATHY
  Basic Principles
  Echocardiographic Approach
  Limitations/Technical Considerations
  Clinical Utility
  Alternate Approaches
HYPERTENSIVE HEART DISEASE
  Basic Principles
  Echocardiographic Approach
    Ventricular Hypertrophy
    Diastolic Function
    Systolic Function
    Other Echocardiographic Findings

Limitations/Technical Considerations
Clinical Utility
  Diagnosis and Prognosis
  Choices of Medical Therapy
  Efficacy of Medical Therapy
  Evaluation of Heart Failure Symptoms in a
    Patient with Hypertension
Alternate Approaches
EVALUATION OF THE POST-CARDIAC-TRANSPLANT
PATIENT
  Basic Principles
  Echocardiographic Approach
    Normal Findings after Cardiac Transplantation
    Evaluation of Abnormal Findings
    Echocardiographic Diagnosis of Transplant
      Rejection
    Echocardiographic Diagnosis of Transplant
      Coronary Artery Disease
  Limitations/Technical Considerations/Alternate
    Approaches
PULMONARY HEART DISEASE
  Chronic versus Acute Pulmonary Disease
  Echocardiographic Approach
    Pulmonary Pressures
    Right Ventricular Pressure Overload
    Secondary Tricuspid Regurgitation
  Limitations/Technical Considerations
  Clinical Utility
  Alternate Approaches
SUGGESTED READING

Cardiomyopathy is defined as a primary disease of the myocardium, excluding myocardial dysfunction due to ischemia or chronic valvular disease. There are several possible approaches to classification of cardiomyopathies, such as etiology or anatomy, but a physiologic classification is most useful clinically. The three basic physiologic categories of cardiomyopathy are dilated, hypertrophic, and restrictive. The disease process in an individual patient may correspond closely with one of these physiologic categories; however, overlap between these categories (particularly between dilated and restrictive) can occur. Echocardiographic evaluation focuses on confirming the diagnosis and type of cardiomyopathy present and on defining the physiologic consequences of the disease process in that individual (Table 8–1).

TABLE 8–1	Typical Features of the Three Physiologic Types of Cardiomyopathy		
	Dilated	**Hypertrophic**	**Restrictive**
LV systolic function	Moderately to severely ↓	Normal	Normal
LV diastolic function	May be abnormal	Abnormal	Abnormal
LV hypertrophy	↑ LV mass due to left ventricular dilation with normal wall thickness	Asymmetric LV hypertrophy	Concenric LV hypertrophy
Chamber dilation	All four chambers	Left and right atrial dilation if mitral regurgitation is present	Left and right atrial dilation
Outflow tract obstruction	Absent	Dynamic LV outflow tract obstruction may be present	Absent
Left ventricular end-diastolic pressure	Elevated	Elevated	Elevated
Pulmonary artery pressures	Elevated	Elevated	Elevated

LV = Left ventricular; ↓ = decreased; ↑ = increased.

While hypertensive and pulmonary heart disease, strictly speaking, are not cardiomyopathies, they are included in this chapter because their clinical and echocardiographic presentation may mimic a cardiomyopathy. In addition, evaluation of the post-cardiac-transplant patient is included.

DILATED CARDIOMYOPATHY

Basic Principles

Dilated cardiomyopathy is characterized by four-chamber enlargement with impaired systolic function of both ventricles. The list of possible etiologies is long and includes postviral, toxins (e.g., alcohol), parasitic diseases (e.g.,

TABLE 8–2	Examples of Potential Causes of Dilated Cardiomyopathy

Idiopathic

Toxins (alcohol, medications, cobalt, snake bites)

Metabolic (thiamine deficiency, acromegaly)

Peripartum

Infections (Chagas' disease, postviral)

Systemic diseases (e.g., immune-mediated injury)

Inherited disorders (Duchenne's muscular dystrophy, sickle cell anemia)

Chagas' disease), peripartum, and idiopathic (Table 8–2). The physiology of dilated cardiomyopathy is characterized predominantly by impaired contractility of the left ventricle with reduced cardiac output and elevated left ventricular end-diastolic pressure. Clinically, patients most often present with heart failure, with initial complaints ranging from symptoms of pulmonary or systemic venous congestion to symptoms of low forward cardiac output. Coexisting mitral regurgitation frequently is present secondary to left ventricular and mitral annular dilation. In addition, pulmonary hypertension develops in most patients in response to the chronic elevation in left atrial pressure. Left ventricular diastolic dysfunction often coexists with systolic dysfunction but typically is not the predominant feature of this disease.

Echocardiographic Approach (Table 8–3)

Two-dimensional (2D) imaging from standard windows allows evaluation of the size and function of all four cardiac chambers (Figs. 8–1 and 8–2). Qualitative evaluation of right ventricular size and systolic function and quantitative evaluation of left ventricular size and systolic function provide important clinical data. In addition to 2D imaging, other signs of poor left ventricular systolic function include the M-mode findings of an increased mitral E-point to septal separation due to ventricular dilation, and reduced anteroposterior aortic root motion

TABLE 8–3	Echocardiographic Approach to the Patient with a Suspected Cardiomyopathy		
		Qualitative	**Quantitative**
2D/M-mode imaging		Chamber dimensions	LV-EDV, LV-ESV
		Degree and pattern of LV hypertrophy	LV mass
		Evidence for dynamic outflow tract obstruction	
		SAM of mitral valve	
		Aortic valve midsystolic closure	
LV systolic function		Visual estimate of EF	Apical biplane EF
Doppler echo		Associated valvular regurgitation	Maximum and mean ΔP
		Pattern of LV diastolic filling	PA pressures
		Pattern of LA filling (pulmonary venous inflow)	
		Velocity curve of dynamic outflow tract obstruction	
		Localization of the level of obstruction	

2D = Two-dimensional; LA = left atrial; LV = left ventricular; EDV = end-diastolic volume; ESV = end-systolic volume; SAM = systolic anterior motion; ΔP = pressure gradient; PA = pulmonary artery; EF = ejection fraction.

reflecting reduced left atrial filling and emptying (Fig. 8–3). Doppler findings may include a reduced aortic ejection velocity and velocity-time integral, indicating a reduced stroke volume, although compensatory mechanisms (including left ventricular dilation) result in a normal stroke volume at rest in many individuals. A slow rate of rise in velocity of the mitral regurgitant jet indicates a reduced rate of rise in left ventricular pressure in early systole *(dP/dt)*.

Associated atrioventricular valve regurgitation can be assessed with Doppler techniques

FIGURE 8–1. Schematic diagram of the key features of dilated cardiomyopathy in an apical four-chamber view. All four chambers are enlarged with reduced left and right ventricular (LV and RV) systolic function. *Dashed lines* indicate the limited extent of endocardial motion between end-diastole and end-systole. An apical thrombus is present. Secondary mitral and tricuspid regurgitation are indicated by the *arrows* (LA = left atrium; RA = right atrium).

FIGURE 8–2. 2D images in a patient with dilated cardiomyopathy. In the parasternal long-axis view *(above)*, left ventricular and atrial enlargement is seen. A pleural effusion is present posteriorly. A Swan-Ganz catheter is seen in the enlarged right ventricular outflow tract. In the apical four-chamber view *(below)*, dilation of all four chambers is seen. In real time, right and left ventricular systolic function is severely reduced (DA = descending aorta).

FIGURE 8–3. M-mode findings in dilated cardiomyopathy. There is increased mitral *E*-point septal separation (EPSS) and a "B-bump" *(left)* and decreased aortic root motion with early closure of the aortic valve *(right).*

(see Chap. 11) and often is moderate in severity (Fig. 8–4). Pulmonary pressures usually are elevated and can be estimated from the velocity in the tricuspid regurgitant jet, as described in Chapter 5.

The pattern of left ventricular diastolic filling can be evaluated with Doppler recordings of left ventricular inflow. Early in the disease course, a reduced *E* velocity and increased *A* velocity consistent with impaired early diastolic relaxation may be observed. However, once left ventricular function has deteriorated significantly, the pattern changes to that of an increased *E* velocity and reduced *A* velocity. In this situation, the high ratio of *E* to *A* velocity most likely indicates a high left atrial pressure (increased gradient from left atrium to left ventricle at mitral valve opening) and a high left ventricular end-diastolic pressure (reduced *A* velocity) (Fig. 8–5). This pattern of mitral inflow, often termed "pseudonormalization," can be distinguished from a normal inflow pattern by the pulmonary venous inflow signal, which shows an increased atrial reversal velocity signal and an increased ratio of antegrade diastolic to systolic flow. Another echocardiographic finding that correlates with an elevated end-diastolic pressure is the M-mode finding of a delayed rate of mitral valve, termed a "B-bump" or "AC-shoulder" (see Fig. 8–3).

When significant left ventricular systolic dysfunction is present (ejection fraction ≤35%), a careful search for apical left ventricular thrombus is indicated (Fig. 8–6). Details on the technical aspects of identifying a left ventricular thrombus are given in Chapter 7.

Limitations/Technical Considerations

Echocardiography rarely can establish the *etiology* of a dilated cardiomyopathy, even though it is instrumental both in confirming the diagnosis and in providing prognostic data. The echocardiographic appearance of a dilated cardiomyopathy is fairly uniform despite a wide range of disease processes. One exception is Chagas' heart disease; these patients typically have a left ventricular apical aneurysm with minimal involvement of the ventricular septum. In patients with endomyocardial fibrosis due to Chagas' disease, there is apical obliteration with a small ventricular chamber, atrial en-

FIGURE 8–4. Color Doppler of mitral and tricuspid regurgitation due to ventricular dilation and systolic dysfunction in a patient with a dilated cardiomyopathy. (See Color Plate 7, p. 274.)

FIGURE 8–5. Doppler findings in dilated cardiomyopathy. Left ventricular diastolic inflow shows a high *E* velocity and low *A* velocity suggestive of "pseudonormalization" due to an elevated end-diastolic pressure *(left)*. The mitral regurgitant jet shows a slow rate of rise in velocity consistent with a reduced *dP/dt (right)*.

largement, and atrioventricular valve regurgitation. While Chagas' disease is rare in North America and Europe, it is endemic in South and Central America and may be diagnosed in immigrants from those areas. Recognition of the echocardiographic features of this disease may prompt the correct diagnosis in a nonendemic area.

In most patients with dilated cardiomyopathy, an exact etiology cannot be identified, even when all diagnostic modalities are used. The most useful additional data are a careful patient history to uncover possible precipitating factors.

An endomyocardial biopsy is rarely diagnostic except when an infiltrative process (e.g., amyloid, sarcoid, hemochromatosis) is present. Findings of "myocarditis" are nonspecific and usually do not change the therapeutic approach.

Clinical Utility

Echocardiographic evaluation is indicated at the initial presentation of a patient with symptoms consistent with dilated cardiomyopathy. If an echocardiogram performed in a patient with a suspected dilated cardiomyopathy shows no significant impairment of left ventricular systolic dysfunction, a careful search is needed for other causes of heart failure symptoms, such as pericardial constriction, restrictive or hypertrophic cardiomyopathy, ischemic disease, or valvular disease (Table 8–4).

FIGURE 8–6. Left ventricular apical thrombus *(arrow)* in an apical four-chamber view in a patient with dilated cardiomyopathy.

TABLE 8–4	Echocardiographic Differential Diagnosis of "Heart Failure"

Ischemic disease

Valvular disease

Hypertensive heart disease

Cardiomyopathy
  Dilated
  Hypertrophic
  Restrictive

Pericardial disease
  Constriction
  Tamponade

Pulmonary heart disease

If the echocardiogram is consistent with the clinical diagnosis of dilated cardiomyopathy, detailed information on ventricular function, chamber sizes, associated valvular disease, and pulmonary artery pressures is obtained.

While "routine" follow-up studies are not indicated, repeat echocardiograms may be needed if a significant change in clinical status occurs suggesting an interval change in ventricular function. Since ventricular function is a strong predictor of outcome, assessment of the patient's current status allows appropriate tailoring of medical therapy. A severe decrease in

FIGURE 8–7. Calculation of stroke volume in a patient with dilated cardiomyopathy. Outflow tract diameter is measured from a parasternal long-axis view for calculation of a circular cross-sectional area (CSA_{LVOT}). The left ventricular outflow tract velocity-time integral (VTI_{LVOV}) is recorded just proximal to the aortic valve from an apical approach using a pulsed Doppler sample volume length of 5 to 10 mm. Stroke volume (SV) is calculated as VTI × CSA. Cardiac output is stroke volume times heart rate.

ventricular systolic function may prompt consideration of cardiac transplantation.

In the intensive care unit, echocardiographic evaluation can be helpful in patients with dilated cardiomyopathy to assess left ventricular function, pulmonary artery pressures, the degree of coexisting mitral regurgitation, and to estimate left ventricular filling pressure. Evaluation of an individual patient's response to afterload reduction therapy can be performed by repeat 2D echo ejection fraction measurements or by sequential measurements of stroke volume and cardiac output using Doppler and 2D echo techniques (see Chap. 5 and Fig. 8–7).

Alternate Approaches

If measurement of pulmonary vascular resistance is needed (e.g., in a heart transplant candidate), cardiac catheterization is indicated. Although echocardiographic measures of pulmonary pressure are accurate, calculation of pulmonary vascular resistance currently is not reliable enough for clinical decision making.

HYPERTROPHIC CARDIOMYOPATHY

Basic Principles

Hypertrophic cardiomyopathy is an autosomal dominant inherited disease of the myocardium (with variable penetrance) related to abnormalities in the β-myosin heavy-chain gene. Predominant anatomic features of this disease are (1) asymmetric hypertrophy of the left ventricle, (2) normal ventricular systolic function, and (3) impaired diastolic left ventricular function (Fig. 8–8). Subaortic dynamic obstruction to left ventricular outflow is present in some individuals. Other important clinical features of this disease are a high risk of sudden death (especially during exertion); symptoms of angina, exercise intolerance, and syncope; and a systolic murmur on cardiac auscultation.

The *pattern* of left ventricular hypertrophy in patients with hypertrophic cardiomyopathy can be quite variable, ranging from "classic" septal hypertrophy to isolated apical hypertrophy. In addition, the *degree* of myocardial thickening is quite variable, even within a family. Hypertrophy may be confined to the anterior segment of the ventricular septum (type I) or may involve the anterior and posterior segments of the septum (type II) with sparing of the lateral, posterior, and inferior walls. Some patients have extensive ventricular hypertrophy

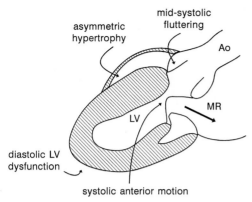

FIGURE 8–8. Schematic diagram of the typical features of hypertrophic cardiomyopathy in a parasternal long-axis view. There is midsystolic closure and coarse fluttering of the aortic valve leaflets, asymmetric septal hypertrophy with sparing of the basal posterior wall, normal left ventricular systolic function with impaired diastolic function, dynamic outflow tract obstruction with systolic anterior motion of the mitral valve leaflets, and mitral regurgitation.

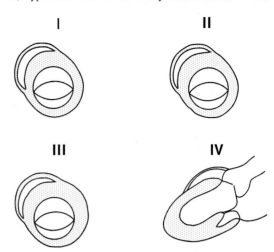

FIGURE 8–9. Schematic diagram of patterns of ventricular hypertrophy in hypertrophic cardiomyopathy in a parasternal basal short-axis view. Type I = hypertrophy confined to anterior septum; type II = anterior and posterior septum involved; type III = extensive hypertrophy sparing only the basal posterior wall; type IV = apical hypertrophy (in a long-axis schematic view).

with normal wall thickness seen only in the basal segment of the posterior wall (type III). An unusual pattern of hypertrophy is *apical hypertrophic cardiomyopathy* (type IV), which is of particular note to the echocardiographer because it can be missed if the marked displacement of the apical endocardium is not recognized. Clinically, the clue to an apical pattern of hypertrophy is inverted precordial T waves on the electrocardiogram (Fig. 8–9). The common feature of all these hypertrophy patterns is normal thickness (or "sparing") of the basal posterior left ventricular wall. In the parasternal long- and short-axis views, this region is seen at the base (between the papillary muscle and mitral annulus) posterior to the mitral valve leaflets.

In patients with subaortic obstruction, apposition of the anterior leaflet of the mitral valve against the hypertrophied ventricular septum is seen in systole. This obstruction is *dynamic* rather than fixed, both in the sense that it occurs only in mid to late systole and in the sense that the presence and severity of obstruction can be altered by loading conditions. These features contrast with the relatively fixed obstruction of aortic valve stenosis, which persists from the onset to the end of ejection and in which the severity of the stenosis is relatively insensitive to changes in loading conditions. Dynamic outflow obstruction in hypertrophic cardiomyopathy typically has a pattern of onset in midsystole, with the maximum left ventricular to

aortic pressure gradient occurring in late systole (Figs. 8–10 and 8–11). Controversy persists regarding (1) the mechanism of dynamic obstruction and (2) the lack of a clear relationship between clinical status and hemodynamic findings. Of note, late systolic obstruction occurs after the majority of the stroke volume has been ejected, thus minimally affecting forward stroke volume in most patients.

Obstruction can be diminished by maneuvers that increase ventricular volume—an increase in preload or a decrease in contractility—or by maneuvers that increase afterload. Conversely, the degree of obstruction is increased by a reduction in preload, an increase in contractility, or a decrease in afterload. All these conditions are similar in that they reduce left ventricular volume. Some patients with no or minimal evidence of outflow obstruction at rest develop obstruction with maneuvers performed during the physical examination or with echocardiography. Clinically useful maneuvers include examination during a postpremature contraction beat (increased contractility), with Valsalva maneuver (decreased preload), or after inhalation of amyl nitrate (decreased afterload and preload). All of these maneuvers lead to an increase in the degree of dynamic obstruction with a louder murmur and an increased Doppler velocity.

Dynamic outflow obstruction usually is as-

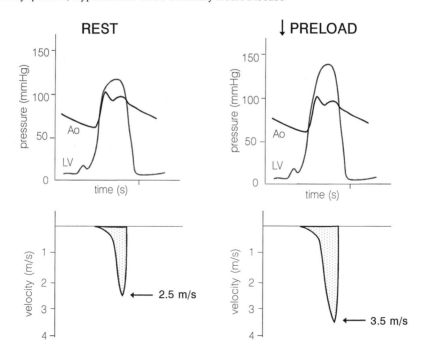

FIGURE 8–10. Schematic diagrams of the pressure gradient and velocity curve in dynamic outflow obstruction due to hypertrophic cardiomyopathy. At rest, a small gradient is present only in late systole between the left ventricle (LV) and aorta (Ao). The continuous-wave Doppler curve shows a late-peaking velocity of 2.5 m/s, with the origin of this velocity being the subaortic region. With alterations in loading conditions (decreased preload), the degree of obstruction increases dramatically. A late-peaking, high-velocity (3.5 m/s) Doppler curve now is obtained.

sociated with mitral regurgitation, since the systolic anterior motion of the leaflets in systole disrupts normal coaptation. A posteriorly directed mitral regurgitant jet of mild to moderate severity originates at the malcoapted segment of the leaflets (Fig. 8–12).

Left ventricular systolic function typically is normal in patients with hypertrophic cardiomyopathy. However, left ventricular diastolic function is abnormal, accounting for many of the heart failure symptoms in patients with hypertrophic cardiomyopathy. The thickened myocardium exhibits impaired relaxation and decreased compliance.

FIGURE 8–12. Color flow image of mitral regurgitation in a patient with hypertrophic cardiomyopathy showing a posteriorly directed jet originating from the malcoapted segment of the mitral leaflets in association with systolic anterior motion. Turbulence in the outflow tract is seen due to subaortic dynamic obstruction. (See Color Plate 7, p. 274.)

FIGURE 8–11. Continuous-wave Doppler in a patient with hypertrophic cardiomyopathy shows the characteristic late-peaking high-velocity curve due to dynamic outflow tract obstruction.

Echocardiographic Approach

Left Ventricular Asymmetric Hypertrophy

Evaluation of the pattern and extent of left ventricular hypertrophy is made from multiple tomographic views. In the parasternal long-axis view, particular attention is focused on the posterobasal wall between the papillary muscle and the mitral annulus. Although the wall in this region is not thickened in patients with hypertrophic cardiomyopathy, it is thickened in patients with concentric hypertrophy due to other etiologies (e.g., hypertension, restrictive cardiomyopathy). Two-dimensionally guided M-mode tracings provide the best endocardial definition for measurement of septal and posterior wall thickness, although 2D measurements can be used when image quality is adequate. Two-dimensional imaging in both long- and short-axis views is used to ensure that the M-mode beam is perpendicular to the left ventricular walls and to avoid inclusion of right ventricular trabeculation in the septal wall thickness.

The parasternal long-axis view also offers the best opportunity to define the exact relationship between the pattern of septal hypertrophy and the outflow tract (Fig. 8–13). This is important when a surgical approach, such as myotomy-myectomy, is being considered, since surgical visualization usually is retrograde across the aortic valve, allowing only limited direct inspection of the septal endocardium and little information on the extent of septal thickening or the degree of septal curvature. Parasternal short-axis views from base to apex allow assessment of the lateromedial extent of the hypertrophic process.

It is important to recognize that some degree of bulging of the septum into the left ventricular outflow tract, often called a septal "knuckle," is seen in normal older individuals. This apparent septal prominence most likely is due to increased tortuosity of the aorta resulting in a more acute angle between the basal septum and aortic root. There is no evidence that this septal contour pattern is inherited or associated with clinical events so that these patients should not be considered to have hypertrophic cardiomyopathy.

Apical views again allow visualization of the pattern and extent of hypertrophy. Diagnosis of apical hypertrophy can be difficult, since endocardial definition may be poor and the endocardial surface (which may be located up to one-third the distance from the apical epicardium to the base) may be missed if image quality is sub-

FIGURE 8–13. Two-dimensional images of hypertrophic cardiomyopathy in a parasternal long-axis view at end-diastole *(above)* and end-systole *(below)*. Systolic anterior motion of the mitral valve is seen *(arrow)*.

optimal. In some cases, the epicardium may be mistaken for the apical endocardium. A careful examination, when the referring physician has alerted the echocardiographer to this possible diagnosis, avoids this potential pitfall. Color or pulsed Doppler examination is helpful in demonstrating the absence of blood flow in the "apical" region, which is occupied by the hypertrophied myocardium.

Qualitative and quantitative evaluation of left ventricular systolic function is performed using standard approaches (see Chap. 5).

Left Ventricular Diastolic Function

Left ventricular diastolic function is evaluated from the Doppler inflow velocity curve recorded at the mitral valve leaflet tips. The *E* velocity, the *A* velocity, the *E/A* ratio, and the early diastolic deceleration slope can be measured. Sequential studies, in conjunction with clinical data, allow inferences about left ventricular diastolic function (see Chap. 6). Typical changes in patients with hypertrophic cardiomyopathy include a prolonged isovolumic relaxation time, reduced *E* velocity, and enhanced *A* velocity; however, there is marked patient variability. Changes in the filling pattern after medical or surgical therapy may be seen consistent with improved diastolic filling.

Dynamic Outflow Tract Obstruction

2D/M-Mode Imaging. In a patient with dynamic left ventricular outflow tract obstruction, the parasternal long-axis view shows systolic anterior motion of the mitral valve leaflets. This can be appreciated better on M-mode recordings showing the systolic anterior motion and apposition between the anterior mitral leaflet and the septum in mid to late systole. Note that with pathologic systolic anterior motion, the rate of anterior leaflet motion is more rapid than the anterior motion of the posterior wall in systole (Fig. 8–14). A "contact lesion" on the ventricular septum at the site of mitral leaflet impingement may be seen on 2D long- and short-axis imaging in some patients.

Short-axis parasternal views also show the systolic anterior motion of the mitral valve leaflets. Frame-by-frame analysis shows the cross-sectional area of the outflow tract throughout systole.

Apical 2D views are helpful for demonstrating the abnormal mitral leaflet motion, especially the apical long-axis and the anteriorly angulated four-chamber views. Note that the degree of systolic anterior motion may not be uniform from medial to lateral across the mitral leaflets, so imaging in multiple planes with slight adjustments in transducer angulation may be needed to demonstrate the presence and extent of dynamic outflow obstruction.

The aortic valve shows normal leaflet opening in early systole, followed by midsystolic abrupt partial closure with coarse fluttering of the aortic valve leaflets in late systole due to the late systolic dynamic outflow obstruction. Again, these rapid leaflet movements are best documented on M-mode recordings (Fig. 8–15). The aortic leaflets themselves may be sclerotic because of the long-term effect of a turbulent jet as a result of subaortic obstruction, and some degree of coexisting aortic regurgitation may be noted.

Doppler Evaluation. Doppler studies provide a more direct evaluation of the presence, location, and degree of dynamic subaortic obstruction than do 2D or M-mode techniques. With conventional pulsed or color flow imaging, the site of obstruction is identified based on the location of the poststenotic turbulence. Both parasternal and apical long-axis views are useful for this examination.

Using pulsed Doppler from an apical approach, the sample volume is slowly moved from the apex progressively toward the base, recording the velocity curve at each step. Proximal to the outflow obstruction, velocities are normal. At the site of obstruction, the velocity increases abruptly to a velocity reflecting the

FIGURE 8–14. M-mode at the mitral valve level *(left)* in a patient with dynamic outflow obstruction due to hypertrophic cardiomyopathy showing the classic septal hypertrophy and systolic anterior motion *(SAM)* of the mitral leaflets *(arrows)*.

FIGURE 8–15. An M-mode view at the aortic valve level (in the same patient as in Fig. 8–14) shows midsystolic closure of the aortic valve *(arrow)* followed by coarse fluttering of the leaflets.

FIGURE 8–16. Example of the use of a stepwise pulsed-Doppler examination to localize the level of outflow tract obstruction. With the sample volume at the mitral valve level in the outflow tract *(top left)*, pulsed Doppler shows a marked increase in velocity with signal aliasing *(upper right)*. This velocity can be resolved with high pulse repetition frequency Doppler *(lower right)* or with continuous-wave Doppler ultrasound (as shown in Fig. 8–11).

degree of obstruction (as stated in the Bernoulli equation). This approach, using stepwise evaluation with pulsed Doppler ultrasound, is advantageous in that intracavity gradients due to apical hypertrophy or apposition of the papillary muscle with the septum will be recognized and not mistaken for *subaortic* dynamic obstruction (Fig. 8–16).

Continuous-wave Doppler from an apical approach typically shows a late-peaking high-velocity systolic jet in patients with dynamic left ventricular outflow tract obstruction. The shape of this curve is distinctive, corresponding to the temporal course of the left ventricular to aortic pressure gradient (see Fig. 8–10). Again, since continuous-wave Doppler measures velocities along the entire length of the ultra-

sound beam, other techniques are needed to confirm the depth of origin of the signal. In patients with hypertensive heart disease or hypovolemia, the combination of left ventricular hypertrophy and hyperdynamic systolic function may result in a similar late-peaking high-velocity systolic waveform. However, in these patients the site of obstruction is *not* subaortic; it is closer to the apex, at the midventricular level.

When features suggestive of hypertrophic cardiomyopathy are present and there is no evidence for outflow obstruction at rest, maneuvers to "provoke" outflow obstruction may be performed in order to make a definite diagnosis or to relate the patient's symptoms to the echocardiographic findings. When only a modest degree of obstruction is seen at rest, interventions to increase the degree of obstruction may be performed for similar reasons.

A spontaneous premature ventricular contraction (PVC) results in an increased degree of obstruction on the post-PVC beat due to increased left ventricular contractility. Alternatively, the strain phase of the Valsalva maneuver increases obstruction by decreasing preload (smaller left ventricular cavity size) but is difficult to perform simultaneously with echocardiography due to changes in cardiac position and lung interference as the patient performs the maneuver. A simple and reasonably safe method to provoke dynamic outflow obstruction in the echocardiography laboratory is amyl nitrate inhalation under direct physician supervision. This medication results in a brief decrease in preload (venodilation) and decrease in afterload (arterial dilation), both of which increase the degree of obstruction. A moderate degree of tachycardia may occur, but the duration of action of this inhaled medication is brief. The sonographer records the continuous-wave Doppler signal in the left ventricular outflow tract before, during, and after administration of amyl nitrate by the physician to document the effects of the medication on the degree of outflow obstruction. Attention is needed to maintain a parallel intercept angle between the ultrasound beam and the high-velocity jet, particularly with respect to the phase of the respiratory cycle. The physician monitors heart rate, rhythm, symptoms, and blood pressure. Care is needed to ensure that only the patient (and not the other individuals in the room) are exposed to the medication.

Mitral Valve Abnormalities

The mitral valve is anatomically and functionally abnormal in the majority of patients with hypertrophic cardiomyopathy. Functionally, mitral regurgitation results from systolic anterior motion of the leaflets into the outflow tract leading to late systolic failure of coaptation and a consequent posteriorly directed regurgitant jet. However, anatomic abnormalities are present as well. Both autopsy and echocardiographic studies demonstrate that the mitral leaflets have an increased surface area and a longer length (particularly the anterior leaflet) compared to normal subjects. In addition, the degree of coaptation is excessive, and the coaptation plane is displaced posteriorly. About 10% of patients have anomalous papillary muscle anatomy with direct insertion of the papillary muscle into the leaflet.

Limitations/Technical Considerations

As discussed earlier, it is important to distinguish hypertrophic cardiomyopathy with dynamic subaortic obstruction associated with systolic anterior motion of the mitral leaflet from a concentrically hypertrophied ventricle due to other disease processes (such as hypertension). In some situations, the hypertrophied ventricle may be hyperdynamic, with midcavity obliteration resulting in an intracavity gradient. The distinction between hypertrophic cardio-

FIGURE 8–17. Example of a concentrically hypertrophied hyperdynamic left ventricle with midcavity obliteration at end-systole *(above)* resulting in a late-peaking high-velocity outflow tract Doppler curve *(below)*. This condition must be distinguished from the dynamic subaortic obstruction seen in hypertrophic cardiomyopathy. SV = sample volume.

myopathy and a hyperdynamic concentrically hypertrophied ventricle can be made by careful attention to the 2D images (sparing of the basal posterior wall in hypertrophic cardiomyopathy) and M-mode findings (characteristic aortic and mitral valve motion) and by evaluation of the depth of origin of the high-velocity jet using conventional pulsed, high pulse repetition frequency (HPRF), and color Doppler techniques (Fig. 8–17).

Another difficult problem is separating the degree of outflow obstruction due to dynamic subaortic obstruction from that due to valvular aortic stenosis in the rare patient with both conditions. In the presence of serial stenoses, an accurate measure of the pressure drop across each narrowing may not be possible, since the simplified Bernoulli equation applies to a single stenosis. However, HPRF Doppler may allow examination of velocities at each site, indicating the relative contribution of each site to the total degree of obstruction to ventricular outflow. Occasionally, a patient with valvular aortic stenosis and a hypertrophied ventricle will demonstrate dynamic subaortic obstruction only *after* aortic valve replacement. Some of these patients have hypertrophic cardiomyopathy that is "unmasked" by the afterload reduction of valve replacement. Others have a hyperdynamic ventricle with a midcavity pressure gradient that may resolve as the degree of left ventricular hypertrophy decreases postoperatively.

Clinical Utility

Diagnosis and Screening

Echocardiography is the procedure of choice for accurate diagnosis of hypertrophic cardiomyopathy. Since this is an inherited disorder, screening with echocardiography is indicated for all first-degree relatives of the affected individual. This diagnosis significantly changes clinical management even in asymptomatic individuals, given the high risk of sudden death with exertion, and has important implications for genetic counseling.

Evaluation of Medical Therapy

In patients with a definite diagnosis of hypertrophic cardiomyopathy, Doppler findings can be used to assess the impact of medical therapy. Specifically, the pattern of left ventricular diastolic filling after institution of therapy to improve diastolic function (such as beta blockers or calcium channel blockers) may show an improvement in early diastolic filling. The degree

of dynamic outflow obstruction also may show improvement on medical therapy.

Surgical Therapy

Preoperative and intraoperative echocardiographic evaluation of the patient undergoing surgical treatment for hypertrophic cardiomyopathy is essential. Preoperative knowledge of the extent, distribution, and curvature of septal hypertrophy guides the surgeon in terms of the location and size of the muscle segment to be removed. Intraoperative monitoring allows evaluation of the adequacy of the procedure in relieving outflow tract obstruction, using both 2D imaging and Doppler techniques. Images are obtained at baseline and immediately following the procedure (after cardiopulmonary bypass is discontinued). Note that while transesophageal imaging provides adequate images of the myectomy site in some cases, epicardial imaging often is preferable, since the septum is located anteriorly relative to the esophagus. Color flow imaging from a transesophageal or transepicardial approach allows evaluation of the flow pattern in the left ventricular outflow tract as an indicator of residual obstruction. Since the degree of obstruction is influenced dramatically by loading conditions, the postbypass study should be performed under hemodynamic conditions as similar as possible to the baseline state. It may be difficult to obtain an accurate continuous-wave Doppler recording of the degree of outflow obstruction in the operating room because the transesophageal approach rarely provides a transgastric apical view from which the beam can be aligned parallel to the jet. An epicardial apical position may not be obtainable with a median sternotomy because the transducer often is too large to fit under the ribs at the apex. Placement of a sterile transducer on the ascending aorta with inferior angulation toward the outflow tract may allow a parallel intercept angle in some patients.

Postmyectomy complications that are detectable by intraoperative echocardiography include a ventricular septal defect at the site of the myectomy as well as residual outflow tract obstruction.

Alternate Approaches

Usually, echocardiography provides all the data needed for clinical management of a patient with suspected or diagnosed hypertrophic cardiomyopathy. Alternate tomographic imaging techniques can provide data on the anatomic pattern of hypertrophy but do not allow evaluation of abnormal diastolic filling or the presence and degree of dynamic outflow tract obstruction.

When the echocardiographic findings and clinical presentation are discrepant, cardiac catheterization may be helpful. First, evaluation of coronary anatomy may be indicated, since coexisting epicardial coronary artery disease may explain some symptoms in a patient with hypertrophic cardiomyopathy. Second, recordings of left ventricular and aortic pressures at rest and after provocative maneuvers to increase or decrease dynamic outflow obstruction and with slow "pullback" across the outflow tract and aortic valve allow more detailed hemodynamic evaluation. This is particularly helpful in the patient with sequential stenoses in the subaortic region and at the aortic valve level.

In the operating room, direct left ventricular and aortic pressure measurements after myectomy may be helpful if residual obstruction is suspected.

RESTRICTIVE CARDIOMYOPATHY

Basic Principles

Restrictive cardiomyopathy is characterized by normal left ventricular systolic function with impaired diastolic function due to a stiff, hypertrophied left ventricle. Heart failure symptoms are due to the resultant elevation in left ventricular end-diastolic pressure and the inability to increase cardiac output with exercise due to impaired diastolic filling. Note that *heart failure*—defined as the inability to maintain a normal cardiac output or maintenance of a normal cardiac output *only* with an elevated left ventricular end-diastolic pressure—can occur with normal systolic function. In many patients with restrictive cardiomyopathy, right-sided failure predominates initially with symptoms of peripheral edema and ascites.

As the disease process progresses, an individual patient may progress from an anatomic/ hemodynamic pattern consistent with restrictive cardiomyopathy to a pattern showing some features of dilated cardiomyopathy, ending with a picture indistinguishable from dilated cardiomyopathy.

The etiology of restrictive cardiomyopathy includes infiltrative processes such as amyloidosis and hemochromatosis and inflammatory diseases such as sarcoidosis (Table 8–5). Compared with dilated cardiomyopathy, restrictive cardiomyopathy is a rare diagnosis. An unusual cause of restrictive cardiomyopathy is the hypereosinophilic syndrome. This systemic dis-

TABLE 8–5	Etiology of Restrictive Cardiomyopathy (Examples)

Amyloidosis

Hemochromatosis

Sarcoidosis

Hypereosinophilic syndrome (Löffler's endocarditis)

Glycogen storage diseases

ease is characterized by hypereosinophilia with involvement of the lungs, bone marrow, brain, and heart. Cardiac involvement is typical and exhibits unique echocardiographic features. In this syndrome, left ventricular thrombus formation occurs *in the absence of an underlying wall motion abnormality* (particularly in the apex), resulting in gradual apical "obliteration" (as seen on angiography) or filling in of the apex with an echogenic mass (on echocardiography). Thrombus formation also occurs under the posterior mitral valve leaflet, leading to adherence of the posterior leaflet to the endocardium and significant mitral regurgitation.

Echocardiographic Approach

Two-dimensional echocardiographic imaging in patients with restrictive cardiomyopathy typically shows a nondilated, thick-walled left ventricle with normal systolic function and abnormal diastolic function. The right ventricular free wall often is thickened as well, and biatrial

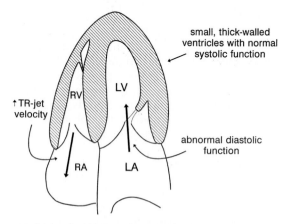

FIGURE 8–18. Schematic diagram of the typical features of restrictive cardiomyopathy, which include a thick-walled, small left ventricle (LV) with impaired diastolic function, left and right atrial enlargement (LA, RA), and signs of secondary pulmonary hypertension, including paradoxical septal motion and a high-velocity tricuspid regurgitant (TR) jet.

enlargement is seen. Secondary signs of moderate pulmonary hypertension may be present, including paradoxic septal motion and tricuspid regurgitation (Figs. 8–18 and 8–19).

Doppler evaluation confirms moderate pulmonary hypertension based on the (1) time to peak velocity in the pulmonary artery, and (2) tricuspid regurgitant jet velocity plus an estimate of right atrial pressure (see Chap. 5). Note that in the untreated patient, right atrial

FIGURE 8–20. Tricuspid regurgitant jet velocity of 2.7 m/s in a patient with restrictive cardiomyopathy *(above)*. Right atrial pressure estimated from the size and respiratory motion of the inferior vena cava *(below)* was 20 mmHg. Estimated pulmonary artery systolic pressure then is 49 mmHg.

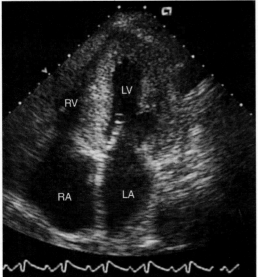

FIGURE 8–19. Parasternal long-axis *(above)* and apical four-chamber *(below)* 2D echocardiographic images in a patient with a restrictive cardiomyopathy due to amyloidosis. There is biventricular hypertrophy, biatrial enlargement, and both systolic and diastolic dysfunction of the left ventricle (DA = descending aorta).

pressure usually is high, so the inferior vena cava is dilated with reduced respiratory variation (Fig. 8–20).

The pattern of left ventricular diastolic filling parallels the abnormalities in left ventricular diastolic function in this disease. However, interpretation is complicated both by the numerous confounding factors that affect left ventricular diastolic filling (see Chap. 6) and by temporal changes in diastolic filling as the disease progresses in an individual patient. Early in the disease course, impaired diastolic relaxation of the left ventricle results in impaired *early* diastolic filling. The Doppler left ventricular inflow curve shows a reduced *E* velocity, increased *A* velocity, prolonged isovolumic relaxation time, and decreased early diastolic deceleration slope

(Fig. 8–21). With impaired ventricular relaxation, the pulmonary vein flow curve shows a reduced diastolic filling phase and normal systolic filling phase, resulting in a decreased ratio of systolic to diastolic pulmonary venous flow.

EARLY

PSEUDO-NORMAL

LATE

FIGURE 8–21. Schematic diagrams of left ventricular diastolic filling in restrictive cardiomyopathy. Early in the disease course ventricular relaxation abnormalities predominate, and the E velocity and early deceleration slope are reduced while the isovolumic relaxation time and A velocity are increased. Pseudonormalization occurs as left ventricular end-diastolic pressure rises, resulting in relatively normal E and A velocities. With advanced (late) disease, ventricular compliance decreases, resulting in a high E velocity, steep deceleration slope, short isovolumic relaxation time, and reduced A velocity.

As the disease progresses, left atrial pressure rises, resulting in an increased pressure gradient from the left atrium to left ventricle at mitral valve opening. Along with reduced diastolic compliance of the left ventricle, this increased mitral opening pressure leads to an increased E velocity and a rapid deceleration slope. The A velocity is reduced due to a combination of increased left ventricular end-diastolic pressure and reduced atrial contractile function (Fig. 8–22). Thus the pattern of diastolic filling in advanced restrictive cardiomyopathy (which may coincide with the initial clinical presentation) is similar to the "big E, little A" pattern seen in normal young individuals. This "pseudonormal" pattern can be distinguished from normal by (1) the rapid early diastolic deceleration slope, (2) the patient's age, clinical presentation, and associated echocardiographic

FIGURE 8–22. Left ventricular diastolic filling in a patient with a restrictive cardiomyopathy shows an increased E velocity and reduced A velocity consistent with pseudonormalization *(above)*. This pattern is distinguished from normal by a pulmonary venous inflow pattern *(below)* showing reduced systolic flow, increased antegrade diastolic flow (D), and a prominent atrial (A) reversal signal.

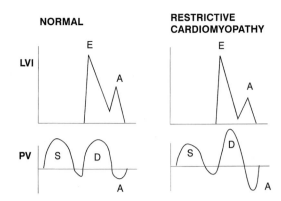

FIGURE 8–23. Schematic diagrams of left ventricular inflow (LVI) and pulmonary vein (PV) Doppler flow patterns with normal diastolic function and in restrictive cardiomyopathy. Although the inflow patterns are similar superficially, the "pseudonormal" pattern has a steeper deceleration slope and lower A velocity. The pulmonary vein flow shows increased diastolic filling and a prominent A reversal compared with the normal pattern.

findings, and (3) the pattern of pulmonary venous inflow into the left atrium. With a pseudonormal left ventricular inflow pattern, pulmonary venous inflow in diastole is normal or increased as blood flows in a conduit from the pulmonary veins to left ventricle while systolic filling is decreased. When atrial contraction occurs, the increased resistance to left ventricular filling results in an increase in the velocity and duration of the atrial flow reversal in the lower resistance pulmonary veins. Thus pulmonary venous flow shows an increased diastolic phase, reduced systolic phase, and prominent *a*-wave flow reversal. This is in contrast to the normal pattern of nearly equal systolic and diastolic pulmonary venous inflow curves (Fig. 8–23) and a small *a* wave.

Examination of right atrial filling by recording hepatic vein (or superior vena cava) flow patterns also can be helpful. These patterns correspond to the physical findings of the neck vein pulsations seen in patients with restrictive cardiomyopathy. Using this analogy, the hepatic vein flow pattern typically shows a prominent reverse flow phase with atrial contraction (*a* wave) followed by a rapid filling curve in systole (*x* descent). The diastolic phase of right atrial filling is blunted corresponding to a diminished *v* wave and *y* descent. These findings correspond to the pattern of right atrial pressure recordings at catheterization; the *x* descent represents the "dip," and the blunted systolic filling phase represents the "plateau" of the dip-and-plateau pattern.

Limitations/Technical Considerations

Differentiation of restrictive cardiomyopathy from constrictive pericarditis is problematic. Both have a similar clinical presentation, and both are characterized by preserved left ventricular systolic function with impaired diastolic filling. Features that distinguish these two conditions include the patterns of atrial and ventricular diastolic filling, the presence or absence of pericardial thickening, and the degree of associated pulmonary hypertension. However, no single feature is diagnostic of either condition (see Table 8–5).

Attention to technical details is necessary in recording Doppler atrial and ventricular filling patterns, particularly their relationship to the phase of respiration. Respiratory variation is assessed most reliably using a respirometer to mark the onsets of inspiration and expiration. Prior to recording Doppler signals, 2D and color flow imaging is used to convince the sonographer that there is no significant respiratory variation in the angle between the ultrasound beam and the direction of blood flow since respiratory changes in intercept angle could result in apparent changes in velocity even under constant-flow conditions due to the erroneous assumption that cos θ remains 1 in the Doppler equation. Once a constant intercept angle is ascertained, recordings of left ventricular diastolic inflow are made with the sample volume positioned first at the mitral annulus level and then at the mitral leaflet tips.

Recording right atrial filling patterns is straightforward using a subcostal approach with the pulsed Doppler sample volume positioned in the central hepatic vein. This vein connects directly to the inferior vena cava and right atrium, with no intervening venous valve, and conveniently lies parallel to the direction of the ultrasound beam from the subcostal window.

Left atrial filling is more technically challenging to record due to signal attenuation at the depth of the pulmonary veins from an apical approach. Other transthoracic acoustic windows rarely allow interrogation of pulmonary vein flow at a near-parallel intercept angle. A transesophageal approach is helpful if recordings of pulmonary vein flow are inadequate on transthoracic interrogation and are needed for patient management.

Clinical Utility

In a patient with symptoms of heart failure, a diagnosis of restrictive cardiomyopathy may not have been suspected on clinical grounds. In some cases, echocardiographic findings may provide the first clues pointing toward this diagnostic possibility. In a patient with known restrictive cardiomyopathy, echocardiography can be used to follow disease progression. A meticulous examination with careful attention to technical details and with integration of 2D, Doppler, and clinical data may allow differentiation of restrictive cardiomyopathy from constrictive pericarditis.

Alternate Approaches

Diagnostic evaluation of the patient with probable restrictive cardiomyopathy may include cardiac catheterization with measurement of intracardiac pressures at rest and with volume loading, endomyocardial biopsy, and chest computed tomographic imaging (to detect pericardial calcification or thickening). In some cases, constrictive pericarditis may remain a diagnostic possibility despite the results of these tests. The diagnosis of constrictive pericarditis is critical, since it can be treated by removal of the adherent pericardial layers. In patients in whom there is a high level of suspicion but nondiagnostic test results, thoracotomy may be indicated to confirm (and treat) or exclude a diagnosis of pericardial constriction.

In the future, tissue characterization based on analysis of the backscattered acoustic signal may prove helpful in evaluation of infiltrative cardiomyopathies.

HYPERTENSIVE HEART DISEASE

Basic Principles

Hypertensive heart disease is an end-organ consequence of systemic hypertension. Chronic systemic pressure overload results in left ventricular hypertrophy to maintain normal wall stress. Initially, diastolic function is impaired, while systolic function remains normal. With long-standing hypertension, systolic dysfunction and ventricular dilation can occur. Other cardiac abnormalities associated with chronic hypertension include aortic root dilation, aortic valve sclerosis, mitral annular calcification, left atrial enlargement, and atrial fibrillation.

Echocardiographic Approach

Ventricular Hypertrophy (Table 8–6)

Standard 2D views demonstrate concentric left ventricular hypertrophy with increased wall thickness and a nondilated chamber (Fig. 8–24). In contrast to hypertrophic cardiomyopathy, the pattern of hypertrophy is symmetric, including involvement of the basal posterior wall. M-mode recordings confirm an increased end-diastolic wall thickness (>11 mm). Left ventricular mass can be calculated from the M-mode data, assuming hypertrophy is symmetric, but preferably is calculated from 2D data (Fig. 8–25; also see Chap. 5).

TABLE 8–6	Conditions with Increased Left Ventricular Wall Thickness		
	Hypertensive Heart Disease	Hypertrophic Cardiomyopathy	Restrictive Cardiomyopathy
LV hypertrophy	+	+	+
Pattern of hypertrophy	Concentric	Asymmetric	Concentric
Clinical history of hypertension	+	Absent	Absent
Outflow obstruction	Midventricular cavity obliteration	Dynamic subaortic obstruction	Absent
RV hypertrophy	Absent	May be present	+
Pulmonary hypertension	Mild	Mild	Moderate
LV systolic function	Normal initially but may be reduced late in disease course	Normal	Normal initially but may be reduced late in disease course
LV diastolic function	Abnormal	Abnormal	Abnormal

+ = Present; LV = left ventricular; RV = right ventricular.

FIGURE 8–24. Schematic diagram of hypertensive heart disease in an anteriorly angulated apical four-chamber view. Note concentric left ventricular hypertrophy (LVH), mitral annular calcification (MAC), left atrial enlargement (LAE), aortic (Ao) valve sclerosis, aortic root dilation, and impaired early diastolic relaxation (E < A).

FIGURE 8–25. Two-dimensional echo views needed for left ventricular mass determination in a hypertensive patient. Parasternal short-axis *(above)*, apical four-chamber *(above right)*, and two-chamber *(right)* views at end-diastole are shown. Epicardial and endocardial borders in the short-axis view and an apical length measurement are needed to calculate left ventricular mass using Eq. (5.22).

Diastolic Function

Left ventricular diastolic function is characterized by impaired early diastolic relaxation. This results in a prolonged isovolumic relaxation time (IVRT), reduced E velocity, reduced E/A ratio, and prolonged deceleration slope. Interestingly, in individuals with physiologic hypertrophy (due to physical conditioning), diastolic dysfunction is not seen even when increased wall thickness is present. In pathologic hypertrophy (due to hypertension), diastolic dysfunction often is the first evidence of end-organ damage, usually antedating clear evidence of anatomic hypertrophy.

Systolic Function

Typically, systolic function is preserved early in the disease course. Segmental wall motion abnormalities are not seen unless coexisting coronary artery disease is present. With a small, hypertrophied, normally functioning left ventricular chamber, midcavity obliteration at end-systole may be seen with an associated Doppler velocity curve showing a brief, late-systolic high-velocity signal (see Fig. 8–17). The duration of this intracavity gradient is briefer than that seen with hypertrophic cardiomyopathy, the level of obstruction is midventricular rather than subaortic, and systolic anterior motion of the mitral leaflets is not seen. Midcavity obliteration is exacerbated by hypovolemia or increased contractility.

Other Echocardiographic Findings

Aortic root dilation often is present in hypertensive patients and is associated with increased tortuosity of the ascending aorta, arch, and descending aorta. Increased irregular echogenicity of the aortic walls, representing atherosclerosis, also may be noted. In uncomplicated hypertension, the aortic annulus itself is not dilated. The aortic valve leaflets usually show fibrocalcific changes and associated mild aortic regurgitation. Mitral annular calcification frequently is present in patients with chronic hypertension and is one cause of mild to moderate mitral regurgitation in these patients. Left atrial enlargement is due to a combination of a chronically elevated left ventricular end-diastolic pressure and mitral regurgitation.

Limitations/Technical Considerations

Left ventricular mass determinations are dependent on optimal image quality with clear definition of endocardial and epicardial surfaces and on correct endocardial border tracing at end-diastole and end-systole. It remains controversial whether 2D or M-mode mass calculations are optimal, especially given cost considerations in large patient populations. Differentiation of hypertensive heart disease from hypertrophic or restrictive heart disease is based on the pattern of hypertrophy, associated echocardiographic findings, and integration of the echocardiographic and clinical data.

Clinical Utility

Diagnosis and Prognosis

Left ventricular mass, measured by echocardiography, is a strong predictor of clinical outcome in patients with hypertension. In subjects with borderline hypertension, increased left ventricular mass identifies a subgroup of patients with a poor prognosis without medical therapy. In patients with definite hypertension, the degree of left ventricular hypertrophy reflects the chronic elevation of systemic pressure, in theory serving as an index of the temporally averaged blood pressure over long periods of time. Thus left ventricular mass may be a more accurate method for assessing the severity of hypertension than occasional blood pressure recordings in the physician's office or even 24-hour recordings of blood pressure.

Choices of Medical Therapy

Some hypertension clinics tailor medical therapy in individual patients based on noninvasive Doppler echo evaluation of hemodynamics. Since blood pressure equals cardiac output times systemic vascular resistance, hypertension can be due to elevation of either one or both of the components of this equation. To assess hemodynamics noninvasively in hypertensive patients, cardiac output is measured using Doppler recordings of ascending aortic flow and 2D aortic diameter measurements (see Chap. 5). Systemic vascular resistance then is calculated from the cuff blood pressure and Doppler cardiac output. Appropriate medications are chosen based on the specific hemodynamics in each patient.

Efficacy of Medical Therapy

Determination of left ventricular mass also is useful in assessing the long-term effect of medical therapy. Again, rather than measuring blood pressure at rare intervals in the disease course, the chronic end-organ effects of hypertension on the left ventricle are measured. It seems plausible that effective antihypertensive therapy should reverse end-organ changes; specifically, it should result in regression of left ventricular hypertrophy.

Evaluation of Heart Failure Symptoms in a Patient with Hypertension

In a patient with chronic hypertension, heart failure symptoms may be due to diastolic or systolic left ventricular dysfunction, superimposed coronary artery disease, or superimposed valvular disease. Early in the disease course, pathologic hypertrophy is associated with impaired early diastolic filling. Impaired ventricular filling leads to elevated left atrial pressures and pulmonary venous hypertension, resulting in dyspnea. Diagnosis of diastolic dysfunction with preserved systolic function can be made by echocardiography and has important clinical implications, since the therapy for heart failure symptoms is quite different for diastolic versus systolic dysfunction.

An extreme form of preserved systolic function with left ventricular hypertrophy and heart failure symptoms has been observed in hypertensive patients and has been termed *hypertensive hypertrophic cardiomyopathy*. This condition is characterized by normal to hyperdynamic systolic function, concentric hypertrophy, diastolic dysfunction, and a midventricular late systolic gradient due to cavity obliteration. Strictly speaking, this combination of findings is not a "cardiomyopathy" but simply represents severe end-organ damage due to hypertension. However, awareness of this specific clinical picture results in consideration of this diagnosis in patients in whom hypertrophic or restrictive cardiomyopathy otherwise might be suspected.

With long-standing hypertension, impairment of left ventricular contractility can occur, even in the absence of coexisting coronary artery disease. Physiologically, elevated afterload (as in valvular aortic stenosis) is the proximate cause of systolic dysfunction. However, systolic function may not improve even with aggressive antihypertensive therapy when systolic dysfunction is long-standing, suggesting that irreversible changes in ventricular contractility have occurred. End-stage hypertensive heart disease has an echocardiographic appearance similar to end-stage dilated cardiomyopathy.

Alternate Approaches

The need for routine echocardiographic evaluation of patients with hypertension is controversial. Medical management based on intermittent office blood pressure measurements remains standard practice at most medical centers. When needed, estimates of the chronicity of blood pressure elevation can be obtained by 24-hour blood pressure monitors or evaluation of other end-organ damage (e.g., renal function, retinal examination). While electrocardiographic estimates of left ventricular hypertrophy are less accurate and precise than echocardiographic measurements, there is a substantial cost differential between these diagnostic tests.

EVALUATION OF THE POST-CARDIAC-TRANSPLANT PATIENT

Basic Principles

Echocardiographic evaluation of the post-cardiac-transplant patient typically is directed toward one of three goals: (1) assessment of cardiac anatomy and physiology prompted by a specific clinical problem, (2) the elusive goal of noninvasive diagnosis of early rejection of the transplanted heart, or (3) diagnosis of post-transplant coronary artery disease.

Clinical problems encountered in the post-cardiac-transplant patient include:

1. Pericardial effusion, particularly early postoperatively.
2. Right ventricular systolic dysfunction due to inadequate myocardial preservation at the time of transplantation, persistently elevated pulmonary vascular resistance, or transplant rejection.
3. Left ventricular systolic dysfunction due to inadequate myocardial preservation, acute rejection early after transplantation, or superimposed coronary artery disease at a longer interval after transplantation.

Primary valvular disease, of course, is uncommon due to screening of donor hearts before transplantation. However, mitral or tricuspid regurgitation secondary to ventricular dysfunction and annular dilation may be seen. Diastolic dysfunction clearly occurs and may be a marker of early rejection. Unfortunately, evaluation of diastolic function after cardiac transplantation is fraught with difficulty due to the confounding effects of loading conditions, heart rate, patient age, coexisting mitral regurgitation, and other factors, as detailed in Chapter 6.

Echocardiographic Approach

Normal Findings after Cardiac Transplantation

Typically, right and left ventricular size, wall thickness, and systolic function are normal in the absence of perioperative complications or rejection. However, abnormal septal motion is the norm with anterior motion of the septum in systole with a slight decrease in the extent of systolic thickening of the septal myocardium. Valvular anatomy and function are normal, with small amounts of mitral, tricuspid, and pulmonic regurgitation present at a prevalence similar to that in normal individuals. The suture lines in the aorta and pulmonary artery may be difficult to appreciate, depending on the distance of the suture lines from the valve planes. A small pericardial effusion is seen early in the postoperative period but rarely persists beyond a few weeks. Pulmonary artery pressures may show some degree of persistent elevation as calculated from the velocity in the tricuspid regurgitant jet and estimates of right atrial pressure.

If the surgical approach included anastomoses of the normal and donor atrium, a normal echocardiogram after cardiac transplantation will show biatrial enlargement (Fig. 8–26) with an variably prominent ridge between the donor and recipient portions of both right and left atrium. The atrial suture line should not be mistaken for an abnormal atrial mass (Fig. 8–27). When transplantation is performed with anastomosis of the superior and inferior vena cava for the right atrium and a cuff of tissue with the pulmonary veins for the left atrium,

FIGURE 8–27. Parasternal long-axis *(above)* and apical four-chamber view *(below)* in a posttransplant patient showing biatrial enlargement with a prominent suture line *(arrows)*.

there is little atrial enlargement and the suture lines may not be evident.

Evaluation of Abnormal Findings

The echocardiographic approach to the posttransplant patient with suspected cardiac dysfunction is similar to that in any patient, with the proviso that the expected findings after transplantation (such as the atrial suture line) are recognized.

Pericardial effusions often are loculated due to postoperative pericardial adhesions, so careful examination in multiple tomographic planes

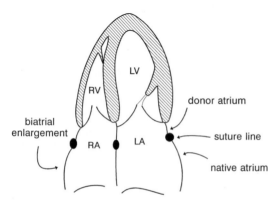

FIGURE 8–26. Schematic diagram of the posttransplant heart. Note the suture line between the donor and native atria resulting in an appearance of biatrial enlargement. Right and left ventricular size and systolic function are normal.

from parasternal, apical, and subcostal windows is essential when this diagnosis is suspected.

Echocardiographic Diagnosis of Transplant Rejection

With acute rejection, echocardiography shows increased left ventricular mass, decreased systolic function, and an increase in the echogenicity of the myocardium. In addition, a new or increasingly pericardial effusion may accompany acute rejection.

With mild or early rejection, 2D echocardiographic changes are subtle and are not accurate or reproducible enough to allow adjustment of immunosuppressive medications in individual patients. Instead, proposed echocardiographic approaches to diagnosis of early rejection have focused on measures of diastolic function, specifically measures of early diastolic relaxation. Approaches have included assessment of diastolic filling based on digitized M-mode posterior wall motion, Doppler recording of right and left ventricular diastolic inflow, Doppler recordings of superior vena cava flow, and M-mode or Doppler recordings of the interval between aortic valve closure and mitral valve opening (IVRT). In general, transplant rejection is associated with a "restrictive" filling pattern with a decreased IVRT, an increased early diastolic filling velocity, a shortened pressure half-time (more rapid early diastolic deceleration), and a loss of forward systolic flow in the superior vena cava. Although some centers have found these measures clinically useful, they have not yet gained wide acceptance for patient management. More refined approaches to ultrasonic tissue characterization also appear promising, since they may detect interstitial edema early in the course of rejection.

Echocardiographic Diagnosis of Transplant Coronary Artery Disease

As survival after cardiac transplantation has improved, increasing numbers of patients are seen with posttransplant coronary artery disease. Transplant coronary disease differs from typical atherosclerosis in that both epicardial vessels and the microvasculature are diffusely involved and the disease course often is accelerative. Echocardiographic exercise stress testing has a higher prevalence of false-negative results due to the diffuse disease process masking regional wall motion abnormalities. Dobutamine stress echocardiography may be more accurate in this patient population. However, coronary angioplasty usually is needed for accurate diag-

nosis, often with concurrent intravascular ultrasound examination of the coronary arteries.

Limitations/Technical Considerations/ Alternate Approaches

The standard method for evaluation of transplant rejection remains transvenous endomyocardial biopsy. Some centers use echocardiographic (rather than fluoroscopic) guidance for this procedure. Since echocardiographic images are tomographic, any segment of the biotome shaft going through the image plane will appear to be the "tip." Thus it is crucial to identify the open forceps of the biotome for correct identification of the biopsy site. A subcostal window often is most practical, since, with the patient supine, clear views of the right ventricle and septum are obtained, and the sonographer is clear of the sterile field (usually the right internal jugular vein approach is used). In some cases, the apical view also may be helpful.

PULMONARY HEART DISEASE

Chronic versus Acute Pulmonary Disease

Chronic pulmonary hypertension, whether due to intrinsic lung disease, recurrent pulmonary emboli, or primary pulmonary hypertension, results in a group of clinical signs and symptoms termed *cor pulmonale*. The underlying pathophysiology of this clinical syndrome is chronic pressure overload of the right ventricle as it ejects into a high-resistance pulmonary vascular bed. Initially, compensatory hypertrophy of the right ventricle occurs with preserved systolic function. Over time, right ventricular contractility deteriorates, and right ventricular dilation, moderate to severe tricuspid regurgitation, and consequent right atrial enlargement are seen (Fig. 8–28).

Acute pulmonary embolism also can affect right-sided heart function due to the sudden onset of elevated pulmonary vascular resistance. Echocardiographic evaluation may be helpful in assessing pulmonary artery pressures and right ventricular function in patients with either chronic or acute pulmonary hypertension.

Echocardiographic Approach

Pulmonary Pressures

Standard approaches for noninvasive evaluation of pulmonary pressures (PAP), as described in Chapter 5, are applicable to the patient with suspected or known pulmonary hypertension. The most reliable approach is to

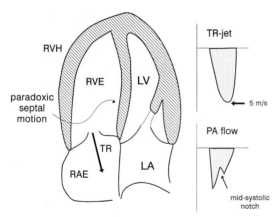

FIGURE 8–28. Schematic diagram of the key features of pulmonary heart disease. Right ventricular hypertrophy (RVH) and enlargement (RVE) are seen with paradoxic septal motion. Secondary tricuspid regurgitation (TR) and right atrial enlargement (RAE) are common. Elevated pulmonary artery pressures will be reflected in the high-velocity tricuspid regurgitant jet velocity and midsystolic notching in the pulmonary artery velocity curve.

record the maximum tricuspid regurgitant jet velocity (V_{TR}) for calculation of the right ventricular to right atrial systolic pressure difference (Fig. 8–29). Care is needed to interrogate the tricuspid regurgitant jet from multiple acoustic windows (apical, parasternal) with careful transducer angulation to obtain a parallel intercept angle between the ultrasound beam and jet. Right atrial pressure (RAP) is estimated from the size and respiratory variation in the inferior vena cava. Then pulmonary artery systolic pressure (in the absence of pulmonic stenosis) is calculated as

$$PAP = 4V_{TR}^2 + RAP$$

Pulmonary mean pressure can be estimated from the time to peak velocity of the pulmonary artery or right ventricular outflow tract velocity curve. Diastolic pulmonary artery pressure can be estimated from the velocities in the pulmonic regurgitant Doppler curve.

Indirect signs of pulmonary hypertension often are seen on echocardiography which indicate the presence, but not the exact severity, of pulmonary hypertension. An M-mode recording through the pulmonic valve shows a reduced *a* dip and midsystolic closure of the valve. This pattern has a reasonably high specificity (>90%) for detecting pulmonary hypertension but a low sensitivity (30% to 60%). This motion pattern is paralleled by the Doppler velocity curve, which shows an abrupt midsystolic deceleration of flow (Fig. 8–30). Signs of right ventricular pressure overload, including abnormal ventricular septal motion, may be valuable clues suggesting the presence of pulmonary hypertension, as detailed in the following section.

Right Ventricular Pressure Overload

The response of the right ventricle to chronic pressure overload is concentric hypertrophy. This increase in thickness of the right ventricular free wall is best seen on the subcostal view. Ventricular septal motion is abnormal or "paradoxical" with anterior motion of the septum during systole both on M-mode and 2D imaging. A rational explanation for this pattern of septal motion is based on the concept that the septum moves toward the center of mass of the heart during systole. With right ventricular hy-

FIGURE 8–29. Tricuspid regurgitant jet in a patient with pulmonary heart disease. The maximum velocity of 4 m/s indicates a right ventricular to right atrial pressure difference of 64 mmHg. Right atrial pressure was elevated at 15 mmHg, so estimated pulmonary artery systolic pressure is 79 mmHg.

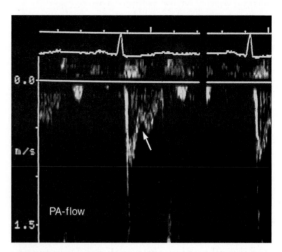

FIGURE 8–30. Pulmonary artery velocity curve showing midsystolic notching *(arrow)* due to severe pulmonary hypertension.

pertrophy, the center of mass is shifted anteriorly, so the septum moves toward the center of the right ventricle instead of the normal pattern of motion toward the center of the left ventricle. On 2D imaging, the curvature of the septum is reversed in both systole and in early to middiastole. In contrast, right ventricular volume overload is characterized by diastolic flattening of the septum in late diastole with a normal curvature in systole, due to increased volume flow into the right ventricle (compared with the left ventricle) in diastole but normal ventricular pressures in systole (Figs. 8–31 and 8–32).

With long-standing or acute pulmonary hypertension, right ventricular systolic dysfunction can occur, with secondary dilation serving as a compensatory mechanism to maintain forward stroke volume. However, right ventricular dilation leads to tricuspid regurgitation due to annular dilation and malalignment of the papillary muscles. This superimposed volume overload results in further right ventricular dilation and more tricuspid regurgitation. Right atrial dilation is due to both pressure (*v* wave) and volume (tricuspid regurgitation) overload of the right atrium.

Secondary Tricuspid Regurgitation

Tricuspid regurgitation secondary to pulmonary hypertension and/or right ventricular systolic dysfunction can be evaluated with color Doppler flow imaging from parasternal, apical, and subcostal views. Severe regurgitation results in systolic flow reversal in the inferior vena cava and hepatic veins. Careful attention to tricuspid valve anatomy is needed to ensure that other etiologies of tricuspid regurgitation (e.g., vegetation, rheumatic, Ebstein's anomaly) are not present.

The intensity of the continuous-wave Doppler tricuspid regurgitant jet relates to the severity of regurgitation, but the *velocity* relates to the right ventricular to right atrial pressure difference. With acute tricuspid regurgitation, a rapid falloff in velocity in late systole may be seen consistent with a right atrial *v* wave.

Limitations/Technical Considerations

The major limitation of echocardiography in evaluation of cor pulmonale is poor ultrasound tissue penetration resulting in poor image quality and low Doppler signal strength. Hyperexpanded lungs obscure the standard acoustic windows in many patients with chronic lung disease. However, adequate image quality may be obtained by careful patient positioning.

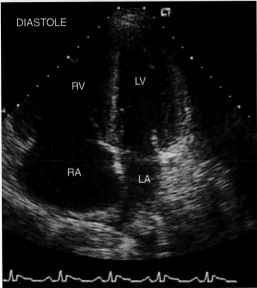

FIGURE 8–31. Apical four-chamber view at end-diastole *(above)* and end-systole *(below)* in a patient with cor pulmonale. There is right ventricular enlargement, right ventricular hypertrophy, paradoxical septal motion, and reduced systolic function of the right ventricle.

Assessment of the severity of pulmonary hypertension depends on obtaining a parallel intercept angle between the ultrasound beam and tricuspid regurgitant jet. Underestimation of pulmonary artery pressures should be considered in all patients, especially when Doppler signal strength is suboptimal or when the Doppler data and clinical setting are discrepant. The absence of a recordable tricuspid

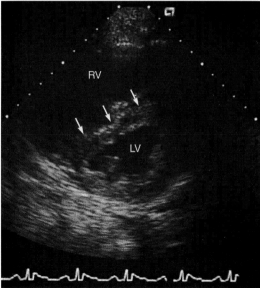

FIGURE 8–32. Parasternal views in the same patient with pulmonary hypertension seen in Figure 8–31 show flattening of the ventricular septum in diastole and right ventricular enlargement. A Swan-Ganz catheter (with reverberation artifact) is seen in the right ventricular outflow tract.

regurgitant jet does *not* indicate normal pulmonary pressures. In this situation, the echocardiographer should indicate that the data are inadequate and alternate diagnostic approaches should be considered.

Clinical Utility

Echocardiography allows confirmation of a clinical diagnosis of cor pulmonale, assess-ment of the degree of pulmonary hypertension, and evaluation of right ventricular size and systolic dysfunction. In addition, it offers at least the potential for evaluating changes in pulmonary pressures with therapeutic interventions.

In the patient with an acute pulmonary embolus, imaging may show a residual thrombus originating from or in transit through (from a deep vein thrombosis) the right side of the heart. Transesophageal imaging can demonstrate thrombus in the main, right, or left pulmonary artery. However, the sensitivity of echocardiography for *diagnosis* of pulmonary embolism based on demonstrating a thrombus is *low* because the thrombus is lodged more distally in the pulmonary vasculature in most cases. In addition, adequate visualization of the pulmonary artery bifurcation is not possible in all patients due to interposition of the air-filled trachea and bronchi.

Indirect signs of pulmonary embolism include evidence of acute right ventricular pressure overload with elevated pulmonary artery pressures, right ventricular dilation and dysfunction, and tricuspid regurgitation. Similar findings may be seen in patients with chronic recurrent pulmonary emboli. The possibility of pulmonary embolism should be strongly considered in patients with these findings even when a different working clinical diagnosis or "reason for echo" was entertained. Often patients in whom pulmonary embolism is subsequently diagnosed are initially referred for nonspecific indications including "chest pain," "dyspnea," or "heart failure."

Alternate Approaches

Cardiac catheterization allows direct measurement of right ventricular and pulmonary artery pressures and calculation of pulmonary vascular resistance. Right ventricular size and systolic function can be evaluated by angiography.

Clinically, the standard approach for diagnosis of pulmonary embolism is a radionuclide lung ventilation-perfusion scan. These data often are combined with a radionuclide or vascular diagnostic evaluation for deep venous thrombus. In some cases, pulmonary angiography is needed with injection of contrast material directly into the main pulmonary artery. The risk of pulmonary angiography is relatively high, especially in patients with pulmonary hypertension, so noninvasive approaches are preferable whenever possible.

SUGGESTED READING

General

1. Lewis JF: Doppler and two-dimensional echocardiographic evaluation in acute and long-term management of the heart failure patient. *In* Otto CM (ed): The Practice of Clinical Echocardiography. Philadelphia, WB Saunders, 1997, pp. 433–448.

   Summary of the echocardiographic findings and the clinical implications of the echocardiographic data in terms of further diagnostic evaluation, therapy, and long-term prognosis.

2. Waller BF: Pathology of the cardiomyopathies. *J Am Soc Echocardiogr* 1:4–19, 1988.

   Review of the pathology and pathophysiology of cardiomyopathies. Excellent illustrations.

3. Acquatella H, Schiller NB: Echocardiographic recognition of Chagas' disease and endomyocardial fibrosis. *J Am Soc Echocardiogr* 1:60–68, 1988.

   Review of the echocardiographic findings in Chagas' disease.

4. Tei C, Nishimura RA, Seward JB, Tajik AJ: Noninvasive Doppler derived myocardial performance index: Correlation with simultaneous measurements at cardiac catheterization. *J Am Soc Echocardiogr* 10:169–178, 1997.

   An overall assessment of both systolic and diastolic left ventricular function can be expressed as the myocardial performance index (MPI):

   $$MPI = (IVCT + IVRT)/ET$$

   where IVCT = isovolumic contraction time, IVRT = isovolumic relaxation time, and ET = ejection time. This proposed Doppler index correlates with simultaneously recorded +dP/dt, −dP/dt, and tau. This calculation also can be made using the interval from cessation to onset of transmitral flow (which equals IVRT + IVCT + ET) as:

   $$MPI = (interval\ between\ transmitral$$
   $$flows - ET)/ET$$

   A normal MPI is 0.39 ± 0.04 with elevated values indicating combined systolic and diastolic dysfunction.

Dilated Cardiomyopathy

5. Vanoverschelde J-LJ, Raphael DA, Robert AR, Cosyns JR: Left ventricular filling in dilated cardiomyopathy: Relation to functional class and hemodynamics. *J Am Coll Cardiol* 15:1288–1295, 1990.

   In patients with dilated cardiomyopathy (n = 34), more severe symptoms were associated with a higher E velocity, lower atrial filling fraction, higher E/A ratio, shorter IVRT, and shorter time to peak filling rate. Severely symptomatic patients also had a higher pulmonary artery wedge pressure, lower cardiac output, and more severe mitral regurgitation. Diastolic parameters of left ventricular function correlated better than systolic parameters with functional class.

6. Shen W-F, Tribouilloy C, Rey JL, et al: Prognostic significance of Doppler-derived left ventricular diastolic filling variables in dilated cardiomyopathy. *Am Heart J* 124:1524–1533, 1992.

   In 62 consecutive patients with dilated cardiomyopathy, the E/A ratio was the only significant Doppler predictor of clinical outcome at 31 ± 14-month follow-ups (27 cardiac events, 23 deaths, and 4 cardiac transplants). The cardiac event rate was 77% with an E/A ratio >2 versus 19% for E/A ≤2 (P < .001). Clinical functional improvement was associated with normalization of left ventricular filling parameters.

7. Lapu-Bula R, Robert A, DeKock M, et al: Risk stratification in patients with dilated cardiomyopathy: Contribution of Doppler-derived left ventricular filling. *Am J Cardiol* 82:779–785, 1998.

   In 197 consecutive patients with dilated cardiomyopathy, multivariate predictors of outcome (death or cardiac transplantation) were New York Heart Association functional class, left ventricular ejection fraction, E/A ratio, and systolic blood pressure. These data emphasize the importance of diastolic dysfunction in predicting clinical outcome in heart failure patients.

8. Simonson JS, Schiller NB: Descent of the base of the left ventricle: An echocardiographic index of left ventricular function. *J Am Soc Echocardiogr* 2:25–35, 1989.

   The extent of apical motion of the mitral annulus in systole is a simple measure of left ventricular systolic function. A "descent of the base" (annular apical motion) of <8 mm in the apical four-chamber view corresponded to an ejection fraction <50% with a sensitivity of 98% and specificity of 82%.

9. Douglas PS, Morrow R, Ioli A, Reichek N: Left ventricular shape, afterload and survival in idiopathic dilated cardiomyopathy. *J Am Coll Cardiol* 13:311–315, 1989.

   In 36 patients with dilated cardiomyopathy, poorer survival was related to a more spherical left ventricle (overall cavity shape or ratio of short- to long-axis dimensions), but not to systolic cavity dimensions, wall thickness, or fractional shortening.

10. Lewis JF, Webber JD, Sutton LL, et al: Discordance in degree of right and left ventricular dilation in patients with dilated cardiomyopathy: Recognition and clinical implications. *J Am Coll Cardiol* 21:649–654, 1993.

    In 67 patients with dilated cardiomyopathy, patients with greater involvement of the left than the right ventricle had a better outcome than those with equal degrees of dilation and systolic dysfunction of right and left ventricles.

11. Juilliere Y, Barbier G, Feldmann L, et al: Additional predictive value of both left and right ventricular ejection fraction on long-term survival in idiopathic dilated cardiomyopathy. *Eur Heart J* 18:276–280, 1997.

    Multivariate analysis identified only left and right ventricular ejection fractions as predictors of clinical outcome (death or heart transplantation) in 62 consecutive patients with dilated cardiomyopathy followed for 2.2 ± 1.3 years. This finding again emphasizes the importance of right ventricular function in patients with dilated cardiomyopathy.

12. Isaaz K, Pasipoularides A: Noninvasive assessment of intrinsic ventricular load dynamics in dilated cardiomyopathy. *J Am Coll Cardiol* 17:112–121, 1990.

    A new method to evaluate the net force of ejection using noninvasive Doppler data is proposed. Net force F of ejection is

$$F = A \cdot dv/dt + B \cdot v^2$$

    where v is ejection velocity and A and B are variables related to left ventricular chamber and outflow tract geometry. In patients with dilated cardiomyopathy, maximal ejection force, peak local acceleration, and outflow velocity were depressed compared with normal.

13. Wong M, Johnson G, Shabetai R, et al: Echocardiographic variables as prognostic indicators and therapeutic monitors in chronic congestive heart failure: Veterans Affairs Cooperative Studies V-HeFT I and II. *Circulation* 87(suppl VI):65–70, 1993.

    Echocardiographic variables including E-point septal separation, systolic left ventricular interval dimension, and the ratio of ventricular radius to wall thickness were shown to be predictors of mortality in patients with congestive heart failure in a large randomized trial (V-HeFT).

Hypertrophic Cardiomyopathy

14. Wei KS, Wigle ED, Rakowski H: Echocardiography in the evaluation and management of patients with hypertrophic cardiomyopathy. *In* Otto CM (ed): The Practice of Clinical Echocardiography. Philadelphia, WB Saunders, 1997, pp. 449–472.

    This chapter details the echocardiographic findings in hypertrophic cardiomyopathy and correlates the echocardiographic data with clinical, genetic, and pathophysiologic aspects of the disease process.

15. Wiegle ED, Rakowski H, Kimball BP, Williams WG: Hypertrophic cardiomyopathy: Clinical spectrum and treatment. *Circuation* 92:1680–1692, 1995.

    Review of hypertrophic cardiomyopathy including pathophysiology, clinical presentation, natural history, complications, treatment, and echocardiographic findings. 209 references.

16. Solomon SD, Wolff S, Watkins H, et al: Left ventricular hypertrophy and morphology in familial hypertrophic cardiomyopathy associated with mutations of the beta-myosin heavy chain gene. *J Am Coll Cardiol* 22:498–505, 1993.

    Two-dimensional echocardiograms were compared in 39 genetically affected and 30 unaffected family members. The spectrum of abnormal findings in genetically affected individuals was broad, with a maximal left ventricular wall thickness ranging from 11 to 40 (mean 24) mm. In the affected group, 62% had systolic anterior motion of the mitral leaflet, 79% had reversed septal curvature, and 77% had a septal/free wall ratio >1.3.

17. Klues HG, Maron BJ, Dollar AL, Roberts WC: Diversity of structural mitral valve alterations in hypertrophic cardiomyopathy. *Circulation* 85:1651–1660, 1992.

    Detailed anatomic study of mitral valve abnormalities seen in hypertrophic cardiomyopathy. Abnormalities were present in 66% of 94 valves and included increased leaflet area, elongation of the leaflets, and anomalous direct insertion of the anterior mitral leaflet into the papillary muscle.

18. Schwammenthal E, Nakatani S, He S, et al: Mechanism of mitral regurgitation in hypertrophic cardiomyopathy, mismatch of posterior to anterior leaflet length and mobility. *Circulation* 98:856–865, 1998.

    These authors propose that the mechanism of mitral regurgitation in patients with hypertrophic cardiomyopathy and systolic anterior motion of the valve is inadequate mobility and coaptation of the posterior leaflet.

19. Stewart WJ, Schiavone WA, Salcedo EE, et al: Intraoperative Doppler echocardiography in hypertrophic cardiomyopathy: Correlations with the obstructive gradient. *J Am Coll Cardiol* 10:327–335, 1987.

    Evaluation of the accuracy of intraoperative assessment of the degree of dynamic outflow obstruction before and after myectomy. Of note, a parallel intercept angle between the jet and Doppler beam was obtained by placing a sterile continuous-wave transducer directly on the ascending aorta with angulation toward the outflow tract. Careful positioning was required to obtain the highest-velocity signal.

20. Grigg LE, Wigle ED, Williams WG, et al: Transesophageal Doppler echocardiography in obstructive hypertrophic cardiomyopathy: Clarification of pathophysiology and importance in intraoperative decision making. *J Am Coll Cardiol* 20:42–52, 1992.

    Discussion of the utility of intraoperative transesophageal echocardiography in planning the extent of myotomy/myectomy, assessing the immediate results of the procedure, and evaluating for any potential complications. Abnormalities of the mitral valve also are described. Note that accurate assessment of the subaortic pressure gradient may be difficult from a transesophageal approach due to a nonparallel intercept angle between the jet and the ultrasound beam.

21. Marwick TH, Stewart WJ, Lever HM, et al: Benefits of intraoperative echocardiography in the surgical management of hypertrophic cardiomyopathy. *J Am Coll Cardiol* 20:1066–1072, 1992.

    In 50 patients, the impact of the combined use of preoperative transthoracic and intraoperative transesophageal echocardiography on patient management are discussed. In 10 patients (20%), a persistent outflow gradient >50 mmHg or increased moderate mitral regurgitation prompted reinstitution of cardiopulmonary bypass for further myectomy or mitral valve repair.

22. Franke A, Schondube FA, Kuhl HP, et al: Quantitative assessment of the operative results after extended myectomy and surgical reconstruction of the subvalvular mitral apparatus in hypertrophic obstructive cardiomyopathy using dynamic three-dimensional transesophageal echocardiography. *J Am Coll Cardiol* 31:1641–1649, 1998.

Three-dimensional echocardiography allows detailed evaluation of left ventricular outflow tract geometry and obstruction both before and after surgical myectomy.

23. Nagueh SF, Lakkis NM, He ZX, et al: Role of myocardial contrast echocardiography during nonsurgical septal reduction therapy for hypertropic obstructive cardiomyopathy. *J Am Coll Cardiol* 32:225–229, 1998.

    Selective contrast injection into the septal perforator arteries with simultaneous transthoracic echocardiography allows delineation of the myocardial area supplied by those vessels. This allows more precise control of the extent of myocardial loss induced by injection of ethanol to provide nonsurgical septal reduction in patients with obstructive hypertrophic cardiomyopathy.

Restrictive Cardiomyopathy

24. Leung DY, Klein AL: Restrictive cardiomyopathy: Diagnosis and prognostic implications. *In* Otto CM (ed): The Practice of Clinical Echocardiography. Philadelphia, WB Saunders, 1997, pp. 473–494.

    Detailed discussion of the importance of echocardiography in the diagnosis, management, and evaluation of prognosis in patients with restrictive cardiomyopathies.

25. Gottdiener JS, Maron BJ, Schooley RT, et al: Two-dimensional echocardiographic assessment of the idiopathic hypereosinophilic syndrome: Anatomic basis of mitral regurgitation and peripheral embolization. *Circulation* 67:572–578, 1983.

    Cardiac manifestations of the hypereosinophilic syndrome include (1) mitral regurgitation due to posterior leaflet thickening and adherence to the posterior left ventricular wall, and (2) apical left ventricular thrombi in the absence of abnormal wall motion.

26. Klein AL, Hatle LK, Taliercio CP, et al: Prognostic significance of Doppler measures of diastolic function in cardiac amyloidosis: A Doppler echocardiography study. *Circulation* 83:808–816, 1991.

    Left ventricular diastolic filling in cardiac amyloidosis is characterized by reduced early diastolic filling and an enhanced atrial contribution to filling early in the disease course, with progression to rapid early filling and a reduced atrial contribution late in the disease course ("pseudonormalization"). The Doppler pattern of left ventricular diastolic filling was predictive of clinical outcome in 63 consecutive patients. Those with a deceleration time ≤150 ms had a 1-year probability of survival of 49% compared with 76% in those with a deceleration time >150 ms (P < .001).

Hypertensive Heart Disease

27. Devereux RB, de Simone G, Ganau A, et al: Left ventricular hypertrophy and hypertension. *Clin Exp Hypertens* 15:1025–1032, 1993.

    Review of the left ventricular response to chronic hypertension emphasizing the value of ventricular mass in predicting outcome in patients with hypertension, the role of echocardiography in assessing the degree of end-organ damage, and the potential role of echocardiographic data in clinical decision making in hypertensive patients.

28. Gottdiener JS: Hypertension: Left ventricular hypertrophy, hypertensive heart disease, and the impact of echocardiographic data on treatment options, prognosis and assessment of therapy. *In* Otto CM (ed): The Practice of Clinical Echocardiography. Philadelphia, WB Saunders, 1997, pp. 521–546.

    This chapter reviews approaches to evaluation of left ventricular mass in population-based studies with emphasis on technique reproducibility and cost. The clinical relevance of echocardiography in determining the prognosis and in tailoring medical therapy in the hypertensive patient is discussed.

29. Ren JF, Panchoby SB, Iskandrian AS, et al: Doppler echocardiographic evaluation of the spectrum of left ventricular diastolic dysfunction in essential hypertension. *Am Heart J* 127:906–913, 1994.

    In 41 patients with essential hypertension, left ventricular mass was inversely correlated with the normalized peak filling rate (r = −0.89). In patients with concentric hypertrophy, the normalized peak filling rate was decreased despite normal end-diastolic and end-systolic volumes, suggesting that diastolic dysfunction occurs early in the clinical course of hypertensive heart disease and may precede evidence of systolic dysfunction.

30. Karam R, Lever HM, Healy BP: Hypertensive hypertrophic cardiomyopathy or hypertrophic cardiomyopathy with hypertension? A study of 78 patients. *J Am Coll Cardiol* 13:580–584, 1989.

    These authors emphasize that the clinical and echocardiographic features of elderly hypertensive patients with "hypertensive hypertrophic cardiomyopathy" are similar to those of normotensive patients with hypertrophic cardiomyopathy alone.

Evaluation after Heart Transplantation

31. Valentine HA, Schnittger I: Role of echocardiography in the evaluation of patients after heart transplantation. *In* Otto CM (ed): The Practice of Clinical Echocardiography. Philadelphia, WB Saunders, 1997, pp. 753–772.

    An approach to evaluation of the posttransplant patient in which echocardiographic data are key is presented. The role of echocardiography in detection of transplant rejection and in diagnosis of transplant coronary artery disease is reviewed.

32. Miller LW, Labovitz AJ, McBride LA, et al: Echocardiographically guided endomyocardial biopsy. A 5-year experience. *Circulation* 78:99–102, 1988.

    Description of utility of echocardiography for guiding endomyocardial biopsy in 4700 individual biopsies in 58 patients. Only two complications occurred.

33. Desruennes M, Corcos T, Cabrol A, et al: Doppler echocardiography for the diagnosis of acute cardiac allograft rejection. *J Am Coll Cardiol* 12:63–70, 1988.

    On serial studies in 55 consecutive patients, a 20% decrease in pressure half-time had a sensitivity of 88% and a specificity of 87% for diagnosis of acute rejection using endomyocardial biopsy as the standard of reference.

34. Simmonds MB, Lythall DA, Slorach C, et al: Doppler examination of superior vena caval flow for the detection of acute cardiac rejection. *Circulation* 86(suppl II):259–266, 1992.

In 30 patients, a forward systolic flow velocity <17 cm/s had a sensitivity of 100% and a specificity of 80% for diagnosis of acute rejection. The postulated mechanism of this observation was diminished long-axis shortening of the right ventricle.

Pulmonary Heart Disease

35. Comess, KA: Echocardiographic findings in acute and chronic pulmonary disease: Differentiation from primary cardiac disease. *In* Otto CM (ed): The Practice of Clinical Echocardiography. Philadelphia, WB Saunders, 1997, pp. 565–584.

The technical aspects of noninvasive measurement of pulmonary pressures are reviewed followed by a discussion of the clinical utility of echocardiography in patients with pulmonary disease including acute pulmonary embolism, chronic obstructive pulmonary disease, primary pulmonary hypertension, and evaluation before and after lung transplantation.

36. Come PC: Echocardiographic evaluation of pulmonary embolism and its response to therapeutic interventions. *Chest* 101(suppl 4):151S–162S, 1992.

Review of echocardiographic findings in pulmonary embolism emphasizing that with an acute event, pressures are only moderately elevated (about 40 mmHg mean pulmonary artery pressure). Thus higher right-sided pressures suggest chronic or recurrent disease.

37. Hunter JJ, Johnson KR, Karagianes TG, Dittrich HC: Detection of massive pulmonary embolus-in-transit by transesophageal echocardiography. *Chest* 100:1210–1214, 1991.

Description of the visualization of pulmonary emboli "in transit" through the right side of the heart using transesophageal echocardiography.

Pericardial Disease: Two-Dimensional Echocardiographic and Doppler Findings

9

NORMAL PERICARDIAL ANATOMY AND PHYSIOLOGY
PERICARDITIS
  Basic Principles
  Echocardiographic Approach
  Clinical Utility
PERICARDIAL EFFUSION
  Basic Principles and Tamponade Physiology
  Echocardiographic Approach to Diagnosis of
    Pericardial Effusion
    Diffuse Effusion
    Loculated Effusion
    Distinguishing from Pleural Fluid
  Echocardiographic Approach to Pericardial
    Tamponade
    Right Atrial Systolic Collapse
    Right Ventricular Diastolic Collapse
    Reciprocal Changes in Ventricular Volumes

    Respiratory Variation in Diastolic Filling
    Plethora of the Inferior Vena Cava
  Limitations/Alternate Approaches
  Clinical Utility
    Diagnosis of Pericardial Effusion
    Echo-Guided Pericardiocentesis
PERICARDIAL CONSTRICTION
  Basic Principles
  Echocardiographic Approach
    2D/M-Mode Imaging
    Doppler Examination
    *Comparison of Pericardial Tamponade,
      Constrictive Pericarditis, and Restrictive
      Cardiomyopathy*
  Limitations/Alternate Approaches
  Clinical Utility
SUGGESTED READING

NORMAL PERICARDIAL ANATOMY AND PHYSIOLOGY

The pericardium consists of two serous surfaces surrounding a closed, complex, saclike potential space. The visceral pericardium is continuous with the epicardial surface of the heart. The parietal pericardium is a dense but thin fibrous structure that is closely apposed to the pleural surfaces laterally and blends with the central tendon of the diaphragm inferiorly. Around the right and left ventricles and the ventricular apex, the pericardial space is a simple ellipsoid structure conforming to the shape of the ventricles. Around the systemic and pulmonary venous inflows and around the great vessels, the parietal and visceral pericardia meet to close the "ends" of the sac—these areas often are referred to as *pericardial reflections*. The pericardial space encloses the right atrium and right atrial appendage anteriorly and laterally, with pericardial reflections around the superior and inferior vena cava near their junction with the right atrium. Superiorly, the pericardium extends a short distance along the great vessels,

with a small "pocket" of pericardium surrounding the great arteries posteriorly—the *transverse sinus*. The pericardial space extends lateral to the left atrium, and a blind pocket of the pericardium extends posterior to the left atrium, between the four pulmonary veins—the *oblique sinus* (Fig. 9–1). The pericardial space normally contains a small amount (5 to 10 ml) of fluid that may be detectable by echocardiography.

Anatomically, the pericardium isolates the heart from the rest of the mediastinum and from the lungs and pleural spaces. In addition, it may serve a lubricating function to allow normal rotation and translation of the heart during the cardiac cycle. However, the normal physiologic function of the pericardium is unclear. Some investigators suggest that the pericardium exerts a "restraining" effect on normal cardiac filling, while others argue that the pericardium has no significant hemodynamic function. In either case, the importance of the pericardium becomes clear with disease processes such as inflammation, infection, or malignancy.

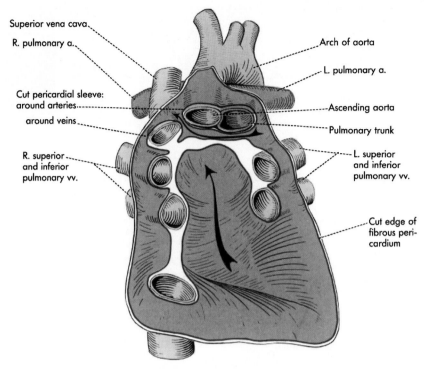

FIGURE 9–1. The posterior wall of the pericardial sac after the heart has been removed by severing its continuity with the great arteries and veins and by cutting the two pericardial sleeves that surround the arteries and veins. The parietal serous pericardium is dark gray; the fibrous pericardium is white; the *horizontal arrow* is in the transverse sinus; the *vertical arrow* is in the oblique sinus of the pericardium. (Reprinted with permission from Rosse C, Goddum-Rosse P: Hollinshead's Textbook of Anatomy, 5th ed. Philadelphia, Lippincott-Raven, 1997.)

PERICARDITIS

Basic Principles

Pericarditis is inflammation of the pericardium, and it can be due to a wide variety of causes, including bacterial or viral infection, trauma, uremia, and transmural myocardial infarction (Table 9–1). Clinically, the diagnosis is based on the characteristic triad of chest pain, electrocardiographic changes, and the presence of a pericardial rub on auscultation. While it is probable that most patients with pericarditis have a pericardial effusion at some point in the disease course, a pericardial effusion is not a necessary criterion for diagnosis of pericarditis, nor does the presence of an effusion indicate a diagnosis of pericarditis. Interestingly, there is no correlation between the size of the pericardial effusion and the presence or absence of a pericardial "rub" on physical examination.

Echocardiographic Approach

In a patient with suspected pericarditis, the echocardiogram may show a pericardial effusion of any size or pericardial thickening with or without an effusion, or it may be entirely nor-

TABLE 9–1	Differential Diagnosis of Pericardial Effusion/ Pericarditis

I. Infections
 A. Postviral pericarditis
 B. Bacterial
 C. Tuberculosis

II. Malignant
 A. Metastatic disease (e.g., lymphoma, melanoma)
 B. Direct extension (lung carcinoma, breast carcinoma)
 C. Primary cardiac malignancy

III. "Inflammatory"
 A. Postmyocardial infarction (Dressler's syndrome)
 B. Uremia
 C. Collagen vascular disease
 D. Postcardiac surgery

IV. Intracardiac-Pericardial Communications
 A. Blunt or penetrating chest trauma
 B. Postcatheter procedures (electrophysiology studies, percutaneous coronary intervention, valvuloplasty)
 C. Left ventricular rupture postmyocardial infarction

mal. A pericardial effusion is recognized as an echolucent space around the heart, as described in detail in the following sections (Fig. 9–2).

Pericardial thickening is evidenced by increased echogenicity of the pericardial reflection on two-dimensional (2D) imaging and as multiple parallel reflections posterior to the left ventricle on M-mode recordings (Fig. 9–3). However, since the pericardium typically is the most echogenic structure in the image, it can be difficult to distinguish normal from thickened pericardium.

A careful echocardiographic examination from several windows is needed when pericarditis is suspected, since effusion or thicken-

FIGURE 9–3. Pericardial thickening on M-mode echocardiography appears as multiple parallel dense echos posterior to the left ventricular epicardium *(arrows)*.

ing can be localized and may be seen in only certain tomographic views. If a pericardial effusion is present, the possibility of tamponade physiology should be considered. If pericardial thickening is present, examination for evidence of constrictive physiology should be considered (see following sections).

Clinical Utility

Pericarditis is a clinical diagnosis that cannot be made independently by echocardiography. The goal of the echocardiographic examination is to evaluate for pericardial effusion or thickening.

PERICARDIAL EFFUSION

Basic Principles and Tamponade Physiology

A wide variety of disease processes can result in a pericardial effusion with a differential diagnosis similar to that for pericarditis (see Table 9–1). The physiologic consequences of fluid in the pericardial space depend both on the volume and rate of fluid accumulation. A slowly expanding pericardial effusion can become quite large (>1000 ml) with little increase in pericardial pressure, whereas rapid accumulation of even a small volume of fluid (50 to 100 ml) can lead to a marked increase in pericardial pressure (Fig. 9–4).

Tamponade physiology occurs when the pressure in the pericardium exceeds the pressure in the cardiac chambers, resulting in impaired cardiac filling. As pericardial pressure increases, filling of each cardiac chamber is sequentially impaired, with lower-pressure cham-

FIGURE 9–2. Parasternal long- and short-axis views of a large posterior pericardial effusion (PE).

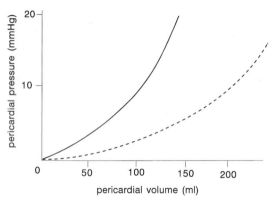

FIGURE 9–4. Schematic graph of pericardial pressure versus pericardial volume for an acute effusion (*solid line,* with a steep pressure-volume relationship) and for a chronic effusion (*dashed line,* where large volumes may lead to only mild pressure elevation).

bers (atria) affected before higher-pressure chambers (ventricles). The compressive effect of the pericardial fluid is seen most clearly in the phase of the cardiac cycle when pressure is lowest in that chamber—systole for the atrium, diastole for the ventricles. Filling pressures become elevated as a compensatory mechanism to maintain cardiac output. In fully developed tamponade, diastolic pressures in all four cardiac chambers are equal (and elevated) due to exposure of the entire heart to the elevated pericardial pressure.

Clinically, tamponade physiology is manifested as low-cardiac-output symptoms, hypotension, and tachycardia. Jugular venous pressure is elevated and pulsus paradoxus (an inspiratory decline >10 mmHg in systemic

blood pressure) is present on physical examination. The clinical finding of pulsus paradoxus is closely related to the echo findings of reciprocal respiratory changes in right and left ventricular filling and emptying (Fig. 9–5).

Echocardiographic Approach to Diagnosis of Pericardial Effusion

Diffuse Effusion

A pericardial effusion is recognized on 2D echocardiography as an echolucent space adjacent to the cardiac structures. In the absence of prior pericardial disease or surgery, pericardial

FIGURE 9–5. Schematic graph showing the relationship between pericardial pressure (PP), right atrial pressure (RAP), mean arterial pressure (MAP), and cardiac output (CO). Note that when pericardial pressure exceeds right atrial (RA) pressure, blood pressure and cardiac output fall. When right ventricular (RV) pressure is exceeded *(at the arrow),* cardiac output and mean arterial pressure fall further.

FIGURE 9–6. Pericardial effusion seen from an apical four-chamber view *(above)* and from a subcostal view *(below).*

effusions usually are diffuse and symmetric with clear separation between the parietal and visceral pericardium (Fig. 9–6). A relatively echogenic area anteriorly, in the absence of a posterior effusion, most likely represents a pericardial fat pad. M-mode recordings are helpful, especially with a small effusion, showing the flat posterior pericardial echo reflection and the moving epicardial echo with separation between the two in both systole and diastole.

In patients with recurrent or long-standing pericardial disease, fibrinous stranding within the fluid and on the epicardial surface of the heart may be seen (Fig. 9–7). When a malignant effusion is suspected, it is difficult to distinguish this nonspecific finding from metastatic disease. Features suggesting the latter include a nodular appearance, evidence of extension into the myocardium, and the appropriate clinical setting.

The size of the pericardial effusion is considered to be small when the separation between parietal and visceral pericardium is <0.5 cm, moderate when it is 0.5 to 2 cm, and large when it is >2 cm. More quantitative measures of the size of the pericardial effusion rarely are needed in the clinical setting.

Loculated Effusion

In the postoperative patient or the patient with recurrent pericardial disease, a *loculated* pericardial effusion can occur. In this situation,

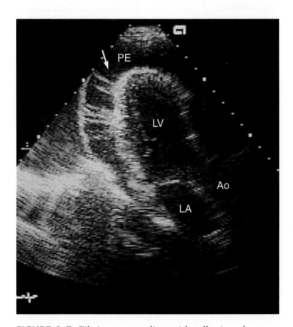

FIGURE 9–7. Fibrinous stranding with adhesions between the visceral and parietal pericardia in a chronic effusion seen on an apical long-axis view.

FIGURE 9–8. Apical four-chamber view showing a localized pericardial thrombus *(arrows)* compressing the right ventricle and atrium, leading to tamponade physiology in this postoperative patient.

the effusion is localized by adhesions to a small area of the pericardial space or consists of several separate areas of pericardial effusion, separated by adhesions. Recognition of a loculated effusion is especially important because hemodynamic compromise can occur with even a small, strategically located fluid collection. In addition, drainage of a loculated effusion may not be possible from a percutaneous approach (Fig. 9–8).

Distinguishing from Pleural Fluid

In order to reliably exclude the possibility of a loculated pericardial effusion, echocardiographic evaluation requires a careful examination from multiple acoustic windows. The parasternal approach demonstrates the extent of the fluid collection at the base of the heart in both long- and short-axis views. Note that pericardial fluid may be seen posterior to the left atrium (in the oblique sinus), as well as posterior to the left ventricle. Care should be taken that the coronary sinus or descending thoracic aorta is not mistaken for pericardial fluid. In fact, these structures can help in distinguishing pericardial from pleural fluid, since a left pleural effusion will extend posterolateral to the descending aorta, whereas a pericardial effusion will track anterior to the descending aorta (see Figs. 8–2 and Fig. 9–9).

In the apical views, the lateral, medial, and apical extent of the effusion can be appreciated.

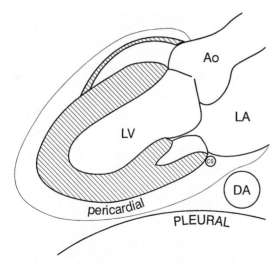

FIGURE 9–9. Schematic diagram of the relationship between a pericardial effusion and the descending aorta (DA) compared with a left pleural effusion. Pericardial fluid tracks posterior to the left atrium (LA) in the oblique sinus of the pericardium, anterior to the descending aorta.

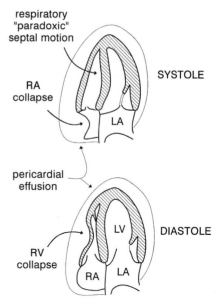

FIGURE 9–10. Schematic diagram of 2D echo findings with tamponade physiology.

In the apical four-chamber view, an isolated echo-free space superior to the right atrium most likely represents pleural fluid. The subcostal view demonstrates fluid between the diaphragm and right ventricle and is particularly helpful in echo-guided pericardiocentesis. The sensitivity and specificity of echocardiography for detection of a pericardial effusion are very high.

Echocardiographic Approach to Pericardial Tamponade (Fig. 9–10)

When cardiac tamponade occurs with a diffuse moderate to large pericardial effusion, the associated physiologic changes are evident on echocardiographic and Doppler examination (Table 9–2).

Right Atrial Systolic Collapse

When intrapericardial pressure exceeds right atrial systolic pressure (lowest point of the atrial pressure curve), inversion or collapse of the right atrial free wall occurs. Since the right atrial free wall is a thin, flexible structure, brief right atrial wall inversion can occur in the absence of tamponade physiology. However, the longer the duration of right atrial inversion relative to the cycle length, the greater is the likelihood of cardiac tamponade. Inversion for greater than a third of systole has a sensitivity of 94% and a specificity of 100% for the diagnosis of tamponade. Careful frame-by-frame 2D-image analysis is needed for this evaluation (Fig. 9–11).

Right Ventricular Diastolic Collapse

Right ventricular diastolic collapse occurs when intrapericardial pressure exceeds right ventricular diastolic pressure *and* when the right ventricular free wall is normal in thickness

TABLE 9–2	Pericardial Tamponade

Clinical Findings
Low cardiac output

Elevated venous pressures

Pulsus paradoxus

Hypotension

2D Echo
Moderate to large pericardial effusion

Right atrial systolic collapse (duration $>\frac{1}{3}$ systole)

Right ventricular diastolic collapse

Reciprocal changes in right and left ventricular volumes (varying pattern of septal motion) with respiration

Inferior vena cave plethora (indicator of elevated right atrial pressure)

Doppler
Respiratory variation in right and left ventricular diastolic filling

Increased right ventricular filling on first beat after inspiration

Decreased left ventricular filling on first beat after inspiration

FIGURE 9–11. Apical four-chamber view showing systolic collapse on the right atrial free wall *(arrow)* in a patient with clinical tamponade. PE = pericardial effusion.

FIGURE 9–12. Parasternal long-axis *(above)* and short-axis *(below)* views showing right ventricular diastolic collapse *(arrows)*.

and compliance. The presence of right ventricular hypertrophy or infiltrative diseases of the myocardium may allow development of a pressure gradient between the pericardial space and right ventricular chamber without inversion of the normal contour of the free wall. Right ventricular diastolic collapse is best appreciated in the parasternal long-axis view or from a subcostal window. If the timing of right ventricular wall motion is not clear on 2D imaging, an M-mode recording through the right ventricular free wall is helpful. The presence of right ventricular diastolic collapse is somewhat less sensitive (60% to 90%) but more specific (85% to 100%) than brief right atrial systolic collapse for diagnosing tamponade physiology (Fig. 9–12).

Reciprocal Changes in Ventricular Volumes

Reciprocal respiratory variation in right and left ventricular volumes may be seen on 2D imaging when tamponade is present. In the apical four-chamber view, an increase in right ventricular volume with inspiration (shift in septal motion toward the left ventricle in diastole and toward the right ventricle in systole) and a decrease during expiration (normalization of septal motion) can be appreciated. This pattern of motion corresponds to the physical finding of pulsus paradoxus. The proposed explanation for this observation is that total pericardial volume (heart chambers plus pericardial fluid) is fixed in tamponade so that as intrathoracic pressure becomes more negative during inspiration, enhanced right ventricular filling limits left ventricular diastolic filling. This pattern reverses during expiration (Fig. 9–13).

Respiratory Variation in Diastolic Filling

Doppler recordings of right and left ventricular diastolic filling in patients with tamponade physiology show a similar pattern. With inspiration, the right ventricular early diastolic filling velocity is augmented, while left ventricular diastolic filling diminishes (Figs. 9–14 and 9–15). In addition, the flow velocity integral in the pulmonary artery increases with inspiration, while the aortic flow velocity integral decreases. In the acutely ill patient, these changes can be difficult to demonstrate in part due to respiratory changes in the intercept angle

FIGURE 9–13. M-mode tracing showing reciprocal changes in right and left ventricular volumes with respiration when tamponade is present.

FIGURE 9–15. Doppler recording of left ventricular inflow in a patient with tamponade showing reduced filling during respiration.

between the Doppler beam and the flow of interest causing artifactual apparent velocity changes. Differentiating the normal respiratory variation in diastolic filling from the excessive variation (>25%) seen in tamponade may be subtle in borderline cases. Tamponade physiology is not an all-or-none phenomenon; a patient may exhibit varying degrees of hemodynamic impairment as the degree of pericardial compression (pericardial pressure) increases.

Plethora of the Inferior Vena Cava

Inferior vena cava plethora, a dilated inferior vena cava with <50% inspiratory reduction in diameter near the inferior vena cava–right atrium junction, also has been proposed as a sensitive (97%), albeit nonspecific (40%), indicator of tamponade physiology. This simple

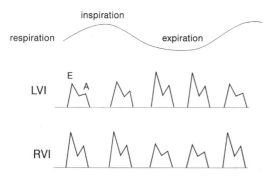

FIGURE 9–14. Schematic diagram of left and right ventricular diastolic inflow (RVI and LVI). Doppler curves with tamponade physiology showing enhanced right ventricular (and reduced left ventricular) diastolic filling with inspiration and a reversal of this pattern during expiration.

finding reflects the elevated right atrial pressure seen in tamponade.

Limitations/Alternate Approaches

Echocardiography is very sensitive for the diagnosis of pericardial effusion, even when loculated, if care is taken to examine the heart in multiple tomographic planes from multiple acoustic windows. Loculated effusions can be difficult to assess in certain locations, particularly if localized to the atrial region, since the effusion itself may be mistaken for a normal cardiac chamber.

The etiology of the pericardial effusion is not always evident on echocardiographic examination. Irregular pericardial or epicardial masses in a patient with a known malignancy certainly raise the possibility of a malignant effusion, but this appearance can be mimicked by fibrinous organization of a long-standing pericardial effusion. Masses adjacent to the cardiac structures (in the mediastinum) resulting in pericardial effusion can be missed by echocardiography. Wide-view tomographic imaging procedures, such as computed tomography (CT) or magnetic resonance imaging (MRI), are helpful in these cases.

Obviously, whether a pericardial effusion is infected or inflammatory in etiology cannot be determined by echocardiography. Depending on the associated clinical findings in each case, diagnostic pericardiocentesis and/or pericardial biopsy may be indicated to establish the correct diagnosis.

With cardiac rupture, either due to myocardial infarction or to trauma, the site of rupture itself rarely can be detected, so a high level of suspicion is needed when this diagnosis is a possibility. In some cases, the site of left ventricular rupture is "contained" by pericardial adhesions, resulting in formation of a pseudo-aneurysm. A *pseudoaneurysm* is defined as a saccular structure communicating with the ventricle with walls composed of pericardium (Fig. 9–16). In contrast, the walls of a "true" aneurysm are composed of thinned, scarred myocardium. A pseudoaneurysm can be distinguished from a true aneurysm by echocardiography based on (1) an abrupt transition from normal thickness of myocardium to the thin-walled sac, (2) an acute angle between the contour of the aneurysm and the left ventricle, and (3) a narrow opening ("neck") between the ventricular chamber and the aneurysm with a ratio of the neck diameter to maximum aneurysm diameter <0.5. This distinction is important because pseudoaneurysms are prone to rupture and require surgical correction, whereas a diagnosis of a true aneurysm does not mandate surgical intervention.

Clinical Utility

Diagnosis of Pericardial Effusion

Echocardiography is the procedure of choice for diagnosis of pericardial effusion. When

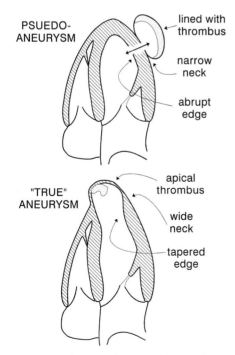

FIGURE 9–16. Schematic diagram of a pseudoaneurysm versus a true aneurysm.

transthoracic images are inadequate, as occasionally occurs (especially in postoperative patients), transesophageal imaging or an alternate tomographic imaging procedure (MRI, CT) may be needed. Echocardiography can be helpful in establishing a diagnosis of pericardial tamponade but requires integration with other clinical data.

In evaluating a patient for cardiac tamponade, it is essential to remember that tamponade is a clinical and hemodynamic diagnosis. Furthermore, varying degrees of tamponade physiology may be seen. The most important finding on echocardiography in a patient with suspected pericardial tamponade is whether or not a pericardial effusion is present. The absence of a pericardial effusion *excludes* the diagnosis, again taking care that a loculated effusion is not missed. Only rarely does tamponade physiology result from other mediastinal contents under pressure (i.e., air due to barotrauma or a compressive mass). Conversely, in a patient with convincing clinical evidence for tamponade, the presence of a moderate to large pericardial effusion on echocardiography *confirms* the diagnosis.

In intermediate cases, either when the clinical diagnosis has not been considered or when the clinical evidence is equivocal, 2D findings of chamber collapse and inferior vena cava plethora and Doppler findings showing marked respiratory variation in right and left ventricular filling may be helpful. Since none of these findings has a positive predictive value of 100%, each needs to be considered in conjunction with the clinical data. Another diagnostic test that is helpful in making this diagnosis is right-sided heart catheterization showing a depressed cardiac output and equalization of right atrial, right ventricular diastolic, and pulmonary artery wedge pressures.

Echo-Guided Pericardiocentesis

The success rate without complications of percutaneous needle pericardiocentesis can be enhanced by using echocardiographic guidance. With the patient in the position planned for the procedure, the optimal transcutaneous approach is identified based on the location of the effusion, the distance from the chest wall to the pericardium, and the absence of intervening structures. The transducer angle and pericardial depth are noted, and the transducer position is marked prior to prepping the site for the procedure. After the procedure, the residual amount of pericardial fluid is assessed using standard tomographic views. If monitoring during the procedure is needed, an acoustic window that allows visualization of the effusion but does not compromise the sterile field is identified. (Alternatively, a sterile sleeve is used for the transducer.) Note that with *tomographic* imaging it is difficult to identify the *tip* of the needle, since any segment of the needle passing through the image plane may appear to be the tip. Scanning in both superoinferior and lateromedial directions during imaging helps minimize this source of error. Confirmation that the needle tip is in the pericardial space can be made by injecting a *small* amount of agitated sterile saline solution through the needle to achieve an echo-contrast effect.

PERICARDIAL CONSTRICTION

Basic Principles

In constrictive pericarditis, the visceral and parietal layers of the pericardium are adherent, thickened, and fibrotic, resulting in impairment of diastolic ventricular filling. Pericardial constriction can occur after repeated episodes of pericarditis, after cardiac surgery, after radiation therapy, and from a variety of other causes. The diagnosis often is delayed because clinical symptoms are nonspecific—fatigue and malaise due to low cardiac output—and physical findings either are subtle (elevated jugular venous pressure, distant heart sounds) or occur only late in the disease course (ascites and peripheral edema).

The physiology of constrictive pericarditis is characterized by impaired diastolic cardiac filling due to the abnormal pericardium surrounding the cardiac structures, acting like a rigid "box" (Fig. 9–17). Early diastolic filling is rapid, with an abrupt cessation of ventricular filling as diastolic pressure rises—when the "box" is "full." Pressure tracings typically show (1) a brief, rapid fall of ventricular pressure in early diastole followed by a high early diastolic pressure plateau (*dip-plateau* or *square-root sign*), (2) a rapid descent of right atrial pressure with the onset of ventricular filling (*y* descent), (3) only modest elevation of right ventricular and pulmonary artery systolic pressures, (4) a right ventricular diastolic pressure plateau that is a third or more of systolic pressure, and (5) equalization of diastolic pressures in the right ventricle and left ventricle even after volume loading (Fig. 9–18).

Echocardiographic Approach (Table 9–3)

2D/M-Mode Imaging

Typically, left ventricular wall thickness, internal dimensions, and systolic function are normal in the patient with constrictive pericarditis. Left atrial enlargement is seen due to chronic left atrial pressure elevation. Pericardial thickening may be evident on 2D imaging as increased echogenicity in the region of the pericardium (Fig. 9–19). Careful examination from several acoustic windows is needed because the spatial distribution of pericardial thickening may be asymmetric. From the parasternal approach, an M-mode recording shows multiple dense echos, posterior to the left ventricular epicardium, moving parallel with each other. These echos persist even at a low-gain setting. M-mode recordings also may demonstrate an

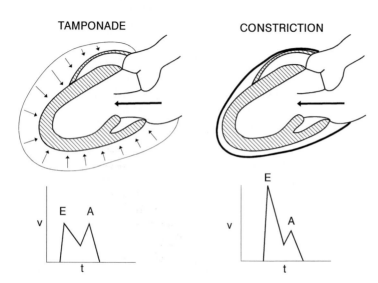

FIGURE 9–17. Schematic diagram of pericardial tamponade compared with pericardial constriction. With tamponade, diastolic filling is impaired in both early and late diastole due to the elevated pericardial pressures "compressing" the heart. With constriction, early diastolic filling is rapid but ends abruptly when the volume limits of the rigid pericardial space are reached.

Constrictive Pericarditis

Pericardial Tamponade

FIGURE 9–18. Typical pressure tracings in tamponade and constriction.

TABLE 9–3	Echo Doppler Findings in Constrictive Pericarditis

M-Mode/2D

Pericardial thickening

Normal left ventricular size and systolic function

Left atrial enlargement

Flattened diastolic wall motion

Abrupt posterior motion of the ventricular septum in early diastole

Dilated inferior vena cava and hepatic veins

Doppler

Prominent *y* descent on hepatic vein or superior vena cava flow pattern

Left ventricular inflow shows prominent *E* velocity with a rapid early diastolic deceleration slope and a small or absent *A* velocity

Increase in LV-IVRT by >20% on first beat after inspiration

Respiratory variations in right ventricular/left ventricular diastolic filling (difference >25%) with increase in right ventricular filling and decrease in left ventricular filling with inspiration

Pulmonary venous flow shows prominent *a* wave and blunting of systolic phase of left atrial filling

LV-IVRT = Left ventricular isovolumic relaxation time.

FIGURE 9–19. Constrictive pericarditis from a parasternal short-axis and apical four-chamber view. Note the thickened pericardium *(arrow)*, biatrial enlargement, and small ventricles.

FIGURE 9–20. M-mode in constrictive pericarditis showing rapid anterior motion of the septum *(arrow)* with atrial contraction before the QRS on the ECG.

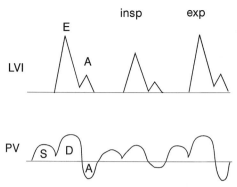

FIGURE 9–21. Schematic diagram of the Doppler flow patterns in constrictive pericarditis. Left ventricular inflow shows reduced early diastolic filling with inspiration, while the pulmonary vein shows a prominent *a* wave and blunting of the systolic filling phase.

abrupt posterior motion of the ventricular septum in early diastole, with flat motion in middle diastole and abrupt anterior motion following atrial contraction (Fig. 9–20). This pattern of motion appears to be due to initial rapid right ventricular diastolic filling, followed by equalization of filling of right and left ventricles as the "plateau" phase of the pressure curve is reached, and increased right ventricular filling after atrial contraction. The left ventricular posterior wall endocardium shows little posterior motion during diastole (<2 mm from early to late diastole) due to the impairment of diastolic filling resulting in a "flat" pattern of diastolic posterior wall motion. On subcostal views, the inferior vena cava and hepatic veins are dilated, reflecting the elevated right atrial pressure.

Doppler Examination

The Doppler findings in constrictive pericarditis reflect the abnormal hemodynamics in this condition (Fig. 9–21). Pulsed Doppler recordings of hepatic vein flow (from a subcostal approach) measure right atrial filling and show a prominent *a* wave and a deep *y* descent (Fig. 9–22). Similarly, pulsed Doppler recordings of pulmonary vein flow (transthoracic apical four-chamber view or transesophageal approach) indicate left atrial filling and again show a prominent *a* wave, prominent *y* descent, and blunting of the systolic phase of atrial filling.

Both right and left ventricular diastolic filling show a high *E* velocity due to rapid early diastolic filling occurring simultaneously with the initial high atrial to ventricular pressure difference during the brief early diastolic "dip" in

ventricular pressure. As left ventricular pressure rises, filling abruptly ceases, reflected in a short deceleration time of the *E*-velocity curve. Little ventricular filling occurs in late diastole due to the elevated left ventricular diastolic pressure (the "plateau") and the constrictive effect of the thickened pericardium. Doppler recordings of ventricular inflow thus show a very small *A*-velocity following atrial contraction.

Marked reciprocal respiratory variations in right and left ventricular diastolic inflow veloc-

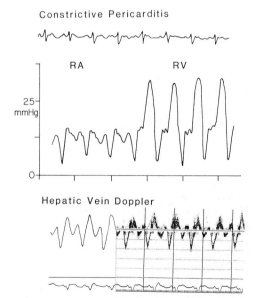

FIGURE 9–22. Pressure tracing and hepatic vein flow in a patient with constrictive pericarditis. Note the prominent *a* wave, flat diastolic segment, and prominent *y* descent, all consistent with the "square-root sign" or dip and plateau in the pressure tracings.

ities are seen due to the differing effects of changes in intrapleural pressure on filling of the two ventricles. With inspiration, intrapleural pressure becomes more negative, resulting in augmentation of right ventricular diastolic filling and inflow velocity. Left ventricular filling velocities *decrease* with inspiration and *increase* with expiration. Similar directional changes occur in normal individuals, with the respiratory changes being more marked (variation >25%) with constrictive pericarditis. The left ventricular isovolumic relaxation time—measured from the aortic closure to the mitral opening click on Doppler recordings—increases by a mean of 20% with inspiration in patients with constrictive pericarditis.

Comparison of Pericardial Tamponade, Constrictive Pericarditis, and Restrictive Cardiomyopathy (Table 9–4)

Although the hemodynamics of pericardial tamponade and pericardial constriction have some similarities, differentiating between these two diagnoses usually is straightforward based on the presence or absence of a pericardial effusion. Differentiating constrictive pericarditis from a restrictive cardiomyopathy is more difficult. Both are characterized by clinical signs and symptoms of elevated venous pressure and low cardiac output, and both show a normal-sized left ventricular chamber with normal systolic function on 2D echocardiography. Pericardial thickening may be difficult to appreciate, and other 2D and M-mode findings may not reliably differentiate between these two diagnoses. A difference (>25%) in maximum *E* velocity from expiration to inspiration has been suggested as a useful method for distinguishing constrictive pericarditis from restrictive cardiomyopathy. These characteristic Doppler findings may favor one clinical diagnosis over another and, in conjunction with other clinical data, may be definitive in some cases. However, Doppler data are far from absolutely accurate due to overlap between groups in the Doppler findings and due to differing hemodynamics in

TABLE 9–4	Comparison of Pericardial Tamponade, Pericardial Constriction, and Restrictive Cardiomyopathy		
	Pericardial Tamponade	**Constrictive Pericarditis**	**Restrictive Cardiomyopathy**
Hemodynamics			
Right atrial pressure	↑	↑	↑
Right/left ventricular filling pressures	↑, RV = LV	↑, RV = LV	↑, LV > RV
Pulmonary artery pressures	Normal	Mild elevation (35 to 40 mmHg systolic)	Moderate to severe elevation (≥60 mmHg systolic)
Right ventricular diastolic pressure plateau		>$^1/_3$ peak RV pressure	<$^1/_3$ peak RV pressure
Radionuclide Diastolic Filling		Rapid early filling, impaired late filling	Impaired early filling
2D Echo	Moderate-large PE	Pericardial thickening without effusion	Left ventricular hypertrophy Normal systolic function
Doppler Echo	Reciprocal respiratory changes in right and left ventricular filling Inferior vena cava plethora	*E* > *a* on LV inflow Prominent *y* descent in hepatic vein Pulmonary venous flow = prominent *a* wave, reduced systolic phase Respiratory variation in IVRT and in *E* velocity	(1) Early in disease *e* < A on LV inflow (2) Late in disease *E* > *a* (3) Constant IVRT (4) Absence of significant respiratory variation
Other Diagnostic Tests	Therapeutic/diagnostic pericardiocentesis	CT or MRI for pericardial thickening	Endomyocardial biopsy

CT = Computed tomography; IVRT = isovolumic relaxation time; LV = left ventricle; MRI = magnetic resonance imaging; PE = pericardial effusion; RV = right ventricular.

FIGURE 9–23. In a patient with tuberculous constrictive pericarditis, chest CT *(left)* shows thickening of visceral and parietal pericardial layers surrounding consolidated caseous material as alternating bands of light and dark anterior to the right ventricle *(arrows)*. In a second patient with constrictive pericarditis, the chest MRI *(right)* shows pericardial thickening as a low signal band *(dark area)* anterior to the right ventricle *(arrow)*. Epicardial fat is high signal *(white)* with the right coronary artery (RCA) indicated.

patients with restrictive cardiomyopathy depending on disease stage (see Chap. 8). One of the most helpful findings on Doppler examination is estimation of pulmonary artery systolic pressure from the tricuspid regurgitant jet velocity. Patients with restrictive cardiomyopathy typically have moderate to severe pulmonary hypertension, while those with constrictive pericarditis have only mild elevations in pulmonary pressures.

Limitations/Alternate Approaches

When the diagnosis of constrictive pericarditis is in question, several alternate approaches may be helpful. Chest fluoroscopy shows calcification of the pericardium in about 50% of cases of constrictive pericarditis. Either chest CT or MRI scanning is more definitive for detection of pericardial thickening, especially when it is asymmetric (Fig. 9–23). Evaluation of early diastolic ventricular filling on frame-by-frame angiography or by radionuclide techniques also has been proposed as a method to distinguish constrictive pericarditis from restrictive cardiomyopathy. Endomyocardial biopsy occasionally will confirm a diagnosis of restrictive cardiomyopathy due to an infiltrative process.

Right- and left-sided heart catheterization with recording of intracardiac pressures and waveforms, including simultaneous recording of right ventricular and left ventricular diastolic pressures after volume loading, remains the standard of reference for diagnosis of constrictive pericarditis. However, even with this technique some cases will be missed, so exploratory thoracotomy may be needed to make a defini-

tive diagnosis. If present, pericardial constriction then can be relieved by surgical removal of the pericardium.

Clinical Utility

The diagnosis of pericardial constriction remains problematic, with no single diagnostic feature on echocardiographic or Doppler examination. However, the conjunction of several findings in a patient in whom the level of clinical suspicion is high increases the likelihood of this diagnosis and may be definitive in some cases. Conversely, the echo and Doppler findings may provide the first clues for this diagnosis in a patient in whom it was not previously considered, for example, a patient presenting with ascites and no prior cardiac history.

SUGGESTED READING

Pericardial Effusion

1. Markiewicz W, Brik A, Brook G, et al: Pericardial rub in pericardial effusion: Lack of correlation with amount of fluid. *Chest* 77:643–646, 1980.

   In 76 patients with a pericardial effusion, a rub was noted on auscultation in 4 of 13 (30%) with a small effusion, 23 of 40 (58%) with a moderate effusion, and 10 of 23 (43%) patients with a large effusion. These findings suggest that the size of the effusion cannot be predicted from the presence or absence of a rub.

2. Markiewicz W, Monakier I, Brik A, et al: Clinical-echocardiographic correlations in pericardial effusion. *Eur Heart J* 3:260–266, 1982.

   Of 100 patients with an effusion on echocardiography, 49 had a clinical course consistent with acute pericarditis (idiopathic in 23, postradiation therapy in 7, Dressler's syndrome in 7, purulent in 4, and other in 7). In the 51 patients with chronic pericarditis, the etiology was carcinoma in 20, heart disease in 12, uremia in 7, rheumatoid arthritis in 5, chronic idiopathic pericarditis in 4, and other in 3 patients.

3. Permanyer-Miralda G, Sagrista-Sauleda J, Soler-Soler J: Primary acute pericardial disease: A prospective series of 231 consecutive patients. *Am J Cardiol* 56:623–630, 1985.

   Of 231 patients with primary acute pericarditis, "therapeutic pericardiocentesis" was performed in 44 for tamponade physiology, while 32 had a "diagnostic" pericardiocentesis for suspected purulent pericarditis. The diagnostic yield was 29% for therapeutic and 6% for diagnostic pericardiocentesis. The overall diagnostic yield of pericardial biopsy was 22%.

4. Drummond JB, Seward JB, Tsang TS, et al: Outpatient two-dimensional echocardiography-guided pericardiocentesis. *J Am Soc Echocardiogr* 11:433–435, 1998.

   Discussion of patient selection and the approach to pericardiocentesis using echocardiographic guidance.

Tamponade Physiology

5. Gillam LD, Guyer DE, Gibson TC, et al: Hydrodynamic compression of the right atrium: A new echocardiographic sign of cardiac tamponade. *Circulation* 68:294–301, 1983.

   Right atrial free wall systolic inversion that persists for a third or more of the cycle length had a sensitivity of 94% and specificity of 100% for the diagnosis of tamponade physiology in 127 patients (19 with tamponade).

6. Leimgruber P, Klopfenstein HS, Wann LS, Brooks HL: The hemodynamic derangement associated with right ventricular diastolic collapse in cardiac tamponade: An experimental echocardiographic study. *Circulation* 68:612–620, 1983.

   In an experimental model, right ventricular diastolic collapse occurred when intrapericardial pressure exceeded right ventricular diastolic pressure and was associated with a 21% reduction in cardiac output (but no change in mean aortic pressure). Of note, right ventricular diastolic collapse did not occur in the presence of right ventricular hypertrophy.

7. Reddy PS, Curtiss EL, Uretsky BF: Spectrum of hemodynamic changes in cardiac tamponade. *Am J Cardiol* 55:1487–1491, 1990.

   The range of hemodynamic compromise that can be seen with tamponade physiology is emphasized in this study of 77 consecutive patients with >150 ml of pericardial fluid. In group I, intrapericardial pressures were less than right atrial and pulmonary artery wedge pressures. In group II, intrapericardial and right atrial pressures had equaled. In group III, intrapericardial, right atrial, and pulmonary artery wedge pressures were equal. All subjects improved after pericardiocentesis, with the greatest improvement seen in group III.

8. Gonzalez MS, Basnight MA, Appleton CP: Experimental cardiac tamponade: A hemodynamic and Doppler echocardiographic reexamination of the relation of right and left heart ejection dynamics to the phase of respiration. *J Am Coll Cardiol* 18:243–252, 1991.

   In this model, there was an inverse relationship between peak left and right ventricular systolic pressures and ejection times, and between pulmonary and aortic flow velocities, when tamponade physiology was present. This suggests that the mechanism of pulsus paradoxus is the reciprocal changes in right and left ventricular filling due to a "fixed" total cardiac volume in tamponade.

9. Gonzalez MS, Basnight MA, Appleton CP: Experimental pericardial effusion: Relation of abnormal respiratory variation in mitral flow velocity to hemodynamics and diastolic right heart collapse. *J Am Coll Cardiol* 17:239–248, 1991.

   Respiratory changes in left ventricular diastolic filling are exaggerated in tamponade, with this variation occurring before equalization of intracardiac pressures and definite right-sided heart collapse. The presence of excessive respiratory variation, but not its magnitude, is predictive of tamponade physiology.

10. Leeman DE, Levine MJ, Come PC: Doppler echocardiography in cardiac tamponade: Exaggerated respiratory variation in transvalvular blood flow velocity integrals. *J Am Coll Cardiol* 11:572–578, 1988.

    Exaggerated respiratory variation in left ventricular filling on Doppler examination was noted in 13 patients with tamponade physiology, with resolution of these changes after pericardiocentesis.

11. Picard MH, Sanfilippo AJ, Newell JB, et al: Quantitative relation between increased intrapericardial pressure and Doppler flow velocities during experimental cardiac tamponade. *J Am Coll Cardiol* 18:234–242, 1991.

    In contrast to Suggested Reading 9, these authors did note a quantitative relationship between the degree of increase in intrapericardial pressure and the percentage change in inflow/outflow patterns with respiration.

12. Chuttani K, Pandian NG, Mohanty PK, et al: Left ventricular diastolic collapse: An echocardiographic sign of regional cardiac tamponade. *Circulation* 83:1999–2006, 1991.

    Loculated effusions, especially after cardiac surgery, can cause compression of individual cardiac chambers leading to tamponade physiology. Conventional signs of tamponade may be absent on echocardiography in these cases.

13. Himelman RB, Kircher B, Rockey DC, Schiller NB: Inferior vena cava plethora with blunted respiratory response: A sensitive echocardiographic sign of cardiac tamponade. *J Am Coll Cardiol* 12:1470–1477, 1988.

    Dilation of the inferior vena cava reflects an elevated right atrial pressure. Plethora of the inferior vena cava had a sensitivity of 97% but a specificity of only 40% for the diagnosis of pericardial tamponade. False-positive results occurred in patients with right ventricular failure, tricuspid regurgitation, and pulmonary hypertension.

14. Eisenberg MJ, Schiller NB: Bayes' theorem and the echocardiographic diagnosis of cardiac tamponade. *Am J Cardiol* 68:1242–1244, 1991.

    Using Bayes' theorem, the predictive values of right ventricular collapse, right atrial collapse, and inferior vena cava plethora for the diagnosis of tamponade were calculated (using published sensitivities and specificities for these variables). When the pretest probability of tamponade is high (50%), both right atrial and right ventricular collapse have high positive and negative predictive values. With a medium (10%) or low (1%) pretest likelihood, all three variables have a high (~97%) negative predictive value (i.e., tamponade can be excluded if absent) but a low positive predictive value.

15. Levine MJ, Lorell BH, Diver DJ, Come PC: Implications of echocardiographically assisted diagnosis of pericardial tamponade in contemporary medical patients: Detection before hemodynamic embarrassment. *J Am Coll Cardiol* 17:59–65, 1991.

   Echocardiography identified right heart chamber collapse in the presence of an effusion (i.e., tamponade) in patients with minimal evidence of hemodynamic compromise. Symptoms persisted even with hemodynamic improvement after pericardiocentesis in many patients. When malignancy was the cause of tamponade, 1-year survival was only 17%.

Constrictive Pericarditis

16. Schnittger I, Bowden RE, Abrams J, Popp RL: Echocardiography: Pericardial thickening and constrictive pericarditis. *Am J Cardiol* 42:388–395, 1978.

   Description of echocardiographic diagnosis of pericardial thickening and correlation with surgical, autopsy, and catheterization findings.

17. von Bibra H, Schober K, Jenni R, et al: Diagnosis of constrictive pericarditis by pulsed Doppler echocardiography of the hepatic vein. *Am J Cardiol* 63:483–488, 1989.

   In patients with constrictive pericarditis, hepatic vein flow showed abrupt reversal in late systole and in mid-diastole, similar to the "W pattern" seen on physical examination of the neck veins. This hepatic vein flow pattern had a sensitivity of 68% and a specificity of 100% for the diagnosis of constrictive pericarditis in 51 patients (13 with constrictive pericarditis, 13 controls, 12 with right ventricular pressure overload, and 12 with right ventricular pressure and volume overload).

18. Hatle LK, Appleton CP, Popp RL: Differentiation of constrictive pericarditis and restrictive cardiomyopathy by Doppler echocardiography. *Circulation* 79:357–370, 1989.

   Patients with constrictive pericarditis showed marked respiratory variation in left and right ventricular inflow velocities and isovolumic relaxation times, while patients with restrictive cardiomyopathy did not have respiratory variation. With constrictive pericarditis, the first beat after inspiration showed a decrease in left ventricular inflow velocity, an increase in right ventricular inflow velocity, and an increase in left ventricular isovolumic relaxation time. These changes resolve after pericardiectomy.

19. Aroney CN, Ruddy RD, Dighero H, et al: Differentiation of restrictive cardiomyopathy from pericardial constriction: Assessment of diastolic function by radionuclide angiography. *J Am Coll Cardiol* 13:1007–1014, 1989.

   Diastolic filling curves were evaluated using radionuclide techniques. In patients with constrictive pericarditis, the rate of early diastolic filling and the time to peak filling rate were increased, while the atrial contribution to left ventricular filling was decreased compared with patients with restrictive cardiomyopathy and normal individuals.

20. Garcia MJ, Rodriquez L, Ares M, et al: Differentiation of constrictive pericarditis from restrictive cardiomyopathy: Assessment of left ventricular diastolic velocities in longitudinal axis by Doppler tissue imaging. *J Am Coll Cardiol* 27:108–114, 1996.

   The peak velocity of longitudinal axis expansion, measured with Doppler tissue imaging, is reduced in patients with restrictive cardiomyopathy due to intrinsic myocardial disease. In contrast, longitudinal axis expansion is normal with constrictive pericarditis, as elastic recoil of the myocardium is not affected by extrinsic pericardial compression.

21. Oh JF, Tajik AJ, Appleton CP, et al: Preload reduction to unmask the characteristic Doppler features of constrictive pericarditis: A new observation. *Circulation* 95:3799–3800, 1997.

   Increased filling pressures can mask the reciprocal changes in right and left ventricular diastolic filling seen in patients with constrictive pericarditis. If this diagnosis is suspected on clinical grounds, repeat recordings of ventricular filling after decreasing filling volumes is warranted (for example, in the sitting rather than supine position).

22. Oki T, Tabata T, Yamada H, et al: Right and left ventricular wall motion velocities as diagnostic indicators of constrictive pericarditis. *Am J Cardiol* 81:465–470, 1998.

   Doppler tissue imaging demonstrates an abrupt outward motion of the ventricular walls immediately after the early diastolic filling velocity in patients with constrictive pericarditis compared to normal subjects. This finding has potential value for diagnosis of constrictive pericarditis.

Left Ventricular Pseudoaneurysm

23. Catherwood E, Mintz GS, Kotler MN, et al: Two-dimensional echocardiographic recognition of left ventricular pseudoaneurysm. *Circulation* 62:294–303, 1980.

   Characteristic echocardiographic findings in left ventricular pseudoaneurysm are presented.

24. Gatewood RP Jr, Nanda NC: Differentiation of left ventricular pseudoaneurysm with two-dimensional echocardiography. *Am J Cardiol* 46:869–878, 1980.

   Characteristic echocardiographic findings in left ventricular pseudoaneurysm are presented.

Valvular Stenosis: Diagnosis, Quantitation, and Clinical Approach 10

BASIC PRINCIPLES
  Approach to Evaluation of Valvular Stenosis
  Fluid Dynamics of Valvular Stenosis
    High-Velocity Jet
    Relationship Between Pressure Gradient and
      Velocity
    Distal Flow Disturbance
    Proximal Flow Patterns
AORTIC STENOSIS
  Diagnostic Imaging of the Aortic Valve
    Calcific Aortic Stenosis
    Bicuspid Aortic Valve
    Rheumatic Aortic Stenosis
    Congenital Aortic Stenosis
    Differential Diagnosis
  Quantitation of Stenosis Severity
    Pressure Gradients
    Continuity Equation Valve Area
    Velocity Ratio and Other Measures of Stenosis
      Severity
    Technical Considerations and Potential Pitfalls
  Coexisting Valvular Disease
  Response of the Left Ventricle to Valvular Aortic
    Stenosis
  Clinical Applications in Specific Patient Populations
    Symptomatic Adults with Valvular Aortic Stenosis
      Being Considered for Surgical Intervention
    Disease Progression and Prognosis in
      Asymptomatic Aortic Stenosis
    Evaluation of Aortic Stenosis with Left
      Ventricular Systolic Dysfunction

    Assessment of a Systolic Murmur
  Case Examples
MITRAL STENOSIS
  Diagnostic Imaging of the Mitral Valve
    Rheumatic Disease
    Mitral Annular Calcification and Calcific Mitral
      Stenosis
    Differential Diagnosis
  Quantitation of Mitral Stenosis Severity
    Pressure Gradients
    Mitral Valve Area
    Technical Considerations and Potential Pitfalls
  Coexisting Lesions in Mitral Stenosis
    Left Atrial Enlargement and Thrombus
    Pulmonary Hypertension
    Mitral Regurgitation
    Other Coexisting Valvular Disease
    Left Ventricular Response
  Clinical Applications in Specific Patient Populations
    Diagnosis, Hemodynamic Progression, and Timing
      of Intervention
    Pre- and Post-Percutaneous Commissurotomy
    Evaluation of the Pregnant Patient with
      Pulmonary Congestion
  Case Examples
TRICUSPID STENOSIS
PULMONIC STENOSIS
SUGGESTED READING

BASIC PRINCIPLES

Approach to Evaluation of Valvular Stenosis

Narrowing, or stenosis, of a cardiac valve can be due to a congenitally abnormal valve, a postinflammatory process (e.g., rheumatic), or degenerative calcification. As the degree of valve opening decreases, the increasing obstruction to blood flow results in an increased flow velocity and pressure gradient across the valve. In isolated valve stenosis, clinical symptoms typically occur when the valve orifice is reduced to one-quarter its normal size. In mixed stenosis and regurgitation, symptoms can occur when each lesion, if isolated, would be considered only moderate in severity.

Secondary changes in patients with valvular stenosis include the response of the specific cardiac chambers affected by pressure overload. The ventricular response to pressure overload is hypertrophy; the atrial response is dilation. Chronic pressure overload also can lead to irreversible changes in other upstream cardiac chambers and in the pulmonary vascular bed (e.g., in mitral stenosis).

Complete echocardiographic evaluation of the patient with valvular stenosis includes (1) diagnostic imaging of the valve to define the etiology of stenosis, (2) quantitation of stenosis severity, (3) evaluation of coexisting valvular lesions, (4) assessment of left ventricular systolic function, and (5) the response to chronic pressure overload of other upstream cardiac chambers and the pulmonary vascular bed. This echocardiographic evaluation then is integrated with pertinent clinical data for a complete evaluation of the patient.

Fluid Dynamics of Valvular Stenosis

High-Velocity Jet

The fluid dynamics of a stenotic valve are characterized by the formation of a laminar, high-velocity jet in the narrowed orifice. The flow profile in cross section at the origin of the jet is relatively blunt (or flat) and remains blunt as the jet reaches its narrowest cross-sectional area in the vena contracta, slightly downstream from the anatomic orifice (Fig. 10–1). Thus the narrowest cross-sectional area of flow (physiologic orifice area) is smaller than the anatomic orifice area. The magnitude of this difference between physiologic and anatomic area depends on orifice geometry and the Reynold's number (a descriptor of the inertial and shear stress properties of the fluid). The ratio of the physiologic to anatomic orifice area is known as the *discharge coefficient*.

The length of the high-velocity jet is dependent on orifice geometry as well and can be variable in the clinical setting with, for example, a very short jet across a deformed, irregular, calcified aortic valve and a longer jet across a smoothly tapering, symmetric, rheumatic mitral valve or a congenitally stenotic semilunar valve (Fig. 10–2).

Relationship Between Pressure Gradient and Velocity

The pressure gradient across the stenotic valve is related to the velocity in the jet, according to the unsteady Bernoulli equation:

$$\text{Bernoulli equation} \qquad (10.1)$$
$$\Delta P = 1/2\rho(v_2{}^2 - v_1{}^2) + \rho\left(\frac{dv}{dt}\right)dx + R(v)$$

Convective acceleration	Local acceleration	Viscous resistance

where ΔP is the pressure gradient across the stenosis (mmHg), ρ is the mass density of blood (1.06×10^3 kg/m^3), v_2 is velocity in the stenotic jet, v_1 is velocity proximal to the stenosis, $(dv/dt)dx$ is the time-varying velocity at each distance along the flowstream, and R is a constant describing the viscous losses for that fluid and orifice. Historically, the first description of this equation was proposed about 1738 by Daniel Bernoulli from studies of steady water flow in rigid tubes. The concepts were later expanded and refined by Euler. Of note, these equations may not be strictly applicable to pulsatile blood flow in compliant chambers and

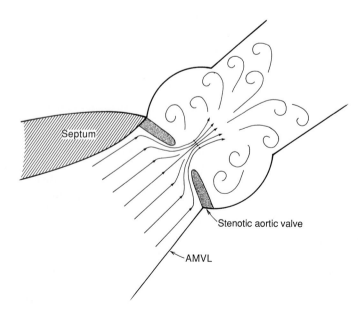

FIGURE 10–1. Schematic illustration of the fluid dynamics of the stenotic aortic valve in systole. The left ventricular outflow tract (LVOT) is bounded by the septum and anterior mitral valve leaflet (AMVL). As LVOT flow accelerates and converges, a relatively flat velocity profile occurs proximal to the stenotic valve, as indicated by the *arrowheads*. Flow accelerates in a spatially small zone adjacent to the valve as blood enters the narrowed orifice. In the stenotic orifice, a high-velocity laminar jet is formed with the narrowest flowstream (vena contracta, indicated by the dots) occurring downstream from the orifice. Beyond the jet, flow is disturbed, with blood cells moving in multiple directions and velocities. (Reprinted with permission from Judge KW, Otto CM: *Cardiol Clin* 8:203, 1990.)

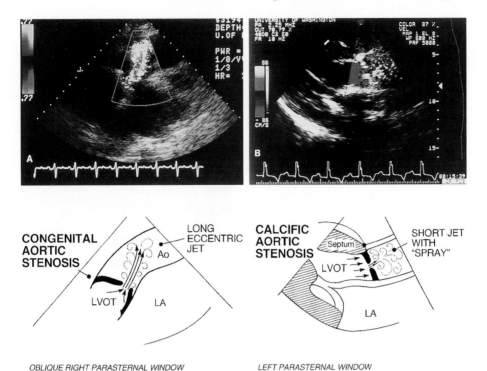

FIGURE 10–2. Color flow imaging in congenital valvular aortic stenosis *(left)* from an oblique high right parasternal window and in calcific aortic stenosis *(right)* from a left parasternal window, with corresponding line drawings below. In the congenital case, note the domed valve with a long, eccentric jet; in the calcific case, note the short jet with a diffuse "spray" (LV = left ventricle; Ao = aorta, LA = left atrium). (See Color Plate 7, p. 274.) (Reprinted with permission from Judge KW, Otto CM: *Cardiol Clin* 8:203, 1990.)

vessels, although clinical studies have shown that remarkably accurate pressure-gradient predictions can be made with this approach. This equation was first applied to Doppler data from stenotic mitral valves by Dr. Holen in 1976 and from stenotic aortic valves by Dr. Hatle in 1979.

Eliminating the terms for viscous losses and acceleration, substituting known values for the mass density of blood, and adding a conversion factor for measuring velocity in units of meters per second (m/s) and pressure gradient in millimeters of mercury (mmHg), the Bernoulli equation can be reduced to

$$\Delta P = 4(v_2^2 = v_1^2) \qquad (10.2)$$

If the proximal velocity is ≤1 m/s, as is commonly the case for stenotic valves, it becomes even smaller when squared [for example, $(0.8)^2 = 0.64$]. Thus the proximal velocity often can be ignored in the clinical setting so that:

Simplified Bernoulli equation
$$\Delta P = 4v^2 \qquad (10.3)$$

This equation allows highly accurate and reproducible calculation of maximum pressure gradients (from maximum velocity) and mean pressure gradients (by integrating the instantaneous pressure difference over the flow period).

Distal Flow Disturbance

Distal to the stenotic jet, the flowstream becomes disorganized with multiple blood flow velocities and directions, although fully developed turbulence, as strictly defined in fluid dynamic terms, may not occur. The distance that this flow disturbance propagates downstream is related to stenosis severity. In addition, the *presence* of a downstream flow disturbance can be extremely useful in defining the exact anatomic site of obstruction, e.g., allowing differentiation of subvalvular outflow obstruction (flow disturbance on the ventricular side of the valve) from valvular obstruction (flow disturbance only distal to the valve).

Proximal Flow Patterns

Proximal to a stenotic valve, flow is smooth and organized (laminar) with a normal flow velocity. The spatial flow velocity profile proximal to a stenotic valve depends on valve anatomy, inlet geometry, and the degree of flow acceleration. For example, in calcific aortic stenosis, the acceleration of blood flow by ventricular systole coupled with a tapering outflow tract geometry results in a relatively uniform flow velocity (a "flat" flow profile) across the outflow tract just proximal to the stenotic valve. Immediately adjacent to the valve orifice there is acceleration as flow converges to form the high-velocity jet, but this region of proximal acceleration is spatially small. The flow profile differs slightly for congenital aortic stenosis in that the proximal acceleration region under the domed leaflets in systole is larger than with calcific stenosis. However, proximal flow patterns are similar regardless of disease etiology in that a relatively flat velocity profile is present at the aortic annulus.

In contrast, the flow pattern proximal to the stenotic mitral valve is quite different (Figs. 10–3 and 10–4). Here, the left atrial to left ventricular pressure gradient drives flow passively from the large inlet chamber (the left atrium) abruptly across the stenotic orifice. Proximal flow acceleration is prominent over a large region of the left atrium. The three-dimensional (3D) velocity profile is curved; that is, flow velocities are faster adjacent to and in the center of a line continuous with the jet direction through the narrowed orifice and slower at increasing radial distances from the valve orifice. The proximal velocity profile of an atrioventricular valve thus is hemi-elliptical), unlike the more flattened velocity profile proximal to a stenotic semilunar valve. Any 3D surface area

FIGURE 10–4. Color flow of a mitral stenosis jet. A well-defined proximal isovelocity surface area is seen. (See Color Plate 8, p. 274.)

proximal to a narrowed orifice at which all the blood velocities are equal can be referred to as a *proximal isovelocity surface area* (PISA).

The clinical importance of these flow patterns is that stroke volume can be calculated proximal to a stenotic valve based on knowledge of the cross-sectional area of flow and the spatial mean flow velocity over the period of flow, as described in Chapter 5. This concept applies to the flat flow profile proximal to a stenotic aortic valve (used in the continuity equation), to the proximal flow patterns seen in mitral stenosis, and to the PISAs seen with regurgitant lesions (see Chap. 11).

AORTIC STENOSIS

Diagnostic Imaging of the Aortic Valve
(Fig. 10–5)

Calcific Aortic Stenosis

The most common etiology of valvular aortic stenosis in adults is degenerative calcification of an apparently normal trileaflet valve. Calcification occurs slowly over many years and may be seen on two-dimensional (2D) echo as aortic valve "sclerosis"—areas of increased echogenicity, typically at the base of or on the valve leaflets, without significant obstruction to left ventricular outflow. Clinically significant obstruction tends to occur at the ages of 70 to 85 years. When obstruction is present, 2D imaging shows a marked increase in echogenicity of the leaflets consistent with fibrocalcific disease and reduced systolic opening. When

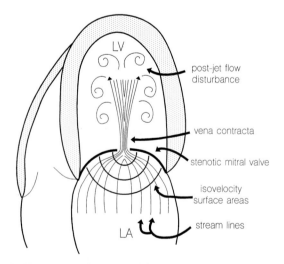

FIGURE 10–3. Schematic diagram of the fluid dynamics of rheumatic mitral stenosis. The stream lines of flow accelerate as they approach the stenotic orifice, with several curved proximal isovelocity surface areas indicated. The mitral stenosis jet is long, with the postjet flow disturbance occurring adjacent and distal to the laminar jet.

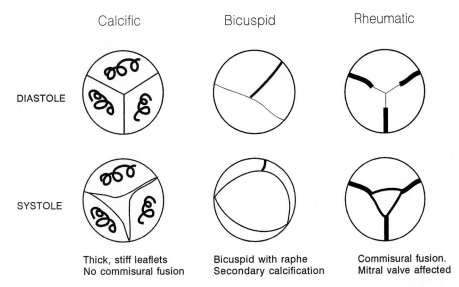

| Calcific | Bicuspid | Rheumatic |

DIASTOLE

SYSTOLE

Thick, stiff leaflets
No commisural fusion

Bicuspid with raphe
Secondary calcification

Commisural fusion.
Mitral valve affected

FIGURE 10–5. Schematic diagram of the three most common causes of valvular aortic stenosis. *Calcific* aortic stenosis is characterized by lipocalcific masses on the aortic side of the leaflet that result in increased leaflet stiffness without commissural fusion. A *congenital* bicuspid valve undergoes secondary degenerative changes. The diagnostic features of *rheumatic stenosis* are commissural fusion and mitral valve involvement.

aortic stenosis is suspected, a systolic leaflet separation of 15 mm or more by 2D or 2D-guided M-mode echocardiography reliably excludes severe obstruction. When the leaflets are abnormal and systolic separation is less than 15 mm, the degree of obstruction may be mild, moderate, or severe, depending on the cross-sectional area of the narrowed orifice. Direct measurement of valve area on short-axis 2D imaging is possible in some patients either with excellent transthoracic images or from a transesophageal approach. However, directly planimetered aortic valve areas should be interpreted with caution due to the complex 3D anatomy of the orifice in calcific degenerative stenosis. It is critical to ensure that the image plane is aligned at the narrowest orifice of the valve, although if the orifice is nonplanar, planimetry of valve area may be misleading. Even when carefully performed, 2D valve area reflects anatomic valve area, whereas Doppler data provide functional valve area.

Bicuspid Aortic Valve

Secondary calcification of a bicuspid aortic valve can be difficult to distinguish from calcification of a trileaflet valve once stenosis becomes severe. Average age at symptom onset is younger for adults with bicuspid valve stenosis, with presentation typically at the ages of 45 to 65 years.

Earlier in the disease course a bicuspid valve can be identified on 2D parasternal short-axis views by demonstrating that there are only two open leaflets in systole (Fig. 10–6). Long-axis views show systolic bowing of the leaflets into the aorta, resulting in a "domelike" appearance. M-mode recordings may help in identifying a bicuspid valve if an eccentric closure line is present but can be misleading in terms of the degree of leaflet separation if the M-mode is taken through the base, rather than the tips, of the bowed leaflets. Similarly, 2D planimetry of valve area may be erroneous if the image plane is not aligned with the narrowest point at the leaflet tips.

Typically, the two leaflets are unequal in size, with the anterior (if the leaflet opening is anteroposterior) or rightward (if the leaflet opening is lateromedial) leaflet being larger. Many bicuspid valves have a raphe in the larger leaflet so that the closed valve in diastole appears trileaflet; accurate identification of the number of aortic valve leaflets can be made only in systole. Doppler interrogation of the aortic valve should be performed whenever a bicuspid valve is suspected to evaluate for stenosis and/or regurgitation.

Rheumatic Aortic Stenosis

Rheumatic valvular disease preferentially involves the mitral valve, so rheumatic aortic stenosis is diagnosed when aortic disease occurs concurrently with rheumatic mitral valve disease. The rheumatic disease process results in commissural fusion of the aortic leaflets, similar to the pathology seen in rheumatic mitral

FIGURE 10–6. Bicuspid aortic valve with diastolic *(above)* and systolic *(below)* frames shown in parasternal long-axis *(left)* and short-axis *(right)* views. Note the diastolic sagging and systolic doming of the leaflets in the long-axis view. In short-axis view, only two leaflets are seen to open in systole with the commissures at 4- and 10-o'clock positions.

stenosis. Two-dimensional imaging may show increased echogenicity along the leaflet edges, commissural fusion, and systolic doming of the aortic leaflets. Often, however, the echocardiographic images appear similar to those of calcific aortic stenosis (other than the presence of rheumatic mitral valve disease).

Congenital Aortic Stenosis

Congenital aortic stenosis usually is diagnosed in childhood, but some patients may not become symptomatic until young adulthood or may present with restenosis after surgical valvotomy performed in childhood or adolescence. These patients most often have a unicuspid valve with a single eccentric orifice and prominent systolic doming.

Differential Diagnosis (Table 10–1)

The differential diagnosis of left ventricular outflow obstruction includes fixed subvalvular obstruction (a subaortic membrane or a muscular subaortic stenosis), dynamic subaortic obstruction (hypertrophic cardiomyopathy), and supravalvular stenosis. In a patient with a clinical diagnosis of valvular aortic stenosis, the echocardiographic study should demonstrate whether the obstruction is, in fact, valvular or if one of these other diagnoses accounts for the clinical presentation (Fig. 10–7).

A subaortic membrane should be suspected in young adults when the valve anatomy is not clearly stenotic, yet Doppler examination reveals a high transaortic pressure gradient. Since the membrane may be poorly visualized on a

TABLE 10–1	Echocardiographic Differential Diagnosis of Left Ventricular Outflow Tract Obstruction

Valvular Aortic Stenosis
Calcific aortic stenosis
Bicuspid valve with secondary calcification
Rheumatic aortic stenosis
Congenital aortic stenosis (e.g., unicuspid or fused trileaflet valve)

Subaortic Stenosis
Membranous
Muscular
Dynamic (e.g., hypertrophic cardiomyopathy)

Supravalvular Stenosis

VALVULAR AORTIC STENOSIS

SUBAORTIC MEMBRANE

HYPERTROPHIC CARDIOMYOPATHY

FIGURE 10–7. Examples of the shape of the continuous-wave Doppler velocity curve in valvular aortic stenosis, fixed subvalvular obstruction due to a subaortic membrane, and dynamic obstruction due to hypertrophic cardiomyopathy. Note that the continuous-wave curves for subvalvular and valvular aortic stenosis are similar, although coarse fluttering of the valve with subvalvular obstruction results in a "rough" appearance of the systolic velocity curve. These can be distinguished by 2D and color flow imaging. The shape of the curve with dynamic obstruction is distinctly different with velocity peaking in late systole.

transthoracic study, transesophageal imaging should be considered when this diagnosis is suspected. The spatial orientation of the jet and the shape of the continuous-wave Doppler velocity curve are similar for fixed obstructions, whether sub-, supra-, or valvular, but careful pulsed Doppler or color flow imaging allows localization of the level of obstruction by detection of the poststenotic flow disturbance.

In dynamic outflow obstruction, the timing and shape of the late-peaking continuous-wave Doppler velocity curve are distinctive. In addition, the degree of obstruction changes dramatically with provocative maneuvers, as detailed in Chapter 8. In the occasional patient with both subvalvular *and* valvular obstruction, high-pulse-repetition-frequency Doppler ultrasound can be helpful in defining the maximum velocities at each site of obstruction.

Quantitation of Stenosis Severity

The severity of valvular aortic stenosis can be determined accurately using equations derived from our understanding of the fluid dynamics of a stenotic valve.

Pressure Gradients

Maximum transaortic pressure gradient (ΔP_{max}) can be calculated from the maximum aortic jet velocity (V_{max}) using the simplified Bernoulli equation (Fig. 10–8):

$$\text{Maximum gradient}$$
$$\Delta P_{max} = 4v_{max}^2 \qquad (10.4)$$

Mean pressure gradient (ΔP_{mean}) can be calculated by digitizing the aortic jet velocity curve (where $v_1, \ldots v_n$, are instantaneous velocities) and averaging the instantaneous gradients over the systolic ejection period:

$$\text{Mean gradient}$$
$$\Delta P_{mean} = \frac{4v_1^2 + 4v_2^2 + 4v_3^2 + \cdots + 4v_n^2}{n} \qquad (10.5)$$

Interestingly, in native aortic valve stenosis, transaortic pressure gradient correlates closely and linearly with maximum transaortic gradient so that mean gradient can be approximated from published regression equations as

$$\text{Mean gradient}$$
$$\text{regression equation}$$
$$\Delta P_{mean} = \frac{(\Delta P_{max})}{1.45} + 2 \text{ mmHg} \qquad (10.6)$$

or (from a different study):

$$\Delta P_{mean} = 2.4(v_{max})^2 \qquad (10.7)$$

FIGURE 10–8. Continuous-wave Doppler recording of an aortic stenosis jet recorded from an apical *(top)* and a high right parasternal *(center)* approach in a 56-year-old man with a systolic murmur. The highest-velocity jet (right parasternal in this case) is used because it represents the most parallel intercept angle between the direction of blood flow and the stenotic jet. Maximum pressure gradient is calculated as $\Delta P = 4v^2$, with mean pressure gradient determined by integrating the instantaneous gradients over the systolic ejection period. Severe concentric left ventricular hypertrophy also was present *(bottom)*.

TABLE 10–2	Selected Studies Validating Doppler Pressure Gradients in Valvular Stenosis (in vivo simultaneous data)				

First Author/Year	N	Study Group/Model	R	Range (mmHg)	SEE (mmHg)
Callahan/1985	120	Supravalvular constriction (canines)	0.99 (ΔP_{max})	7–179	5.2
			0.98 (ΔP_{mean})	N/A	4.3
Smith/1985	88	Supravalvular constriction (canines)	0.98 (ΔP_{max})	5–166	5.3
			0.98 (ΔP_{mean})	5–116	3.3
Currie/1985	100	Adults with valvular aortic stenosis	0.92 (ΔP_{max})	2–180	15
			0.92 (ΔP_{mean})	0–112	10
Smith/1986	33	Adults with valvular aortic stenosis	0.85 (ΔP_{max})	27–138	N/A
Simpson/1985	24	Adults with valvular aortic stenosis	0.98 (ΔP_{max})	0–120	N/A
Burwash/1993	98	Chronic valvular aortic stenosis (canines)	0.95 (ΔP_{max})	10–128	8.4
			0.91 (ΔP_{mean})	5–77	5.3

SEE = Standard error of the estimate.
Data from Callahan et al: Am J Cardiol 56:989–993, 1985; Smith et al: JACC 6:1306–1314, 1985; Currie et al: Circ 71:1162–1169, 1985; Smith et al: Am Heart J 111:245–252, 1986; Simpson et al: Br Heart J 53:636–639, 1985; Burwash et al: Am J Physiol 265 (Heart Circ Physiol 34): H734–H1743, 1993.

Note that these two equations give similar results.

With careful attention to technical details, Doppler-determined pressure gradients are accurate, as has been demonstrated in numerous in vitro and animal models and in clinical studies (Table 10–2). Although Doppler maximum gradients correspond to maximum instantaneous gradients by catheter measurement and Doppler mean gradients correspond to catheter-measured mean gradients, neither Doppler gradient correlates with the peak-to-peak gradient reported at catheterization. In fact, peak aortic and peak left ventricular pressures do not occur simultaneously, so none of the instantaneous velocities recorded with Doppler ultrasound are strictly comparable with this clinical measurement. Potential confusion about Doppler pressure gradient data in an individual patient can be avoided by clearly identifying the specific type of gradient measured, for example "maximum instantaneous" or "mean systolic" (Fig. 10–9).

Physiologic changes in pressure gradient should be taken into consideration when comparing nonsimultaneous data recordings and in patient management decisions. Pressure gradients depend on volume flow rate, as well as the degree of valve narrowing, so in an individual patient the pressure gradient will rise when transaortic stroke volume increases (e.g., anxiety, exercise) and will fall when stroke volume decreases (e.g., sedation, hypovolemia).

The dependence of pressure gradients on volume flow rate can lead to erroneous conclusions about stenosis severity in adult patients with either a chronically elevated or depressed transaortic stroke volume. For example, a patient with coexisting aortic regurgitation will have a high transaortic pressure gradient with only a moderate degree of valve narrowing. Conversely, a patient with left ventricular systolic dysfunction or coexisting mitral regurgitation may have a low transaortic pressure gradient despite severe aortic stenosis. These coexisting conditions are common in adults with valvular aortic stenosis, so determination of the stenotic orifice area is essential for complete evaluation of disease severity (Figs. 10–10 and 10–11).

Continuity Equation Valve Area

Aortic valve area can be calculated based on the principle of continuity of flow (Table 10–3). Specifically, the stroke volume (SV) just proximal to the aortic valve (SV_{LVOT}) and that in the stenotic valve orifice (SV_{Ao}) are equal:

$$SV_{LVOT} = SV_{Ao} \qquad (10.8)$$

If flow is laminar with a spatially flat velocity profile,

$$SV = CSA \times VTI \qquad (10.9)$$

where CSA is the cross-sectional area of flow (cm^2), SV is stroke volume (cm^3), and VTI is the velocity-time integral (cm). Since flow both

FIGURE 10–9. Example of left ventricular (LV) and aortic (Ao) pressures measured with fluid-filled catheters in a patient with severe valvular aortic stenosis. Note that the maximum instantaneous gradient is greater than the peak-to-peak gradient. Mean gradient is indicated by the shaded area.

proximal to and in the aortic jet itself is laminar with a reasonably flat velocity profile,

$$CSA_{LVOT} \times VTI_{LVOT} = CSA_{Ao} \times VTI_{Ao} \quad (10.10)$$

All the variables in this equation can be measured with 2D or Doppler echo except CSA_{Ao}, which is the stenotic aortic valve area (AVA) itself. Rearranging the equation,

Continuity equation
$$AVA = CSA_{LVOT} \times (VTI_{LVOT}/VTI_{Ao}) \quad (10.11)$$

Thus, the measurements needed to calculate valve area with the continuity equation are (Fig. 10–12):

1. The circular outflow tract cross-sectional area (CSA), calculated from outflow tract diameter measured on a 2D parasternal long-axis midsystolic image.
2. The velocity-time integral in the outflow tract, recorded with pulsed Doppler echocardiography from an apical approach.
3. The velocity-time integral in the aortic stenosis jet, recorded with continuous-wave Doppler ultrasound.

For clinical use, the continuity equation can be simplified by substituting maximum velocities (V) for velocity-time integrals. Since the shape and timing of outflow tract and aortic jet velocity curves are similar, their ratios are nearly identical:

Velocity ratio
$$VTI_{LVOT}/VTI_{Ao} \approx V_{LVOT}/V_{Ao} \quad (10.12)$$

The simplified continuity equation then is:

Simplified continuity equation
$$AVA = CSA_{LVOT} \times (V_{LVOT}/V_{Ao}) \quad (10.13)$$

Attempts to further simplify the continuity equation by eliminating the need to measure outflow tract diameter have been unsuccessful. While the group mean outflow tract diameter is smaller in women than in men, there is substantial overlap in the range of diameters in men and women. Although outflow tract diameter correlates with body size when people of all ages from infancy to adulthood are considered, in the adult population, the relationship between body size (either body surface area, height, or weight) and outflow tract diameter is weak. Thus outflow tract diameter must be measured in each patient for accurate valve area calculations. On the other hand, outflow tract diameter tends to remain constant in a given adult patient over time. Apparent differences in diameter at follow-up visits are more likely to represent measurement error than an actual interval anatomic change. Thus the ratio of outflow tract velocity to aortic jet velocity can be used to follow disease progression in individual patients.

Velocity Ratio and Other Measures of Stenosis Severity

Although not strictly comparable to valve area, the velocity ratio also may be a useful measure of stenosis severity that, in effect, is "indexed" for body size. Obviously, normal valve area is dependent on body size—infants and children have smaller valve areas than adults and large adults are expected to have larger valve areas than small adults. One way to take the effect of body size into account is to "index" valve area by dividing it by body surface area (BSA):

$$\text{Aortic valve index} = \frac{\text{AVA}}{\text{BSA}} \quad (10.14)$$

An alternate approach is to define the "normal" valve area for that individual as the cross-sectional area of the outflow tract. Then, the increase in velocity from outflow tract to aortic jet reflects stenosis severity regardless of body size. If

$$\text{"Normal" AVA} = \text{CSA}_{\text{LVOT}} \text{ and}$$

$$\text{Actual AVA} \cong \text{"Normal" AVA} \times \frac{V_{\text{LVOT}}}{V_{\text{Ao}}} \quad (10.15)$$

then $\dfrac{\text{Actual AVA}}{\text{"Normal" AVA}} \cong \dfrac{V_{\text{LVOT}}}{V_{\text{Ao}}}$

FIGURE 10–10. Left ventricular outflow tract diameter and velocity in a patient with low transaortic volume flow. Pressure gradients alone will underestimate stenosis severity in this setting. (Reprinted with permission from Judge KW, Otto CM: *Cardiol Clin* 8:203, 1990.)

FIGURE 10–11. Left ventricular outflow tract diameter and velocity in a patient with mixed moderate aortic stenosis and moderate aortic regurgitation. Both the outflow tract velocity and aortic jet velocity are elevated due to the elevated transaortic volume flow rate. Calculation of valve area remains accurate in this setting. (Reprinted with permission from Judge KW, Otto CM: *Cardiol Clin* 8:203, 1990.)

A velocity ratio near 1 indicates little obstruction, a velocity ratio of 0.5 indicates a valve area that is one-half normal, and a velocity ratio of 0.25 indicates a valve area reduced to one-quarter its normal value.

Several alternative measures of aortic stenosis severity have been proposed. Valve resistance, which assumes a linear relationship between flow and pressure gradient, is calculated as the ratio of mean pressure gradient to flow. Stroke work loss reflects the amount of work lost in ejection of blood across the stenotic orifice and is expressed as the ratio of aortic to left ventricular systolic pressure (calculated from

| TABLE 10–3 | Selected Studies of Aortic Valve Area Determination |

First Author/Year	Comparison	N	Study Group	R*	Range (cm²)	SEE* (cm²)
Hakki/1981	Simplified vs original Gorlin formula	60	Aortic stenosis	0.96	0.2–2	0.10
Skjaerpe/ 1985	Cont eq vs Gorlin	30	Aortic stenosis	0.89	0.4–2.4	0.12
Zoghbi/ 1986	Cont eq vs Gorlin	39	Aortic stenosis	0.95	0.4–2	0.15
Otto/1988	Cont eq vs Gorlin	103	Aortic stenosis	0.87	0.2–3.7	0.34
Teirstein/ 1986	Cont eq vs Gorlin	30	Aortic stenosis	0.88	0.3–1.6	0.17
Oh/1988	Cont eq vs Gorlin	100	Aortic stenosis	0.83	0.2–1.8	0.19
Danielson/ 1989	Cont eq vs Gorlin	100	Aortic stenosis	0.96	0.4–2	—
Cannon/ 1985	Gorlin vs videotape of valve opening	42	Porcine valves in pulsatile flow model	0.87	0.6–2.5	0.28
	New formula vs actual orifice area	42	Porcine valves in pulsatile flow model	0.98	0.6–2.5	0.11
Segal/ 1987	Cont eq vs actual valve area		In vitro pulsatile flow with orifice plates	0.99	0.05–0.5	0.016
	Gorlin formula vs actual valve area			0.87		0.047
Cannon/ 1988	Gorlin vs known valve area	135	Prosthetic aortic valves	0.39	0.6–2.3	—
Nishimura/ 1988	Cont eq vs Gorlin	55	Pre-BAV	0.72	0.2–0.9	0.10
			Post-BAV	0.61	0.5–1.3	0.17
Desnoyers/ 1988	Cont eq vs Gorlin	42	Pre-BAV	0.74	0.3–1.3	—
Tribouilloy/ 1994	TEE vs cont eq	54	Aortic stenosis	0.96	0.3–2	0.11
	TEE vs Gorlin			0.90		0.12
Cormier/ 1996	TEE vs Gorlin	45	Aortic stenosis	0.74	0.5–1.4	—
Kim/1997	TEE vs Gorlin	81	Aortic stenosis	0.89	0.4–2	0.04

AS = Aortic stenosis; BAV = balloon aortic valvuloplasty; Cont eq = continuity equation; Gorlin = Gorlin formula valve area; TEE = planimetered 2D valve area on transesophageal echocardiography.

*If not stated in the publication, statistics were calculated from the raw data provided in tables. A blank indicates that data for this calculation were not available.

Data from Hakki et al: Circ 63:1050–1055, 1981; Skjaerpe et al: Circ 72:810–818, 1985; Zoghbi et al: Circ 73:452–459, 1986; Otto et al: Arch Intern Med 148:2553–2560, 1988; Teirstein et al: JACC 8:1059–1065, 1986; Oh et al: JACC 11:1227–1234, 1988; Danielson et al: Am J Cardiol 63:1107–1111, 1989; Cannon et al: Circ 71:1170–1178, 1985; Segal et al: JACC 9:1294–1305, 1987; Cannon et al: Am J Cardiol 62:113–116, 1988; Nishimura et al: Circ 78:791–799, 1988; Desnoyers et al: Am J Cardiol 62:1078–1084, 1988; Tribouilloy et al: Am Heart J 128:526–532, 1994; Cormier et al: Am J Cardiol 77:882–885, 1996; Kim KS et al: Am J Cardiol 79:436–441, 1997.

FIGURE 10–12. Continuity equation aortic valve area (AVA) calculations require measurement of left ventricular outflow tract diameter on a parasternal long-axis view for circular cross-sectional area (CSA) calculation *(above, left)*, pulsed Doppler recording of the left ventricular outflow tract velocity-time integral (VTI) from an apical approach *(above, right)*, and continuous-wave Doppler recording of the aortic stenosis velocity-time integral *(VTI AS-jet)* from whichever window gives the highest-velocity signal.

$$SV_{LVOT} = SV_{AS\text{-}Jet}$$

$$CSA_{LVOT} \times VTI_{LVOT} = AVA \times VTI_{AS\text{-}Jet}$$

$$AVA = (VTI_{LVOT} \times CSA_{LVOT})/VTI_{AS\text{-}Jet}$$

the systolic blood pressure and transaortic pressure difference). Neither of these measures has gained widespread clinical acceptance.

Technical Considerations and Potential Pitfalls (Table 10–4)

Continuity equation valve areas have been well validated in comparison with Gorlin formula valve areas calculated from invasive measurements of pressure gradient and cardiac output. Some of the discrepancies between Doppler echo and invasive measurements of valve area are due to measurement variability for the invasive data and to limitations of the Gorlin formula itself. However, technical considerations in recording the Doppler and 2D echo data and the mea-surement variability of the noninvasive technique also are important.

With careful attention to technical details, an experienced laboratory can obtain accurate noninvasive data for calculation of transaortic pressure gradients and valve areas in nearly all adults with valvular aortic stenosis. However, accurate noninvasive quantitation of aortic stenosis severity is a technically demanding procedure, and a significant learning-curve effect is seen in each laboratory for this clinical application. There are several potential pitfalls in the Doppler approach, as detailed below. Each laboratory should confirm the accuracy of its data by comparison with those of an experienced echocardiography laboratory or with other diagnostic tests.

TABLE 10–4	Pitfalls in Echocardiographic Evaluation of Aortic Stenosis

Technical
Acoustic access
Intercept angle between aortic stenosis jet and ultra-
  sound beam
Outflow tract diameter imaging
Respiratory motion
Learning-curve effect

Interpretation
Identification of flow signal origin (AS vs MR)
Beat-to-beat variability (AF, PVCs)
Intraobserver and interobserver measurement
  variability
Calculation errors

Physiology
Interim changes in heart rate or stroke volume
Dependence of velocity and ΔP on volume flow rate
Progression of AS severity

Standards of Reference
Maximum vs peak-to-peak ΔP
Continuity vs Gorlin formula valve areas

AS = Aortic stenosis; MR = mitral regurgitation; AF = atrial fibrillation; PVCs = premature ventricular contraction.

The Aortic Jet. Owing to the high velocities seen in aortic stenosis (usually 3 to 7 m/s), continuous-wave Doppler ultrasound is needed for accurate measurement of the aortic jet signal. High-pulse-repetition-frequency Doppler echo also can be used but is more time-consuming and technically demanding, since sample volume depth as well as beam direction must be optimized. When aortic stenosis is suspected, the examination should include use of a nonimaging, dedicated continuous-wave Doppler transducer. The smaller "footprint" of the dedicated transducer allow optimal positioning and angulation of the ultrasound beam. In addition, a dedicated continuous-wave transducer has a higher signal-to-noise ratio than a combined imaging and Doppler transducer.

In recording the aortic jet velocity signal, a search is made for the highest-frequency shift. This signal then is assumed to represent a near-parallel intercept angle (θ) between the ultrasound beam and the direction of the jet. In this situation, $\cos\theta$ equals 1 and thus can be ignored in the Doppler equation (see Chap. 1). Any deviation from a parallel intercept angle will result in underestimation of jet velocity. For example, an intercept angle of 30° will result in a measured velocity of 4.3 m/s when the actual velocity is 5 m/s. Underestimation of velocity, which is squared in the Bernoulli equation, results in a large error in calculated pressure gradient. However, intercept angles within 15° of parallel will result in an error in velocity measurement of 5% or less.

The direction of the aortic jet often is eccentric relative to both the plane of the aortic valve and the long axis of the aorta and rarely can be predicted from the 2D images. Occasionally, jet direction can be visualized with color flow imaging, but, more often, the direction of the short jet of calcific stenosis cannot be identified. Even when jet direction is seen in a single tomographic plane, the orientation of the jet in the elevational plane remains unknown.

Pragmatically, the solution to the problem of aligning the ultrasound beam parallel to an aortic jet of unknown direction is to perform a careful search from several acoustic windows with optimal patient positioning and multiple transducer angulations. The highest-velocity signal obtained then is assumed to represent the most parallel intercept angle. At a minimum, the aortic jet should be interrogated from an apical approach with the patient in a steep left lateral decubitus position on an examination bed with an apical cutout, from a high right parasternal position with the patient in a right lateral decubitus position, and from the suprasternal notch with the patient supine and the neck extended. Even then, the possibility of underestimation of jet velocity due to a nonparallel intercept angle cannot be excluded. In some cases, the highest-velocity signal may be recorded from a subcostal or left parasternal window.

When the continuous-wave beam is aligned with the aortic jet, a smooth velocity curve is seen with a well-defined peak velocity and spectral darkening along the outer edge of the velocity curve. Audibly, the signal is high

TABLE 10–5	Other High-Velocity Systolic Jets that May Be Mistaken for Aortic Stenosis

Subaortic obstruction (fixed or dynamic)

Mitral regurgitation

Tricuspid regurgitation

Ventricular septal defect

Pulmonic or branch pulmonary artery stenosis

Peripheral vascular stenosis (e.g., subclavian artery)

frequency and tonal. The spectral recording should be made with an appropriate velocity scale (at least 1 m/s higher than the observed maximum jet velocity), with wall filters set at a high level, and with gain adjustment to provide clear definition of the maximum velocity. Maximum velocity is measured at the edge of the dark velocity envelope. The velocity-time integral is measured by digitizing the velocity curve over systole.

Care is needed to correctly identify the origin of the high-velocity jet. Other high-velocity systolic jets (Table 10–5 and Fig. 10–13) may be mistaken for aortic stenosis if inadequate attention is paid to timing, shape, and associated

FIGURE 10–13. From an apical approach, three different high-velocity systolic jets directed away from the transducer were recorded in this patient with mild to moderate aortic stenosis, severe mitral stenosis with mild mitral regurgitation, and severe pulmonary hypertension. These three flow signals can be differentiated on the basis of timing, shape, and associated diastolic flow signals.

diastolic flow curves. In some cases, 2D-"guided" continuous-wave Doppler may be helpful in correct identification of the jet, followed by recording with a nonimaging transducer for optimal signal quality.

Outflow Tract Diameter. Left ventricular outflow tract diameter is measured in midsystole, just proximal to and parallel with the plane of the stenotic aortic valve, from the inner edge of the septal endocardial echo to the leading edge of the base of the anterior mitral leaflet. A parasternal long-axis view provides the most accurate measurement because it depends on the axial (rather than lateral) resolution of the ultrasound beam. Outflow tract cross-sectional area (CSA) is assumed to be circular so that:

$$\text{Outflow tract CSA}$$
$$\text{CSA}_{\text{LVOT}} = \pi(D/2)^2 \qquad (10.16)$$

Note that small errors in outflow tract diameter measurement may lead to large errors in calculated cross-sectional area. Furthermore, of the measurements made for evaluating aortic stenosis severity, outflow tract diameter shows the greatest intraobserver and interobserver variability. Several measurements should be averaged to minimize this potential source of error.

Outflow Tract Velocity. The outflow tract systolic velocity signal is recorded from an apical approach using pulsed Doppler echo. Either an anteriorly angulated four-chamber view or an apical long-axis view can be used. A sample volume 5 to 10 mm in length is positioned just proximal to the region of acceleration into the stenotic jet. Correct positioning is ensured by starting with the sample volume *in* the jet and slowly repositioning it apically until a smooth velocity curve with a well-defined peak velocity and little spectral broadening is seen. The presence of an aortic valve closing (but not opening) click indicates that the sample volume is immediately adjacent to the valve. A transducer position is chosen initially that indicates a parallel alignment between the ultrasound beam and the long axis of the outflow tract on 2D imaging. Then, transducer position and angulation are adjusted, based on the audible Doppler signal and the velocity curve, to record the highest-velocity signal proximal to the flow acceleration region. In addition, the sample volume is moved laterally across the outflow tract in each apical view to document a flat flow velocity profile.

The rationale for this protocol for sample volume positioning is that the outflow tract diameter and velocity signals need to be recorded *at the same* anatomic site for accurate transaortic stroke volume calculations. Necessarily, these two recordings are made nonsimultaneously from different acoustic windows because of the need for a parallel orientation between the Doppler beam and the direction of blood flow for accurate velocity measurement versus a perpendicular orientation between the 2D echo beam and the outflow tract for accurate diameter measurement. Measuring both immediately adjacent to the stenotic valve provides a reference point that ensures that both measurements are made at the same spatial location.

The maximum outflow tract velocity is measured at the edge of the most intense spectral signal. The time-velocity integral is measured by tracing the modal velocity of the systolic flow curve. Wall filters are set low enough that the systolic ejection period is clearly defined.

Coexisting Valvular Disease

A high percentage (about 80%) of patients with predominant aortic stenosis also have aortic regurgitation, most often mild or moderate in severity. The degree of regurgitation can be evaluated as described in Chapter 11. Although coexisting aortic regurgitation will result in an increase in the transaortic pressure gradient (due to increased transaortic volume flow), valve area calculations will be accurate because the stroke volume in the continuity equation represents transaortic stroke volume.

Coexisting mitral regurgitation also is common due to mitral annular calcification in adults with calcific aortic stenosis. Again, mitral regurgitant severity can be evaluated as described in Chapter 11. Particular attention should be directed toward aortic valve area calculations when mitral regurgitation is present. Otherwise, severe aortic stenosis may be missed if the transaortic pressure gradient is low due to low transaortic volume flow.

Patients with rheumatic aortic stenosis may have significant mitral stenosis, mitral regurgitation, or mixed mitral disease. Evaluation of aortic stenosis severity is unaffected by these coexisting lesions other than the aforementioned potential for a low transaortic pressure gradient if the transaortic volume flow rate is depressed.

Response of the Left Ventricle to Valvular Aortic Stenosis

The left ventricular response to the chronic pressure overload of valvular aortic stenosis is concentric hypertrophy—an increase in left ventricular mass due to increased wall thickness without chamber dilation. Hypertrophy tends to normalize left ventricular wall stress, since:

$$\text{Left ventricular wall stress}$$
$$\text{Wall stress} \cong (r/t) \times P \quad (10.17)$$

where r is ventricular radius, t is wall thickness, and P is left ventricular pressure. The relative wall thickness (the ratio of wall thickness to radius) is a useful and simple measure of the degree of hypertrophy. Left ventricular mass (which can be indexed for body size) can be calculated from tracings of endocardium and epicardium at end-diastole, as described in Chapter 5.

In aortic stenosis, left ventricular systolic function tends to be preserved until late in the disease course. When left ventricular systolic dysfunction does occur, it may be due to the increased afterload of outflow obstruction and thus is reversible after valve replacement. Ventricular systolic function can be evaluated qualitatively or quantitatively, as described in Chapter 5. Even a qualitative evaluation has significant prognostic implications in unoperated adults with aortic stenosis.

Interestingly, there appear to be gender differences in the response of the left ventricle to aortic stenosis. Women tend to have more hypertrophied, smaller ventricles with preserved systolic function, while men tend to show less increase in wall thickness, more left ventricular dilation, and a higher prevalence of systolic dysfunction.

Clinical Applications in Specific Patient Populations (Table 10–6)

Symptomatic Adults with Valvular Aortic Stenosis Being Considered for Surgical Intervention

Doppler echocardiography is the diagnostic test of choice for symptomatic adults with suspected aortic stenosis in whom valve replacement is being considered. A complete echocardiographic examination includes evaluation of stenosis severity, assessment of left ventricular systolic function, and evaluation of coexisting valvular lesions, as described above. While all the clinical and Doppler echo data should be considered in clinical decision making for each individual patient, a generalized diagnostic approach based on the Doppler data can be derived for this patient population. As for any generalization, exceptions do occur in clinical practice, so this diagnostic approach serves more as a useful frame of reference than as a rigid patient management scheme (Fig. 10–14).

TABLE 10–6	Echocardiographic Approach to Valvular Aortic Stenosis

1. Valve anatomy, etiology of stenosis
2. Exclude other causes of left ventricular outflow obstruction
3. Stenosis severity
   a. Jet velocity
   b. Mean pressure gradient
   c. Continuity equation valve area
4. Degree of coexisting aortic regurgitation
5. Left ventricular hypertrophy and systolic function

For initial evaluation of aortic stenosis severity, aortic jet maximum velocity is the simplest and most useful quantitative measure. This is not surprising, since maximum velocity is predictably related to maximum pressure gradient (via the simplified Bernoulli equation), which, in turn, is linearly related to mean pressure gradient in native valvular aortic stenosis. Thus maximum velocities, maximum gradients, and mean gradient measurements are redundant, simply describing the same data in different ways.

When the aortic jet velocity is >4 m/s, the presence of severe aortic valve disease is confirmed, and valve replacement is needed. Note that some subjects with a jet velocity >4 m/s may have only moderate stenosis with coexist-

ing moderate regurgitation. However, if symptoms consistent with aortic valve disease are present, the high jet velocity confirms the clinical diagnosis, and valve replacement for mixed stenosis and regurgitation is needed. In these subjects, findings at cardiac catheterization are similar, with a high pressure gradient despite only a moderate reduction in valve area.

When the aortic jet velocity is <3 m/s, significant aortic valve disease is not present, and valve replacement is not needed. Caution is needed in this situation to ensure that the jet velocity measurement is accurate—a nonparallel intercept angle between the aortic jet and the Doppler beam can result in underestimation of jet velocity and the erroneous conclusion that severe stenosis is not present. If severe left ventricular systolic dysfunction is present, severe aortic stenosis may be present despite a low velocity (and low gradient). In these patients, calculation of valve area is needed.

In symptomatic adults with an aortic jet velocity between 3 and 4 m/s, further evaluation of stenosis severity is needed. These patients may have only moderate stenosis with normal transaortic volume flow, mild stenosis with coexisting aortic regurgitation, or severe stenosis with low transaortic volume flow. In aortic stenosis, low transaortic volume flow is not necessarily identifiable by 2D imaging. For example, a hypertrophied left ventricle with normal systolic function but a small ventricular chamber will have a small stroke volume. Thus calculation of aortic valve area with the continuity equation is especially important in patients with only a moderate increase in jet velocity (3 to 4 m/s) and a corresponding modest mean pressure gradient (20 to 40 mmHg). In addition, evaluation of the degree of coexisting aortic regurgitation is needed because valve replacement may be warranted in the symptomatic patient with only mild to moderate aortic stenosis and significant aortic regurgitation.

This diagnostic approach has been shown to be accurate and cost-effective in evaluating symptomatic adults with valvular aortic stenosis. Again, it must be emphasized that this approach is only as accurate as the Doppler echo data upon which it is based. Careful attention to technical details is needed during the Doppler examination. In cases where the clinical situation is discrepant with the echo findings, other diagnostic tests such as cardiac catheterization may be helpful. Coronary angiography is needed in most patients if valve replacement is planned (for possible coronary artery bypass grafting) and often is needed if

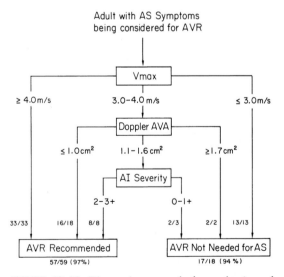

FIGURE 10–14. Diagnostic approach for evaluation of adults with aortic stenosis symptoms being considered for valve replacement. The number of subjects in each group (denominator) and the number in whom this echo approach was correct (numerator) are shown. Overall diagnostic accuracy of this approach is 96%. (From Otto CM, Pearlman AS: *Arch Intern Med* 148:2553–2560, 1988; copyrighted 1988, American Medical Association.)

valve replacement is *not* planned to evaluate alternate etiologies for the patient's symptoms.

Disease Progression and Prognosis in Asymptomatic Aortic Stenosis

In following individual patients over time, the reproducibility of a technique, as well as its accuracy, is important. Reproducibility of Doppler echo data includes recording variability (e.g., intercept angle, wall filters, signal strength, acoustic window), measurement variability (e.g., identification of the maximum velocity, outflow tract diameter), and physiologic variability (e.g., interim changes in heart rate, stroke volume, or pressure gradient). Aortic jet maximum velocity measurement is reproducible as described by the mean coefficient of variation with an intraobserver variability of 3.2% and an interobserver variability of 3.1%. Outflow tract velocity, recorded by two experienced sonographers, also is reproducible with intraobserver and interobserver variability of 3% and 3.9%. Measurement of outflow tract diameter shows the greatest variability, with intraobserver and interobserver mean coefficients of variation of 5.1% and 7.9%. These variabilities indicate that for values at the middle of the range, a change greater than measurement variability is >0.2 m/s for maximum jet velocity, >0.1 m/s for outflow tract velocity, >0.2 cm for outflow tract diameter, and >0.15 cm² for aortic valve area.

Doppler echo has been used to follow disease progression in asymptomatic adults with valvular aortic stenosis. Several observations from these studies are noteworthy. First, prognosis depends on the presence or absence of clinical symptoms and not on hemodynamic severity per se. There is significant overlap in all measures of hemodynamic severity between symptomatic and asymptomatic adults, and it is not unusual to see asymptomatic individuals with a jet velocity >4 m/s. Second, the rate of hemodynamic progression is variable from patient to patient. However, on average, jet velocity increases by 0.3 m/s per year, mean pressure gradient increases by about 7 mmHg per year, and valve area decreases by about 0.1 cm² per year. To date, no baseline characteristics have been identified that predict the rate of progression in individual patients. Third, while hemodynamic progression may present as an increase in aortic jet velocity (and transaortic pressure gradient), disease progression can occur with no change in jet velocity if there is a

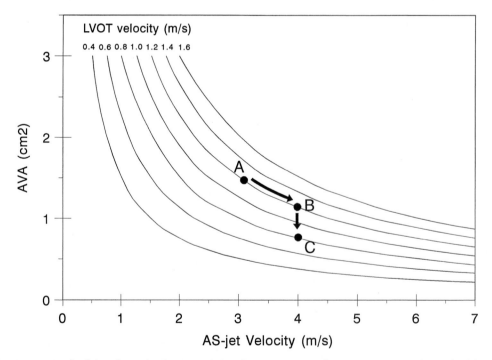

FIGURE 10–15. Graph of the relationship between aortic valve area (AVA) and aortic stenosis jet velocity for left ventricular outflow tract (LVOT) velocities ranging from 0.4 to 1.6 m/s. In the example shown, a patient initially has a jet velocity of 3 m/s and a valve area of 1.5 cm² *(A)*. As stenosis severity increases, jet velocity increases to 4.0 m/s and valve area decreases to 1.2 cm² *(B)*. However, with further disease progression *(C)*, jet velocity was unchanged at 4 m/s, but valve area decreased to 0.8 cm² in the setting of decreased transaortic volume flow (LVOT velocity 1.2 to 0.8 m/s).

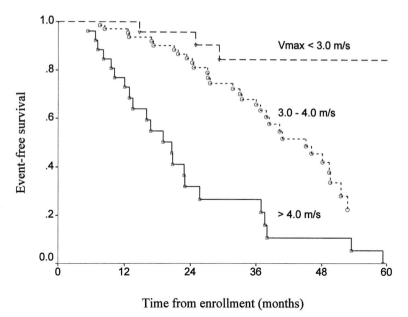

FIGURE 10–16. Cox regression analysis showing event-free survival in aortic stenosis groups defined by aortic jet velocity at entry ($P < .0001$ by log rank test). (From Otto CM, Burwash IG, Legget ME, et al: *Circulation* 95: 2262–2270, 1997.)

concurrent decrease in transaortic volume flow rate (Fig. 10–15).

In patients with asymptomatic aortic stenosis, clinical outcome is highly dependent on Doppler jet velocity. In those with an initial jet velocity <3 m/s, the rate of death or symptom onset requiring valve replacement is 8% per year, compared to 17% per year for those with a jet velocity between 3 and 4 m/s and 40% per year for those with a jet velocity <4 m/s (Fig. 10–16). Although it could be argued that once the baseline examination has established the diagnosis, the patient can be followed only clinically, since the timing of valve replacement is determined by symptom onset, adults with aortic stenosis often have significant comorbid disease and knowledge of hemodynamic severity can be important in patient management. Thus in the clinically stable patient, repeat echocardiography every 2 to 3 years is indicated when the jet velocity is <3 m/s, with annual examinations appropriate in those with higher jet velocities.

Evaluation of Aortic Stenosis with Left Ventricular Systolic Dysfunction

In the patient with significant left ventricular systolic dysfunction and aortic valve stenosis, evaluation of stenosis severity is problematic. Pressure gradients are low due to the low transaortic volume flow rate. In addition,

while valve area is less flow-dependent than pressure gradients, there is compelling evidence that valve area can vary in parallel with flow rate and thus may appear to be reduced when ventricular dysfunction is present, even if stenosis is not severe. Several approaches to this difficult problem have been proposed. One approach is to assess the degree of change in valve area with an increase in flow rate, for example, with dobutamine stress echocardiography. The hypothesis is that an increase in valve area reflects flexible leaflets, whereas a fixed valve area indicates stiff leaflets that cannot open any further. However, this approach has several limitations including interpretation of the data if flow rate is unchanged and the lack of outcome studies. A more detailed discussion of this problem can be found in Suggested Readings 16 to 19.

Assessment of a Systolic Murmur

Echocardiography for evaluation of a systolic murmur allows a correct anatomic diagnosis, determination of the etiology of disease, and evaluation of hemodynamic severity. Evaluation is particularly useful in certain clinical situations.

In the pregnant woman with valvular aortic stenosis, echocardiography can be used to optimize management during pregnancy and to plan the optimal approach to labor and delivery in terms of hemodynamic monitoring, anesthesia, induction of labor, and mode of delivery.

In the patient with a systolic murmur undergoing noncardiac surgery, echocardiographic evaluation can be used to determine the potential need for aortic valve replacement prior to other surgery or may allow a more conservative approach with careful perioperative hemodynamic monitoring given an accurate assessment of aortic stenosis severity.

Case Examples

Case 1

A 39-year-old woman presented with syncope followed by cardiac arrest and was successfully resuscitated. She had a history of aortic valve disease but had refused surgical treatment in the past. Physical examination showed a IV/VI aortic stenosis murmur, a I/VI aortic regurgitation murmur, and bibasilar rales. Echocardiography showed:

2D echo: Aortic valve thickened with systolic doming and reduced systolic opening
Left ventricular hypertrophy with normal systolic function
Left ventricular outflow tract diameter = 2 cm

Doppler: Aortic stenotic jet = 5.9 m/s (Figs. 10–17 and 10–18)
Left ventricular outflow tract velocity = 0.9 m/s
Aortic regurgitation: 1+, Mitral regurgitation: 2+

FIGURE 10–17. Aortic stenosis jet recorded with continuous-wave Doppler from a suprasternal notch approach in a 39-year-old woman with syncope. These data provide a definitive diagnosis in this clinical setting.

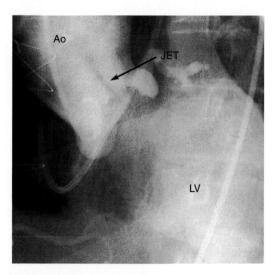

FIGURE 10–18. Supravalvular aortogram in the same patient as in Figure 10–17 with a jet of unopacified blood from the left ventricle highlighted against the background of contrast material in the aortic root.

From these data, outflow tract cross-sectional area is:

$$CSA_{LVOT} = \pi(2/2)^2 = 3.14 \text{ cm}^2$$

Aortic valve area, calculated with the simplified continuity equation, is:

$$AVA = (3.14 \text{ cm}^2 \times 0.9 \text{ m/s}) \times 5.9 \text{ m/s} = 0.5 \text{ cm}^2$$

and the velocity ratio is:

$$\text{Velocity ratio} = 0.9/5.9 = 0.15$$

At surgery, the patient had a severely stenotic and thickened unicuspid aortic valve. Aortic valve replacement was performed, and the patient has done well.

Case 2

A 56-year-old man presented with nephrolithiasis, a III/VI systolic murmur on auscultation, and no cardiac symptoms. Echocardiography showed:

2D echo: Abnormal aortic valve (probably bicuspid) with severe fibrocalcific changes
Severe left ventricular hypertrophy

Doppler: Left ventricular outflow tract diameter = 2.4 cm
Aortic stenotic jet = 7.4 m/s (see Fig. 10–8)
Left ventricular outflow tract velocity = 1.2 m/s
AR: 2+

From these data,

$$\Delta P_{max} = 4(7.4)^2 = 219 \text{ mmHg}$$

$$\Delta P_{mean} = 2.4(7.4)^2 = 131 \text{ mmHg}$$

$$\text{Velocity ratio} = 1.2/7.4 = 0.16$$

$$\text{CSA}_{LVOT} = \pi(2.4/2)^2 = 4.5 \text{ cm}^2$$

$$\text{AVA} = 4.5 \text{ cm}^2 \times (1.2/7.4) = 0.7 \text{ cm}^2$$

Case 3

A 69-year-old man presented with severe congestive heart failure. Examination showed a soft systolic murmur but a single S_2. Echocardiography showed:

2D echo: Calcified trileaflet aortic valve with reduced systolic opening

FIGURE 10–19. Left ventricular outflow tract (LVOT) velocity *(above)* and stenosis jet *(below)* in an elderly patient with severe aortic stenosis with a low V_{max} of 3.2 m/s and coexisting left ventricular systolic dysfunction with a low stroke volume.

Moderate left ventricular dilation with moderately reduced systolic function and global left ventricular hypokinesis

Doppler: Aortic stenotic jet = 3.2 m/s (Fig. 10–19)
Left ventricular outflow tract diameter = 2 cm
VTI_{AO} = 70 cm
Left ventricular outflow tract velocity = 0.9 m/s
VTI_{LVOT} = 20.1 cm

From these data,

$$\Delta P_{max} = 4(3.2)^2 = 41 \text{ mmHg}$$

$$\Delta P_{mean} = 2.4(3.2)^2 = 25 \text{ mmHg}$$

$$\text{Stroke volume} = \text{CSA}_{LVOT} \times \text{VTI}_{LVOT} = \pi(2/2)^2 \times 20.1 = 63 \text{ ml}$$

$$\text{Cardiac output} = \text{SV} \times \text{HR} = 63 \times 80 \text{ bpm} = 5 \text{ L/min}$$

$$\text{AVA (using VTIs)} = \text{CSA}_{LVOT} \times (20.1/70) = 0.9 \text{ cm}^2$$

$$\text{AVA (using velocities)} = \text{CSA}_{LVOT} \times (0.9/3.2) = 0.9 \text{ cm}^2$$

MITRAL STENOSIS

Diagnostic Imaging of the Mitral Valve

Rheumatic Disease

Rheumatic disease predominantly affects the mitral valve and is the most common cause of mitral stenosis. Rheumatic valvular disease is characterized by commissural fusion, which results in bowing or doming of the valve leaflets in diastole (Fig. 10–20). The base and midsections of the leaflets move toward the ventricular apex, while the motion of the leaflet tips is restricted due to fusion of the anterior and posterior leaflets along the medial and lateral commissures. Thickening at the leaflet tips occurs frequently, but the remainder of the leaflets can show variable degrees of thickening and/or calcification. If the base and midportions of the leaflets are relatively thin, leaflet mobility is normal other than the fused commissures. The rheumatic process also typically affects the subvalvular region with fusion, shortening, fibrosis, and calcification of the mitral chordae.

In rheumatic mitral stenosis, 2D echo allows detailed evaluation of mitral valve morphology,

Mitral Stenosis

FIGURE 10–20. Schematic diagram of the 2D echo findings in mitral stenosis. In the parasternal long-axis view (PLAX), commissural fusion with diastolic doming of the mitral leaflets is seen, as well as chordal thickening and fusion. In a parasternal short-axis view (PSAX), at the mitral valve orifice, the area of opening can be planimetered. The plane of the short-axis view is indicated by a *dashed line* on the long-axis image.

including assessment of leaflet thickness, leaflet mobility, the degree of calcification, and the extent of subvalvular involvement on transthoracic parasternal and apical views (Fig. 10–21). Occasionally, if transthoracic images are suboptimal, transesophageal imaging may be needed for evaluation of mitral valve anatomy, although definition of subvalvular disease may be limited due to shadows and reverberations from calcification of the mitral valve and annulus.

Mitral Annular Calcification and Calcific Mitral Stenosis

Mitral annular calcification is a common incidental finding on echocardiography in elderly subjects. Mild annular calcification appears as an isolated area of calcification on the left ventricular side of the posterior annulus, near the base of the posterior mitral leaflet. In more severe mitral annular calcification, increased echogenicity is seen in a hemielliptical pattern involving the entire posterior annulus. The area of fibrous continuity between the anterior mitral leaflet and the aortic root rarely is involved. The etiology of mitral annular calcification is considered to be a "degenerative" age-related process. It can result in mild to moderate mitral regurgitation due to increased rigidity of the

mitral annulus. Occasionally, the calcification extends into the base of the mitral leaflets themselves, resulting in functional mitral stenosis due to narrowing of the diastolic flow area. Calcific mitral stenosis can be distinguished from rheumatic disease by careful imaging techniques to demonstrate thin and mobile mitral leaflet tips without commissural fusion.

Differential Diagnosis (Table 10–7)

In patients referred for echocardiography with suspected mitral stenosis, the initial differential diagnosis includes other causes of pulmonary congestion. Standard echo Doppler evaluation will reveal whether left ventricular systolic dysfunction, aortic valve disease, or mitral regurgitation is present. The possibility of

FIGURE 10–21. Parasternal long-axis view *(above)* of a patient with mild rheumatic mitral stenosis showing the typical doming of the anterior mitral leaflet due to commissural fusion. Left atrial enlargement is present. The short-axis view *(below)* allows accurate planimetry of the mitral orifice (MVO) area if care is taken to identify the smallest opening by scanning slowly from apex toward the base.

TABLE 10–7	Echocardiographic Differential Diagnosis of Left Ventricular Inflow Obstruction

Mitral valve stenosis
 Rheumatic mitral stenosis
 Calcific mitral stenosis (rare)
 Congenital mitral stenosis

Left atrial tumor (myxoma)

Left atrial thrombus

Left ventricular diastolic dysfunction

Congenital disease
 Congenital mitral stenosis
 Cor triatriatum

diastolic left ventricular dysfunction also should be considered. The rare case of an atrial myxoma or other atrial tumor obstructing left ventricular inflow, thus mimicking the clinical presentation of mitral stenosis, can easily be diagnosed by 2D imaging (see Chap. 14). Rarely, a patient with mild obstruction due to cor triatriatum may present as an adult.

Quantitation of Mitral Stenosis Severity

Pressure Gradients (Fig. 10–22)

The mean diastolic transmitral pressure gradient can be determined from the transmitral velocity curve using the simplified Bernoulli equation:

$$\text{Mean mitral } \Delta P = 4(v_1^2 + v_2^2 + v_3^2 + \cdots v_n^2)/n \quad (10.17)$$

With severe stenosis, the mean pressure gradient may be as high as 20 to 30 mmHg, but it may be as low as 5 to 15 mmHg. The variability in pressure gradients in severe mitral stenosis is due to the dependence of pressure gradients on volume flow rate as well as valve area. Severe mitral stenosis may be associated with a low stroke volume (due to the limitation of left ventricular diastolic filling), resulting in a relatively low mean gradient. If volume flow rate increases, for example with exercise, an increase in transmitral gradient is seen. As for other types of valvular stenosis, calculation of valve area, taking both pressure gradient and volume flow rate into account, is helpful in quantitation of mitral stenosis severity.

Mitral Valve Area

2D Echo Valve Area (Fig. 10–23). Compared with valvular aortic stenosis, the 3D anatomy

of rheumatic mitral stenosis is simpler with a planar elliptical orifice that is relatively constant in position in mid-diastole. Thus 2D short-axis imaging of the diastolic orifice allows direct planimetry of valve area. This approach has been well validated compared with measurement of valve area at surgery and in comparison with catheterization-determined valve areas. Since the shape of the mitral valve inflow region is similar to a funnel, with the narrowest cross-sectional area at the leaflet tips, it is important to begin the 2D scan at the apex, slowly moving the image plane toward the mitral valve to identify the smallest orifice. With a low overall 2D gain setting, the inner edge of the black-white interface is traced. Given the accuracy of this technique, 2D echo mitral valve area (MVA) should be measured in patients with mitral stenosis whenever image quality is adequate.

Pressure Half-Time Valve Area (Figs. 10–24 and 10–25). Calculation of mitral valve area by the pressure half-time method is based on the concept that the *rate* of pressure decline across the stenotic mitral orifice is determined by the cross-sectional area of the orifice: the smaller the orifice, the slower is the rate of pressure decline. The influence of left atrial and left ventricular compliance on the rate of pressure decline is assumed to be negligible—an assumption that is not always warranted, especially immediately after percutaneous commissurotomy.

The pressure half-time is defined as the time interval (in milliseconds) between the maxi-

FIGURE 10–22. Transmitral flow curve in the same patient as in Figure 10–21. Using this velocity curve, pressure gradients can be calculated with the Bernoulli equation and valve area by the pressure half-time method. Note the well-defined maximal velocity and the clearly defined, linear deceleration slope. An *A* velocity is seen because sinus rhythm is present.

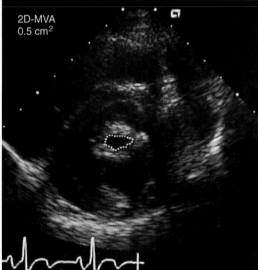

FIGURE 10–23. Long-axis *(above)* and short-axis *(below)* views of severe mitral stenosis in a 13-year-old Ethiopian male. Note the diastolic doming and severe commissural fusion (best seen in the short-axis image). Valve area by 2D planimetry is 0.5 cm². In addition, severe left atrial enlargement is present.

mum early diastolic transmitral pressure gradient and the time point where the pressure gradient is half the maximum value. Initially, the pressure half-time concept was evaluated using invasive measurements of left atrial and left ventricular pressure. Pressure half-time was found to be constant for a given individual, even with exercise-induced changes in volume flow rate, suggesting that this measurement is a constant measure of stenosis severity for a given valve area.

FIGURE 10–24. Pressure half-time measurement in the patient with severe mitral stenosis shown in Figure 10–23. The pressure half-time of 422 ms corresponds to a valve area of 0.52 cm².

This concept then was adapted to transmitral Doppler flow velocity curves. Given the quadratic relationship between velocity and pressure gradients, the half-time is determined from a Doppler spectral velocity curve as the time interval from the maximum mitral velocity (V_{max}) to the point where the velocity has fallen

FIGURE 10–25. Schematic diagram of the relationship between left atrial and left ventricular pressures and the Doppler velocity curve in mitral stenosis. Maximum velocity and the diastolic slope are identified as shown, yielding a pressure half-time of 226 ms corresponding to a mitral valve area of 1 cm². There is no *a* wave because atrial fibrillation is present.

to $V_{max}/\sqrt{2}$ (Fig. 10–24). Initial studies comparing Doppler half-time data with invasively determined Gorlin valve areas found a linear relationship, with a half-time of about 220 ms corresponding to a valve area of 1 cm². The empirical formula

Pressure half-time MVA
$$MVA = 220/T_{1/2} \qquad (10.18)$$

was proposed and has been shown to correlate well with invasive valve areas in several clinical studies (Table 10–8).

Continuity Equation Mitral Valve Area. The continuity principle for calculation of valve area also can be applied to the mitral orifice:

Continuity equation MVA
$$MVA = \text{transmitral } SV/VTI_{MS\text{-jet}} \qquad (10.19)$$

where SV is stroke volume (cm³), VTI is the velocity-time integral (cm) in the mitral stenosis jet, and MVA (cm²) is the mitral valve area. Stroke volume can be determined from the left ventricular outflow tract cross-sectional area and velocity-time integral (in the absence of aortic regurgitation) or from the pulmonary artery diameter and velocity-time integral. Note that stroke volume measured at either of these sites will represent transmitral volume flow accurately only if there is no significant mitral regurgitation.

Proximal Isovelocity Surface Area Method. In theory, transmitral volume flow rate can be calculated accurately in mitral stenosis even when mitral regurgitation is present using the proximal isovelocity surface area method. The color Doppler flow parameters are adjusted to demonstrate a well-defined hemispherical alias-

| TABLE 10–8 | Selected Studies of Mitral Valve Area Determination |

First Author/Year	Comparison	N	Study Group	R	Range (cm²)	SEE (cm²)
Gorlin/1951	MVA by Gorlin formula vs direct autopsy or surgery	11	Mitral stenosis	0.89	0.5–1.5	0.15
Libanoff/1968	$T_{1/2}$ at rest vs exercise	20	Mitral valve disease	0.98	20–340 ms	21 ms
Henry/1975	2D echo vs direct measurement at surgery	20	MS pts undergoing surgery	0.92	0.5–3.5	—
Holen/1977	MVA by Doppler vs Gorlin	10	Mitral stenosis	0.98	0.6–3.4	0.18
Hatle/1979	$T_{1/2}$ vs Gorlin MVA	32	Mitral stenosis	−0.74	0.4–3.5	—
Smith/1986	2D echo vs Gorlin	37	MS alone	0.83	0.4–2.3	0.26
		35	Prior commissurotomy	0.58		0.28
	$T_{1/2}$ MVA vs Gorlin	37	MS alone	0.85		0.22
		35	Prior commissurotomy	0.90		0.14
Come/1988	$T_{1/2}$ MVA vs Gorlin	37	Pre-MBC	0.51	0.6–1.3	—
			Post-MBC	0.47	1.2–3.8	—
	Gorlin vs Gorlin		Repeat catheterization	0.74	0.4–1.4	—
Thomas/1988	Predicted vs actual $T_{1/2}$	18	Pre-MBC	0.93–0.96		
			Post-MBC	0.52–0.66		
Chen/1989	$T_{1/2}$ MVA vs Gorlin	18	Pre-MBC	0.81	0.4–1.2	0.11
			Immediately post-MBC	0.84	1.3–2.6	0.20
			24–48 h post-MBC	0.72	1.3–2.6	0.49
Faletra/1996	2D echo vs direct measurement	30	Mitral stenosis undergoing surgical mitral valve replacement	0.95	0.6–2	0.06
	$T_{1/2}$ vs direct measurement	30		0.80		0.09
	Continuity equation vs direct measurement	30		0.87		0.09
	Flow area vs direct measurement	30		0.54		0.10

MBC = Mitral balloon commissurotomy; Gorlin = Gorlin formula valve area; MS = mitral stenosis; MVA = mitral valve area; 2D = two-dimensional; $T_{1/2}$ = pressure half-time.

Data from Gorlin et al: Am Heart J 41:1–29, 1951; Libanoff et al: Circ 38:144–150, 1968; Henry et al: Circ 51:827–831, 1975; Holen et al: Acta Med Scand 201:83–88, 1977; Hatle et al: Circ 60:1096–1104, 1979; Smith et al: Circ 73:100–107, 1986; Come et al: Am J Cardiol 61:817–825, 1988; Thomas et al: Circ 78:980–993, 1988; Chen et al: JACC 13:1309–1313, 1989; Faletra F et al: J Am Coll Cardiol 28:1190–1197, 1996.

ing surface area on the left atrial side of the mitral orifice. The velocity at this location equals the Nyquist limit (the "aliasing" velocity). The cross-sectional area of the aliased boundary can be calculated as the surface area of a hemisphere with diameter measured from the color flow image. Multiplying cross-sectional area times the known velocity yields the volume flow rate, which then can be used in conjunction with the transmitral velocity time interval in the continuity equation. One difficulty with this approach is that the volume flow rate must be integrated over the diastolic filling period; a single color image yields only the volume flow rate at one time point in diastole. Because of this problem, the proximal isovelocity method has not been widely applied for evaluation of mitral valve area.

Technical Considerations and Potential Pitfalls (Table 10–9)

Currently, assessment of the severity of mitral stenosis in an individual patient typically includes calculation of the mean transmitral pressure gradient, planimetry of the 2D echo valve area, and calculation of the pressure half-time valve area. Besides the physiologic limitations of pressure gradient and valve area measurements in mitral stenosis, potential technical problems deserve attention and in specific instances, other approaches to evaluating stenosis severity may be used. Evaluation of coexisting lesions also is important.

As for any intracardiac blood flow, accurate pressure gradient calculations depend on accurate velocity measurements, which require a near-parallel intercept angle between the direction of blood flow and the Doppler beam. The mitral stenosis jet nearly always can be recorded from an apical approach, but careful transducer positioning and angulation are needed to record an optimal signal. Color flow imaging may be helpful in defining the jet direction in a given tomographic plane. Depending on the maximum jet velocity, the velocity curve can be recorded with conventional pulsed, high-pulse-repetition-frequency, or continuous-wave Doppler ultrasound. Pulsed Doppler recordings may show better definition of the maximum velocity and early diastolic slope than continuous-wave Doppler recordings because of a better signal-to-noise ratio.

Direct planimetry of mitral valve area on 2D short-axis images has proven to be a valid technique in most clinical situations. However, definition of valve area may be difficult if image quality is poor or if there is extensive distortion of the valve anatomy. Valve area can be underestimated if gain settings are too high and can be overestimated if the smallest area at the leaflet tips is not recorded. Low gain settings and careful scanning in a short-axis plane from the apex toward the base help avoid these potential problems.

Pressure half-time valve area calculations have significant limitations in certain clinical settings. When coexisting aortic regurgitation is present, left ventricular filling occurs both antegrade across the mitral valve and retrograde across the aortic valve. This may result in a more rapid rise in left ventricular diastolic pressure than if there were no aortic regurgitation, resulting in a shorter half-time measurement. Conversely, if severe aortic regurgitation impairs mitral leaflet opening, functional mitral stenosis may be superimposed on anatomic mitral stenosis, with lengthening of the half-time measurement. In clinical practice, if the 2D echo shows rheumatic mitral stenosis and only mild to moderate aortic regurgitation is present, the half-time method remains a useful approach for evaluation of stenosis severity. If aortic regurgitation is severe, or if the mitral valve anatomy is atypical, the potential influence of coexisting lesions should be considered.

TABLE 10–9	Pitfalls in Evaluation of Mitral Stenosis Severity

Pressure Gradient
Intercept angle between mitral stenosis jet and ultrasound beam
Beat-to-beat variability in atrial fibrillation
Dependence on transvalvular volume flow rate (e.g., exercise, coexisting mitral regurgitation)

2D Valve Area
Image orientation
Tomographic plane
2D gain settings
Intraobserver and interobserver variability in planimetry of orifice
Poor acoustic access
Deformed valve anatomy post-valvuloplasty

$T_{1/2}$ Valve Area
Definition of V_{max} and early diastolic slope
Nonlinear early diastolic velocity slope
Sinus rhythm with a wave superimposed on early diastolic slope
Influence of coexisting aortic regurgitation
Changing left ventricular and left atrial compliances immediately after commissurotomy

Continuity Equation Mitral Valve Area
Accurate measurement of transmitral stroke volume

$T_{1/2}$ = Pressure half-time; V_{max} = maximum velocity.

FIGURE 10–26. In this patient with mitral stenosis, the diastolic deceleration slope is nonlinear on some beats *(left)* with a steeper early than mid-diastolic slope. If attempts to record a more linear slope *(center)* are unsuccessful, the mid-diastolic slope should be measured.

A major assumption of the half-time method is that left atrial and left ventricular compliances do not significantly affect the rate of pressure gradient decline across the stenotic orifice. While this assumption appears to be warranted in clinically stable patients with mitral stenosis, it is *not* justified in the period immediately after catheter mitral valvuloplasty. After relief of mitral stenosis, the fall in left atrial pressure and the increase in left ventricular filling are accompanied by directionally opposite changes in left atrial and left ventricular compliance. During the 24 to 72 hours after the procedure, equilibrium has not been reached, and the pressure half-time may not be an accurate reflection of orifice area. After this adjustment period, compliances stabilize, and the pressure half-time method again provides useful information.

Even under physiologically stable conditions, accurate pressure half-time measurements require careful recording of the mitral stenosis velocity curve. While a parallel intercept angle is somewhat less important than for pressure gradient calculations (since the *shape* of the curve is the same even at a nonparallel angle), it is important that the intercept angle be *constant* throughout diastole to avoid artifactual distortion in the shape of the curve. The maximum early diastolic velocity and the early diastolic deceleration slope should be well defined. In addition, pressure half-times are most easily and reproducibly measured if the deceleration slope is linear. If a linear slope cannot be obtained even after careful adjustment of transducer position and angulation, the half-time measurement should be made using the mid-diastolic slope of the curve (Fig. 10–26).

In atrial fibrillation, several beats are averaged, since mean gradient will vary with the RR

interval. While the half-time will be relatively constant despite variation in the length of diastole, only beats where the diastolic filling period is long enough to show the early diastolic slope clearly are appropriate for measurement. Although the pressure half-time method is accurate when sinus rhythm is present, the increase in velocity due to atrial contraction may obscure the early diastolic slope, particularly at high heart rates, so that half-time measurements may not be possible unless a slow heart rate allows clear definition of the middiastolic slope.

Continuity equation mitral valve area determinations are most accurate in patients without significant coexisting mitral regurgitation. In this subgroup, continuity equation mitral valve area calculations provide a useful alternative to the pressure half-time method, especially in situations of altered chamber compliances. The accuracy of the continuity equation method, as in aortic stenosis, depends on a parallel intercept angle between the mitral stenotic jet and the ultrasound beam and a careful stroke volume calculation from diameter and velocity recordings. Accurate pulmonary artery diameter measurement for stroke volume calculations can be difficult in adult patients due to poor acoustic access. Left ventricular outflow tract diameter nearly always can be imaged reliably. However, many patients with mitral stenosis have some degree of coexisting aortic or mitral regurgitation so that transaortic stroke volume does not equal transmitral stroke volume.

The proximal isovelocity surface area method avoids the problem of measuring transmitral stroke volume when coexisting regurgitant lesions are present because it measures transmitral volume flow directly. However, there are significant methodologic problems with this approach, specifically accurate calculation of the surface area of the aliasing signal and temporal averaging of the volume flow calculation. Although this method is not widely used because of these problems, it remains a theoretically sound approach to valve area determination.

Coexisting Lesions in Mitral Stenosis

Left Atrial Enlargement and Thrombus

Chronic pressure overload of mitral stenosis leads to gradual enlargement of the left atrium. Left atrial size can become extremely large in long-standing severe mitral stenosis. In conjunction with a low volume flow rate due to the stenotic valve, left atrial enlargement results in stasis of blood flow and thrombus formation. Thrombi are located preferentially in the left atrial appendage but also can occur in the body of the atrium as protruding or as laminated thrombus along the atrial wall or interatrial septum (Fig. 10–27). Left atrial thrombi are most common when atrial fibrillation is present but may occur even in sinus rhythm.

Transthoracic echo has a high specificity for detection of left atrial thrombus (i.e., if it is visualized, it most likely is a real finding), but the sensitivity is less than 50%. In part, this relates to the difficulty of imaging the left atrial appendage in adults. Sometimes the left atrial appendage can be visualized in laterally angulated parasternal short-axis views at the aortic valve level or from apical two-chamber views angulated slightly superiorly; however, often the atrial appendage cannot be visualized at all. When the atrial appendage is seen, image quality often is too poor to allow reliable exclusion of atrial thrombus due to poor ultrasound tissue penetration and beam width artifact at the depth of the left atrium from surface imaging.

Transesophageal echo has a high sensitivity (>99%) and specificity (>99%) for detection of left atrial thrombus. The left atrial appendage can be well visualized in multiple images planes using a multiplane probe. In addition, the higher transducer frequencies (5 to 7 MHz) and lower imaging depths result in high-resolution images. While thrombus in the appendage often protrudes into the chamber, laminated thrombus in the body of the atrium may be more difficult to recognize, especially along the interatrial septum.

FIGURE 10–28. Tricuspid regurgitant jet of 3.1 m/s in the patient with severe mitral stenosis shown in Figure 10–23. This indicates a right ventricular to right atrial pressure difference of 38 mmHg. Given a normal right atrial pressure, this corresponds to a pulmonary systolic pressure of about 40 to 45 mmHg.

Pulmonary Hypertension

In mitral stenosis, increased left atrial pressure results in pulmonary venous hypertension and consequent pulmonary artery hypertension. Initially, the increase in pulmonary artery pressure is "passive"—the pressure difference across the pulmonary bed (pulmonary artery minus left atrial pressure) is normal. In this situation, although pulmonary pressures are elevated, pulmonary vascular resistance is normal, and pulmonary pressures will fall toward normal after relief of mitral stenosis. With longstanding pulmonary venous hypertension, irreversible changes in the pulmonary vascular bed occur, leading to elevated pulmonary vascular resistance and persistent pulmonary hypertension after relief of mitral stenosis.

The presence of pulmonary hypertension can be suspected in mitral stenosis when there is midsystolic partial closure (or "notching") of the pulmonic valve M-mode, a short interval between the onset of flow and maximum velocity, or midsystolic abrupt deceleration in the right ventricular outflow velocity curve. With severe pulmonary hypertension, 2D echo may show right ventricular hypertrophy and enlargement, paradoxical septal motion, and tricuspid regurgitation secondary to annular dilation.

The degree of pulmonary hypertension can be quantitated from the velocity in the tricuspid regurgitant jet and the appearance of the inferior vena cava. The simplified Bernoulli equation is used to calculate the right ventricular to right atrial maximum systolic pressure difference (Fig. 10–28) from the continuous-wave Doppler tricuspid regurgitant jet recording. This difference is added to an estimate of right atrial pressure based on the size and respiratory

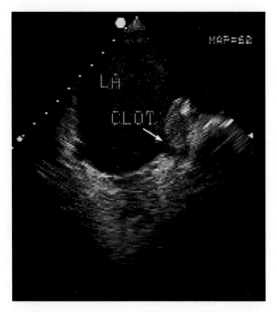

FIGURE 10–27. Clot in the atrial appendage of a patient with mitral stenosis, seen on transesophageal imaging.

variation of the inferior vena cava as it enters the right atrium as described in Chapter 5. While pulmonary vascular resistance cannot be determined with Doppler echo techniques (since an absolute measure of left atrial pressure is not available), pulmonary hypertension out of proportion to the degree of mitral stenosis raises the possibility of a coexisting pulmonary disease process.

Mitral Regurgitation

Some degree of coexisting mitral regurgitation is common in patients with mitral stenosis. Mitral regurgitant severity can be evaluated using standard techniques (see Chap. 11) and is an important factor in deciding on appropriate therapy. For example, significant mitral regurgitation is a contraindication to surgical or percutaneous commissurotomy. Coexisting mitral regurgitation elevates the transmitral pressure gradient (due to increased transmitral volume flow rate), but both 2D echo and pressure half-time valve area measurements remain accurate.

Other Coexisting Valvular Disease

The rheumatic disease process also can affect the aortic valve (second in frequency to the mitral valve) and, less commonly, the tricuspid valve. Aortic valve involvement may result in stenosis and/or regurgitation that can be evaluated with appropriate 2D and Doppler echo techniques. Evaluation of aortic regurgitation by color flow imaging may be complicated in the presence of mitral stenosis due to merging of the two diastolic flow disturbances in the left ventricle. Imaging the aortic regurgitant jet in short axis just proximal to the aortic valve and using other Doppler methods for evaluation of regurgitant severity will avoid this potential problem.

Rheumatic tricuspid stenosis may be difficult to appreciate on 2D imaging. Doppler flow patterns are similar to mitral stenosis, and the same quantitative methods for evaluation of stenosis severity can be applied. Even in the absence of rheumatic involvement of the tricuspid valve, significant tricuspid regurgitation is common (due to pulmonary hypertension and annular dilation) in patients with mitral stenosis. Careful evaluation of tricuspid regurgitation severity is especially important preoperatively in case tricuspid annuloplasty is needed at the time of mitral valve surgery.

Left Ventricular Response

The left ventricle in mitral stenosis is small with normal wall thickness and normal systolic function, although diastolic function is impaired due to the restriction of flow across the mitral orifice. The presence of left ventricular dilation suggests that significant coexisting mitral or aortic regurgitation or primary myocardial dysfunction (cardiomyopathy or ischemic disease) is present.

Clinical Applications in Specific Patient Populations (Table 10–10)

Diagnosis, Hemodynamic Progression, and Timing of Intervention

Echo Doppler is the standard clinical method for evaluation of the presence and severity of valvular mitral stenosis. Disease progression can be followed and the timing of intervention can be determined using Doppler echo and clinical data alone. Evaluation by cardiac catheterization rarely is needed.

Pre- and Post-Percutaneous Commissurotomy

In the potential candidate for percutaneous balloon mitral commissurotomy, echo Doppler evaluation of mitral valve morphology is important in patient selection both in terms of predicted hemodynamic results and in terms of the risk of procedural complications. Mitral valve morphology may be described by a qualitative assessment, an additive scoring system (Table 10–11), or quantitative measurements of leaflet mobility. Whatever approach is used, the important features to consider are leaflet mobility, leaflet thickness, leaflet and commissural calcification, and subvalvular involvement. In general,

TABLE 10–10	Echocardiographic Approach to Mitral Stenosis

1. Valve morphology
2. Exclude other causes of clinical presentation
3. Mitral stenosis severity
   a. Mean transmitral pressure gradient
   b. 2D valve area
   c. $T_{1/2}$ valve area
4. Coexisting mitral regurgitation
5. Left atrial enlargement
6. Pulmonary artery pressure (from TR jet and IVC)
7. TEE for evaluation of left atrial clot if MBC is planned
8. Coexisting tricuspid regurgitation severity

MBC = Mitral balloon commissurotomy; IVC = inferior vena cava; TR = tricuspid regurgitation; TEE = transesophageal echocardiography; $T_{1/2}$ = pressure half-time.

TABLE 10–11	Mitral Valve Morphology* by 2D Echocardiography	
Morphology		**Score**
Mobility		
Highly mobile valve with only leaflet tips restricted		1
Leaflet middle and base portions have normal mobility		2
Valve continues to move forward in diastole, mainly from the base		3
No or minimal forward movement of the leaflets in diastole		4
Leaflet Thickening		
Leaflets near normal in thickness (4–5 mm)		1
Midleaflets normal, marked thickening of margins (5–8 mm)		2
Thickening extending through the entire leaflet (5–8 mm)		3
Marked thickening of all leaflet tissue (>8–10 mm)		4
Subvalvular Thickening		
Minimal thickening just below the mitral leaflets		1
Thickening of chordal structures extending up to one-third of the chordal length		2
Thickening extending to the distal third of the chordal length		3
Extensive thickening and shortening of all chordal structures		4
Calcification		
A single area of increased echo brightness		1
Scattered areas of brightness confined to leaflet margins		2
Brightness extending into the mid portion of the leaflets		3
Extensive brightness throughout much of the leaflet tissue		4
Total score is obtained by adding the scores for each of the four features		

*Massachusetts General Hospital System; see Suggested Reading 31.

the best hemodynamic results are seen with thin, mobile leaflets that have commissural fusion but little calcification or subchordal thickening. However, some patients with a relatively unfavorable morphology do have relief of mitral stenosis with percutaneous commissurotomy. It is noteworthy that patients with the most heavily calcified and deformed valves (and the most severe stenosis) are more likely to suffer procedure-related morbidity and mortality.

Another factor to consider in this patient population is the degree of coexisting mitral regurgitation, since percutaneous commissurotomy is contradicted if moderate or severe regurgitation is present. In addition, since any left atrial thrombi may be dislodged by the catheters during the procedure, transesophageal echocardiography is needed to evaluate for left atrial thrombus prior to the procedure.

After percutaneous commissurotomy, echo Doppler allows identification of complications, permits assessment of hemodynamic results, and provides a baseline for future disease progression. Potential complications include (1) an increase in the severity of mitral regurgitation and (2) the presence of an atrial septal defect (usually small) at the transseptal catheter puncture site (Fig. 10–29). Hemodynamic results can be evaluated with standard echo Doppler techniques, again with an awareness of the potential

inaccuracies in the half-time method in the immediate postcommissurotomy period. Doppler evaluation of postprocedure pulmonary artery systolic pressure also can be helpful.

Evaluation of the Pregnant Patient with Pulmonary Congestion

When echocardiography is requested in a pregnant patient with pulmonary congestion, the possibility of valvular mitral stenosis should

FIGURE 10–29. Small atrial septal defect with left-to-right flow seen on a subcostal view using color flow imaging in a patient after catheter mitral balloon valvuloplasty. (See Color Plate 8, p. 274.)

be considered. Symptoms due to mitral stenosis often occur initially during pregnancy due to increased metabolic demands and volume flow rate, and the murmur may not be appreciated on auscultation. Careful imaging of the valve and recording of the transmitral flow velocity curve allows exclusion or confirmation of this possibility.

Case Examples

Case 1 (Figs. 10–30 and 10–31)

A 56-year-old woman presented with increasing dyspnea on exertion. Echocardiography showed rheumatic mitral stenosis with:

Mitral valve morphology score = 4
Mitral valve area: 2D   1.2 cm²
         $T_{1/2}$ 1.2 cm²
Mitral regurgitation = 2+

Moderate left atrial enlargement

The patient underwent balloon valvuloplasty. At 2-year follow-up she remains asymptomatic with a 2D mitral valve area of 1.9 cm².

Case 2 (Fig. 10–32)

A 61-year-old woman was referred for possible balloon mitral valvuloplasty. Echocardiography showed rheumatic mitral valve disease.

$T_{1/2}$ = 110 ms
MVA = 220/$T_{1/2}$ = 2 cm²
Mitral regurgitation = 4+
Tricuspid regurgitant jet = 3.8 m/s
Estimated right atrial pressure = 10 mmHg
Estimated pulmonary artery systolic pressure = 68 mmHg

Based on these data, it was concluded that valvuloplasty was not appropriate. The patient

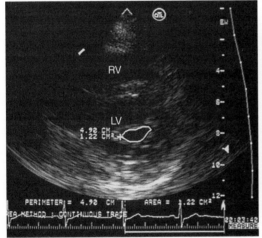

FIGURE 10–30. 2D short-axis mitral valve area before (1.2 cm²) and 2 years after (1.9 cm²) balloon mitral valvuloplasty.

FIGURE 10–31. Doppler velocity curves across a stenotic mitral valve before *(left)* and after *(right)* percutaneous mitral valvuloplasty. Pressure half-time decreased from 297 to 130 ms indicating an increase in valve area from 0.7 to 1.7 cm².

FIGURE 10–32. Left ventricular inflow curve *(upper left)* across the rheumatic mitral valve recorded with pulsed Doppler. The maximum velocity is elevated due to increased transmitral volume flow secondary to mitral regurgitation, but the deceleration slope is only moderately prolonged. The pressure half-time is 110 ms, corresponding to a mitral valve area of 2 cm². The tricuspid regurgitant jet *(lower left)* shows a maximum velocity of 3.8 m/s. Note that the tricuspid regurgitant jet has a longer duration, different shape, lower maximum velocity, and different associated diastolic flow curve than the mitral regurgitant jet *(upper right)* in this patient.

FIGURE 10–33. 2D right ventricular inflow view *(left)* and Doppler flow curve *(right)* views in a patient with rheumatic tricuspid valve disease. The leaflets are thickened, shortened, and immobile, resulting in a fixed orifice in systole and diastole. Right ventricular and right atrial enlargement secondary to volume overload are evident.

underwent mitral valve replacement without complications.

TRICUSPID STENOSIS

Tricuspid stenosis is uncommon in adult patients; in nearly all cases it is due to rheumatic disease in association with rheumatic mitral involvement. Carcinoid heart disease affects both tricuspid and pulmonic valves and can lead either to stenosis or to regurgitation. Right atrial tumors, large vegetations, or a large atrial thrombus (which may have embolized from the venous bed) can obstruct right ventricular inflow and mimic tricuspid stenosis.

2D echo images show thickening and shortening of the tricuspid valve leaflets (Fig. 10–33). Commissural fusion and diastolic bowing indicate rheumatic disease. Doppler recordings of the transvalvular flow velocity allow calculation of mean gradient and pressure half-time valve area as described for the mitral valve (Fig. 10–34).

PULMONIC STENOSIS

Pulmonic stenosis in adults is most often due to congenital disease, either clinically insignificant or residual stenosis after reparative surgery in childhood. Pulmonic stenosis may occur in conjunction with other congenital lesions such as ventricular inversion (congenitally corrected transposition of the great arteries) or tetralogy of Fallot.

2D echo imaging of the pulmonic valve shows thickened leaflets with systolic bowing. On Doppler interrogation, the antegrade velocity is increased with corresponding maximum and mean pressure gradients via the Bernoulli equation. Pulmonic valve area is not usually calculated, but the continuity equation principle can be applied in this situation, using an appropriate intracardiac location for stroke volume determination. Poststenotic pulmonary artery dilation may be present. Differentiation of valvular pulmonic stenosis from subvalvular or supravalvular obstruction can be difficult by 2D echo. Careful examinations with color flow and conventional pulsed Doppler can be very helpful in defining the site of the poststenotic flow disturbance (and thus the site of obstruction) (Fig. 10–35).

FIGURE 10–34. Color flow Doppler of tricuspid regurgitation in the same patient as in Figure 10–33 showing severe tricuspid regurgitation in an apical four-chamber view. (See Color Plate 8, p. 274.)

FIGURE 10–35. M-mode recording *(above)* of the pulmonic valve in a patient with mild pulmonic stenosis showing an increased *a* wave (note timing relative to the QRS complex and P wave). Continuous-wave Doppler from a left parasternal approach shows a pulmonary artery systolic velocity curve with a maximum velocity of 2.4 m/s corresponding to a maximum pressure gradient of 24 mmHg *(below)*.

SUGGESTED READING

Basic Principles of the Fluid Dynamics of Valvular Stenosis

1. Yoganathan AP, Cape EG, Sung H-W, et al: Review of hydrodynamic principles for the cardiologist: Applications to the study of blood flow and jets by imaging techniques. *J Am Coll Cardiol* 12:1344–1353, 1988.

    Review of basic principles of blood flow, including Bernoulli relationships, volume flow calculation, and the fluid dynamics of jets.

2. Pasipoularides A: Clinical assessment of ventricular ejection dynamics with and without outflow obstruction. *J Am Coll Cardiol* 15:859–882, 1990.

    Detailed review of the physiology of left ventricular ejection emphasizing pressure-flow relationships.

3. Thomas JD, Weyman AE: Fluid dynamics model of mitral valve flow: Description with in vitro validation. *J Am Coll Cardiol* 13:221–233, 1989.

    Fluid dynamic model of the mitral valve with emphasis on the implications for Doppler and invasive pressure gradient and valve area calculations.

4. Flachskampf FA, Weyman AE, Guerrero JL, Thomas JD: Influence of orifice geometry and flow rate on effective valve area: An in vitro study. *J Am Coll Cardiol* 15:1173–1180, 1990.

    Further details on transmitral flow dynamics emphasizing variations in the discharge coefficient.

5. Voelker W, Reul H, Neinhaus G, et al: Comparison of valvular resistance, stroke work loss, and Gorlin valve area for quantification of aortic stenosis: An in vitro study in a pulsatile aortic flow model. *Circulation* 91:1196–1204, 1995.

    In vitro model of aortic stenosis demonstrating the flow dependence of resistance and stroke work loss. Of the measures of stenosis severity studied, valve area was the least flow dependent. Includes a discussion of the principles and methods of calculating stroke work loss and resistance.

Aortic Stenosis

6. Hatle L, Angelsen BA, Tromsdal A: Non-invasive assessment of aortic stenosis by Doppler ultrasound. *Br Heart J* 43:284–292, 1980.

    Original description of noninvasive calculation of transaortic pressure gradients from continuous-wave Doppler using the Bernoulli equation in patients with aortic stenosis.

7. Otto CM: Aortic stenosis: Echocardiographic evaluation of disease severity, disease progression and role of echocardiography in clinical decision making. *In* Otto CM (ed): The Practice of Clinical Echocardiography. Philadelphia, WB Saunders, 1997, pp. 405–432.

    Advanced discussion of the echocardiographic approach to evaluation of aortic stenosis severity with a review of the impact of echocardiographic findings on the clinical decision-making process. 150 references.

8. Otto CM: Aortic stenosis. *In* Otto CM (ed): Valvular Heart Disease. Philadelphia, WB Saunders, 1999.

    Clinical review of the pathophysiology, clinical presentation, natural history, therapy and long-term outcome of adults with valvular aortic stenosis. 256 references.

9. Galan A, Zoghbi WA, Quinones MA: Determination of severity of valvular aortic stenosis by Doppler echocardiography and relation of findings to clinical outcome and agreement with hemodynamic measurements determined at cardiac catheterization. *Am J Cardiol* 67:1007–1012, 1991.

    Clinical outcome in relation to noninvasive Doppler findings in a large series of patients with aortic stenosis emphasizing the high degree of accuracy (97%) of this noninvasive approach.

10. Otto CM, Burwash IG, Legget ME, et al: A prospective study of asymptomatic valvular aortic stenosis: clinical, echocardiographic, and exercise predictors of outcome. *Circulation* 95:2262–2270, 1997.

    In a prospective echocardiographic study of 123 adults with initially asymptomatic aortic stenosis, the rate of hemodynamic progression was an increase in mean gradient of 7 ± 7 mmHg/y, an increase in jet velocity of 0.32 ± 0.34 m/s/y, and a decrease in valve area of 0.12 ± 0.19 cm²/y. Kaplan-Meier survival without symptoms prompting valve replacement at 2 years was 84% ± 16% for a jet velocity <3 m/s, 66% ± 13% for a jet velocity of 3 to 4 m/s, and only 21% ± 18% for a jet velocity >4 m/s.

11. Brener SJ, Duffy CI, Thomas JD, Stewart WJ: Progression of aortic stenosis in 394 patients: Relation to changes in myocardial and mitral valve dysfunction. *J Am Coll Cardiol* 25:305–310, 1995.

    The echocardiographic rate of progression of aortic stenosis was an increase in mean gradient of 6.3 mmHg/y and a decrease in valve area of 0.14 cm²/y. An increase in mitral regurgitant severity was associated with left ventricular dilation and worsening systolic function.

12. Faggiano P, Aurigemma GP, Rusconi C, Gaasch WH: Progression of valvular aortic stenosis in adults: Literature review and clinical implications. *Am Heart J* 132:408–417, 1996.

    Concise and complete review of the hemodynamic progression of aortic stenosis as assessed by cardiac catheterization or Doppler echocardiography.

13. Bernard Y, Meneveau N, Vuillemenot A, et al: Is planimetry of aortic valve area using multiplane transesophageal echocardiography a reliable method for assessing severity of aortic stenosis? *Heart* 78:68–73, 1997.

    In this study of 49 adults with valvular aortic stenosis, planimetry of valve area on transesophageal imaging correlated poorly with both Gorlin formula and continuity equation valve areas, with a consistent overestimation of valve area on 2D imaging. Although some centers have shown a better correlation, this study illustrates the potential pitfalls of this approach.

14. Burwash IG, Pearlman AS, Kraft CD, et al: Flow dependence of measures of aortic stenosis severity during exercise. *J Am Coll Cardiol* 24:1342–1350, 1994.

    In 110 exercise Doppler studies in adults with aortic stenosis, volume flow rate increased 24%, mean gradi-

ent increased 36%, valve area increased 14%, valve resistance increased 13%, and stroke work loss increased 17% on average. These findings demonstrate that all measures of stenosis severity are flow-dependent to some extent.

15. Badano L, Cassottano P, Bertoli D, et al: Changes in effective aortic valve area during ejection in adults with aortic stenosis. Am J Cardiol 78:1023–1028, 1996.

Doppler data were used to calculate orifice area at midacceleration, peak velocity, and mid-deceleration. Instantaneous valve area changes during ejection in patients with aortic stenosis, whereas effective valve area is constant in patients with a normal aortic valve.

16. Bermejo J, Garcia Fernandez MA, Torrecilla EG, et al: Effects of dobutamine on Doppler echocardiographic indexes of aortic stenosis. J Am Coll Cardiol 28:1206–1213, 1996.

Low-dose dobutamine (maximum 20 µg/kg/min) increased peak transaortic volume flow rate from 164 ± 48 to 229 ±102 ml/s in 35 patients with aortic stenosis. Valve area increased by 28%, but valve resistance decreased by only 4%. Flow dependence was related to the etiology of aortic stenosis, left ventricular baseline function, and the amount of flow increase induced by dobutamine.

17. deFilippi CR, Willett DL, Brickner ME, et al: Usefulness of dobutamine echocardiography in distinguishing severe from non-severe valvular aortic stenosis in patients with depressed left ventricular function and low transvalvular gradients. Am J Cardiol 75:191–194, 1995.

Dobutamine stress echocardiography in adults with aortic stenosis and left ventricular systolic dysfunction is proposed as a method for distinguishing between severe aortic stenosis with increased left ventricular afterload (valve area will not increase with increased transaortic flow) versus moderate aortic stenosis with primary myocardial dysfunction (valve area will increase with increased transaortic flow). Interpretation of results when there is no change in flow rate is problematic.

18. Lin SS, Roger VL, Pascoe R, et al: Dobutamine stress Doppler. Hemodynamics in patients with aortic stenosis: Feasibility, safety, and surgical considerations. Am Heart J 136:1010–1016, 1998.

Dobutamine stress echocardiography in patients with aortic stenosis and left ventricular dysfunction showed an average increase in valve area of about 0.2 cm². Of note, some patients with severe aortic stenosis confirmed at surgery had an increase in valve area with dobutamine.

19. Bermejo J, Garcia-Fernandez MA, Antoranz JC, et al: Stress echocardiography in aortic stenosis: Insights into valve mechanics and hemodynamics. Echocardiograpy 1999. In press.

Excellent review of the fluid dynamics of aortic stenosis and potential new measures of stenosis severity.

Mitral Stenosis

20. Henry WL, Griffith JM, Michaelis LL, et al: Measurement of mitral orifice area in patients with mitral valve disease by real-time, two-dimensional echocardiography. Circulation 51:827–831, 1975.

Validation of 2D echo planimetry of mitral valve area compared with measurements at operation. 2D echo valve area was within 0.3 cm² of surgical area in 12 of 14 (86%) patients.

21. Smith MD, Handshoe R, Handshoe S, et al: Comparative accuracy of two-dimensional echocardiography and Doppler pressure half-time methods in assessing severity of mitral stenosis in patients with and without prior commissurotomy. Circulation 73:100–107, 1986.

In 74 patients with mitral stenosis, correlations were good for Doppler or 2D echo valve areas versus catheterization (r = 0.80 and 0.83), but Doppler correlated better (r = 0.90) than 2D echo (r = 0.58) in the 35 patients with prior valvuloplasty. Reproducibility was 0.14 cm² for 2D echo and 0.15 cm² for Doppler data.

22. Holen J, Aaslid R, Landmark K, Simonsen S: Determination of pressure gradient in mitral stenosis with a non-invasive ultrasound Doppler technique. Acta Med Scand 199:455–460, 1976.

Original description of Doppler measurement of transmitral pressure gradients.

23. David D, Lang RM, Marcus RH, et al: Doppler echocardiographic estimation of transmitral pressure gradients and correlations with micromanometer gradients in mitral stenosis. Am J Cardiol 67:1161–1164, 1991.

Detailed study of pressure-velocity relations across the stenotic mitral valve.

24. Libanoff AJ, Rodbard S: Evaluation of the severity of mitral stenosis and regurgitation. Circulation 33:218–226, 1966.

Original description of pressure half-time with catheterization data.

25. Hatle L, Angelsen B, Tromsdal A: Noninvasive assessment of atrioventricular pressure half-time by Doppler ultrasound. Circulation 60:1096–1104, 1979.

Application of pressure half-time concept to Doppler data.

26. Thomas JD, Weyman AE: Doppler mitral pressure half-time: A clinical tool in search of theoretical justification. J Am Coll Cardiol 10:923–929, 1987.

Review of theoretical background of pressure half-time concept emphasizing potential effects of left atrial and left ventricular compliance as well as the influence of mitral valve area.

27. Faletra F, Pezzano JA, Fusco R, et al: Measurement of mitral valve area in mitral stenosis: Four echocardiographic methods compared with direct measurement of anatomic orifices. J Am Coll Cardiol 28:1190–1197, 1996.

Careful study demonstrating the accuracy of 2D planimetry, pressure half-time, and proximal flow convergence region methods for calculation of mitral valve area compared to direct measurement of the area of the excised mitral valves.

28. Thomas JD, Wilkins GT, Choong CYP, et al: Inaccuracy of mitral pressure half-time immediately after percutaneous mitral valvotomy: Dependence on transmittal gradient and left atrial and ventricular compliance. *Circulation* 78:980–993, 1988.

Evaluation of pressure half-time before and after mitral balloon valvuloplasty illustrating reciprocal changes in left atrial and left ventricular compliance after valvuloplasty.

29. Reid CL: Echocardiography in the patient undergoing catheter balloon mitral commissurotomy. *In* Otto CM (ed): The Practice of Clinical Echocardiography. Philadelphia, WB Saunders, 1997, pp. 373–388.

Review of the use of echocardiography in patient selection, prediction of hemodynamic results, diagnosis of complications, and long-term outcome after mitral commissurotomy.

30. Iung B, Cormier B, Ducimetiere P, et al: Functional results 5 years after successful percutaneous mitral commissurotomy in a series of 528 patients and analysis of predictive factors. *J Am Coll Cardiol* 27:407–414, 1996.

Stenotic mitral valves were classified by echocardiography as group I (flexible leaflets and mild subvalvular disease), group II (flexible leaflets and extensive subvalvular disease), and group III (calcified valves). Multivariate predictors of long-term functional results after percutaneous commissurotomy were echocardiographic group and cardiothoracic ratio before the procedure and valve area after the procedure.

31. Wilkins GT, Weyman AE, Abascal VM, et al: Percutaneous balloon dilatation of the mitral valve: An analysis of echocardiographic variables related to outcome and the mechanism of dilatation. *Br Heart J* 60:299–308, 1988.

The Massachusetts General Hospital morphology score for mitral stenosis is calculated as the sum of individual 1 to 4+ scores for valve mobility, thickness, calcification, and subvalvular involvement.

32. Dean LS, Mickel MC, Bonan R, et al: Four-year follow-up of patients undergoing percutaneous balloon mitral commissurotomy: A report from the National Heart, Lung, and Blood Institute Balloon Valvuloplasty Registry. *J Am Coll Cardiol* 28:1452–1457, 1996.

Event-free survival after percutaneous commissurotomy was 80% ± 1.5% at 1 year and 66% ± 1.8% at 3 years. Multivariate predictors of mortality were functional class, higher echocardiographic score, and higher postprocedure pulmonary systolic and left ventricular end-diastolic pressures.

33. Cannan CR, Nishimura RA, Reeder GS, et al: Echocardiographic assessment of commissural calcium: A simple predictor of outcome after percutaneous mitral balloon valvotomy. *J Am Coll Cardiol* 29:175–180, 1997.

Commissural calcification on 2D echocardiography predicts a poor outcome after percutaneous commissurotomy.

34. Gordon SP, Douglas PS, Come PC, Manning WJ: Two-dimensional and Doppler echocardiographic determinants of the natural history of mitral valve narrowing in patients with rheumatic mitral stenosis: Implications for follow-up. *J Am Coll Cardiol* 19:968–973, 1992.

Doppler echocardiography in 140 patients with rheumatic mitral stenosis showed an average decrease in valve area of 0.09 ± 0.21 cm^2/y. Predictors of more rapid progression were a higher initial gradient and echocardiographic score. In those with a morphology score ≥8, valve area decreased by 0.3 ± 0.3 cm^2/y compared to 0.0 ± 0.1 cm^2/y in those with a score <8.

35. Sagie A, Freitas N, Padial LR, et al: Doppler echocardiographic assessment of long-term progression of mitral stenosis in 103 patients: Valve area and right heart disease. *J Am Coll Cardiol* 28:472–479, 1996.

In 103 mitral stenosis patients, mitral valve area decreased by 0.09 cm^2/y. Progression was most rapid in those with a larger initial valve area. These findings illustrate the utility of Doppler echocardiography in following disease progression in individual patients.

Valvular Regurgitation: Diagnosis, Quantitation, and Clinical Approach

11

BASIC PRINCIPLES
   Etiology of Valvular Regurgitation
   Fluid Dynamics of Valvular Regurgitation
   Volume Overload
   Detection of Valvular Regurgitation
   Valvular Regurgitation in Normal Individuals
   Approaches to Evaluation of the Severity of
      Regurgitation
      Doppler Flow Mapping
      Continuous-Wave Doppler Approach
      Upstream Flow Reversal
      Volume Flow at Two Intracardiac Sites
      Proximal Isovelocity Surface Area (PISA)
      Jet Momentum
   Alternate Approaches/Technical Considerations
      Etiology of Valve Disease
      Left Ventricular Size and Systolic Function
      Regurgitant Severity
AORTIC REGURGITATION
   Diagnostic Imaging of the Valve Apparatus
   2D/M-Mode Findings in Aortic Regurgitation
   Left Ventricular Response to Aortic Regurgitation
   Evaluation of Aortic Regurgitant Severity
      Doppler Flow Mapping
      Continuous-Wave Doppler
      Holodiastolic Flow Reversal in the Descending
         Aorta
      Volume Flow at Two Intracardiac Sites
   Clinical Utility
      Diagnostic Utility for Aortic Regurgitation

      Timing of Surgical Intervention for Chronic
         Asymptomatic Aortic Regurgitation
      Monitoring the Effect of Medical Therapy
   Alternate Approaches
MITRAL REGURGITATION
   Diagnostic Imaging of the Mitral Valve Apparatus
   Response of the Left Ventricle, Left Atrium, and
      Pulmonary Vasculature to Mitral Regurgitation
   Other 2D/M-Mode Findings in Mitral Regurgitation
   Evaluation of Mitral Regurgitant Severity
      Doppler Flow Mapping
      Pulmonary Vein Flow Reversal
      Continuous-Wave Doppler Evaluation
      Volume Flow at Two Intracardiac Sites
   Clinical Utility
      Diagnosis and Severity of Mitral Regurgitation
      Mitral Valve "Prolapse" Versus Myxomatous
         Mitral Valve Disease
      Follow-up of Chronic Asymptomatic Mitral
         Regurgitation
      Decision Making Concerning Mitral Valve Repair
         or Replacement
      Intraoperative Evaluation of Mitral Valve Repair
TRICUSPID REGURGITATION
   Diagnostic Imaging of the Tricuspid Valve Apparatus
   Right Ventricular and Right Atrial Dilation
   Evaluation of Tricuspid Regurgitation Severity
   Clinical Utility
PULMONIC REGURGITATION
SUGGESTED READING

Echocardiographic evaluation of the patient with valvular regurgitation includes assessment of valve anatomy, the severity of regurgitation, chamber dilation due to the imposed volume overload, ventricular function, and the degree of pulmonary hypertension. In some clinical situations, the clinical significance of valvular regurgitation is related to the *presence* of abnormal regurgitation, regardless of severity. For example, detection of aortic regurgitation in a patient with chest pain and an enlarged aortic root heightens the suspicion of aortic dissection. Detection of regurgitation also may be important in terms of endocarditis risk and the need for prophylactic antibiotics in patients with a cardiac murmur. In other situations (e.g., endocarditis with acute mitral regurgitation), the *severity* of regurgitation is a key factor in clinical decision making regarding surgical intervention. In contrast, in chronic mitral regurgitation due to myxomatous valve disease, the *response of the left ventricle to chronic volume overload*, not regurgitant severity per se, is the most important factor in deciding on the timing of valve surgery.

BASIC PRINCIPLES

Etiology of Valvular Regurgitation

Valvular regurgitation may be due to congenital or acquired abnormalities of the valve leaflets or to abnormalities of the associated supporting structures. For example, aortic root dilation can result in aortic regurgitation even with anatomically normal valve leaflets. Similarly, left ventricular dilation can result in mitral regurgitation even with normal valve leaflets and chordae. Echocardiographic examinations allow definition of the etiology of valvular regurgitation in most cases. Even when a single definite etiology is not evident, the differential diagnosis of the etiology of regurgitation often can be narrowed to the few most likely possibilities. The examination also may provide clues as to whether regurgitation is acute or chronic in duration.

Fluid Dynamics of Valvular Regurgitation (Table 11–1)

The fluid dynamics of a regurgitant valve are, in many ways, similar to the fluid dynamics of a stenotic valve, as described in Chapter 10 (Fig. 11–1). Even though the anatomy of the regurgitant orifice may be quite complex, the regurgitant valve can be thought of as having a regurgitant orifice, which in simple physiologic terms is characterized by a high-velocity laminar jet. The instantaneous velocity in this jet *(v)* is related to the instantaneous pressure difference (ΔP) across the valve, as stated in the simplified Bernoulli equation: $\Delta P = 4v^2$. Recording this high-velocity jet with continuous-wave Doppler allows assessment of the time course of the difference in pressure between the two chambers on either side of the valve.

On the upstream side of the regurgitant valve, flow acceleration proximal to the regurgitant orifice is present, and a proximal isove-locity surface area (PISA) can be defined similar to that seen on the left atrial side of the stenotic mitral valve. This observation provides an alternate method for quantitative evaluation of regurgitant stroke volume as discussed in the following text.

As the high-velocity jet enters the chamber receiving the regurgitant flow, the flow pattern becomes disturbed with nonlaminar flow, multiple blood flow velocities, and multiple blood flow directions. Evaluation of the spatial extent of the flow disturbance *in* the receiving chamber provides a semiquantitative measure of regurgitant severity. Note that the term *jet* is used by some clinicians to refer to the spatial extent of the flow disturbance in the receiving chamber rather than to the high-velocity flow in the regurgitant orifice.

The fluid dynamics of the regurgitant flow disturbance are complex and not fully understood. However, several generalizations are

Valvular Regurgitation

FIGURE 11–1. Schematic drawing of a regurgitant jet showing the proximal isovelocity surface area (PISA), the jet through the regurgitant orifice, and the flow disturbance in the receiving chamber.

TABLE 11–1	Relationship Between Fluid Dynamics of Valvular Regurgitation and Diagnostic Approach

Fluid Dynamic Characteristic	Diagnostic Approach
High-velocity jet in regurgitant orifice	Pressure/velocity relationship of continuous-wave Doppler curve
Proximal acceleration	Proximal isovelocity surface area
Flow disturbance in chamber receiving regurgitant flow	Flow mapping
Increased volume flow across valve	Increased antegrade velocity, volume flow at two sites
Conservation of momentum	Regurgitant orifice area, momentum calculations

possible (Table 11–2). The shape and direction of the regurgitant jet depends on multiple factors, including the anatomy and orientation of the regurgitation orifice, the driving force across the valve, and the size and compliance of the receiving chamber. Jets are "pulled" toward adjacent walls (e.g., mitral regurgitation in the left atrium) if within a critical distance from the wall at the entry site and also are "pulled" toward other flowstreams (e.g., aortic regurgitation and mitral stenosis). Jets that adhere to the wall of the chamber will have a smaller cross-sectional area on tomographic color flow imaging (and a smaller three-dimensional [3D] volume) since entrainment of additional fluid elements into the jet occurs on only one side, instead of on all sides, as with a central jet.

Another approach to quantitation of valvular regurgitation is calculation of the total momentum in the regurgitant jet. *Momentum*, defined as volume flow times velocity, remains constant in any closed fluid system. Thus the total momentum of the regurgitant jet must equal the initial momentum across the narrowed orifice based on the law of conservation of momentum. This observation may prove to be useful in developing new methods for quantitation of regurgitant severity.

Volume Overload

Chronic valvular regurgitation results in progressive volume overload of the ventricle. Volume overload of the left ventricle results in chamber dilation with normal wall thickness so that total left ventricular mass is increased (eccentric hypertrophy). An important clinical feature of chronic left ventricular volume overload is that an irreversible decrease in systolic function can occur in the absence of symptoms. In fact, an irreversible decrease in contractility can occur despite a normal ejection fraction due to the altered loading conditions of the ventricle when regurgitation is present.

In patients with regurgitant valves, the term *total stroke volume* refers to the total volume of blood pumped by the ventricle on a single beat. *Forward stroke volume* is the amount of blood delivered to the peripheral circulation, and *regurgitant volume* is the amount of backflow across the abnormal valve (Fig. 11–2).

Detection of Valvular Regurgitation

Valvular regurgitation can be detected with either conventional pulsed Doppler, color flow imaging, or continuous-wave Doppler ultrasound. While two-dimensional (2D) imaging provides detailed information about valve anat-

TABLE 11–2	Factors that Affect Regurgitation Jet Size and Shape

Physiologic
Regurgitant volume

Driving pressure

Size and shape of regurgitant orifice

Receiving chamber constraint

Wall impingement

Timing relative to the cardiac cycle

Influence of coexisting jets or flowstreams

Technical
Ultrasound system gain

Pulse repetition frequency

Transducer frequency

Frame rate

Image plane

Depth

Signal strength

Mitral Regurgitation

Total SV = Forward SV + Regurgitant SV

FIGURE 11–2. When mitral regurgitation is present, total stroke volume is the sum of the regurgitant (RSV) and forward stroke volumes (FSV).

omy and chamber dilation and function, it provides only indirect evidence for the presence or absence of valvular incompetence. The finding of an anatomically abnormal mitral valve in the presence of left atrial and left ventricular dilation suggests that mitral regurgitation may be present, but Doppler examination is necessary for direct confirmation or exclusion of the diagnosis. Although a few M-mode findings have been shown to be specific for diagnosing valvular regurgitation (e.g., high-frequency fluttering of the anterior mitral leaflet in aortic regurgitation), these findings are not sensitive enough to reliably exclude regurgitation when suspected on clinical grounds.

With color flow imaging, detection of regurgitation is based on identification of the flow disturbance on the upstream side of the valve. When instrument settings and examination technique are optimal, color flow imaging is extremely sensitive (about 90%) and specific (nearly 100%) for diagnosing valvular regurgitation as compared with angiography. In fact, color flow imaging is so sensitive that regurgitation often is detected that is not audible by auscultation. These cases most often are true positives, as evidenced by angiographic confirmation. False-positive results can occur with color flow imaging when the origin or timing of the flow signal is mistaken. For example, normal pulmonary venous inflow may be mistaken for mitral regurgitation. False-negative results occur when signal strength is poor due to poor acoustic access or attenuation due to the depth of interrogation. False-negative results also occur if color flow processing parameters are set incorrectly or if the examiner fails to study the valve in multiple tomographic planes. Additional parameters important in detection of valvular regurgitation with color flow imaging include gray-scale setting, frame rate, and the color map chosen.

With conventional pulsed Doppler ultrasound, a small sample volume is placed on the immediate upstream side of the closed valve; the flow disturbance is identified both audibly and on the spectral display. Care is needed to ensure that the sample volume is correctly positioned (e.g., on the left ventricular side of the aortic valve in *diastole* and on the left atrial side of the mitral valve in *systole*), since considerable motion of the valve planes occurs during the cardiac cycle. Mild regurgitation may not extend throughout systole (for atrioventricular valve regurgitation) or diastole (for semilunar valve regurgitation) (Fig. 11–3). Conventional pulsed Doppler evaluation of valvular regurgitation has largely been replaced by color flow imaging but may still be a useful confirmatory approach when the timing or origin of the color flow signal is in doubt.

Continuous-wave Doppler detection of valvular regurgitation is based on identification of the high-velocity jet through the regurgitant orifice. An advantage of continuous-wave Doppler is that beam width is broad at the level of the valves when studied from an apical approach. Identification of the regurgitant signal uses the

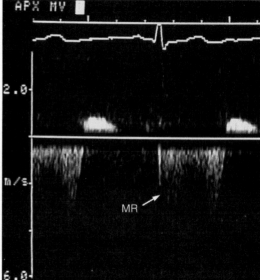

FIGURE 11–3. Example of "physiologic" mitral regurgitation recorded with color *(above)* and continuous-wave *(below)* Doppler in a normal individual. Note the low signal strength compared with antegrade flow and the incomplete systolic signal. (See Color Plate 8, p. 274.)

velocity, shape, timing, and associated antegrade flow signal to correctly identify the origin of the signal.

Valvular Regurgitation in Normal Individuals

Given the high sensitivity of Doppler ultrasound for detection of regurgitation, it has become apparent that a small degree of regurgitation is present in a high percentage of otherwise normal individuals. Typically, regurgitation detected in otherwise normal individuals is spatially restricted to the area immediately adjacent to valve closure, may be short in duration, and represents only a small regurgitant volume (see Fig. 11–3). When meticulously searched for, mitral regurgitation can be detected in 70% to 80%, tricuspid regurgitation in 80% to 90%, and pulmonic regurgitation in 70% to 80% of normal individuals. Thus a small degree of regurgitation of these three valves is normal and appears to have no adverse clinical implications. Aortic regurgitation is found in only a small percentage (5%) of young individuals with an otherwise normal echocardiographic study, but the prevalence of detectable aortic regurgitation increases with age. The clinical significance of a small amount of aortic regurgitation is unknown.

Approaches to Evaluation of the Severity of Regurgitation (Table 11–3)

Doppler Flow Mapping

Semiquantitative evaluation of regurgitant severity is extremely useful in patient management. Often the clinical question is whether only mild regurgitation or hemodynamically significant regurgitation is present. In these settings, precise quantitation of the severity of regurgitation may be unnecessary.

Flow mapping is evaluation of the extent of the flow disturbance in the chamber receiving the regurgitant jet. Although initially developed using conventional pulsed Doppler ultrasound, flow mapping now typically is performed using color flow imaging. For flow mapping of regurgitant jets, color flow imaging has the advantages compared to conventional pulsed Doppler that Doppler velocity signals across a tomographic plane can be sampled simultaneously

TABLE 11–3	Approaches to Evaluation of Regurgitation Severity

Semiquantitative
Flow mapping (pulsed or color)

Continuous-wave Doppler signal intensity

Distal flow reversals

Quantitative
Volume flow at two sites

Descending aortic flow reversal

Proximal isovelocity surface area

Jet momentum

and the visual format is easily understood by referring physicians. For each tomographic image plane, it is noted whether an abnormal flow signal with appropriate timing (i.e., systole for mitral regurgitation, diastole for aortic regurgitation) is present or absent. By integrating data from multiple tomographic planes, the 3D size and shape of the regurgitant jet can be estimated. The overall 3D extent of the regurgitant jet then is described on a 0 to 4+ scale, where 1+ is mild regurgitation (a small jet), 2 to 3+ is moderate regurgitation, and 4+ is severe regurgitation (a jet that nearly fills the receiving chamber) (Figs. 11–4 and 11–5).

Since color flow imaging basically is pulsed Doppler ultrasound with somewhat different signal processing and display formats, it is important to remember that signal aliasing still occurs. However, flow mapping depends on the timing and spatial location of the Doppler signals and *not* absolute blood flow velocity. Thus, signal aliasing does not limit the utility of flow mapping and, in fact, may enhance the appreciation of abnormal flow patterns due to the presence of variance in the color flow signal. In addition, flow mapping can be performed from windows where the intercept angle between the ultrasound beam and the direction of regurgitant flow is nonparallel. Moreover, these windows often allow a shorter distance from the transducer to the flow region of interest, resulting in a better signal-to-noise ratio. For example, aortic regurgitation is best evaluated in the parasternal short-axis view. Similarly, while the direction of an aortic regurgitant jet in the parasternal long-axis view is nearly perpendicular to the ultrasound beam, multiple flow directions within the jet allow detection of the diastolic flow disturbance. Of course, an accurate blood velocity determination cannot be made both because of the nonparallel intercept angle and because the velocity exceeds the Nyquist limit of the pulsed Doppler mode.

The appearance of a regurgitant jet with color flow imaging will vary depending on the ultrasound system, transducer frequency, and specific instrument settings. Correct visual interpretation depends on experience with a particular instrument and knowledge of the influence of instrument settings on the visual display. On most systems, a "variance" color scale results in a green regurgitant signal superimposed on the normal red-blue flow patterns. A "velocity" scale results in a mosaic of red, blue, and white pixels in the regurgitant jet. Since the goal of this application is to identify the location and timing of abnormal flow sig-

Flow Mapping for AR

Long-axis

Short-axis just
below aortic valve

FIGURE 11–4. Semiquantitation of aortic regurgitant severity using color flow mapping in parasternal long- and short-axis views. The depicted jet areas are only rough guides. In the clinical setting, multiple views are used, and jets often are eccentric in direction and asymmetric in shape.

Flow Mapping for MR

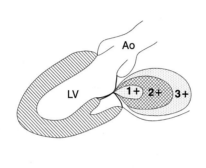

Apical 4-chamber

Parasternal long-axis

FIGURE 11–5. Mitral regurgitation semiquantitative flow mapping. Again, multiple views are used during the examination, and jet geometry is considered in conjunction with jet area in grading the degree of regurgitation. Severe (4+) mitral regurgitation is associated with systolic flow reversal in the pulmonary veins.

nals in a tomographic format, the exact color scale used is not particularly important so long as it displays the boundaries of the flow disturbance accurately.

With either a variance or a velocity color flow scale, it is obvious that an abnormal color pattern is not synonymous with abnormal flow given the physics of pulsed Doppler color flow imaging. An abnormal color pattern can be seen even with normal intracardiac flow patterns. For example, the normal antegrade flow velocity of laminar flow across the aortic valve exceeds the Nyquist limit, resulting in aliasing and an "abnormal" color pattern. Conversely, abnormal flow signals may not demonstrate variance or a mosaic pattern if the flow velocities are within the Nyquist limit for that interrogation depth. For example, the low velocities seen in pulmonic regurgitation result in a uniform color display even though the flow pattern is abnormal. Since the specific color scale chosen is somewhat arbitrary and has not been shown to affect the accuracy of semiquantitative flow mapping, each physician and sonogra-

pher should choose a scale that they find highlights the potential abnormalities most clearly. Interpretation of the color images will be most consistent from study to study if instrument settings and flow maps are standardized for each laboratory.

Evaluation of the exact timing of a flow signal in relation both to valve closing and to the QRS complex can be helpful in correct identification of the signal. With conventional pulsed Doppler, the spectral output of velocity versus time provides high temporal resolution. The mitral regurgitant signal, for example, can be distinguished from the immediately adjacent aortic outflow signal based on its timing: mitral regurgitation starts with mitral valve closure, while aortic outflow starts slightly later, after isovolumic contraction (Fig. 11–6). With 2D color flow imaging, temporal resolution is sacrificed for spatial resolution with color flow imaging frame rates far lower than the sampling rate of pulsed or continuous-wave Doppler. If the origin of a color flow velocity signal is unclear, use of 2D-guided color "M-mode" may be helpful by providing higher time resolution. With color M-mode Doppler the signal is displayed at each depth along a single line of interrogation (*y* axis) versus time (*x* axis) at a higher sampling rate (Fig. 11–7). Thus, the color M-mode tracing allows evaluation of the timing of the flow disturbance in relation to valve opening and closing.

Continuous-Wave Doppler Approach

Several types of information regarding the severity of valvular regurgitation can be derived from the spectral display of the continuous-wave Doppler signal. First, signal intensity is proportional to the number of blood cells contributing to the regurgitant signal. Since the ultrasound beam is relatively broad and signals from the entire length of the beam are recorded, much of the regurgitant jet can be encompassed in the beam with appropriate adjustment of beam direction. It is particularly helpful to compare the intensity of the regurgitant signal to antegrade flow across the same valve as a qualitative estimate of regurgitant severity. A weak signal reflects mild regurgitation, whereas a signal nearly equal in intensity to antegrade flow reflects severe regurgitation. Moderate regurgitation has an intermediate signal strength relative to antegrade flow.

Second, the associated antegrade velocity across the regurgitant valve provides useful information. Regurgitation results in an increase in the antegrade volume flow rate across the valve, which is reflected in an increase in the antegrade velocity across the valve. The greater the severity of regurgitation, the higher is the

antegrade velocity. Of course, the possibility of coexisting valvular stenosis also must be considered.

Third, the shape of the velocity curve depends on the time-varying pressure gradient across the regurgitant valve. Each instantaneous velocity is related to the instantaneous pressure gradient across the valve, as stated in the Bernoulli equation. Normal left ventricular systolic pressure is 100 to 140 mmHg and normal left atrial pressure is 5 to 15 mmHg, so the left ventricular to left atrial pressure difference in systole is 85 to 135 mmHg. Thus the mitral regurgitant velocity curve typically shows a maximum velocity of 5 to 6 m/s. When ventricular function is normal, there is rapid acceleration to peak velocity, with a maintained high velocity in systole and with rapid deceleration prior to diastolic opening of the mitral valve. An increase in end-systolic left atrial pressure (*v wave*) results in a late-systolic decline in the

FIGURE 11–7. Color M-mode of aortic (*above*) and mitral (*below*) regurgitation shows the high time resolution of this approach. (See Color Plate 8, p. 274.)

FIGURE 11–6. Relative timing of mitral regurgitation (MR) and left ventricular outflow tract (LVOT) flow signal. Mitral regurgitation extends from the onset of isovolumic contraction to the end of isovolumic relaxation. Left ventricular outflow is shorter in duration, occurring only during ejection.

instantaneous pressure gradient and in the instantaneous velocity (Fig. 11–8).

Similarly, the shape of the aortic regurgitant velocity curve depends on the time course of the diastolic pressure difference across the aortic valve. When left ventricular end-diastolic pressure is low and aortic end-diastolic pressure is normal or mildly reduced, a large pressure difference (and high velocity) across the valve is present throughout diastole with a slow rate of pressure decline (Fig. 11–9). Acute regurgitation results in more rapid equalization of left ventricular and aortic pressures with a more rapid velocity decline in diastole.

Upstream Flow Reversal

When atrioventricular valve regurgitation is severe enough that a significant volume of blood is displaced by the regurgitant jet, flow reversal is seen in the veins entering the atrium. With severe tricuspid regurgitation, the normal pattern of systolic inflow into the right atrium from the superior and inferior vena cava is reversed. This can be demonstrated with a pulsed Doppler sample volume positioned in the cen-

tral hepatic vein (Fig. 11–10). Severe mitral regurgitation results in reversal of the normal patterns of systolic inflow into the left atrium from the pulmonary veins. This may be difficult to demonstrate on a transthoracic study due to signal attenuation at the depth of the pulmonary vein but is easily recorded from a transesophageal approach (Fig. 11–11).

Regurgitation of a semilunar valve results in reversal of flow in the associated great vessel as blood flows from the great vessel, across the incompetent valve, and into the ventricle. The distance from the valve plane that this flow reversal extends in the great vessel is proportional to regurgitant volume.

Volume Flow at Two Intracardiac Sites

Regurgitant stroke volume can be calculated from the difference between total and forward stroke volume. Total stroke volume is calculated from antegrade flow across the regurgitant valve as the cross-sectional area of flow times the velocity-time integral of transvalvular flow (see discussion of stroke volume calculation in Chap. 5). Forward stroke volume is cal-

FIGURE 11–8. Left ventricular (LV) and left atrial (LA) pressures and the Doppler velocity curve in chronic *(solid lines)* and acute *(dashed lines)* mitral regurgitation are shown. Note that the shape of the velocity curve reflects the shape of the pressure difference between the left ventricle and the left atrium so that a late-systolic rise in left atrial pressure (*v* wave) is seen as a more rapid decrease in velocity in late systole on the Doppler curve.

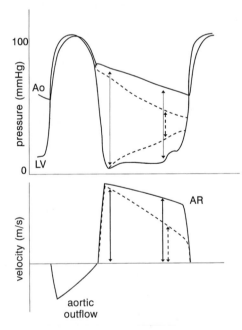

FIGURE 11–9. Left ventricular (LV) and central aortic (Ao) pressures and the corresponding Doppler velocity curve are shown for chronic *(solid lines)* and acute *(dashed lines)* aortic regurgitation. Again, the shape of the velocity curve is related to the instantaneous pressure differences across the valve, as stated in the Bernoulli equation. With acute aortic regurgitation, aortic pressure falls more rapidly and ventricular diastolic pressure rises more rapidly, resulting in a steeper deceleration slope on the Doppler curve.

FIGURE 11–11. With severe mitral regurgitation, systolic flow reversal in the right superior pulmonary vein Doppler velocity curve *(above)* and blunting of systolic flow in the left superior pulmonary vein *(below)* are seen on transesophageal imaging in a patient with an eccentric, anteromedially directed regurgitant jet. D = diastolic flow; A = atrial reversal.

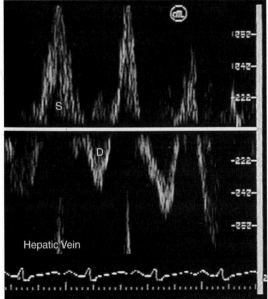

FIGURE 11–10. With the sample volume (SV) positioned in the central hepatic vein from a subcostal approach, systolic (S) flow reversal in the hepatic vein Doppler velocity curve is seen when severe tricuspid regurgitation is present. Forward flow into the right atrium in diastole (D) also is seen.

where CSA is cross-sectional area, VTI is the velocity-time integral, and LVOT is the left ventricular outflow tract. Forward stroke volume is represented by left ventricular inflow (LVI) across the mitral valve, since the amount of blood filling the ventricle equals the amount of blood delivered to the body on each beat, and can be calculated as:

$$SV_{forward} = CSA_{LVI} \times VTI_{LVI} \qquad (11.2)$$

With aortic regurgitation, alternate sites for measurement of forward stroke volume are the pulmonary artery and right ventricular inflow region. Then, regurgitant stroke volume is:

Regurgitant stroke volume
$$SV_{regurgitant} = SV_{total} - SV_{forward} \qquad (11.3)$$

and regurgitant fraction (RF) is:

Regurgitant fraction
$$RF = SV_{regurgitant}/SV_{total} \qquad (11.4)$$

Proximal Isovelocity Surface Area (PISA)

Another approach for determining regurgitant stroke volume is to examine the flow pattern on the upstream side of the valve (proximal to the regurgitant orifice). Acceleration of flow occurs proximal to the valve plane with,

culated as antegrade flow across a different (and nonregurgitant) valve (Fig. 11–12).

For example, with aortic regurgitation, transaortic stroke volume (SV) represents total left ventricular stroke volume and can be calculated as:

$$SV_{total} = CSA_{LVOT} \times VTI_{LVOT} \qquad (11.1)$$

conceptually, a series of isovelocity "surfaces" leading to the high-velocity jet in the regurgitant orifice. Immediately adjacent to the orifice, these surfaces are small with high-velocity flow; at increasing distances from the orifice, areas are larger and velocities are lower. Based on the principle of volume flow calculation by Doppler techniques, the volume flow rate (in this case, regurgitant flow) for any of these surfaces, when averaged over the temporal flow period, is (Fig. 11–13)

$$\text{Regurgitant volume} = \text{PISA} \times \text{Velocity} \qquad (11.5)$$

The velocity for a PISA can be determined from the color flow image as the aliasing velocity where a distinct red-blue interface is seen (Fig. 11–14). At this interface, the velocity is known, being equivalent to the Nyquist limit on the velocity color scale. The size of the PISA can be maximized to allow more accurate regurgitant flow rate calculations by decreasing the velocity range and/or by shifting the velocity baseline.

The shape of the isovelocity surface proximal to a regurgitant valve typically is hemispherical with a tendency toward a hemielliptical shape closer to the orifice (Fig. 11–14). Assuming a hemispherical shape, the PISA is calculated from measurements of the distance from the aliasing velocity to the regurgitant orifice as:

$$\text{PISA} = 2\pi r^2 \qquad (11.6)$$

Note that the PISA method for calculating regurgitant volume is analogous to calculation of stroke volume proximal to a stenotic valve.

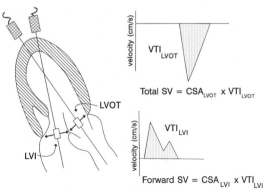

Regurg. SV = Total SV - Forward SV

FIGURE 11–12. Calculation of aortic regurgitant stroke volume (SV) by measurement of transvalvular volume flow rate at two intracardiac sites is illustrated. Transaortic flow, representing total stroke volume, is calculated from the cross-sectional area (CSA) and velocity-time integral (VTI) of the left ventricular outflow tract (LVOT). Transmitral flow, representing forward stroke volume, is calculated from the cross-sectional area and velocity-time integral of left ventricular inflow (LVI) across the mitral annulus. Regurgitant stroke volume is the difference between total and forward stroke volume.

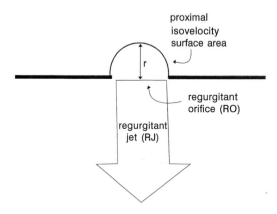

regurg. volume = PISA x velocity

RO area= regurg. volume/VTI$_{RJ}$

FIGURE 11–13. Proximal to a regurgitant orifice, flow accelerates resulting in concentric proximal isovelocity surface areas (PISAs). The color Doppler aliasing velocity allows identification of one of these PISAs, which then can be used to calculate the regurgitant volume based on the aliasing velocity. The radius (r) is used to calculate the PISA. In combination with the velocity-time integral (VTI) of the continuous-wave Doppler recording of the regurgitant jet (RJ), regurgitant orifice area (RO) can be calculated.

FIGURE 11–14. Color flow image of a proximal isovelocity surface area in mitral regurgitation seen on transesophageal imaging. The aliasing velocity is 61 cm/s. (See Color Plate 9, p. 274.)

Color Plate 5

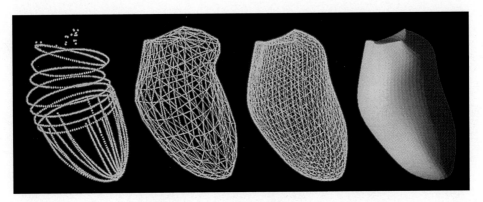

FIGURE 4–15. For legend, see page 95.

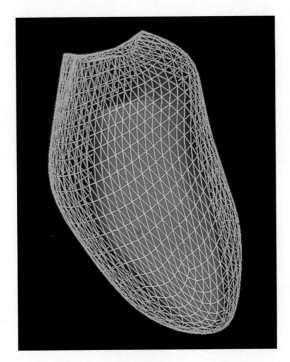

FIGURE 4–16. For legend, see page 95.

Color Plate 6

FIGURE 7–18. For legend, see page 168.

FIGURE 7–22. For legend, see page 172.

Color Plate 7

FIGURE 7–25. For legend, see page 174.

FIGURE 8–4. For legend, see page 186.

FIGURE 8–12. For legend, see page 190.

FIGURE 10–2. For legend, see page 231.

Color Plate 8

FIGURE 10–4. For legend, see page 232.

FIGURE 10–29. For legend, see page 258.

FIGURE 10–34. For legend, see page 261.

FIGURE 11–3. For legend, see page 268.

FIGURE 11–7. For legend, see page 271.

Color Plate 9

FIGURE 11–14. For legend, see page 274.

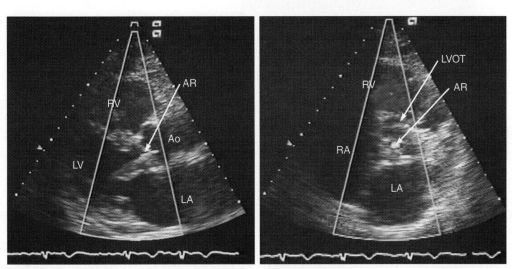

FIGURE 11–19. For legend, see page 282.

FIGURE 11–20. For legend, see page 283.

Color Plate 10

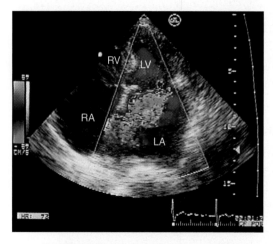

FIGURE 11–29. For legend, see page 289.

FIGURE 11–30. For legend, see page 289.

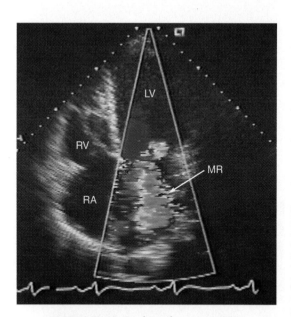

FIGURE 11–31. For legend, see page 290.

FIGURE 11–34. For legend, see page 294.

Color Plate 11

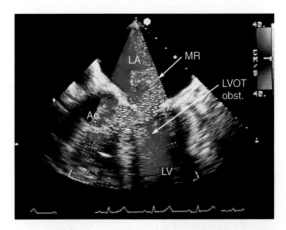

FIGURE 11–36. For legend, see page 295.

FIGURE 11–38. For legend, see page 296.

FIGURE 11–40. For legend, see page 297.

Color Plate 12

FIGURE 12–2. For legend, see page 303.

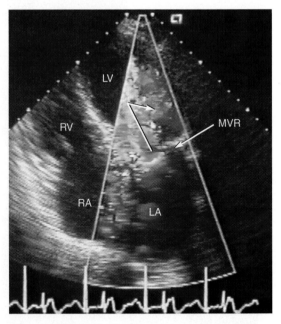

FIGURE 12–3. For legend, see page 303.

FIGURE 12–5. For legend, see page 305.

Color Plate 13

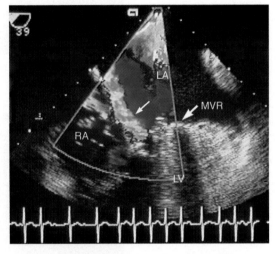

FIGURE 12–19. For legend, see page 317.

FIGURE 12–18. For legend, see page 317.

FIGURE 12–20. For legend, see page 318.

Color Plate 14

FIGURE 13–9. For legend, see page 335.

FIGURE 13–11. For legend, see page 336.

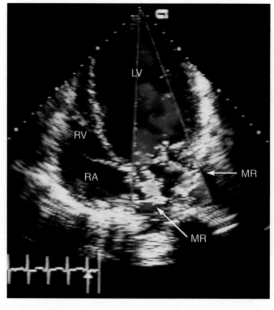

FIGURE 13–17. For legend, see page 340.

Color Plate 15

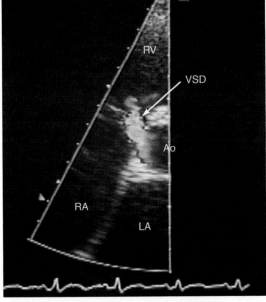

FIGURE 13–18. For legend, see page 341.

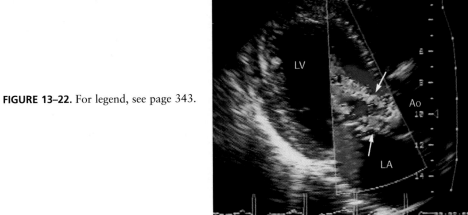

FIGURE 13–20. For legend, see page 342.

FIGURE 13–22. For legend, see page 343.

Color Plate 16

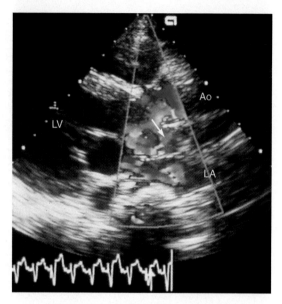

FIGURE 13–24. For legend, see page 345.

FIGURE 13–25. For legend, see page 345.

FIGURE 14–10. For legend, see page 358.

FIGURE 14–13. For legend, see page 359.

The differences between these approaches are (1) the differing shapes of the proximal velocity stream lines, (2) the use of color flow, rather than pulsed Doppler, to measure velocity at a given location, and (3) the need for temporal averaging when color data from single images are used.

The PISA method can be combined with the velocity-time integral of continuous-wave Doppler recording through the regurgitant orifice (VTI_{RO}) to calculate regurgitant orifice area based on the principle of conservation of mass (the continuity equation). Since the regurgitant volume (RV) proximal to and *in* the regurgitant orifice are equal,

$$RV = ROA \times VTI_{RO} \qquad (11.7)$$

so that, solving for regurgitant orifice area:

$$ROA = RV/VTI_{RO} \qquad (11.8)$$

Of course, any method for measuring regurgitant stroke volume can be used in this equation.

Some clinicians use a simplified PISA approach by setting the aliasing velocity at a known value (such as 30 cm/s), measuring the radius of the PISA and then using precalculated tables of the corresponding regurgitant orifice area. However, this approach assumes a normal peak regurgitant jet velocity and is inaccurate if orifice geometry or jet direction are atypical. If the PISA method is used, it is prudent to measure the peak jet velocity as well as the aliasing velocity and surface area.

Jet Momentum

Yet another approach to quantification of the severity of valvular regurgitation is based on the principle of conservation of momentum. Momentum is defined as the product of volume flow rate *(Q)* and velocity *(v)*:

$$Momentum = Q \times v \qquad (11.9)$$

At any cross-sectional plane perpendicular to a regurgitant jet, momentum is equal to any other plane perpendicular to the jet (including at the orifice). In simple terms, this means that as the volume of the jet increases distal to the regurgitant valve, velocity decreases accordingly.

Since volume flow rate equals cross-sectional area times velocity,

$$Q = Area \times v \qquad (11.10)$$

substituting Eq. (11.10) for Q in Eq. (11.9) yields:

$$Momentum = Area \times v^2 \qquad (11.11)$$

Thus momentum can be calculated in the regurgitant orifice by multiplying the regurgitant orifice area (using Eq. 11.8) by the square of the continuous-wave (CW) Doppler jet velocity. Alternatively, momentum can be calculated from measurement of the color flow jet cross-sectional area and velocity measured with pulsed Doppler (PD) at any plane perpendicular to the long axis of the jet.

If regurgitant orifice area is unknown, it can be calculated from determinations of momentum at some point in the jet distal to the orifice plus the continuous-wave Doppler signal, since:

$$Momentum_{orifice} = Momentum_{jet} \qquad (11.12)$$

Using Eq. (11.11),

$$ROA \times v^2_{cw} = Area\ of\ jet \times v^2_{PD} \qquad (11.13)$$

So

$$ROA = (Area\ of\ jet \times v^2_{PD})/v^2_{cw} \qquad (11.14)$$

Several investigators have hypothesized that jet momentum and regurgitant orifice area may be useful descriptors of regurgitant severity and have shown that color regurgitant jet areas correlate well with momentum or regurgitant orifice area. While promising research tools, these methods are tedious and prone to error in the clinical setting and as yet have not gained wide acceptance.

Alternate Approaches/ Technical Considerations

Etiology of Valve Disease

If transthoracic images are suboptimal or nondiagnostic for evaluation of aortic or mitral valve anatomy and the etiology of regurgitation, transesophageal imaging may be helpful. With aortic root disease, visualization of the ascending aorta may be suboptimal on transthoracic imaging, so transesophageal echocardiography, gated computed tomographic scanning, magnetic resonance imaging, or aortography may be needed to fully define the extent and severity of disease.

Left Ventricular Size and Systolic Function

While serial echocardiographic evaluation of left ventricular size in chronic aortic or mitral regurgitation has become a standard method of clinical evaluation, two factors potentially limit the reliability of this approach. First, suboptimal image quality or recording techniques may result in erroneous measurements. Care is needed to ensure that the dimensions are measured perpendicular to the long and short axes of the left ventricle, and instrument settings must be adjusted for optimal endocardial definition. Accurate tracing of endocardial borders for calculation of ventricular volumes depends on clear endocardial definition, standard image planes without foreshortening of the long axis of the ventricle, and a trained and experienced individual tracing the borders at end-diastole and end-systole. Whether 3D echocardiographic techniques will obviate some of the limitations of M-mode and 2D imaging has not yet been demonstrated for routine clinical use.

Second, the reproducibility of left ventricular measurements must be considered. Overall reproducibility includes variation in *recording* the data, variation in *measuring* the data, and *physiologic* variation (such as heart rate and loading conditions) that may affect the measurement. Reproducibility of 2D-guided M-mode measurements of the left ventricle suggests that an interval change of >8 mm in end-systolic or end-diastolic dimensions represents a definite clinical change.

Similar concerns apply to serial qualitative or quantitative evaluations of left ventricular systolic function, such as ejection fraction. While accurate when carefully performed, image orientation and endocardial definition must be carefully optimized, and endocardial border tracing must be performed by an experienced individual. Using 2D echocardiography, a change in ventricular volume or a change in ejection fraction greater than 10% on serial studies performed in the same laboratory indicates a significant change. Alternate methods for evaluation of left ventricular size and systolic function include radionuclide or angiographic ventriculography.

Regurgitant Severity

Doppler evaluation of valvular regurgitant severity has become a standard clinical tool; however, these methods have numerous potential pitfalls and limitations. Doppler flow mapping provides only a semiquantitative estimate of regurgitant severity. Attempts to refine this approach by measurement of jet area or even 3D jet volume are fraught with difficulty due to the complex fluid dynamics of valvular regurgitation. First, the size and shape of the regurgitant jet depend not only on regurgitant volume but also on regurgitant orifice shape and orientation, the shape and compliance of the receiving chamber, entrainment into the jet of static blood within the receiving chamber, deflection of the jet toward adjacent walls, and confluence with other flowstreams within the chamber

(e.g., left ventricular inflow and aortic regurgitation). Second, the size and shape of the jet vary temporally during the cardiac cycle. Third, transducer frequency, depth of interrogation, instrument settings, and recording parameters all affect the appearance of the regurgitant jet on color flow images.

The utility of the continuous-wave Doppler curve depends, in large part, on technical factors in data recording as well as on correct data interpretation. The high-velocity regurgitant signal is optimized when the high-pass ("wall") filter is set at the maximum level, and the gain and velocity scale are adjusted to show the peak velocities clearly. Accurate pressure gradient calculations assume a near-parallel intercept angle between the direction of the ultrasound beam and the regurgitant jet, thus requiring examination from multiple acoustic windows with careful transducer angulation to obtain this parallel alignment. Use of a dedicated, small, continuous-wave transducer often facilitates the examination and provides a better signal-to-noise ratio than 2D-guided continuous-wave Doppler. In addition, the 2D image may distract the examiner from searching for the highest-velocity signal. Color flow imaging is of limited value for locating the best continuous-wave signal because it provides only 2D information; jet direction in the elevational plane remains unknown. Temporal factors also affect data quality, and caution is needed in interpreting the shape of the velocity curve if jet direction (and thus Doppler-jet intercept angle) varies during the regurgitant flow period.

Again, the continuous-wave Doppler signal provides only a semiquantitative evaluation of stenosis severity. Signal intensity is judged subjectively and may underestimate regurgitant severity if ultrasound tissue penetration is suboptimal. Attempts to quantitate regurgitant severity based on the diastolic slope of the velocity curve have been frustrated by the numerous other physiologic abnormalities that affect this measurement.

Calculation of regurgitant volume and regurgitant fraction from volume flow at two intracardiac sites has been shown to be accurate in animal models and in selected patient series. However, wide clinical application of this technique has been limited by the difficulty of measuring 2D diameters accurately, particularly from acoustic windows where the structure of interest is not perpendicular to the ultrasound beam. Small errors in diameter measurement lead to large errors in cross-sectional area calculations due to the quadratic relationship be-

TABLE 11–4	Comparison of Information Derived at Catheterization Versus Echocardiography in Valvular Regurgitation	
	Catheterization	**Echocardiography**
Semiquantitative severity index	Angiographic (0 to 4+)	Flow mapping (0 to 4+)
Quantitative regurgitant stroke volume	Forward versus total stroke volume	Volume flow at two sites
Hemodynamics	Direct pressure measurement	Shape of continuous-wave Doppler curve
Left ventricular size and systolic function	Left ventricular angiography	2D echo

tween the two ($CSA = \pi r^2$). Other potential pitfalls in volume flow measurement are discussed in detail in Chapter 5. This method clearly can provide accurate quantitation of regurgitant severity when image quality is excellent; in other cases, it is helpful to compare the antegrade velocity-time integral (or peak velocity) for the regurgitant valve to the antegrade flow across a competent valve as an indicator of their relative stroke volumes.

Perhaps the most important problem with quantitation of regurgitant severity is the failure of *any* measure (Doppler or angiographic) to provide specific prognostic data or data that affect clinical decision making. Once a diagnosis of "hemodynamically significant" regurgitation is confirmed, it is the patient's symptoms and the left ventricular response to chronic volume overload that dictate medical therapy and the timing of surgical intervention rather than regurgitant severity per se. Given this situation, current Doppler methods remain valuable diagnostic tools mainly because they allow differentiation of mild, moderate, and severe aortic regurgitation. The diagnostic value of the echocardiographic study is increased when the interpretation integrates data from several potential measures of regurgitant severity into a summary statement. Rather than being redundant, the different approaches to regurgitant severity serve as cross-checks on each other. Errors or limitations of one approach will be recognized when other approaches, with better data quality, show discrepant results (Table 11–4). When echocardiographic data are suboptimal, other approaches, such as contrast angiography, should be considered (see Fig. 11–17).

AORTIC REGURGITATION

The echocardiographic approach to the patient with aortic regurgitation includes not only evaluation of the presence of regurgitation but also determination of the etiology and severity of regurgitation along with the effect of the regurgitant lesion on ventricular size and function and any other associated abnormalities (Table 11–5).

Diagnostic Imaging of the Valve Apparatus

Aortic regurgitation may be due either to abnormalities of the aortic root or to abnormalities of the leaflets themselves (Table 11–6). The disease processes that cause valvular aortic stenosis *(congenital bicuspid valve, calcific valve disease,* and *rheumatic disease)* also can result in aortic regurgitation due to alterations in leaflet flexibility or shape leading to inadequate diastolic coaptation of the leaflets. The 2D echocardiographic findings for these diagnoses are discussed in Chapter 10.

Other diseases that cause aortic regurgitation include *myxomatous valve disease,* which can affect the aortic valve as well as the mitral valve. The leaflets are thickened and redundant on 2D echocardiography with slight sagging of the leaflets into the left ventricular outflow tract in diastole (Fig. 11–15). The normal hemicylindrical configuration of each leaflet in diastole is distorted so that the short-axis view intersects the center of the leaflet *en face,* resulting in the

TABLE 11–5	Echocardiographic Approach to Aortic Regurgitation

1. Valve anatomy/etiology of regurgitation
2. Severity of aortic regurgitation
   a. Flow mapping (color or pulsed)
   b. Continuous-wave Doppler
   c. Descending aortic diastolic flow reversal
   d. Volume flow at two sites
3. Left ventricular response
   a. Left ventricular dilation (*end-systolic* dimension)
   b. Left ventricular systolic function
4. Associated abnormalities

TABLE 11–6	Etiology of Aortic Regurgitation (Examples)

Leaflet Abnormalities

Congenital bicuspid valve

Calcific valve disease

Rheumatic valve disease

Myxomatous valve disease

Endocarditis

Nonbacterial thrombotic endocarditis

Aortic Root Abnormalities

Hypertensive aortic root dilation

Cystic medial necrosis

Marfan's syndrome

Aortic dissection

FIGURE 11–15. Parasternal long-axis view in a patient with aortic regurgitation due to bicuspid aortic valve disease with prolapse of the right coronary cusp in diastole resulting in inadequate leaflet coaptation.

false appearance of an ill-defined echogenic "mass."

Endocarditis results in aortic regurgitation either by leaflet perforation due to the infectious process or to deformity of diastolic leaflet closure due to the presence of a valvular vegetation. Less common abnormalities of the aortic valve leaflets leading to aortic regurgitation include congenital leaflet fenestrations, involvement by nonbacterial thrombotic endocarditis (Libman-Sachs vegetations in systemic lupus erythematosus), infiltrative diseases (e.g., amyloid), and collagen-vascular disorders, mucopolysaccharidosis, or glycogen storage diseases. An increased prevalence of mild aortic

regurgitation has been seen in patients taking the anorectic agents fenfluramine or dexfenfluramine.

Abnormalities of the aortic root can result in aortic regurgitation, even when the leaflets themselves are normal, by alterations in the geometry of the structures supporting the leaflets. The aortic annulus is not a discrete planar ring of fibrous tissue but rather a complex crown-shaped structure where the leaflets attach to the aortic valve with the three "points" of the crown at the commissures and the three lowest points at the midsection of each leaflet. Dilation of this area at the base of the aortic root—often termed *annular dilation*—results in aortic regurgitation due to inadequate coaptation of the stretched leaflets. Note that adjacent leaflets normally overlap (apposition zone) so that mild degrees of annular dilation may not result in valvular incompetence. Annular dilation may be due to a variety of causes, including chronic *hypertension, cystic medial necrosis,* or the *Marfan syndrome.* The Marfan syndrome is characterized by effacement of the normal sinotubular junction with dilation of the annulus and sinuses of Valsalva (see Chap. 15). In cystic medial necrosis, the sinotubular junction usually is identifiable, although dilation may involve the base of the root as well as the ascending aorta. Many other diseases cause aortic root dilation, with consequent aortic regurgitation, including rheumatoid arthritis, Reiter's syndrome, syphilitic aortitis, and mycotic aneurysm. Aortic regurgitation due to syphilitic aortitis is rare in the United States. When present, it typically is characterized by extensive calcification of the dilated aortic root. *Aortic dissection* can result in aortic regurgitation either by annular dilation resulting in inadequate coaptation or by the false channel of the dissection undermining the aortic annulus and resulting in a flail leaflet (see Chap. 15).

The *differential diagnosis* for the echocardiographer in evaluation of a patient referred for suspected aortic regurgitation depends on the specific indications for the examination. If a diastolic murmur has been noted on auscultation, differential diagnoses include pulmonic regurgitation, mitral or tricuspid stenosis, and (rarely) a coronary arteriovenous fistula. In some cases, only the diastolic portion of a continuous murmur (e.g., a patent ductus arteriosus) may have been appreciated. If aortic regurgitation is suspected because of a concern for aortic dissection, the differential diagnosis should focus on examination of the ascending aorta.

2D/M-Mode Findings in Aortic Regurgitation (Table 11–7)

In addition to anatomic abnormalities of the aortic valve and the secondary left ventricular dilation that occurs in response to volume overload, several 2D and M-mode echocardiographic findings are seen in patients with aortic regurgitation. If the regurgitant jet impinges on the anterior mitral valve leaflet, it causes impaired leaflet opening, resulting in an increased distance between the maximal anterior motion of the mitral valve in early diastole (the E point) and the most posterior motion of the interventricular septum (e.g., increased E point septal separation). High-frequency fluttering of the anterior mitral valve leaflet resulting from impingement of the regurgitant jet also may be appreciated on M-mode (with its high sampling rate), although it is rarely appreciated on 2D imaging (due to the relatively low frame rate) (Fig. 11–16).

TABLE 11–7	2D and M-Mode Findings in Aortic Regurgitation

Aortic valve and root anatomic abnormalities

Left ventricular dilation and sphericity

Indirect signs of aortic regurgitation
  Increased E-point septal separation
  High-frequency fluttering of the AMVL
  "Reverse doming" of the AMVL
  Jet lesion on septum or AMVL

AMVL = Anterior mitral valve leaflet.

On 2D long- and short-axis imaging, the anterior mitral leaflet may appear curved in diastole with the concavity toward the ventricular septum, with the region of abnormal curvature corresponding to the direction of the regurgitant jet (Fig. 11–17). In short-axis views, a discrete area of reversed curvature corresponding to the spatial location of the regurgitant jet may be seen. This contrasts with the normal linear appearance of the anterior leaflet in diastole in long-axis views and the normal diastolic curvature toward the ventricular septum in the short-axis view. This observation has been termed *reverse doming*, since the curvature of the anterior leaflet is opposite to that seen in rheumatic mitral stenosis.

With chronic regurgitation, the focal blood flow disturbance impinging on the septum or anterior mitral leaflet may result in a raised fibrotic lesion—identifiable by the pathologist postmortem as a jet lesion—which appears as an area of increased echogenicity on 2D imaging.

While none of these indirect signs of aortic regurgitation provides quantitative data, their presence may suggest a previously unsuspected diagnosis and prompt a directed Doppler examination. Recognition of the impact of aortic regurgitation on mitral leaflet motion and the appearance of jet lesions avoids misinterpretation of these findings.

Left Ventricular Response to Aortic Regurgitation

When exposed to chronic volume overload from aortic regurgitation, progressive dilation and increased sphericity of the left ventricle occur (Fig. 11–18). Initially, left ventricular systolic function remains normal. Note that ejec-

FIGURE 11–16. M-mode tracing showing increased E-point–septal separation, and high-frequency fluttering of the anterior mitral leaflet *(arrow)* due to impingement by an aortic regurgitant jet.

FIGURE 11–17. Left ventricular angiogram at end-systole showing severe mitral regurgitation with complete, dense opacification of the left atrium on the first beat.

FIGURE 11–18. Apical four-chamber view showing that geometric changes, specifically increased sphericity, accompany the left ventricular dilation seen with chronic aortic regurgitation.

TABLE 11–8	Chronic versus Acute Aortic Regurgitation	
	Chronic	**Acute**
Etiology (examples)	Bicuspid valve Hypertension	Endocarditis Aortic dissection
Left ventricular size	Dilated	Normal
Left ventricular end-diastolic pressure	Normal	Elevated
Pulse pressure	Wide	Narrow
Continuous-wave Doppler slope	Flat	Steep

tion fraction remains normal (not hypernormal), since the total left ventricular stroke volume is ejected across the aortic valve into the high-impedance systemic vasculature (unlike the situation with chronic mitral regurgitation). With chronic gradually increasing aortic regurgitation, the left ventricle remains compliant in diastole so that end-diastolic pressure remains normal. Typically, left ventricular size slowly increases over a period of years without impairment of systolic function. However, left ventricular systolic dysfunction eventually occurs in the presence of hemodynamically significant chronic volume overload, and in some individuals, irreversible left ventricular systolic dysfunction supervenes even in the absence of clinical symptoms.

In contrast to chronic regurgitation, in acute aortic regurgitation the short interval from onset of volume overload to clinical presentation means that significant left ventricular dilation has not yet occurred. The physiologic differences between acute and chronic aortic regurgitation are reflected both in the 2D echocardiographic findings and in the Doppler examination (Table 11–8).

Evaluation of Aortic Regurgitant Severity (Table 11–9)

Doppler Flow Mapping

Color Doppler flow mapping allows differentiation of mild, moderate, and severe aortic regurgitation. The 3D extent of the regurgitant jet is examined in multiple image planes to assess its length, width, and height. The aortic jet can be imaged in the apical long-axis view and in a four-chamber view angulated anteriorly, providing two nearly orthogonal views. This window is particularly helpful in assessing jet length.

Parasternal views in both long and short axis also are helpful and may allow identification of the exact origin of the regurgitant jet as well as assessment of its width, height, and direction. In fact, a short-axis view of the regurgitant jet immediately adjacent to the aortic valve may be the single most useful image plane. In this view, mild aortic regurgitation fills only a small area of the left ventricular outflow tract, moderate regurgitation fills one-third to two-thirds, and severe regurgitation nearly completely fills the cross-sectional area of the outflow tract area (Figs. 11–19 and 11–20).

Continuous-Wave Doppler

The continuous-wave Doppler spectral recording of aortic regurgitation has its onset at aortic valve closure (during isovolumic relaxation) with a rapid increase in velocity to a maximum of 3 to 5 m/s, followed by a gradual decline in velocity during diastole. The velocity abruptly decelerates during isovolumic contraction, reaching baseline at aortic valve opening. The intensity of the signal, relative to antegrade velocity, is an indicator of regurgitant severity. In moderate or severe regurgitation, the signal can easily be recorded throughout diastole, whereas mild regurgitation may not appear holodiastolic, with a recordable signal only at the beginning or end of diastole. This observation may be due to low signal strength or vari-

TABLE 11-9

Selected Studies Validating Quantitative Evaluation of Regurgitant Severity Using Doppler Echocardiography

First Author/Year	Method	Standard of Reference	N	R Value	SEE
Downstream Flow Reversal					
Boughner/ 1975	Diastolic flow reversal in descending Ao	Angio LV, Fick CO	15 AR patients	0.91 (RF)	—
Touche/1985	Diastolic flow reversal in descending Ao	Angio LV, TD-CO	30 AR patients	0.92 (RF)	8.8%
Volume Flow at Two Sites					
Ascah/1985	Transmitral vs trans-aortic SV	EM flow	30 flow rates in canine model	0.83 (RF)	—
Kitabatake/ 1985	Transaortic vs trans-pulmonic SV	Angio LV, TD-CO	20 AR patients	0.94 (RF)	—
Rokey/1986	Transmitral vs trans-aortic SV	Angio LV, TD-CO	19 MR and 6 AR patients	0.91 (RF)	7%
Continuous-Wave Doppler					
Teague/1986	AR half-time	Angio LV, Fick CO	32 AR patients	−0.88 (RF)	11%
Masuyama/ 1986	AR half-time	Angio LV, ID-CO	20 AR patients	−0.89 (RF)	—
Jenni/1989	CW Doppler Amplitude-weighted velocity	Angio LV, Fick CO	25 MR patients	0.96 (RF)	6.1%
Color Flow Imaging (Regurgitant Jet)					
Spain/1989	Color jet area	Angio LV, TD-CO	15 MR patients	0.62 (RF)	—
Tribouilloy/ 1992	Regurgitant jet width at origin	Angio LV, TD-CO	31 MR patients	0.85 (RSV)	—
Enriquez-Sarano/1993	Color jet area	Doppler SV at two sites	80 MR patients	0.69 (RF)	4.4 cm²
Proximal Acceleration (Color Flow)					
Recusani/1991	PISA (hemispherical)	Rotometer	In vitro, constant flow	0.94-0.99 (flow rate)	1-1.6 L/min
Utsunomiya/ 1991	PISA (hemispherical)	Actual flow rate stopwatch and cylinder	In vitro, pulsatile flow	0.99 (flow rate)	0.53 L/min
Vandervoort/ 1993	PISA	Actual flow rate	In vitro, steady flow	0.98-0.99 (flow rate)	—
Giesler/1993	PISA	LV angio, Fick CO	16 MR patients	0.88 (RSV)	17 ml
Chen/1993	PISA	Doppler SV at two sites	46 MR patients	0.94 (RSV)	18 ml
Jet Momentum					
Cape/1989	Conservation of momentum	EM flow	In vitro, constant flow	0.98	0.18 L/min

Ao = aortic; AR = aortic regurgitation; CO = cardiac output; EM flow = volume flow rate measured by electromagnetic flowmeter; ID = indicator dilation; LV = left ventricle; MR = mitral regurgitation; PISA = proximal isovelocity surface area method; RF = regurgitant fraction; RSV = regurgitant stroke volume; SEE = standard error of the estimate; SV = stroke volume; TD = thermodilution.

Data from Boughher et al: Circ 52:874–879, 1975; Touche et al: Circ 72:819–824, 1985; Ascah et al: Circ 72:377–383, 1985; Kitabatake et al: Circ 72:523–529, 1985; Rokey et al: JACC 7:1273–1278, 1986; Teague et al: JACC 8:592–599, 1986; Masuyama et al: Circ 73:460–466, 1986; Jenni et al: Circ 79:1294–1299, 1989; Spain et al: JACC 13:585–590, 1989; Tribouilloy et al: Circ 85:1248–1253, 1992; Enriquez-Sarano et al: JACC 21:1211–1219, 1993; Rescusani et al: Circ 83:594–604, 1991; Utsunomiya et al: J Am Soc Echo 4:338–348, 1991; Vandervoort et al: JACC 22:535–541, 1993; Giesler et al: AJC 71:217–224, 1993; Chen et al: JACC 21:374–383, 1993; Cape et al: Circ 79:1343–1353, 1989.

FIGURE 11–19. Color Doppler images in parasternal long- axis *(left)* and short-axis *(right)* views in a patient with mild aortic regurgitation. In long axis, a narrow eccentric jet is seen, which in short axis has a small cross-sectional area at the regurgitant orifice relative to the area of the outflow tract. (See Color Plate 9, p. 274.)

ation in jet direction during diastole resulting in significant intercept angle changes.

The shape of the continuous-wave Doppler time-velocity curve depends on the time-varying instantaneous pressure gradient across the valve in diastole, thus reflecting both severity and chronicity of regurgitation. Chronic severe aortic regurgitation results in an increased aortic pulse pressure with a low end-diastolic aortic pressure. The rapid rate of decline in aortic pressure is reflected in a more rapid decline in the Doppler velocity—that is, a steeper diastolic deceleration slope even if end-diastolic left ventricular pressure remains low (Fig. 11–21). This observation led to the suggestion that the diastolic deceleration slope may provide a quantitative measure of aortic regurgitant severity. While this hypothesis is valid to some extent, other factors that affect either left ventricular or aortic diastolic pressure also affect the course of the pressure difference (and velocity) across the regurgitant valve. With *acute* regurgitation, even if only moderate in severity, left ventricular compliance has not yet adapted, as occurs in response to chronic volume overload, so a significant increase in end-diastolic pressure is seen. In extreme cases, aortic and left ventricular end-diastolic pressure may equalize at end-diastole, resulting in a triangular-shaped continuous-wave velocity signal with a linear deceleration slope from maximum velocity to the baseline. Other factors that affect left ventricular diastolic pressure (e.g., systolic dysfunction, ischemia) or aortic diastolic pressure (e.g., sepsis,

patent ductus arteriosus) also will affect the shape of the aortic regurgitant velocity curve.

The continuous-wave signal for aortic regurgitation usually is best recorded from an apical window in order to obtain a parallel intercept angle between the jet and the blood flow direction. Occasionally, an eccentric jet, directed either anteriorly or posteriorly, will be best recorded from a parasternal approach. If signal strength from the suprasternal notch is adequate, a signal similar to that recorded from the apex (but, of course, inverted) is seen.

Holodiastolic Flow Reversal in the Descending Aorta

With severe aortic regurgitation, holodiastolic flow reversal is seen in the proximal abdominal aorta, recorded from the subcostal window (Fig. 11–22). This observation is analogous to the physical examination finding of diastolic reversal in the femoral arteries (DeRosier's sign). Holodiastolic flow reversal in the abdominal aorta is sensitive (100%) and specific (97%) for diagnosing severe aortic regurgitation. False-positive results may be due to the presence of a patent ductus arteriosus, where the diastolic flow is from aorta to pulmonary artery rather than to the left ventricle. More proximal holodiastolic flow reversal, in the descending thoracic aorta, also is sensitive for detection of severe aortic regurgitation but is less specific, also being seen in some subjects with only moderate regurgitation (Fig. 11–23).

Volume Flow at Two Intracardiac Sites

As described above, aortic regurgitant volume and fraction can be calculated as the difference between transaortic and transmitral volume flow (Fig. 11–24). In addition, in the specific case of aortic regurgitation, both forward and total stroke volume can be calculated at a single anatomic site: the proximal descending thoracic aorta. When aortic regurgitation is present, significant systolic expansion of the aorta occurs, so the antegrade flow velocity integral must be multiplied by the systolic cross-sectional area. The flow velocity integral of the reversed flow in diastole is multiplied by diastolic cross-sectional area. Either 2D short-axis imaging or an M-mode through the aortic arch can be used for measurement of systolic and diastolic cross-sectional areas. Note that this quantitative approach is the logical extension of the semiquantitative approach, which relies on the *presence* and spatial extent of holodiastolic flow reversal in the aorta in patients with aortic regurgitation.

Clinical Utility

Diagnostic Utility for Aortic Regurgitation

An echocardiogram may be requested either to confirm or exclude a clinical diagnosis of aortic regurgitation. Given the high sensitivity and specificity of this approach, the resulting

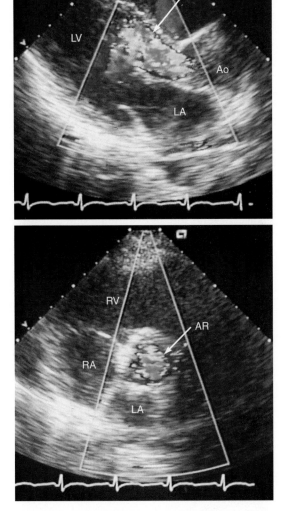

FIGURE 11–20. Color Doppler images in parasternal long- (top) and short-axis (bottom) views in a patient with severe aortic regurgitation. The flow disturbance fills the outflow tract in both views. (See Color Plate 9, p. 274.)

FIGURE 11–21. Continuous-wave Doppler recording in two patients, one with chronic aortic regurgitation (AR) due to calcific aortic valve disease *(above)* and one with acute regurgitation due to aortic dissection *(below)* showing the differences in the deceleration slope in these clinical situations.

FIGURE 11–22. 2D image showing the pulsed Doppler sample volume (SV) position in the descending aorta from a subcostal approach *(above)*. The Doppler velocity curve *(below)* shows holodiastolic flow reversal *(arrows)* consistent with severe aortic regurgitation.

FIGURE 11–23. Recording of flow in the descending thoracic aortic from the suprasternal notch approach *(above)* shows holodiastolic flow reversal *(arrows)*. The systolic flow signal is aliased with the peak velocity appearing at the top of the velocity scale *(open arrow)*.

diagnostic data are highly reliable. In addition, information on the etiology of valve disease, associated conditions, and the degree of left ventricular dilation is obtained.

If aortic regurgitation is detected in the course of an echocardiogram ordered for some other indication, it is incumbent on the echocardiographer to search carefully for the etiology of regurgitation. The finding of regurgita-

MECHANISMS OF MITRAL REGURGITATION

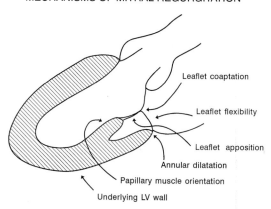

FIGURE 11–24. Schematic diagram illustrating how abnormalities of any part of the complex mitral valve apparatus can result in mitral regurgitation.

tion may be the first clue that aortic root disease or a disease process affecting the aortic leaflets is present.

Timing of Surgical Intervention for Chronic Asymptomatic Aortic Regurgitation

Timing of surgical intervention in the asymptomatic patient is problematic as measures of left ventricular systolic function are dependent on loading conditions, which are altered by the presence of valvular regurgitation. End-systolic volume or dimension provides a relatively load-independent measure of ventricular performance. Several studies examining outcome after valve replacement for aortic regurgitation have shown that a left ventricular end-systolic dimension of less than 55 mm is predictive of preserved (or improved) left ventricular systolic function and an excellent prognosis after valve replacement. While a prospective, randomized trial of surgical intervention in the asymptomatic patient has not been performed, a consensus has developed that surgical intervention is indicated for progressive left ventricular dilation or other evidence of decreased systolic function (see Suggested Reading 17). Annual echocardiography is recommended for evaluation of changes in left ventricle size and systolic function and to optimize the timing of valve replacement in the asymptomatic patient with significant regurgitation. Clearly, end-systolic dimension is not an ideal measure of the left ventricular response to chronic volume overload (since it is afterload-dependent), and continued evaluation of better measures of ventricular contractility is needed. Of note, the relationship between quantitative measures of regurgitant severity (by any diagnostic modality) and clinical outcome has rarely been addressed.

Monitoring the Effect of Medical Therapy

Several recent echocardiographic studies have shown that afterload reduction therapy for patients with chronic asymptomatic aortic regurgitation can prevent progressive left ventricular dilation and hypertrophy. In a randomized trial of nifedipine versus digoxin, afterload reduction reduced the rate of progression to symptoms or left ventricular systolic dysfunction. Thus, echocardiography now is a standard approach to evaluation of the effect of afterload reduction on ventricular dimensions, mass, and systolic function in patients with chronic aortic regurgitation.

In sequential studies, the accuracy of detecting a change in left ventricular dimension is greatest when similar examination techniques are used and when the studies are compared "side by side." With slow disease progression, similar directional changes on serial studies at several time points are more reliable than a single interval change.

Alternate Approaches

Alternate approaches to follow-up in patients with chronic aortic regurgitation include resting and exercise radionuclide ventriculography, magnetic resonance imaging, and cardiac catheterization.

MITRAL REGURGITATION

Diagnostic Imaging of the Mitral Valve Apparatus (Table 11–10)

Functionally, the mitral valve apparatus has several components: the left atrial wall, the mitral annulus, the anterior and posterior leaflets, the chordae, the papillary muscles, and the left ventricular myocardium underlying the papillary muscles. Dysfunction or altered anatomy of any one of these components can result in mitral regurgitation (see Fig. 11–24).

Mitral annular dilation may be due to either left atrial or left ventricular dilation and results in mitral regurgitation because of incomplete leaflet coaptation. The normal mitral apparatus is a saddle-shaped ellipse with its most apical points seen in the apical four-chamber view and its most basal points seen in the long-axis view. As noted for the aortic valve, the mitral leaflets have a normal area of overlap (or apposition) so that some degree of mitral annular dilation may be tolerated without significant regurgitation.

The mitral annulus area normally is smaller in systole than in diastole. Increased rigidity of the annulus, as seen with *mitral annular calcification,* impairs systolic contraction of the annulus leading to mitral regurgitation. Mitral annular calcification has a typical appearance on 2D imaging as an area of increased echogenicity on the left ventricular side of the annulus immediately adjacent to the attachment point of the posterior leaflet (Fig. 11–25).

TABLE 11–10	Etiology and Presumed Mechanisms of Mitral Regurgitation
Etiology	**Presumed Mechanism**
Annular dilation	Inadequate leaflet coaptation
Mitral annular calcification	Increased rigidity of annulus impairing systolic contraction
Myxomatous mitral valve disease	Inadequate coaptation and apposition, flail segments
Rheumatic mitral valve disease	Increased rigidity of leaflets
Endocarditis	Leaflet perforation or deformity
Marfan's syndrome	Anterior leaflet redundancy
Age-related degenerative leaflet changes	Abnormal coaptation
Hypertrophic cardiomyopathy	Abnormal leaflet motion and anatomy
Chordae disruption or elongation	Inadequate systolic support of leaflet
Regional left ventricular dysfunction	Inadequate systolic support of leaflets
Left ventricular dilation	Abnormal papillary muscle orientation
Papillary muscle rupture	Inadequate systolic support of leaflets

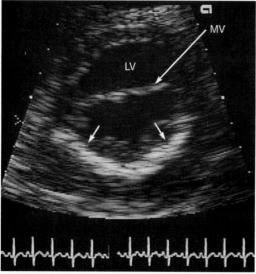

FIGURE 11–25. 2D parasternal long-axis *(top)* and short-axis *(bottom)* views of mitral annular calcification *(arrows)*. Mv = mitral valve leaflet.

Acoustic shadowing, due to the presence of calcium, is seen. In short-axis views, the annular calcium may be focal or extensive, involving the entire U-shaped posterior annulus. The region of anterior mitral leaflet–aortic root continuity is involved only rarely. Mitral annular calcification is commonly seen as an incidental finding in elderly subjects. "Premature" annular calcification is seen in patients with renal failure or hypertension.

Diseases of the mitral valve leaflets include myxomatous disease, rheumatic disease, endocarditis, Marfan's syndrome, and rare disorders such as infiltrative diseases (amyloid, sarcoid, mucopolysaccharidosis) and collagen-vascular disorders (systemic lupus erythematosus, rheu-

matoid arthritis). *Myxomatous* mitral valve disease is characterized by thickened, redundant leaflets and chordae with sagging of portions of the leaflets into the left atrium in systole (Figs. 11–26 and 11–27). The severity of disease is variable, ranging from mitral valve prolapse, in which there is only minimal displacement of the leaflets into the left atrium in systole, to severe involvement of both leaflets by myxomatous disease with frankly prolapsed or flail leaflet segments.

Rheumatic mitral regurgitation, like rheumatic mitral stenosis, is characterized by some degree of commissural fusion and thickening of the leaflet tips. *Endocarditis* results in mitral regurgitation by leaflet destruction, perforation, or deformity. *Marfan's syndrome* is associated with a long redundant anterior leaflet that sags into the left atrium in systole. Infiltrative diseases result in irregular leaflet thickening and inadequate coaptation. Of note, *age-related degenerative changes* in the mitral leaflets often are seen (with or without associated mitral annular calcification) and appear as irregular areas of thickening and increased echogenicity of the mitral leaflets. Obviously, while some conditions with unique anatomic features can be reliably diagnosed by 2D imaging (rheumatic or myxomatous disease), there is considerable overlap in the anatomic features of other conditions (degenerative versus infiltrative leaflet abnormalities). In these cases, the echocardiographer can describe the valve anatomy and indicate the possible etiologies of the findings even though the specific tissue diagnosis remains unknown.

Abnormalities of leaflet motion also can result in mitral regurgitation. The best known example of this phenomenon is *hypertrophic cardiomyopathy.* As the anterior leaflet obstructs the left ventricular outflow tract in systole, coaptation of the anterior and posterior leaflets is disrupted, resulting in a posteriorly directed mitral regurgitant jet. In addition, mitral valve anatomy is abnormal in patients with hypertrophic cardiomyopathy (see Chap. 8).

Chordal disruption or elongation leads to mitral regurgitation because of inadequate tensile support of the closed leaflets in systole. Chordal elongation results in severe bowing of the leaflet, or leaflet segment, into the left atrium, with the tip of the leaflet still directed toward the ventricular apex. With chordal rupture, there is a flail segment of the leaflet such that the leaflet is displaced into the left atrium in systole, with the tip of the leaflet pointing away from the ventricular apex.

Regional left ventricular dysfunction with abnormal contraction of either papillary muscle or the underlying ventricular wall results in mitral regurgitation, presumably due to inadequate support of the closed leaflets in systole. *Abnormal orientation of the papillary muscles,* as seen with dilated cardiomyopathy, also results in mitral regurgitation. Other etiologies of abnormal papillary muscle function or orientation include coronary artery disease, chronic volume overload leading to left ventricular dilation, and systolic dysfunction secondary to other conditions.

Papillary muscle rupture can occur as a complication of acute myocardial infarction. If the entire papillary muscle is disconnected from the underlying left ventricular wall, few patients survive due to acute severe mitral regurgitation. Echocardiographic evaluation in those who do survive shows a mass (the ruptured papillary muscle) attached to flail segments of anterior and posterior leaflets (since each papillary muscle attaches to both leaflets). The ruptured papillary muscle head is seen in the left atrium in systole and in the left ventricle in diastole. Severe mitral regurgitation is present on Doppler examination. Partial rupture of a papillary muscle, defined as rupture of one of several "heads" or as partial disconnection of the base of the papillary muscle, is seen more often than complete rupture as patients are more likely to survive long enough to undergo diagnostic evaluation. In this situation, the echocardiogram shows a thin, attenuated, excessively mobile papillary muscle and, if one head has ruptured, a mass attached to the leaflet with prolapse into the left atrium in systole (see Fig. 7–24).

FIGURE 11–26. Parasternal long-axis *(top)* and M-mode recording *(bottom)* in a young woman with mitral valve prolapse. Posterior leaflet prolapse is seen both on 2D imaging and on M-mode *(arrows)*.

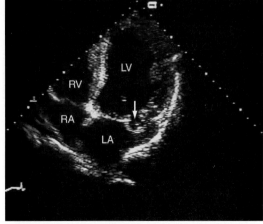

FIGURE 11–27. Diastolic and systolic apical four-chamber views in a patient with myxomatous mitral valve disease and severe prolapse of the posterior leaflet *(arrow)*.

Response of the Left Ventricle, Left Atrium, and Pulmonary Vasculature to Mitral Regurgitation (Table 11–11)

When mitral regurgitation is present, the left ventricle ejects blood both forward into the aorta against systemic vascular resistance and backward into the low-resistance left atrium. Since the left ventricle effectively pumps against a low afterload early in the disease course, the increase in left ventricular stroke volume is achieved mainly by more complete left ventricular emptying (an increased ejection fraction) rather than by left ventricular dilation. Thus the left ventricle is expected to appear hyperdynamic on 2D imaging when mitral regurgitation is present.

With chronic regurgitation, progressive left ventricular dilation eventually occurs as the regurgitant volume (and thus total left ventricular stroke volume) increases. As with aortic regurgitation, an irreversible decline in left ventricular contractility can occur in the absence of symptoms. Given the low left ventricular afterload, apparent "normal" left ventricular systolic function, as assessed qualitatively by 2D imaging or by quantitative ejection fraction measurement, raises the possibility of impaired contractility.

With chronic mitral regurgitation, the left atrium gradually dilates to accommodate the regurgitant volume while maintaining a normal left atrial pressure. Left atrial compliance increases, that is, the left atrial pressure-volume relationship is shifted downward and to the right. With acute mitral regurgitation, the regurgitant volume is delivered into a small, noncompliant left atrium, resulting in a significant increase in left atrial pressure and a *v wave* in the left atrial pressure curve.

TABLE 11–11	Echocardiographic Approach to Mitral Regurgitation

1. Mitral valve apparatus anatomy, etiology of regurgitation
2. Severity of mitral regurgitation
   a. Flow mapping
   b. Continuous-wave Doppler
   c. Pulmonary vein systolic flow reversal
   d. Volume flow at two sites
3. Left atrial dilation
4. Left ventricle
   a. Dilation (*end-systolic* dimension)
   b. Systolic function
5. Pulmonary artery pressures

Pulmonary artery pressure rises passively in response to both the chronic mildly elevated left atrial pressure seen with chronic mitral regurgitation and the acute severe elevation seen with acute regurgitation. When left atrial pressure is chronically elevated, pulmonary vascular resistance may increase. Echocardiographic evaluation of the patient with mitral regurgitation includes noninvasive measurement of pulmonary artery pressure from the tricuspid regurgitant jet velocity and an estimate of right atrial pressure.

Other 2D/M-Mode Findings in Mitral Regurgitation

The anteroposterior motion of the aortic root, as seen on M-mode recordings, reflects left atrial emptying and filling. The left atrium lies between the rigid spinal column posteriorly and the aortic root anteriorly so that an increase in left atrial volume displaces the aortic root anteriorly, while a decrease in left atrial volume allows the aortic root to move posteriorly. Since mitral regurgitation results in increased left atrial volume in systole (due to the regurgitant volume) followed by an abrupt decrease in left atrial volume in diastole (due to the elevated transmitral stroke volume), an increase in aortic root motion is seen on the M-mode recording (Fig. 11–28).

Evaluation of Mitral Regurgitant Severity

Doppler Flow Mapping

Flow mapping of the mitral regurgitant jet is performed with color flow Doppler in several tomographic planes in order to build a mental 3D reconstruction of the extent of the flow disturbance. Based on this evaluation, regurgitation is graded on an 0 to 4+ scale, where 1+ is mild, 2 to 3+ is moderate, and 4+ is severe regurgitation. Apical four-chamber and long-axis views are useful because they are nearly orthogonal to each other, but signal attenuation at the depth of the left atrium may limit their utility if ultrasound penetration is suboptimal. Parasternal long- and short-axis views can be used for flow mapping and may allow identification of the anatomic origin of the regurgitant jet. Imaging of the size of the regurgitant orifice, or the width of the narrowest segment of the jet (the *vena contracta*) also is useful in assessing regurgitant severity.

The shape and direction of the mitral regurgitant jet depend on the regurgitant orifice geometry and thus the etiology of mitral regurgitation. Abnormalities of the posterior leaflet tend to result in an anteriorly directed jet (Fig. 11–29), while anterior leaflet or papillary muscle dysfunction tend to result in a posteriorly directed jet (Fig. 11–30). Dilation of the left ventricle or mitral annulus results in a central, symmetric regurgitant jet (Fig. 11–31).

When evaluation of mitral valve anatomy or the severity of regurgitation is suboptimal from a transthoracic approach, transesophageal imaging may be helpful. Since the transducer frequency, depth of interrogation, and signal strength are quite different for these two approaches, the influence of these factors on the appearance of the regurgitant jet must be considered in the overall evaluation of regurgitation severity (see Chap. 1).

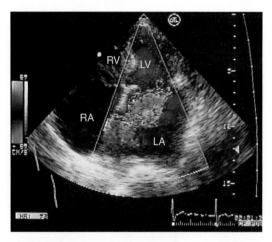

FIGURE 11–29. Color Doppler images in the apical four-chamber view in moderate mitral regurgitation due to myxomatous disease with an anteriorly directed jet. (See Color Plate 10, p. 274.)

FIGURE 11–28. M-mode of increased aortic root motion *(above)*, the mitral valve *(center)* with late-systolic prolapse *(arrow)*, and the hyperdynamic left ventricle *(below)* in a patient with severe mitral regurgitation due to myxomatous mitral valve disease.

FIGURE 11–30. A posteriorly directed mitral regurgitant jet due to papillary muscle dysfunction seen in an apical long-axis view. (See Color Plate 10, p. 274.)

Pulmonary Vein Flow Reversal

As the mitral regurgitant jet enters the left atrium, it necessarily displaces blood that was already in the chamber. When severe regurgitation is present, systolic flow reversal in the pulmonary veins is seen. False-negative results occur when the left atrium is severely enlarged and compliant so that all the excess volume is contained in the left atrium without displacement into the pulmonary veins. False-positive results occur when an eccentric jet is directed into a pulmonary vein, causing flow reversal even when regurgitation is not severe.

Continuous-Wave Doppler Evaluation

The continuous-wave Doppler spectral recording of mitral regurgitation shows a rapid

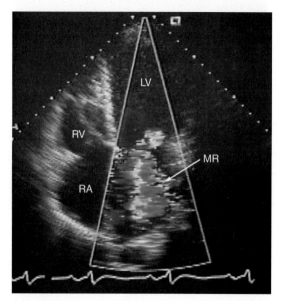

FIGURE 11–31. In an apical four-chamber view, a central mitral regurgitant jet due to dilated cardiomyopathy is seen. (See Color Plate 10, p. 274.)

rise in velocity during isovolumic contraction (proportional to the rate of rise in left ventricular pressure or dP/dt) from baseline to a maximum velocity of 5 to 6 m/s. The velocity stays high throughout systole with a curve paralleling the rise and fall of left ventricular pressure given a normal left atrial pressure. During isovolumic relaxation, the velocity rapidly returns to baseline.

With acute mitral regurgitation (Table 11–12), a rise in left atrial pressure during late systole—a *v wave*—may be present due to a steep pressure-volume relationship of the nondilated left atrium. In this situation, the pressure gradient between the left ventricle and the left atrium is high initially but then begins to equalize in late systole as left atrial pressure rises. The corresponding Doppler velocity curve shows a high initial velocity with a more rapid fall in velocity in mid- to late systole. This pattern of Doppler velocities also is termed a *v wave* (Figs. 11–8 and 11–32).

Signal intensity of the mitral regurgitant signal, in comparison with antegrade flow, is related to mitral regurgitation severity. In addition, significant regurgitation is associated with an increase in the antegrade velocity due to increased transmitral volume flow.

Volume Flow at Two Intracardiac Sites

Mitral regurgitant stroke volume can be calculated from transmitral stroke volume (SV) (total left ventricular stroke volume) and transaortic stroke volume (forward stroke volume) as (Fig. 11–33):

$$\text{Mitral regurgitant SV} = \text{Transmitral SV} - \text{Transaortic SV}$$

Alternate sites for measurement of forward stroke volume are the tricuspid valve and the pulmonary artery.

TABLE 11–12	Chronic Versus Acute Mitral Regurgitation	
	Chronic	**Acute**
Etiology (examples)	Myxomatous valve disease Annular dilation	Endocarditis Papillary muscle rupture Chordal rupture
Left ventricular size	Dilated	Normal
Left ventricular systolic function	Hyperdynamic early; may be normal or depressed with long-standing disease	Hyperdynamic
Left atrial size	Enlarged	Normal
Continuous-wave Doppler curve	High velocity throughout systole	Late systolic velocity decline (*v* wave)

FIGURE 11–32. Continuous-wave Doppler recordings in a patient with chronic mitral regurgitation *(above)* and a patient with more acute regurgitation *(below)* showing a *v* wave *(arrows)*.

FIGURE 11–33. Quantitative evaluation of mitral regurgitant severity by calculation of transmitral and transaortic volume flow rates. Mitral annulus diameter and the velocity-time integral (VTI) of flow across the mitral annulus are used to calculate total stroke volume. Forward stroke volume is determined from the cross-sectional area and velocity-time integral of left ventricular outflow tract flow.

Clinical Utility

Diagnosis and Severity of Mitral Regurgitation

Determination of the etiology of mitral regurgitation using 2D imaging often has important clinical implications. Evaluation of regurgitant severity also is of clinical importance, although a high degree of sophistication in echocardiographic interpretation is needed for this application. In assessing the severity of regurgitation, the echocardiographer should first describe the individual findings and then integrate these findings into a consistent overall interpretation. In addition, the degree of pulmonary hypertension, left atrial size, left ventricular size and systolic function, and any associated abnormalities are added to the

Doppler findings before arriving at a final interpretation.

Examples of clinical situations in which decisions can be based on echocardiographic and Doppler data include acute mitral regurgitation after myocardial infarction, mitral valve endocarditis, and chronic mitral regurgitation due to myxomatous mitral valve disease. The decision whether or not to perform valve surgery (repair or replacement) usually can be made based on clinical and echocardiographic data without invasive studies in these patient groups. Only in cases where there is a discrepancy between the clinical impression and the echocardiographic findings (or when coronary angiography is indicated) are further diagnostic tests warranted.

Mitral Valve "Prolapse" Versus Myxomatous Mitral Valve Disease

Myxomatous mitral valve disease is a pathologic condition characterized histologically by increased mucopolysaccharides, thickening, and disarray of the mitral valve leaflet. Grossly, the leaflets and chordae are thick and redundant but with reduced tensile strength so that they are prone to progressive elongation or rupture. Two-dimensional imaging demonstrates thick, redundant leaflets and chordae with systolic displacement of the leaflets into the left atrium in systole. Over time, a partial flail leaflet due to chordal rupture may develop. Patients with this disease have a high incidence of significant mitral regurgitation and often go on to require mitral valve surgery. Patients with myxomatous mitral valve disease also may have aortic or tricuspid valve involvement.

In contrast, patients with the mitral valve prolapse syndrome typically have a more benign long-term outcome, even though it is likely that this condition represents one end of the spectrum that includes myxomatous mitral valve disease. In order to avoid a false-positive diagnosis of mitral valve prolapse, strict echocardiographic criteria must be used. For example, in an apical four-chamber view, the closure plane of the mitral leaflets may appear "flat" relative to the mitral annulus even in subjects with normal valve leaflets since the most apical points of the saddle-shaped annulus are seen in this view. In addition, normal leaflet closure may appear displaced to the atrial side of the annulus if image planes are oblique relative to the annular plane. Displacement of the leaflets into the left atrium in systole is most reliably assessed in parasternal and apical long-axis views. In addition, it is helpful to describe valve anatomy (leaflet size, thickness, redundancy, chordal involvement) as well as the pattern of valve motion. The clinician then can interpret these findings in conjunction with the patient's symptoms and physical findings. While a few echocardiographic findings are independently diagnostic of mitral valve prolapse, others only support the diagnosis in the appropriate clinical setting. Yet other findings simply represent the range of normal variation in mitral valve anatomy and dynamics (Table 11–13).

Follow-up of Chronic Asymptomatic Mitral Regurgitation

Sequential echocardiographic studies can be used to follow asymptomatic patients with mitral regurgitation. While mitral regurgitation

TABLE 11–13	Guidelines for the Clinical Diagnosis of Mitral Valve Prolapse

Major Criteria*

Auscultation

Mid- to late systolic clicks and late systolic murmur or whoop alone or in combination at the cardiac apex

2D Echocardiogram

Marked superior systolic displacement of mitral leaflets with coaptation point at or superior to annular plane

Mild to moderate superior systolic displacement of mitral leaflets with

    Chordal rupture or

    Doppler mitral regurgitation or

    Annular dilatation

Echocardiogram plus Auscultation

Mild to moderate superior systolic displacement of mitral leaflets with

    Prominent mid- to late systolic clicks at the cardiac apex or

    Apical late systolic or holosystolic murmur in the young or

    Late systolic "whoop"

Minor Criteria*

Auscultation

Loud first heart sound with an apical holosystolic murmur

2D Echocardiogram

Isolated mild to moderate superior systolic displacement of the posterior mitral leaflet

Moderate superior systolic displacement of both mitral leaflets

Echocardiogram plus History

Mild to moderate superior systolic displacement of mitral leaflets with

    Focal neurologic attacks or amaurosis fugax in the young or

    First-degree relatives with major criteria

---

*Major criteria establish the diagnosis. Minor criteria are supportive but not diagnostic.

Reprinted with permission from Perloff JK, Child JS, Edwards JE: New guidelines for the clinical diagnosis of mitral valve prolapse. Am J Cardiol 57:1124–1129, 1986.

severity and mitral valve anatomy are important data, the most important factor in patient evaluation is left ventricular size and systolic function. Current data suggest that evidence of progressive ventricular dilation, an end-systolic dimension ≥ 45 mm, or any reduction in left ventricular systolic function should prompt consideration of surgical intervention regardless of the symptomatic status of the patient to prevent irreversible ventricular dysfunction postoperatively. (See Suggested Reading 17.)

Decision Making Concerning Mitral Valve Repair or Replacement

Once the decision has been made that surgical intervention is needed, the echocardiographic images are invaluable in considering whether mitral valve repair or reconstruction is possible. The study should be reviewed with the surgeon, focusing on the exact etiology of mitral regurgitation, the degree of annular dilation, the relative involvement of anterior and posterior leaflets, the chordal and papillary muscle structural integrity, and overall ventricular size and systolic function. Typically, posterior leaflet prolapse and annular dilation are most amenable to repair, while more complex or extensive disease requires more complex procedures with a lower likelihood of successful repair.

Intraoperative Evaluation of Mitral Valve Repair

In the patient undergoing surgical mitral valve repair, transesophageal echocardiography is used to assess results after the procedure. Baseline transesophageal images are obtained in the operating room to reconfirm regurgitant severity under the loading conditions of general anesthesia and to serve as a baseline for comparison to the postrepair echocardiogram. After valve repair, the patient is weaned from cardiopulmonary bypass, and valve anatomy and mitral regurgitant severity are reassessed. Preferably, regurgitant severity is evaluated under physiologic loading conditions with similar hemodynamics to those recorded during the baseline study (Fig. 11–34). If significant residual mitral regurgitation is present, a second bypass pump run may be done as part of the same procedure to allow a second attempt at repair or mitral valve replacement. Other complications of the valve repair also may be identified, including dynamic left ventricular outflow tract obstruction (Figs. 11–35 and 11–36), functional mitral stenosis, and worsening of left ventricular systolic dysfunction.

TRICUSPID REGURGITATION

Diagnostic Imaging of the Tricuspid Valve Apparatus

Tricuspid regurgitation occurs with abnormalities of the supporting structures (annulus, right ventricle) or the leaflets themselves. Tricuspid regurgitation secondary to *annular dilation* often is due either to primary right ventricular dilation and systolic dysfunction or to *pulmonary hypertension.* Left-sided heart disease leading to pulmonary hypertension—specially mitral stenosis or regurgitation—often results in significant tricuspid regurgitation, presumably on the basis of right ventricular dilation and systolic dysfunction.

Abnormalities of the tricuspid valve leaflets also are a cause of tricuspid regurgitation. *Rheumatic disease* involves the tricuspid valve in about 20% to 30% of cases, nearly always occurring in conjunction with mitral and aortic valve involvement as well. Rheumatic tricuspid disease typically is mild and may be difficult to appreciate on 2D echocardiography unless careful attention is directed toward imaging the valve leaflets and searching for evidence of commissural fusion. Rheumatic tricuspid regurgitation is more common than rheumatic tricuspid stenosis.

Carcinoid heart disease is a rare condition, but the echocardiographic findings are pathognomonic. Carcinoid heart disease (seen with metastatic carcinoid tumor to the liver) is characterized by thickened, shortened, and immobile tricuspid valve leaflets with resultant tricuspid regurgitation or, less often, tricuspid valve stenosis. The pulmonic valve also may be involved. *Endocarditis* may involve the tricuspid valve, resulting in tricuspid regurgitation, and is most common in patients with a history of intravenous drug abuse.

Ebstein's anomaly of the tricuspid valve is a congenital abnormality in which one or more leaflets of the tricuspid valve are displaced from the tricuspid annulus toward the ventricular apex (see Figs. 16–8 and 16–9). Most often, the septal leaflet is involved, either in isolation or in association with apical displacement of posterior and anterior leaflets. The degree of apical displacement is extremely variable. While the normal tricuspid valve insertion plane is slightly more apical than the mitral valve attachment plane, Ebstein's anomaly should be considered when the separation between mitral and tricuspid valve planes is greater than 11 mm. The portion of the right ventricle excluded from the pumping chamber is said to be *atrialized*, since it effectively functions as part of the right atrium. The right atrium may appear severely enlarged due to "atrialization" of the base of the ventricle *plus* dilatation of the atrium due to tricuspid regurgitation. Right ventricular enlargement is seen as well if significant tricuspid regurgitation is present.

FIGURE 11–34. 2D *(left)* and color Doppler *(right)* intraoperative transesophageal images in a patient with myxomatous mitral valve disease before *(above)* and after *(below)* mitral valve repair. Before repair, severe mitral prolapse with a partial flail leaflet segment and moderate to severe mitral regurgitation are present. After repair, only minimal regurgitation is detected at similar loading conditions. A mitral annuloplasty ring *(arrows)* is seen. (See Color Plate 10, p. 274.)

Right Ventricular and Right Atrial Dilation

Hemodynamically significant tricuspid regurgitation results in progressive right ventricular and right atrial enlargement due to volume overload. This dilation may complicate assessment of the etiology of regurgitation because the dilation itself may further increase regurgitant severity.

Right ventricular volume overload is associated with a pattern of abnormal septal motion characterized on M-mode recording by posterior motion of the septum in diastole (since right ventricular filling exceeds left ventricular filling) and anterior motion of the septum in systole, often referred to as *paradoxical septal motion*. On 2D short-axis imaging, the ventricular septum appears "flattened" in diastole as the increased transtricuspid stroke volume fills the right ventricle. In systole, the ventricular septum moves toward the center of gravity of the heart (normally toward the middle of the left ventricle), which is the midline of the right ventricle if severe right ventricular dilation is present.

The differential diagnosis of 2D findings of right ventricular dilation and paradoxical septal motion includes other causes of right ventricular volume overload such as an atrial septal defect, partial anomalous pulmonary venous return, pressure overload due to pulmonic valve disease, or pulmonary hypertension either due to left-sided heart disease or intrinsic lung disease.

Evaluation of Tricuspid Regurgitation Severity

Tricuspid regurgitation can be evaluated with Doppler flow mapping in a manner similar to that described for mitral regurgitation. Mild regurgitation is characterized by a flow disturbance in systole localized to the area adjacent to the valve closure plane (less than a third of the atrial area). Moderate regurgitation fills between one-third and two-thirds of the

right atrium, while severe regurgitation fills more than two-thirds of an enlarged right atrium (Figs. 11–37 and 11–38). Multiple views are needed to fully "map" the flow disturbance because the 3D anatomy of the jet may be asymmetric. Useful views include the right ventricular inflow view, the apical four-chamber view, and the subcostal four-chamber view. Mild to moderate tricuspid regurgitation often is directed along the interatrial septum and must be distinguished from normal caval inflow or from atrial septal defect flow.

Severe tricuspid regurgitation results in systolic flow reversal in the inferior and superior vena cava, analogous to the physical finding of a systolic pulsation in the neck veins. Inferior

FIGURE 11–35. Dynamic left ventricular outflow tract obstruction seen on intraoperative transesophageal imaging immediately after mitral valve repair. The anterior leaflet demonstrates systolic anterior motion (SAM, *arrow*), while a guided continuous-wave Doppler recording (despite a possibly nonparallel intercept angle) shows high-velocity flow across this region that was confirmed by direct manometric measurement of left ventricular and aortic pressures.

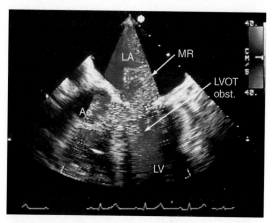

FIGURE 11–36. Color flow imaging in the same patient as in Figure 11–35 shows systolic turbulence in the left ventricular outflow tract distal to the obstruction and persistent severe mitral regurgitation due to the systolic anterior motion of the mitral leaflet. (See Color Plate 11, p. 274.)

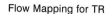

FIGURE 11–37. Schematic diagram of flow mapping for semiquantitative evaluation of tricuspid regurgitant severity. Severe (4+) tricuspid regurgitation is associated with systolic reversal in the hepatic veins.

vena caval flow is best recorded in the central hepatic vein, which provides a flow channel parallel to the ultrasound beam from a subcostal approach and has no venous valves between the recording site and the right atrium.

The absolute value of the maximum velocity in the tricuspid regurgitant continuous-wave Doppler spectral recording reflects the maximum pressure difference across the tricuspid valve and *not* the severity of regurgitation. Severe regurgitation with a normal right ventricular systolic pressure (as seen with tricuspid valve endocarditis) has a low maximum velocity. Mild tricuspid regurgitation in the presence of pulmonary hypertension (as seen with primary pulmonary hypertension) has a high maximum velocity. However, the intensity of the continuous-wave signals relative to the antegrade flow signal intensity does relate to regurgitant severity. In addition, the shape of the velocity-time curve indicates the time course of the instantaneous pressure differences across the valve (Fig. 11–39). A right atrial *v* wave seen in acute regurgitation results in a more rapid decline in velocity in late systole similar to that seen in acute mitral regurgitation.

Clinical Utility

Evaluation of tricuspid regurgitation by Doppler echocardiography is the standard clinical approach to this problem. Even cardiac catheterization is of limited value, since the catheter placed across the tricuspid valve to perform the right ventricular angiogram may itself induce regurgitation.

FIGURE 11–38. Color flow imaging in parasternal right ventricular inflow *(top)* and apical four-chamber *(bottom)* views in a patient with moderate tricuspid regurgitation (TR). (See Color Plate 11, p. 274.)

FIGURE 11–39. Continuous-wave Doppler recording of tricuspid regurgitation in a patient with chronic *(above)* and acute *(below)* tricuspid regurgitation. Note the late systolic velocity decline (*v* wave) in the acute case *(arrow)*.

Evaluation of tricuspid regurgitant severity is particularly important in the patient undergoing mitral valve surgery. Many of these patients have significant coexisting tricuspid regurgitation, and many of the clinical symptoms will persist postoperatively if this condition is not recognized and treated (with tricuspid annuloplasty) at the time of surgery.

In patients undergoing tricuspid valve repair or surgery for endocarditis, intraoperative transesophageal echocardiography can be used to optimize the surgical approach and assess the functional consequences of the repair procedure.

PULMONIC REGURGITATION

Pulmonic regurgitation most often is an incidental benign finding, with a small amount of diastolic backflow across the pulmonic valve seen in most normal individuals (Fig. 11–40). Pathologic pulmonic regurgitation usually is a result of congenital pulmonic valve disease, either untreated mild disease or residual regurgitation after pulmonic valve surgery. Acquired pulmonic regurgitation is rare, being due to endocarditis, carcinoid syndrome, or myxomatous valve disease.

Evaluation of pulmonic valve anatomy may be limited in adult patients by poor acoustic access. With congenital disease, thickened, deformed leaflets are seen. In endocarditis, a valvular vegetation may be identified, although the pulmonic valve is involved least often. Carcinoid syndrome results in shortening and thickening of the pulmonic valve leaflet, similar to the involvement of the tricuspid valve, and may lead to stenosis and/or regurgitation. Myxomatous valve disease is rare, resulting in thickening, redundancy, and systemic sagging of the pulmonic valve leaflets.

Pulmonic regurgitation is diagnosed by documenting a diastolic flow disturbance in the right ventricular outflow tract with conventional pulsed or color Doppler flow imaging. The extent of the flow disturbance provides a semiquantitative index of pulmonic regurgitant severity. The intensity and shape of the continuous-wave Doppler velocity-time spectral output also provide an indication of regurgitant severity, analogous to the findings in aortic regurgitation. Holodiastolic flow reversal may be noted in the main pulmonary artery when significant regurgitation is present and must be distinguished from diastolic flow reversal due to a patent ductus arteriosus.

In adults, evaluation of pulmonic regurgitation is of most importance in patients with un-

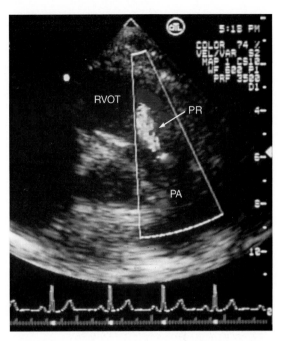

FIGURE 11–40. Color flow imaging in a right ventricular outflow view showing a small amount of pulmonic regurgitation. (See Color Plate 11, p. 274.)

corrected or residual congenital heart disease. In these patients, the severity of pulmonic regurgitation may be a factor in deciding whether to perform further surgical procedures and in the specific design of the surgical procedure.

When pulmonic regurgitation is present, even if only mild in degree, the velocity in the pulmonic regurgitant curve reflects the pulmonary artery to right ventricular diastolic pressure difference. The instantaneous end-diastolic pulmonary artery to right ventricular gradient (calculated as $4v^2$) can be added to an estimate of right ventricular diastolic pressure (from inferior vena cava size and respiratory variation) to provide an estimate of diastolic pulmonary artery pressure. This approach to estimation of pulmonary artery pressure complements systolic pressure estimation from the tricuspid regurgitant jet and serves as an internal validity check when both can be recorded accurately.

SUGGESTED READING

Basic Principles and Quantitative Approaches

1. Perloff JK, Roberts WC: The mitral apparatus: Functional anatomy of mitral regurgitation. *Circulation* 46:227–239, 1972.

  Classic detailed description of the anatomy of the mitral valve apparatus with correlations between the valve anatomy and the mechanism of mitral regurgitation for differing etiologies of mitral valve disease.

2. Vandervoort PM, Thomas JD: New approaches to quantitation of valvular regurgitation. *In* Otto CM (ed): The Practice of Clinical Echocardiography. Philadelphia, WB Saunders, 1997, pp. 307–326.
   Review of newer approaches to quantitation of valvular regurgitation including the proximal isovelocity surface area approach and vena contracta imaging.

3. Rokey R, Sterling LL, Zoghbi WA, et al: Determination of regurgitant fraction in isolated mitral or aortic regurgitation by pulsed Doppler two-dimensional echocardiography. *J Am Coll Cardiol* 7:1273–1278, 1986.
   Calculation of regurgitant volume and regurgitant fraction by Doppler at two intracardiac sites (mitral and aortic) was compared with invasive determinations in 25 patients (r = 0.91, SEE = 7%).

4. Recusani F, Bargiggia GS, Yoganathan AP, et al: A new method for quantification of regurgitant flow rate using color Doppler flow imaging of the flow convergence region proximal to a discrete orifice: An in vitro study. *Circulation* 83:594–604, 1991.
   The proximal isovelocity surface area method was used to calculate volume flow rate and then combined with continuous-wave Doppler data to calculate orifice areas in an in vitro study (r = 0.75–0.96).

5. Utsunomiya T, Ogawa T, Doshi R, et al: Doppler color flow "proximal isovelocity surface area" method for estimating volume flow rate: Effects of orifice shape and machine factors. *J Am Coll Cardiol* 17:1103–1111, 1991.
   The proximal isovelocity surface area method is applicable to noncircular orifices and is insensitive to changes in ultrasound system colorflow settings, including gain, wall filters, frame rate, transmit power, packet size, and aliasing velocity.

6. Reimold SC, Ganz P, Bittl JA, et al: Effective aortic regurgitant orifice area: Description of a method based on the conservation of mass. *J Am Coll Cardiol* 18:761–768, 1991.
   Description of a method for calculating regurgitant orifice area based on the continuity equation using a Doppler catheter system (for regurgitant volume flow measurement) and continuous-wave Doppler recordings of the regurgitant jet (for transvalvular mean velocity measurement) in an in vitro model and in 23 patients.

7. Takenaka K, Dabestani A, Gardin JM, et al: A simple Doppler echocardiographic method for estimating severity of aortic regurgitation. *Am J Cardiol* 57:1340–1343, 1986.
   Holodiastolic flow reversal in the proximal abdominal aorta is a sensitive (100%) and specific (97%) method for separating subjects with 3 to 4+ from those with 0 to 2+ aortic regurgitation. The single false-positive result was in a patient with a patent ductus arteriosus.

8. Grayburn PA, Handshoe R, Smith MD, et al: Quantitative assessment of the hemodynamic consequences of aortic regurgitation by means of continuous wave Doppler recordings. *J Am Coll Cardiol* 10:135–141, 1987.
   Relationship between the shape of the aortic regurgitant jet on continuous-wave Doppler recordings and intracardiac dynamics is explored. All 10 patients with a diastolic decay slope >3 m/s² had 3+ to 4+ aortic regurgitation, although 9 of 21 (43%) of those with a slope <3 m/s² also had severe aortic regurgitation.

9. Heinle SK, Hall SA, Brickner E, et al: Comparison of vena contracta width by multiplane transesophageal echocardiography with quantitative Doppler assessment of mitral regurgitation. *Am J Cardiol* 81:175–179, 1998.
   The vena contracta width could be identified on transesophageal color flow imaging in 97% of patients with native mitral valve regurgitation. A vena contracta width ≥0.5 cm indicates severe mitral regurgitation (regurgitant volume >60 ml and an effective regurgitant orifice area ≥0.4 cm²). Conversely, a vena contracta width ≤0.3 cm indicates mild regurgitation.

10. Seiler C, Aeschbacher BA, Meier B: Quantitation of mitral regurgitation using the systolic/diastolic pulmonary venous flow velocity ratio. *J Am Coll Cardiol* 31:1383–1390, 1998.
    In patients in sinus rhythm and isolated mitral regurgitation (no aortic regurgitation, left ventricular ejection fraction >45%), the ratio of the systolic to diastolic velocity-time integral of flow in the pulmonary vein correlated moderately well with other quantitative measures of regurgitant severity. Although a systolic/ diastolic pulmonary vein flow ratio <0 had a specificity of 96% for identification of severe mitral regurgitation, sensitivity was only 52%.

Color Flow Mapping of Valvular Regurgitation

11. Reimold SC, Maier SE, Fleischmann KE, et al: Dynamic nature of the aortic regurgitant orifice area during diastole in patients with chronic aortic regurgitation. *Circulation* 89:2085–2092, 1994.
    Using 2D/Doppler echocardiography (continuity equation) and cine phase-contrast magnetic resonance imaging, regurgitant orifice area was found to vary directly with regurgitant fraction (r = 0.86) in 17 patients with chronic aortic regurgitation. However, the regurgitant orifice area decreased during diastole in 88% of patients. This dynamic component decreased with increasing regurgitant fraction (r = − 0.90).

12. Taylor AL, Eichhorn EJ, Brickner ME, et al: Aortic valve morphology: An important in vitro determinant of proximal regurgitant jet width by Doppler color flow mapping. *J Am Coll Cardiol* 16:405–412, 1990.
    In an in vitro model using simulated degenerative, rheumatic, and bicuspid aortic valves, although jet width was related to valve area (P = .0001), bicuspid shapes had a smaller proximal jet width than circular, rheumatic, or degenerative orifices.

13. Chen C, Thomas JD, Anconina J, et al: Impact of impinging wall jet on color Doppler quantification of mitral regurgitation. *Circulation* 84:712–720, 1991.
    For the same regurgitant fraction, mitral regurgitant jets that impinge on a left atrial wall have smaller color Doppler jet areas (by 40%) than jets that are "free" within the chamber.

14. Thomas JD, O'Shea JP, Rodriguez L, et al: Impact of orifice geometry on the shape of jets: An in vitro Doppler color flow study. *J Am Coll Cardiol* 17: 901–908, 1991.

    Jet momentum, defined as the product of the volume flow rate across the orifice, and velocity predict the appearance of jets in vitro. However, this approach assumes axial symmetry of the jet. In this article, the authors use an in vitro model to show that jets from irregular orifices became nearly axisymmetric within a few orifice diameters of jet origin.

15. Cape EG, Yoganathan AP, Weyman AE, Levine RA: Adjacent solid boundaries alter the size of regurgitant jets on Doppler color flow maps. *J Am Coll Cardiol* 17:1094–1102, 1991.

    Influence of impinging walls on jet geometry and area is described. Jets deflected toward adjacent walls have smaller jet areas than jets that are centrally located in the receiving chamber.

16. Smith MD, Harrison MR, Pinton R, et al: Regurgitant jet size by transesophageal compared with transthoracic Doppler color flow imaging. *Circulation* 83: 79–86, 1991.

    Color Doppler regurgitant jet areas appear larger from a transesophageal than from a transthoracic approach.

Clinical Applications in Aortic Regurgitation

17. Donovan CL, Starling MR: Role of echocardiography in the timing of surgical intervention for chronic mitral and aortic regurgitation. *In* Otto CM (ed): The Practice of Clinical Echocardiography. Philadelphia, WB Saunders, 1997, pp 327–354

    Detailed review of the literature on the natural history, postoperative outcome, and optimal timing of surgical intervention for chronic valvular regurgitation. Algorithms are proposed for timing of surgical intervention based on a combination of clinical findings, ejection fraction, and end-systolic left ventricular dimension. Additional predictors of outcome also are discussed. 159 references.

18. Biem HJ, Detsky AS, Armstrong PW: Management of asymptomatic chronic aortic regurgitation with left ventricular dysfunction: A decision analysis. *J Gen Intern Med* 5:394–401, 1990.

    Review of the literature on timing of aortic valve replacement in chronic asymptomatic aortic regurgitation emphasizing echo parameters. Convincing decision analysis suggests that an "early surgical approach" (when end-systolic dimension exceeds 55 mm or onset of left ventricular systolic dysfunction) is preferable to "late surgery" (onset of symptoms) based on quality-adjusted life years.

19. Szlachcic J, Massie BM, Greenberg B, et al: Intertest variability of echocardiographic and chest x-ray measurements: Implications for decision making in patients with aortic regurgitation. *J Am Coll Cardiol* 7: 1310–1317, 1986.

    Excellent discussion of the factors affecting intertest variability in sequential examinations of cardiac size. The 95% level prediction limits were ±8 mm for left ventricular dimensions and 12% for fractional shortening, so a difference greater than these limits indicates an interval change between studies.

20. Bonow RO, Lakatos E, Maron BJ, Epstein SE: Serial long-term assessment of the natural history of asymptomatic patients with chronic aortic regurgitation and normal left ventricular systolic function. *Circulation* 84:1625–1635, 1991.

    Clinical study in 104 asymptomatic patients with aortic regurgitation demonstrating that the initial end-systolic dimensions, rate of change in end-systolic dimension, and resting ejection fraction are predictive of long-term outcome.

21. Borer JS, Hochreiter C, Herrold EM, et al: Prediction of indications for valve replacement among asymptomatic or minimally symptomatic patients with chronic aortic regurgitation and normal left ventricular performance. *Circulation* 97:525–534, 1998.

    In 104 asymptomatic patients with aortic regurgitation followed for 7.4 ± 3.7 years, 28 (72%) developed symptoms warranting valve replacement, 7 (18%) developed asymptomatic excessive left ventricular dilation, and 4 (10%) experienced sudden death. The overall rate of endpoints was 6.2% per year with the strongest multivariate predictor of clinical outcome being change in left ventricular ejection fraction from rest to exercise, normalized for the exercise change in end-systolic wall stress.

22. Scognamiglio R, Rahimtoola SH, Fasoli G, et al: Nifedipine in asymptomatic patients with severe aortic regurgitation and normal left ventricular function. *N Engl J Med* 331:689–694, 1994.

    In a randomized trial of 143 asymptomatic patients with aortic regurgitation, after 6 years only 15% ± 3% of the patients receiving afterload reduction (nifedipine) had undergone valve replacement for symptoms or left ventricular dysfunction compared to 34% ± 6% of the patients treated with digoxin.

23. Padial LR, Oliver A, Vivaldi M, et al: Doppler echocardiographic assessment of progression of aortic regurgitation. *Am J Cardiol* 80:306–314, 1998.

    In 127 patients with varying degrees of aortic regurgitation, the ratio of proximal regurgitant jet height to outflow tract diameter increased over a follow-up interval of 21 ± 11 months. Left ventricular volumes and mass increased faster in patients with more severe aortic regurgitation and in those with more rapid progression of aortic regurgitant severity.

24. Reimold SC, Orav EJ, Come PC, et al: Progressive enlargement of the regurgitant orifice in patients with chronic aortic regurgitation. *J Am Soc Echocardiogr* 11:259–265, 1998.

    In a prospective study of 59 patients with audible aortic regurgitation murmurs, aortic regurgitant jet width increased by 0.04 ± 0.01 cm/y and regurgitant orifice area increased by 0.01 ± 0.01 cm^2/y. Rate of progression was not related to the cause of aortic regurgitation, gender, or baseline regurgitant severity.

25. Desjardins VA, Enriquez Sarano M, et al: Intensity of murmurs correlates with severity of valvular regurgitation. *Am J Med* 100:149–156, 1996.

Murmur grade (0 to 5) on physical examination cor-related moderately well with regurgitant severity ex-pressed as Doppler regurgitant fraction or volume. A murmur grade ≥3 for aortic and ≥4 for mitral regurgi-tation predicts severe disease, while a murmur ≤1 for aortic and ≤2 for mitral regurgitation indicates mild disease. However, there is a wide overlap in disease severity in those with intermediate murmur grades.

26. Devereux RB: Appetite suppressants and valvular heart disease. *N Engl J Med* 339:765–766, 1998.
    This editorial discusses the studies showing an asso-ciation between use of the appetite-suppressant drugs, fenfluramine and dexfenfluramine, and valvular heart disease. Although several studies have shown an in-creased risk of aortic regurgitation (usually mild in severity) the magnitude of this risk remains unclear.

Clinical Applications in Patients with Mitral Regurgitation

27. Griffin BP, Stewart WJ: Echocardiography in patient se-lection, operative planning, and intraoperative evalua-tion of mitral valve repair. *In* Otto CM (ed): The Prac-tice of Clinical Echocardiography. Philadelphia, WB Saunders, 1997, pp 355–372.
    Detailed review of the use of echocardiography in patients undergoing mitral valve repair procedures with numerous practical tips and excellent illustrations.

28. Reed D, Abbott RD, Smucker ML, Kaul S: Prediction of outcome after mitral valve replacement in patients with symptomatic chronic mitral regurgitation: The im-portance of left atrial size. *Circulation* 84:23–24, 1991.
    Clinical study in 176 patients who underwent mitral valve replacement shows that preoperative pulmonary rales, left atrial size, and the ratio of end-systolic left ventricular wall thickness to chamber dimension are predictive of mortality postoperatively (follow-up 3.8 ± 0.5 years).

29. Sheikh KH, Bengtson JR, Rankin JS, et al: Intra-opera-tive transesophageal Doppler color flow imaging used to guide patient selection and operative treatment of is-chemic mitral regurgitation. *Circulation* 84:594–604, 1991.
    Use of intraoperative transesophageal echo in 246 pa-tients undergoing surgery for coronary artery disease re-sulted in a change in operative management in 27 patients (11%) due to finding less mitral regurgitation by echo versus catheterization (n = 22) so that valve replacement was not needed or to finding more severe mitral regurgi-tation (n = 5) necessitating valve replacement.

30. Stewart WJ, Currie PJ, Salcedo EE, et al: Intraoperative Doppler color flow mapping for decision-making in valve repair for mitral regurgitation: Technique and re-sults in 100 patients. *Circulation* 81:556–566, 1990.
    Intraoperative echo in 100 patients undergoing mi-tral valve repair showed a satisfactory repair in 92, per-sistent significant mitral regurgitation in 4, dynamic outflow obstruction in 3, and a persistent flail leaflet in 1 patient. Further mitral valve surgery was performed at the same operation in 6 of the 8 patients with unsat-isfactory results; the other 2 required reoperation for persistent regurgitation.

31. Weisenbaugh T, Skudicky D, Sareli P: Prediction of out-come after valve replacement for rheumatic mitral re-gurgitation in the era of chordal preservation. *Circula-tion* 89:191–197, 1994.
    In 61 patients with rheumatic mitral regurgitation, preoperative end-systolic diameter was the only inde-pendent predictor of postoperative death. There was an increased probability of death or severe heart failure with a preoperative end-systolic diameter greater than 50 mm, with a 98% accuracy of this breakpoint for predicting outcome.

32. Tischler MD, Cooper KA, Rowen R, LeWinter MM: Mitral valve replacement versus mitral valve repair: A Doppler and quantitative stress echocardiographic study. *Circulation* 89:132–137, 1994.
    Exercise Doppler and quantitative 2D echocardio-graphic studies were performed in 10 patients pre– and post–mitral valve repair and in 10 matched subjects un-dergoing mitral valve replacement. In patients with mi-tral valve repair, end-systolic circumferential wall stress was lower at rest and with exercise, ejection fraction was higher, and the left ventricle was less spherical than in patients with mitral valve replacement.

33. He S, Fontaine AA, Schwammenthal E, et al: Integrated mechanism for functional mitral regurgitation–leaflet restriction versus coapting force: In vitro studies. *Cir-culation* 96:1826–1834, 1997.
    Use of 3D echocardiography to study the complex interrelationships of the mitral valve apparatus.

34. Leung DY, Griffin BP, Stewart WJ, et al: Left ventricu-lar function after valve repair for chronic mitral regur-gitation: Predictive value of preoperative assessment of contractile reserve by exercise echocardiography. *J Am Coll Cardiol* 28:1198–1205, 1996.
    In a study of 74 patients with severe mitral regurgi-tation the change in left ventricular end-systolic volume index with exercise was the best predictor of postoper-ative outcome.

Alternate Approaches to Evaluation of Valvular Regurgitation

35. Globits S, Higgins CB: Assessment of valvular heart disease by magnetic resonance imaging. *Am Heart J* 129:369–381, 1995.
    Concise review of evaluation of valvular heart dis-ease by magnetic resonance imaging including evalua-tion of valve anatomy, visualization of regurgitant and stenotic jets, measurement of transvalvular pressure gradients, and quantitative evaluation of left ventricular size and function.

36. Baim DS, Grossman W: Cardiac Catheterization, An-giography, and Intervention. Baltimore, Williams & Wilkins, 1996.
    Textbook of cardiac catheterization techniques em-phasizing clinical applications. Chapters on hemody-namic principles and profiles in valvular heart disease are especially helpful.

Echocardiographic Evaluation of Prosthetic Valve Dysfunction

12

BASIC PRINCIPLES
Types of Prosthetic Valves and Fluid Dynamics
Bioprosthetic Valves
Homograft Valves
Mechanical Valves
Valved Conduits
Mechanisms of Prosthetic Valve Dysfunction
Tissue Degeneration
Mechanical Failure
Paraprosthetic Regurgitation
Prosthetic Valve Endocarditis
Technical Aspects of Echo Evaluation
ECHOCARDIOGRAPHIC APPROACH
2D/M-Mode Imaging
Bioprosthetic Valves
Mechanical Valves
Valved Conduits
Doppler Evaluation
Normal Doppler Findings

Prosthetic Valve Stenosis
Prosthetic Valve Regurgitation
Other Echocardiographic Findings in Prosthetic Valve
Dysfunction
TECHNICAL ASPECTS/LIMITATIONS/ALTERNATE
APPROACHES
Echocardiographic Approach to the Patient with a
Prosthetic Valve
Transthoracic Examination
Transesophageal Examination
Limitations and Alternate Approaches
CLINICAL UTILITY
Prosthetic Valve Stenosis
Prosthetic Valve Regurgitation
Prosthetic Valve Endocarditis
Prosthetic Valve Thrombosis
"Routine" Follow-Up of Prosthetic Valve Function
SUGGESTED READING

Echocardiographic evaluation of prosthetic valves is similar, in many respects, to evaluation of native valvular disease. However, there are some important dissimilarities. First, there are several different types of prosthetic valves with differing fluid dynamics for each basic design and differing flow velocities for each valve size. Second, the mechanisms of valve dysfunction are somewhat different from those for native valve disease. Third, the technical aspects of imaging artificial devices—specifically, the problem of acoustic shadowing—significantly affect the diagnostic approach when prosthetic valve dysfunction is suspected (Table 12–1).

Echocardiographers increasingly are asked to evaluate prosthetic valve function, given the increasing number of prosthetic valves implanted annually and the greater longevity of patients with prosthetic valves. Both an understanding of the basic approach to echocardiographic evaluation (as outlined in this chapter) and detailed knowledge of the specific flow dynamic for the size and type of prosthesis in an individual patient (which may require additional reference sources) are needed for appropriate patient management.

BASIC PRINCIPLES

Types of Prosthetic Valves and Fluid Dynamics (Fig. 12–1)

The three basic types of prosthetic valves are (1) tissue valves, or bioprostheses, (2) homograft valves, and (3) mechanical valves (Table 12–2).

Bioprosthetic Valves

Tissue valves are composed of three biologic leaflets with an anatomic structure similar to the native aortic valve. Valve leaflets (heterografts, typically porcine), or pericardium (usually bovine) shaped to mimic normal leaflets are mounted on a cloth-covered metal support that functions as the crown-shaped aortic annulus with a raised "stent" at each of the three commissures. Variations in the support structure

TABLE 12–1	Comparison of Different Valve Types		
Normal	**Native Valve**	**Bioprosthesis**	**Mechanical Valve**
Fluid dynamics	Central orifice, laminar flow, blunt flow profile	Central orifice, laminar flow, blunt flow profile	Complex fluid dynamics depending on valve type
Antegrade velocity	Normal	Increased	Increased
Normal regurgitation	Mild, central	Mild, central	Mild, oblique jets
Mechanisms of dysfunction	Multiple	Tissue degeneration, endocarditis, pannus ingrowth, sewing ring dehiscence	Mechanical failure, endocarditis, pannus ingrowth, thrombus, sewing ring dehiscence
Technical aspects of imaging	Calcification may cause acoustic shadows in some cases	Acoustic shadow from sewing ring	Extensive reverberations and acoustic shadowing

FIGURE 12–1. Photographs of four different prosthetic valves: a ball-cage type valve (Starr-Edward mitral, *above, left*), a tissue valve (Carpentier-Edward aortic, *below, left*), a bileaflet mechanical valve (St. Jude Medical—heart valve, *above, right*), and a tilting-disk valve (Medtronic Hall valve, *below, right*). (Courtesy of Baxter Healthcare Corporation, Santa Ana, California; St. Jude Medical, St. Paul, Minnesota; and Medtronic, Inc., Minneapolis, Minnesota.)

and leaflet types abound in commercially available valves. Examples include Carpentier-Edwards porcine valves, Hancock porcine valves, Ionescu-Shiley bovine pericardial valves, and Carpentier-Edwards pericardial valves. In addition, newer "stentless" bioprosthetic valve

have become available for the aortic position, with the leaflets supported by a flexible cuff consisting of aortic tissue or cloth, with no rigid stents. Examples include the St. Jude Toronto SPV valve and the Carpentier-Edwards freestyle valve.

All these tissue valves are similar in that the trileaflet valve opens to a circular orifice (in systole in the aortic position or in diastole in the mitral position). The normal flow pattern is similar to that of a native valve, specifically, laminar flow with a relatively blunt flow profile. Regardless of valve type, the orientation of a mitral prosthesis valve results in the inflow stream being directed anteriorly and medially toward the ventricular septum in most patients instead of toward the ventricular apex, as is seen for normal native valves (Fig. 12–2). This results in a reversed vortex of blood flow in mid-diastole, as seen in an apical four-chamber view (Fig. 12–3).

Conventional tissue valves also differ from native valves in the presence of the support structure, which both (1) limits acoustic access and (2) results in a "normal" valve area that is smaller than the native valve (with corresponding higher "normal" antegrade flow velocities)

TABLE 12–2	Examples of Valve Types and Names
Homografts	Cryopreserved by tissue bank
Heterografts	
Porcine	Carpentier-Edwards
Bovine	Hancock Ionescu-Shiley
pericardium	
Pericardial	Carpentier-Edwards
Stentless	St. Jude Toronto Stentless
	Porcine Valve (SPV)
	Edwards Freestyle
Mechanical	
Ball-cage	Starr-Edwards
Floating-disk	Beall (no longer used)
Tilting-disk	Omniscience
	Bjork-Shiley
Bileaflet	St. Jude

FIGURE 12–2. Normal left ventricular inflow pattern across a porcine mitral valve replacement (MVR) in the parasternal long-axis view. The flowstream is directed toward the ventricular septum. The flow velocity is greater than the Nyquist limit, so flow toward the transducer is displayed in blue. (See Color Plate 12, p. 274.)

FIGURE 12–3. Apical four-chamber view *(top)* in a patient with a porcine mitral valve replacement (MVR) showing color flow *(bottom)* toward the apex along the ventricular septum with flow toward the base along the lateral wall—the opposite of the normal pattern shown in Figure 2–41. (See Color Plate 12, p. 274.)

due to limitation of the flow area by the supporting structure. These limitations are largely avoided with the newer stentless valves, which appear similar to a normal native valve on 2D imaging and have hemodynamics more closely approximating normal valve function. As is seen with native valves, a small degree of valve regurgitation is found in a high percentage of normally functioning bioprosthetic valves.

Homograft Valves

Homograft valves are cryopreserved human aortic valves harvested at autopsy. Typically, the valve, ascending aorta, and anterior mitral leaflet are preserved as a block, to be trimmed appropriately at the time of implantation. Aortic homografts are used in the aortic or pulmonic position and in valved conduits but are rarely used for an atrioventricular valve replacement (since a supporting prosthetic structure would be needed). While the fluid dynamics of a homograft are similar to those of a native valve, flow velocities are slightly higher and valve areas slightly smaller than for a normal native valve due to the space occupied by the homograft annulus in the patient's outflow tract.

Mechanical Valves

A wide variety of mechanical valves currently are available. In addition, several other types of valves, which were implanted in the past, are still in situ in some patients. The basic types of mechanical valves are (1) a ball-cage valve in which a spherical occluder is contained by a metal "cage" when the valve is open and fills the orifice in the closed position (like on a snorkel), (2) a tilting-disk valve where a single circular disk opens at an angle to the annulus plane, being constrained in its motion by a smaller "cage," a central strut, or a slanted slot in the valve ring, and (3) a bileaflet valve where two semicircular disks hinge open to form two large lateral orifices and a smaller central orifice (Fig. 12–4).

Antegrade Flow Profiles. As might be expected, the spatial flow profiles across each of these valve types vary substantially, and none is analogous to flow across the normal native valve. With a ball-cage valve in the open position, blood flows across the sewing ring and around the ball occluder on all sides. When the valve closes, a small amount of regurgitation is seen circumferentially around the ball as it seats in the sewing ring.

The fluid dynamics of a tilting-disk valve are characterized by two orifices in the open position, one larger than the other (major versus minor), with an asymmetric flow profile as

FIGURE 12–4. Bileaflet mitral valve prosthesis seen in systole *(above)* and diastole *(below)* from a transesophageal approach. In systole, the two leaflets close with a slightly obtuse closure angle. In diastole, the sewing ring and two parallel open leaflets are seen. Reverberations from the leaflets and shadowing from the sewing ring are prominent in both systole and diastole.

blood accelerates along the tilted surface of the open disk. Subtle variations in this flow pattern depend on the shape of the disk (convex versus concave surface) as well as the sewing ring design.

Bileaflet mechanical valves have complex fluid dynamics that affect the Doppler echocardiographic evaluation of these valves. With the leaflets open, there are two large lateral valve orifices and a small narrow central "slitlike" orifice. The flow velocity profile shows three peaks corresponding to these three orifices, with higher velocities in the center of each orifice. Of note, the local acceleration forces within the narrow central orifice result in localized high-pressure gradients in this region of the valve. These local gradients often are substantially higher than the overall pressure gradient across the valve.

Normal Mechanical Valve Regurgitation. With a tilting-disk valve, when the disk closes to occlude the valve annulus, regurgitation occurs at the closure line with the major regurgitant jet directed away from the sewing ring at the edge of the major orifice (Fig. 12–5). Note that the orientation of the prosthetic valve in the annulus can be variable, depending on surgical preference, so that the open disk position and the orientation of the regurgitant jet vary correspondingly. Additional smaller regurgitant jets circumferentially around the annulus normally are present. With a single-disk valve and a central strut (e.g., Medtronic-Hall), a small central jet of regurgitation also occurs around the central hole of the disk, as might be expected. When a bileaflet valve closes, two crisscross jets of regurgitation are seen in the plane parallel to the leaflet opening plane. In the perpendicular plane, two smaller diverging regurgitant jets are seen. The total volume of regurgitation is small with normal prosthetic valve function.

Valved Conduits

Valved conduits are used in congenital heart surgery and in ascending aortic repairs when both a new passageway for blood flow and a valve are needed. The conduit may be biologic (i.e., a homograft) or artificial (i.e., Gore-Tex or Dacron) material. A conduit may incorporate either a tissue or a mechanical valve with fluid dynamics similar to those for a valve implanted in the native annulus.

Mechanisms of Prosthetic Valve Dysfunction

The types of disease processes that affect prosthetic valves are distinctly different from those seen with native valvular heart disease.

Tissue Degeneration

Failure of a bioprosthetic valve to open or close properly (mechanical failure) usually is the result of slowly progressive tissue degeneration with fibrocalcific changes of the leaflets resulting in increased resistance to opening (stenosis) or failure to coapt during valve closure (regurgitation). Acute bioprosthetic valve stenosis is rare. Acute bioprosthetic regurgitation can occur with a leaflet tear, usually adjacent to a region of calcification. Occasionally, these patients present with the sudden onset of a "honking noise in my chest" and no other symptoms.

Mechanical Failure

Failure of a mechanical valve can occur due to faulty design or wear and tear of the prosthetic material resulting in disk escape or incomplete valve closure. More often, mechanical valve stenosis or regurgitation is due to thrombus formation or pannus ingrowth around the valve, impairing disk excursion or closure.

FIGURE 12–5. Color flow image of a bileaflet mitral valve prosthesis in diastole *(above)*, showing acceleration of flow across the valve with two large lateral orifices and a small central orifice. In systole *(below)*, two normal jets of regurgitation are seen. (See Color Plate 12, p. 274.)

Paraprosthetic Regurgitation

With both bioprosthetic and mechanical valves, paravalvular regurgitation can occur around the sewing ring due to loss of suture material postoperatively, most often related to fibrocalcific disease in the valve annulus. The new onset of paravalvular regurgitation late after surgery raises the possibility of an infectious process (endocarditis) resulting in valve dehiscence.

Prosthetic Valve Endocarditis

Infection of a valve prosthesis is a serious clinical problem, so suspected endocarditis is a frequent indication for echocardiography in patients with prosthetic valves. Endocarditis on a bioprosthesis may result in vegetations similar to those seen on a native valve. However, with a mechanical valve, the infection often is paravalvular, and no discrete vegetation may be present.

Technical Aspects of Echo Evaluation

The most technically limiting aspect of echocardiographic evaluation of prosthetic valves is the problem of acoustic shadowing. The sewing rings of both bioprosthetic and mechanical valves and the occluders of mechanical valves are strong echo reflectors, resulting in acoustic shadows and reverberations (Fig. 12–6). These reverberations and shadows obscure the motion of the valve structures themselves and block visualization of two-dimensional (2D) or Doppler abnormalities in the acoustic shadow region. During the examination, considerable effort is directed toward utilizing windows and views that avoid these imaging artifacts. Transesophageal echocardiography is particularly useful in evaluation of prosthetic mitral valves because it provides acoustic access from the left atrial side of the valve.

ECHOCARDIOGRAPHIC APPROACH

2D/M-Mode Imaging

Bioprosthetic Valves

An aortic homograft appears similar to a native aortic valve except for some increased thickness in the left ventricular outflow tract and the ascending aorta at the proximal and distal suture sites (Fig. 12–7). Typically, the homo-

FIGURE 12–7. Aortic valve homograft in a parasternal long-axis view showing an appearance similar to a native valve other than thickening and increased echogenicity of the aortic root. Continuous-wave Doppler shows a mildly increased antegrade velocity across the homograft compared with a native valve. RPA = right pulmonary artery.

FIGURE 12–6. Parasternal short-axis view of a bileaflet mechanical aortic valve in systole. The anterior disk is seen as a clear line. The posterior disk and posterior sewing ring are obscured by reverberations from the valve.

graft is implanted using the mini-root technique with the homograft replacing a segment of the native aorta. This approach necessitates reimplantation of the coronary arteries. In the past, the aortic homograft sometimes was positioned inside the patient's native aorta with appropriate trimming to maintain patency of the coronary ostia. In patients with endocarditis, the attached anterior mitral leaflet of the homograft may be used to patch a ventricular septal defect or abscess cavity. The echocardiographic appearance of a homograft on 2D and M-mode evaluations is very similar to that of a native aortic valve, except for the associated surgical changes. Standard parasternal long- and short-axis image planes provide optimal visualization of valve leaflet anatomy and motion.

Heterograft leaflet or pericardial tissue prosthetic valves have a trileaflet structure similar to a native aortic valve. An M-mode through the leaflets shows the typical "boxlike" opening in systole (for the aortic position) or diastole (for the mitral position) as is seen with a normal native aortic valve. However, with conventional valve designs, the echogenic sewing ring and struts may limit visualization of the leaflets on 2D imaging with the specific 2D echo appearance of the supporting structures depending on the specific model. Since there is marked variability in surgeons' valve preferences, it is helpful to obtain photographs of the valves most commonly encountered at your institution. For example, a Carpentier-Edwards porcine valve has three prominent struts on 2D short-axis imaging (Fig. 12–8). Stentless bioprosthetic aortic valves have an echocardiographic appearance similar to a native aortic valve, other than increased echogenicity in the aortic root in the early postoperative period (Fig. 12–9).

Improved images of the valve leaflets can be obtained from a transesophageal approach, particularly for valves in the mitral position, since the ultrasound beam has a perpendicular orientation to the leaflets with no intervening

FIGURE 12–8. Transesophageal view of a porcine aortic valve replacement in a short-axis view showing the three normal stents that support the valve leaflets.

FIGURE 12–9. Parasternal long-axis *(left)* and short axis *(right)* views of a stentless tissue valve in the aortic position. The valve appearance is similar to a native trileaflet aortic valve other than slightly increased echogenicity in the aortic root.

structures from this approach. Although with aortic valve prostheses the anterior part of the sewing ring shadows the leaflets from a transthoracic approach, transesophageal imaging is less rewarding because now the posterior part of the sewing ring shadows the valve leaflets. When images of the leaflets themselves are suboptimal, Doppler data can provide valuable information.

Conventional bioprosthetic valves have an average longevity of only about 10 years, with slowly progressive tissue failure being the primary reason for reoperation. Typically, the leaflets develop fibrocalcific changes that result in leaflet deformity (leading to regurgitation) and/or increased stiffness (leading to stenosis). Echocardiographically, increased echogenicity and irregularity of the leaflets may be noted, although images of the leaflets often are suboptimal due to shadowing and reverberation.

Mechanical Valves

2D and M-mode imaging of mechanical valves from a transthoracic approach is frustrating because of severe reverberations and acoustic shadowing. While the 2D images may provide clues as to the type of valve prostheses (e.g., "low-profile" bileaflet or tilting-disk valve versus "high-profile" ball-cage valve), obviously it is simpler to ascertain the exact valve type and size from the patient's medical record or valve identification card. Assessing motion of the valve occluder often is difficult. For example, the leading edge of a tilting-disk valve results in a strong reverberation across the 2D image obscuring motion of the disk itself. In addition, an oblique image plane often is obtained relative to the prosthetic valve, since orientation of the prosthesis within the annulus is not standard. With a tomographic plane perpendicular to the open bileaflet valve, the two leaflets can be identified clearly, an image plane that is best identified on multiplane transesophageal imaging.

Technical limitations make identification of prosthetic valve endocarditis or thrombosis problematic because the abnormalities may be obscured by reverberations or hidden by acoustic shadowing. Transesophageal imaging can be helpful in identifying thrombus or infected vegetations on the atrial side of a mitral prosthesis, since the left atrium is "masked" by the prosthetic valve from both parasternal and apical windows. In a patient with a mechanical aortic valve, the subaortic region can be evaluated well from a transthoracic approach from parasternal and apical windows. In this situa-

tion, transesophageal images are less helpful due to shadowing of the outflow tract by the posterior aspect of the prosthesis.

While M-mode patterns of occluder motion have been described for both normally and abnormally functioning mechanical valves, the use of M-mode largely has been supplanted by evaluation of prosthetic valve hemodynamics with Doppler echocardiography. M-mode tracings remain helpful in verifying rapid independent motion of structures attached to the prosthetic valve seen on 2D imaging that may represent vegetations or thrombus formation.

Valved Conduits

The 2D and M-mode evaluation of a bioprosthetic or mechanical valve in a conduit (e.g., right ventricular to pulmonary artery) may be difficult due to ultrasound attenuation by the conduit prosthetic material. Of note, stenosis in a valved conduit can occur as a result of stenosis of the valve prosthesis or fibrotic ingrowth along the length of the conduit. In addition, residual or progressive stenosis at the proximal or distal anastomosis site can occur. Evaluation of narrowing in the conduit is difficult with 2D imaging, but a careful Doppler examination may allow detection of this diagnosis. Continuous-wave Doppler is used to assess the maximum flow velocity, while pulsed Doppler or high-pulse-repetition-frequency (HPRF) Doppler is used to localize the level of obstruction along the length of the conduit.

Doppler Evaluation

Normal Doppler Findings

Prosthetic Valve "Clicks." The motion of the occluder of a mechanical valve (or the tissue leaflets of a biologic valve) creates a brief intense Doppler signal that appears as a dark narrow band of short duration on the spectral display (Fig. 12–10). Audibly, this signal is similar to the valve "click" appreciated on auscultation. However, unlike auscultation, usually both opening and closing valve clicks are seen on spectral Doppler analysis. The Doppler signals associated with valve opening and closing are similar to those seen with native valves but are of greater intensity. The motion of the occluder also may result in color flow artifacts, with color signals covering large areas of the 2D sector that are inconsistent from beat to beat.

Antegrade Velocities/Pressure Gradients. Compared with a normal native valve, all prosthetic

FIGURE 12–10. Left ventricular inflow across a mechanical mitral valve replacement showing an increased antegrade velocity (compared with a native valve) and prominent valve clicks *(arrows)*.

valves are inherently stenotic to some extent. Specifically, the expected antegrade velocities and pressure gradients across a normally functioning prosthetic valve are higher than the corresponding values for a native valve. Similarly, the effective orifice area of a prosthetic valve is smaller than the orifice area of a normal native valve.

The expected velocities, pressure gradients, and valve areas depend on the specific type, size, and position of the prosthetic valve. While manufacturers have data on in vitro flow characteristics for each valve, in vivo echocardiographic data are sparse owing to the large number of valve types and sizes. Even in a large study, only a few patients have the same valve type, position, and size. In the available Doppler studies of normal prosthetic valves, data often are presented in various ways. Some studies report the mean ± 1 SD for each variable; others include the range as well. While compilation of the normal values from all these studies is not possible from the published data, estimates of the expected normal velocities, pressure gradients, and valve areas for several commonly seen prosthetic valves are shown in Tables 12–3 and 12–4.

Note that, in general, the larger the valve size, the lower are the velocities and gradients and the larger is the effective orifice area. In fact, many of the smaller prosthetic valves have hemodynamics that are consistent with clinical stenosis even with normal valve function. Also note the different expected velocities with different valve types. Typically, mechanical valves

have better hemodynamics at small valve sizes (the apparent discrepancies in the data for bileaflet valves are discussed below) than do conventional stented bioprosthetic valves. The significant exceptions are the aortic homograft valve and stentless tissue valves, which have excellent hemodynamics over the entire size range. Finally, note that mitral valve prostheses have lower velocities and pressure gradients than aortic valve prostheses due, in part, to larger valve sizes but also to passive flow at a lower pressure gradient from the atrium into the ventricle in diastole compared with active ejection and a higher left ventricular to aortic pressure gradient in systole.

As indicated by the ranges and standard deviations in the tables, there is a wide range of reported "normal" values for a given prosthetic valve type and size. Anatomic features and the details of implantation in each patient may account for some of this variability. However, the impact of transvalvular volume flow rate on transvalvular velocities and pressure gradients should not be underestimated. Even with a normally functioning prosthesis, a high cardiac output (e.g., postoperative, pregnancy, or sepsis) results in a high velocity and pressure gradient. This variability in "normal" velocities can be compensated for by calculating effective orifice area to "correct" for volume flow rate. Alternatively, a pragmatic approach is to obtain a baseline Doppler echo study in each patient after valve replacement (but not in the immediate postoperative period). The values obtained then serve as the "normal" reference for that patient (Fig. 12–10). This facilitates detection of changes in prosthetic valve function over time, with each patient serving as his or her own control. In some patients with a stentless valve in the aortic position, high velocities are seen early postoperatively with a progressive decline in velocity to the normal range at 1- to 2-year follow-up, presumably related to geometric remodeling of the annulus and outflow tract region.

Normal Regurgitation. Normal prosthetic valve function implies a small degree of valvular regurgitation in virtually all mechanical valves and in a high percentage (30% to 50%) of bioprosthetic valves. The patterns of regurgitation detected corresponds to the fluid dynamics of each valve type (see previous text). Color flow imaging shows the spatial distribution of normal prosthetic regurgitation with patterns specific to each valve type.

On a transthoracic study, it may be difficult to separate normal from pathologic prosthetic

TABLE 12–3	Normal Doppler Data for Prosthetic Aoritc Valves				
Valve Type	Size (mm)	V_{max} (m/s)	Mean Gradient (mmHg)	Velocity Ratio	Aortic Valve Area (cm²)
Bileaflet (St. Jude)	19	3.0 (2.0-4.5)	20 (10-30)	0.37	1.0
	21	2.7 (2.5-3.5)	14 (10-30)	0.40	1.3
	23	2.5 (2.0-3.5)	12 (10-30)	0.37	1.3
	25	2.4 (2.0-3.5)	12 (5-30)	0.42	1.8
	27	2.2 (2.0-3.1)	11 (5-20)	0.46	2.4
	29	2.0 (2.0-2.5)	10 (5-15)	0.49	2.7
	31	2.1 (1.5-2.5)	10 (5-15)	0.49	3.1
Tilting-disk (Bjork-Shiley, Medtronic Hall)	19	21 ± 7			
	21	2.8 ± 0.9	16		
	23	2.6 ± 0.4	14 ± 5		
	25	2.1 ± 0.3	13 ± 3		
	27	1.9 ± 0.2	10 ± 3		
	29	1.9 ± 0.2	7 ± 6		
Ball-cage (Starr-Edwards)		3.1 ± 0.5	24 ± 4		
Porcine tissue (Hancock or Carpentier-Edwards)	19	2.8 ± 0.7	16 ± 2		1.5 ± 0.1
	21	2.6 ± 0.4	15 ± 6		1.8 ± 0.2
	23	2.6 ± 0.4	13 ± 6		2.1 ± 0.2
	25	2.5 ± 0.4	11 ± 2		
	27	2.4 ± 0.4	10 ± 1		
	29	2.4 ± 0.4	12		
Nonstented tissue valves SPV-Toronto (St. Jude)		2.2 ± 0.4	3 (2-20)		1.8-2.3
Aortic homograft		1.8 ± 0.4	7 ± 3		2.2 (1.7-3.1)

Values shown are mean ± 1 SD or mean (range). Velocity ratio = left ventricular outflow velocity/aortic jet velocity.
Data from: Reisner et al: JASE 1:201, 1988; Zabalgoitia et al: Curr Prob Cardiol 5:271, 1992; Sagar et al: JACC 7:68, 1986; Baumgartner et al: Circ 82:1467, 1990; Chafizadeh et al: Circ 83:213, 1991; Jaffe et al: AJC 63:1466, 1989.

TABLE 12–4	Normal Doppler Data for Prosthetic Mitral Valves			
Valve Type	V_{max} (m/s)	Mean Gradient (mmHg)	$T_{1/2}$ (mm/s)	Mitral Valve Area (cm²)
Mechanical				
Bileaflet (St. Jude)	1.6 ± 0.3	4 ± 1	77 ± 17	2.9 ± 0.6
Tilting-disk (Bjork-Shiley)	1.6 ± 0.3	3 ± 2	90 ± 22	2.4 ± 0.6
Ball-cage (Starr-Edwards)	1.9 ± 0.5	5 ± 2	110 ± 27	2.0 ± 0.5
Porcine Tissue				
Ionescu-Shiley	1.5 ± 0.3	3 ± 1	93 ± 25	2.4 ± 0.8
Carpentier-Edwards	1.8 ± 0.2	6 ± 2	90 ± 25	2.5 ± 0.7
Hancock	1.5 ± 0.3	4 ± 2	129 ± 31	1.7 ± 0.4

$T_{1/2}$ = Pressure half time.
Values shown are mean ± 1 SD.
Data from Reisner and Meltzer: JASE 1:201, 1988; Zabalgoitia: Curr Prob Cardiol 5:271, 1992.

regurgitation, especially for the mitral position. On color flow imaging, normal prosthetic regurgitation tends to be a uniform color with little variance, whereas pathologic regurgita- tion shows aliasing and variance with a "confetti-like" appearance to the flow pattern. On continuous-wave Doppler examination, normal prosthetic regurgitation has a low signal strength, may persist through only part of the cardiac cycle, and is spatially localized. Note that pathologic regurgitation may appear "mild" by both continuous-wave and color Doppler criteria due to acoustic shadowing of the flow signal. In some cases, consideration of other echocardiographic and clinical factors may allow differentiation of pathologic from physiologic prosthetic regurgitation. However, if pathologic regurgitation is suspected, transesophageal imaging is needed in many aortic valve and all mitral valve cases.

On transesophageal imaging, the normal patterns of prosthetic regurgitation for each valve type can be identified, keeping in mind that normal regurgitation tends to be relatively uniform in color, even though the jet area may appear relatively large. Pathologic regurgitation is characterized by a flow disturbance with an abnormal spatial pattern of flow indicated by an eccentric or large jet with marked variance on the color flow display. Evaluation of the origin of the jet also is helpful. Physiologic regurgitation originates within the sewing ring with typical patterns for each valve type. Pathologic regurgitation often originates around the valve sewing ring in unpredictable locations. Color flow imaging allows identification of the vena contracta and the proximal flow acceleration region on the left ventricular side of the mitral valve.

Prosthetic Valve Stenosis

Pressure Gradients. The principles applied to evaluation of native valve stenosis also have been used for suspected stenosis of prosthetic valves. From a continuous-wave Doppler recording of the antegrade velocity across the valve, obtained at a parallel intercept angle, maximum instantaneous and mean pressure gradients can be calculated using the Bernoulli equation ($4v^2$). Although the maximum velocity across a prosthetic valve is higher than that for a native valve, the shape of the velocity curve is triangular (in contrast to the rounded contour seen in aortic stenosis). Thus, the calculated mean gradient typically is less for a prosthetic valve than for a native valve with the same maximum antegrade velocity (Fig. 12–11).

Maximum and mean pressure gradients across bioprosthetic valves calculated by Doppler echo compare well with directly measured pressure gradients (Table 12–5). The situation is more complex for mechanical valves because of the differing fluid dynamics of each type of prosthesis. In theory, the pressure gradient across a given degree of stenosis will be identical whether the stenosis consists of a single ori-

fice or multiple orifices, with the Bernoulli relationship being valid for each orifice. Thus a maximum pressure gradient of 36 mmHg will correspond to a single or multiple 3-m/s jets across the valve. However, while this theory holds true when local acceleration and viscous forces can be ignored, local higher-pressure gradients do occur with some valve types. This phenomenon has been studied most thoroughly for the bileaflet valve.

With the valve leaflets open, the bileaflet valve has a narrow, slitlike central orifice flanked by two larger semicircular orifices (Fig. 12–12). The walls of this narrow central orifice are formed by the parallel valve disks, which are nearly perpendicular to the sewing ring of the valve. Within this narrow central flowstream, acceleration forces result in a localized high-pressure gradient (and corresponding high velocity) with rapid pressure recovery distal to the valve. Therefore, the pressure difference measured between the upstream side of the valve and this central orifice is greater than the pressure difference between the upstream and downstream sides of the valve. Since continuous-wave Doppler ultrasound records the highest velocity along the length of the ultrasound beam, it is this higher localized velocity that is recorded. While this high localized gradient is measured correctly, the gradient of interest is the upstream-to-downstream valve gradient. This explains the observation that even though the correlation between Doppler and invasive pressure gradient measurements is high, the slope of the regression line indicates that the Doppler approach consistently "overestimates" the overall transvalvular gradient. This overestimation is large enough

FIGURE 12–11. Antegrade velocity across a normal aortic valve replacement. The antegrade velocity is increased compared with a native valve, the shape of the flow curve is triangular, and prominent prosthetic valve clicks are present.

TABLE 12–5	Validation of Doppler Echo Prosthetic Mean Valve Gradients Compared with Invasive Data (Selected Series)				
First Author/Year	**Valve Type/Position**	**n**	**r**	**SEE (mmHg)**	**Mean Difference**
Sagar/1986	Hancock & BS/mitral	19	0.93	2.5	
Sagar/1986	Hancock & BS/aortic	11	0.94	7.4	
Wilkins/1986	Starr-Edwards, BS/porcine/ mitral	11	0.96	—	
Burstow/1989	Mixed/aortic	20	0.94	3	
	Mixed/mitral	20	0.97	1.2	
Baumgartner/1990	St. Jude	In vitro	0.98	1.9	10 ± 3 mmHg
	Hancock	In vitro	0.98	1.4	2 ± 1 mmHg
Stewart/1991	Bioprosthetic/aortic	In vitro	0.78-0.98		Overestimation by Doppler
Baumgartner/1992	St. Jude	In vitro	0.98	2.0	13 ± 8 mmHg
	Medtronic-Hall	In vitro	0.99	0.5	0.8 ± 0.6
	Starr-Edwards	In vitro	0.97	2.0	8 ± 4 mmHg
	Hancock	In vitro	0.99	1.5	1.9 ± 1.6

BS = Bjork-Shiley tilting-disk mechanical valve.
References as in Suggested Reading.

Bi-leaflet Mechanical Valve

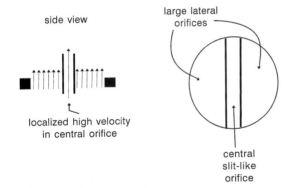

side view

large lateral orifices

localized high velocity in central orifice

central slit-like orifice

FIGURE 12–12. Schematic drawing of a bileaflet mechanical valve in the open position in side *(left)* and frontal *(right)* views. Two large lateral orifices flank a central slit-like orifice that is associated with localized high-velocity flow (and a localized pressure gradient).

that an erroneous diagnosis of severe stenosis might be made if the phenomenon of pressure recovery is not recognized.

Interestingly, the overestimation of pressure gradients across bileaflet valves becomes less significant in the presence of prosthetic valve stenosis. The proposed mechanism for this observation is a gradual reduction in the size of the central orifice as leaflet opening is reduced. Clinically, this poses a dilemma in that a high

velocity across a bileaflet valve might represent overestimation of the pressure gradient with normal valve function or a correct estimate of a high gradient with a stenotic valve. Again, a baseline study in the postoperative period provides a standard of comparison when subsequent valve dysfunction is suspected.

Valve Areas. Even when accurately measured, the physiologic limitation of transvalvular velocities across prosthetic valves is that velocities vary with volume flow rate for a given orifice area. A normally functioning valve prosthesis in an individual patient may have a high transvalvular velocity if cardiac output is elevated (e.g., with exercise, anemia, fever) or a low transvalvular velocity if cardiac output is depressed (e.g., left ventricular dysfunction). For these reasons, a flow-independent measure of prosthetic valve function is more useful clinically.

Aortic. Bioprosthetic aortic valves have fluid dynamics similar to those of a native aortic valve, and it is logical to assume that continuity equation valve area calculations are valid in this situation (Fig. 12–13). In fact, direct comparisons of Doppler echo (AVA_{prost}) and invasive valve areas in patients with suspected stenosis of bioprosthetic aortic valves have shown a reasonable correlation. As for a native aortic valve, the components of the continuity equation are the left ventricular outflow tract velocity-time integral (VTI_{LVOT}), the left ventricular outflow tract cross-sectional area (CSA_{LVOT}), and the aortic jet velocity-time integral (VTI_{Ao}). The continuity equation, then, is

$$AVA_{prost} = (CSA_{LVOT} \cdot VTI_{LVOT})/VTI_{Ao}$$

Left ventricular outflow tract velocity is recorded from an apical approach using pulsed Doppler echo with the sample volume positioned proximal to the prosthetic valve, avoiding the small region of flow acceleration immediately adjacent to the valve. Aortic jet velocity is recorded with continuous-wave Doppler from whichever window gives the highest-velocity signal, as for native valve stenosis. Left ventricular outflow tract diameter is measured in a parasternal long-axis view in midsystole from the septal endocardium to the anterior mitral leaflet parallel to and immediately adjacent to the aortic valve (Fig. 12–14). Direct measurement of outflow tract diameter is preferable to use of the implanted prosthetic valve size, since valve size relates to the external diameter of the sewing ring, not the effective diameter of the subvalvular flow region. As usual, a circular cross-sectional left ventricular outflow tract area is calculated as $\pi(D/2)^2$ from this diameter measurement.

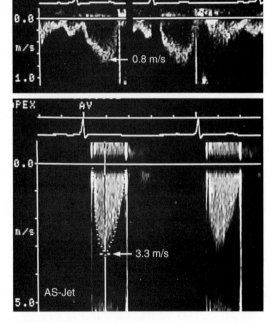

FIGURE 12–13. The continuity equation can be used for calculation of aortic valve area (AVA) for an aortic valve replacement (AVR). Left ventricular outflow tract (LVOT) flow is recorded from an apical approach using pulsed Doppler with the sample volume positioned just proximal to the prosthetic valve. LVOT diameter is measured from a parasternal long-axis view for calculation of a circular cross-sectional area (CSA) of flow. Continuous-wave (CW) Doppler is used to record the flow signal across the prosthetic valve from whichever window yields the highest-velocity jet.

FIGURE 12–14. Continuity equation prosthetic valve area is calculated from a parasternal long-axis midsystolic diameter (2.9 cm) measurement *(above)*, the pulsed Doppler left ventricular outflow tract velocity (0.8 m/s) recorded from an apical approach *(center)*, and the continuous-wave Doppler signal of flow across the valve (3.3 m/s) recorded from whichever window gives the highest velocity *(below)*. Even though the antegrade velocity is increased compared with a native valve, the calculated valve area is 1.6 cm².

The use of the continuity equation for mechanical aortic valves is more problematic. Presumably, if the transvalvular velocity-time integral is an accurate reflection of transvalvular volume flow rate, then calculated valve areas should be accurate. Remember that the continuity equation assumes a flat flow velocity profile *in* the stenotic orifice (or vena contracta), as well as proximal to the valve. Clearly, this assumption is not true for bileaflet valves. The local high velocities in the central orifice will result in a significant error in measurement of volume flow rate across the valve orifice, with a consequent underestimation of valve area. However, for tilting-disk and ball-cage valves, limited data suggest that the continuity equation may be reasonably accurate, despite complex fluid dynamics, because the continuous-wave velocity signal provides an approximation of the spatial mean flow velocity across the valve (Table 12–6).

Another approach to evaluation of suspected prosthetic aortic valve stenosis is to measure the "step-up" in velocity across the valve. The ratio of the outflow tract velocity to aortic jet velocity reflects the degree of stenosis—if no obstruction is present, these velocities will be nearly equal with a ratio close to 1; as the degree of narrowing increases, the aortic jet velocity will increase with no change in outflow tract velocity resulting progressively in a ratio <1. Since all prosthetic valves are inherently stenotic to some degree, the "normal" velocity ratio across an aortic prosthesis ranges from

0.35 to 0.50, compared with 0.75 to 0.90 for a normal native aortic valve.

The advantages of the use of the velocity ratio are (1) it takes volume flow rate into account, (2) it does not require an outflow tract diameter measurement, (3) a baseline "normal" value can be established for comparison on follow-up studies, and (4) it is easily measured and reproducible. Some investigators advocate measuring the velocity ratio with increases in flow rate (e.g., with exercise) to increase its specificity in excluding prosthetic valve stenosis.

Pragmatically, even if Doppler velocities and continuity equation valve areas overestimate the degree of prosthetic valve stenosis, in an individual patient a *change* in velocity or valve area is valuable in patient management decisions. Again, a baseline study at a time when valve function is normal provides a reference point for subsequent studies.

Mitral. Prosthetic mitral valve areas can be estimated using the pressure half-time approach as for native mitral valve stenosis (Fig. 12–15). The expected normal half-time for a prosthetic valve is longer than for a native valve, with the specific value depending on valve type and size. For bioprosthetic mitral valves, valve area can be estimated from the same formula as for native valves:

$$MVA = 220/T_{1/2}$$

where the pressure half-time ($T_{1/2}$) is measured in milliseconds, as described in Chapter 10.

TABLE 12–6	Validation of Doppler Echo Prosthetic Valve Areas (Selected Series)					
First Author/Year	Valve Type/ Position	n	Comparison	r	SEE	Mean Difference
Sagar/1986	Hancock and BS/mitral	12	$T_{1/2}$ vs. Gorlin	0.98	0.1 cm²	
Wilkins/1986	Porcine/mitral	8	$T_{1/2}$ vs. Gorlin	0.65	—	—
Rothbart/ 1990	Bioprosthetic/aortic	22	Cont eq vs. Gorlin at catheterization	0.93	—	—
Chafizadeh/ 1991	St. Jude/aortic	67	Cont eq vs actual orifice area	0.83	Doppler effective orifice area less than actual orifice area	
Baumgartner/ 1992	St. Jude	In vitro	Cont eq vs Gorlin	0.99	0.08	0.4-0.6 cm²
	Medtronic-Hall	In vitro		0.97	0.10	0-0.25 cm²
	Hancock/aortic	In vitro		0.93	0.10	0-0.25 cm²

BS = Bjork-Shiley tilting-disk mechanical valve; Cont eq = continuity equation valve area with Doppler and 2D echo data; Gorlin = Gorlin formula valve area using invasive data; $T_{1/2}$ = Doppler pressure half-time method.
References as in Suggested Reading.

FIGURE 12-15. Pressure half-time for a mitral prosthetic valve is calculated as for a native valve. In this case, the $T_{1/2}$ is 120 ms.

Somewhat surprisingly, the empirical constant 220 also appears to provide a reasonable approximation of mitral valve area for mechanical prostheses. With a bileaflet valve, the higher localized velocities in the central slitlike orifice affect the accuracy of pressure gradient calculations. However, the pressure half-time measurement is less affected because it depends on the *time course* of the velocity decline relative to the maximum velocity rather than on the velocities themselves.

Continuity equation valve area also can be calculated for a mitral prosthesis (in the absence of mitral regurgitation) using the antegrade stroke volume across the aortic or pulmonic valve in the equation.

The antegrade velocity curve across a mitral bioprosthesis may be recorded from an apical approach using pulsed, high pulse-repetition frequency, or continuous-wave Doppler ultrasound. Care in positioning the transducer is needed because inflow may be directed obliquely into the ventricular chamber. Some echocardiographers find it helpful to use the color flow image to aid in alignment of the Doppler beam parallel to the inflow stream. In many patients after mitral valve replacement, the inflow stream is directed anteriorly and medially toward the ventricular septum. In these patients, a low parasternal window may provide an optimal intercept angle for recording antegrade velocity. As for native mitral valve stenosis, Doppler acquisition parameters are adjusted to show a smooth velocity deceleration slope and a band of velocity signals along the edge of the curve.

Prosthetic Valve Regurgitation

Detection of Regurgitation. The echocardiographic approaches described for evaluation of native valve regurgitation in Chapter 11 also apply to evaluation of prosthetic valve regurgitation. The major differences between evaluation of native or prosthetic valves are (1) the prosthetic valve has a higher antegrade velocity, (2) the degree of normal prosthetic regurgitation is greater than the trivial amounts of native valve regurgitation seen in normal individuals, and (3) acoustic shadowing, reverberations, and beam width artifact make evaluation of a prosthetic valve more difficult and decrease the sensitivity of transthoracic echocardiography for detection of prosthetic regurgitation so that transesophageal imaging is needed more frequently.

Transthoracic color Doppler flow imaging for prosthetic valve regurgitation can be helpful, particularly if a view can be obtained where the ultrasound beam has access to the chamber receiving the regurgitant flow without first traversing the valve prosthetic. For the aortic valve, both parasternal and apical views are helpful because the ultrasound signal reaches the left ventricular outflow tract region without intercepting the valve prosthesis, avoiding the problem of acoustic shadowing. For the mitral valve, the parasternal approach may be helpful if a view can be obtained where the left atrial side of the valve is not shadowed by the valve prosthesis. Apical views often are limited due to acoustic shadowing, but occasionally, a paraprosthetic jet can be identified from this approach. In addition to acoustic shadowing, color artifacts are prominent in patients with prosthetic valves, which may obscure detection of abnormal flow signals (Figs. 12–16 and 12–17).

Conventional pulsed Doppler can be used to detect prosthetic regurgitation, but a meticulous examination is needed with persistent repositioning of the sample volume in multiple views to detect the regurgitant signal. However, when a suspicious signal is seen with color flow imaging, its timing can be more carefully assessed using conventional pulsed Doppler ultrasound. Mitral regurgitation starts immediately after mitral valve closure, whereas aortic outflow starts slightly later (after isovolumic contraction). Note that with loud prosthetic valve clicks and a low signal-to-noise ratio, it is easy to mistake normal left ventricular outflow for mitral regurgitation if signal timing is not examined.

Continuous-wave Doppler has the advantage of a wide beam size at the depth of a prosthetic valve and a high signal-to-noise ratio, enhancing the likelihood that a weaker signal or eccentric jet (i.e., paraprosthetic regurgitation) will be identified. Again, the timing of the presumed regurgitant signal is extremely important for correct identification of the origin of

FIGURE 12–16. Continuous-wave Doppler recording of prosthetic mitral regurgitation obtained from an apical window. The regurgitant signal starts immediately after the mitral closure click and continues up to the onset of antegrade flow across the prosthesis in diastole. The jet is eccentric and not parallel with the ultrasound beam, so flow signals appear as both sides of the baseline.

FIGURE 12–17. Continuous-wave Doppler signal from the same patient as in Figure 12–16 from a parasternal window. Again, a high-velocity signal is seen on both sides of the baseline due to an eccentric jet orientation. The patient's presenting complaint was a "honking noise in my chest." The prominent systolic striations in the Doppler signal were due to fluttering of a ruptured porcine valve cusp adjacent to a calcific nodule.

the Doppler signal. Many laboratories find it helpful to examine the prosthetic valve with continuous-wave Doppler starting with the ultrasound beam aligned in the flow direction of the valve and then slowly scanning in progressively larger circles to identify any potential paraprosthetic jets (Fig. 12–17).

Due to the problems of acoustic shadowing and reverberations, even the most carefully performed transthoracic examinations have a low sensitivity for detection and quantitation of prosthetic regurgitation. Especially for the mitral position, the transesophageal approach provides both improved image quality and the opportunity to interrogate the valve from the left atrial side—that is, the acoustic shadow now will obscure the left ventricle rather than the left atrium. Thus, when prosthetic mitral valve regurgitation is suspected, a transesophageal study should be considered. A transthoracic study showing prosthetic regurgitation can be clinically useful (high positive predictive value) but rarely allows for accurate quantitation of mitral regurgitant severity. A transthoracic study that does not show prosthetic regurgitation does not exclude this possibility (low negative predictive value).

Severity and Etiology of Prosthetic Regurgitation. When prosthetic regurgitation is detected, the first step in evaluation and interpretation is whether "normal" or pathologic prosthetic regurgitation is present. While the normal backflow across the valve represents a small volume of blood, the color jets on transesophageal imaging can be fairly large in area. Distinguishing features are the characteristic pattern for each valve type, a uniform color pattern rather than the mosaic flow disturbance seen with pathologic regurgitation, and the absence of other features (increased antegrade velocity, chamber sizes and function, pulmonary hypertension) to suggest significant regurgitation (Figs. 12–18 and 12–19).

Regurgitation of bioprosthetic valves most often is due to degenerative changes of the leaflets. This can be slowly progressive, with gradually increasing severity of a central regurgitant stream, or can occur abruptly, with cusp rupture adjacent to a fibrocalcific nodule. Regurgitant severity is graded as for a native valve by (1) the extent of the flow disturbance in the receiving chamber with color flow imaging, (2) evidence for distal flow reversal (e.g., descending aorta diastolic flow in aortic regurgitation), (3) the intensity and shape of the continuous-wave Doppler signal, and (4) associated Doppler and 2D findings.

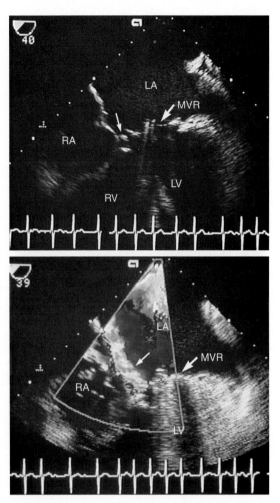

FIGURE 12–18. Transesophageal view of prosthetic mitral regurgitation with an eccentric jet directed laterally into the left atrium seen on color flow imaging *(top)*. Continuous-wave Doppler recorded from the transesophageal approach shows an intense, high-velocity regurgitant jet *(bottom)*. (See Color Plate 13, p. 274.)

FIGURE 12–19. Transesophageal 2D image *(top)* showing discontinuity *(arrow)* at the medial aspect of the sewing ring for a St. Jude mitral valve replacement in a patient with hemolytic anemia. Color flow imaging shows a relatively narrow, eccentric, medially directed mitral regurgitant jet. Notice that a slightly oblique image plane (40° rotation with a multiplane probe) was needed to image the vena contracta where the regurgitant flow crosses the mitral annulus *(arrows)*. (See Color Plate 13, p. 274.)

Mechanical valves can have prosthetic regurgitation due to incomplete closure resulting from pannus ingrowth around the sewing ring or from thrombus formation. Again, the flow disturbance will be larger than that seen with "normal" regurgitation, and severity can be estimated by the usual approaches. Transesophageal imaging is helpful in identifying the etiology as well as the severity of regurgitation for prosthetic valves in the mitral position.

Paraprosthetic regurgitation is most common with mechanical valves but also can occur with bioprosthetic valves. Distinguishing prosthetic from paraprosthetic regurgitation is diffi-cult on transthoracic imaging; in most cases, transesophageal echocardiography is needed. The etiology of paraprosthetic regurgitation may be a scarred and/or calcified annulus resulting in disruption of the sutures securing the valve or a paravalvular abscess with tissue destruction. The regurgitant jet originates external to the sewing ring, with an eccentric jet extending into the receiving chamber (Figs. 12–20 to 12–22). A single or multiple paraprosthetic jets may be present. Color flow imaging may show proximal flow acceleration (on the left ventricular side of the mitral valve) into the regurgitant orifice, facilitating identification of

FIGURE 12–20. 2D *(above)* and color flow *(below)* images in parasternal long-axis *(left)* and short-axis *(right)* views in a patient with aortic valve dehiscence due to endocarditis and paraprosthetic aortic regurgitation. 2D imaging shows an echolucent space anterior to the sewing ring *(arrows)*. Color flow imaging shows abnormal, diastolic flow anterior to the prosthesis in a long-axis view with a circumferential pattern of regurgitation seen in the short-axis view. (See Color Plate 13, p. 274.)

FIGURE 12–21. Continuous-wave Doppler (CWD) in the same patient as in Figure 12–20 shows an aortic regurgitant signal of equal intensity to antegrade flow with a steep deceleration slope consistent with acute, severe aortic regurgitation (AR).

the paraprosthetic origin of the signal. Immediately after implantation, a small degree of paraprosthetic regurgitation may be normal on intraoperative transesophageal echocardiography and usually does not have long-term adverse clinical consequences.

Other Echocardiographic Findings in Prosthetic Valve Dysfunction (Table 12–7)

In addition to direct imaging or Doppler interrogation of the prosthetic valve itself, several other findings on the echocardiographic examination are integrated in the overall interpretation of prosthetic valve function.

1. The response of the cardiac chambers in terms of size, hypertrophy, and systolic function should be considered. For example, persistent left ventricular hypertrophy after aortic

FIGURE 12–22. With a pulsed Doppler sample volume (SV) in the proximal abdominal aorta *(above)* in the same patient as in Figure 12–20, prominent holodiastolic *(arrow)* flow reversal *(below)* is seen, again consistent with severe aortic regurgitation.

TABLE 12–7	**Echocardiographic Signs of Prosthetic Valve Dysfunction**

Increased antegrade velocity across the valve

Decreased valve area (continuity equation or $T\frac{1}{2}$)

Increased regurgitation on color flow

Increased intensity of continuous-wave Doppler regurgitant signal

Progressive chamber dilation

Persistent left ventricular hypertrophy

Recurrent pulmonary hypertension

valve replacement for aortic stenosis raises the possibility of prosthetic valve stenosis. In other cases, left ventricular dilation may suggest aortic or mitral prosthetic regurgitation with resultant volume overload. A hyperdynamic (but previously normal) left ventricle may indicate prosthetic mitral regurgitation. While it may be difficult in some patients to separate persistent postoperative abnormalities from new pathologic findings, a change between examinations is of concern.

2. The antegrade velocity across the prosthetic valve is evaluated. An increase in antegrade velocity may be due to increased volume flow as a result of prosthetic regurgitation rather than prosthetic stenosis. In this case, while the calculated gradient will be higher, the valve area will be unchanged. Alternatively, an increased flow velocity across the prosthetic valve may be due to a high cardiac output state (such as fever, anemia, or anxiety). In this situation, antegrade velocities across the other cardiac valves will be increased proportionately.

3. Pulmonary artery pressures are estimated and compared with previous studies in that patient. While pulmonary hypertension can persist after successful mitral valve surgery, *recurrent* pulmonary hypertension (after an initial postoperative decline) may relate to prosthetic valve dysfunction.

An incidental finding in some patients with a prosthetic valve is the phenomenon of *spontaneous contrast*. This phenomenon is similar to the spontaneous left atrial contrast seen in patients with an enlarged left atrium and low-velocity flow, which has been reported to be associated with a high propensity for thrombus formation. With a prosthetic valve, the appearance of echogenic particles downstream from the valve can occur even in the absence of a low flow state. The presumed mechanism of spontaneous contrast with a prosthetic valve is microcavitation due to impact of the occluder against the sewing ring and this phenomenon is more common with mechanical valves.

TECHNICAL ASPECTS/LIMITATIONS/ALTERNATE APPROACHES

Echocardiographic Approach to the Patient with a Prosthetic Valve

Transthoracic Examination

During the transthoracic echocardiographic examination of the patient with a prosthetic valve, attention is focused on

1. The antegrade velocity across the valve in relation to the size, type, and position of the implanted prosthesis

2. Calculation of mean gradient and valve area when stenosis is suspected

3. A careful search for prosthetic valve regurgitation using both color flow imaging and continuous-wave Doppler

4. Evaluation of chamber sizes, wall thickness, and systolic function

5. Estimation of pulmonary artery pressure

These data then are evaluated in conjunction with clinical data and in comparison with previous examinations.

The echocardiographic windows and technical details of data recording are the same for prosthetic valves as for native valve disease. Thus the antegrade velocity curve across a prosthetic mitral valve typically is recorded from an apical approach with either pulsed or continuous-wave Doppler (although sometimes a parasternal approach provides a more parallel intercept angle), while an aortic prosthesis requires a meticulous examination with continuous-wave Doppler from multiple windows (apical, suprasternal, right parasternal) with careful transducer angulation to obtain the highest-velocity signal.

The approaches used for native valve regurgitation also apply to prosthetic valves. The major technical difference between examination of a native and a prosthetic valve is the problem of acoustic shadowing. This problem may be circumvented by careful image acquisition or the use of unusual image planes (e.g., mitral regurgitation from a suprasternal notch approach), but transesophageal echocardiography clearly is a more sensitive technique in this situation.

Transesophageal Examination

When prosthetic valve dysfunction is suspected on clinical grounds or on the basis of transthoracic echocardiography, transesophageal imaging is indicted. However, both transthoracic and transesophageal imaging are needed for complete clinical evaluation.

Mitral Valve. For a mitral valve prosthesis, 2D images are recorded from a high transesophageal position using a high-frequency transducer with optimization of depth and other instrument settings. Starting from the four-chamber image plane, the image plane is slowly rotated to the long-axis plane, taking care to ensure the valve remains centered in the image plane. Color flow images then are recorded as the image plane is slowly rotated back to the four-chamber plane. Adjustment of transducer position and angulation may be needed to fully demonstrate the extent of an eccentric regurgitant jet. If a regurgitant jet is detected, careful rotation and angulation may allow visualization of the vena contracta and proximal flow acceleration region.

In some cases, images in a short-axis view can be obtained from a low esophageal position and provide a cross-sectional view of the regurgitant jet origin. Transgastric views are rarely helpful due to shadowing of the left atrium by the prosthesis from this approach.

Pulsed Doppler is used from the transesophageal approach to measure the antegrade velocity across the mitral prosthesis for calculation of mean gradient and pressure half-time. Flow in each of the pulmonary veins is recorded to evaluate for systolic flow reversal.

Continuous-wave Doppler allows recording of the mitral regurgitant jet either from the high esophageal position or from a transgastric apical view. Signal strength of the regurgitant jet relative to antegrade flow may be helpful in evaluation of severity. However, accurate measurement of peak velocity and the rate of change in pressure over time *(dP/dt)* should be made from transthoracic recordings as it is difficult to ensure a parallel intercept angle with the regurgitant jet from the limited transducer positions available on transesophageal echocardiography.

In addition to direct evaluation of the mitral prosthesis, the transesophageal examination should include evaluation of right and left ventricular size and systolic function, albeit the left ventricle is now shadowed by the mitral prosthesis. The tricuspid jet may be recorded for estimation of pulmonary pressures but again, the possibility of underestimation of velocity from the transesophageal approach should be considered.

Aortic Valve. Transesophageal imaging is needed less often for suspected aortic valve prosthetic dysfunction as the severity of regurgitation and stenosis can be accurately evaluated on transthoracic imaging since the prosthesis does not shadow the left ventricular outflow tract. Transesophageal imaging is most useful for evaluation of the posterior aspect of the sewing ring and for detection of paravalvular abscess. The aortic prosthesis is evaluated on 2D imaging beginning in an anteriorly angulated four-chamber view and then slowly rotating to the long-axis view. The short-axis view (at about 45°) also is helpful, with movement of the transducer to examine the subvalvular and supravalvular regions. Color flow imaging in each of these views allows evaluation of aortic regurgitant severity, although anterior paravalvular leaks may be missed due to shadowing by the valve prosthesis.

Continuous-wave Doppler recording of the antegrade and retrograde flows across the aortic prosthesis sometimes can be obtained from an anteriorly angulated transgastric apical four-chamber view but underestimation of velocity can occur due to a nonparallel intercept angle. It rarely is possible to adequately evaluate flow reversal in the descending thoracic aorta from the transesophageal approach, so these data should be obtained on transthoracic imaging.

Limitations and Alternate Approaches

As repeatedly emphasized in this chapter, the major limitation of transthoracic echocardiography for evaluation of prosthetic valves is technical, specifically reverberations, artifacts, and acoustic shadowing. The last of these problems can be circumvented to some extent with the transesophageal approach by casting the shadow in the opposite direction. Reverberations and other ultrasound artifacts remain a problem with both approaches.

Other limitations are overestimation of transvalvular pressure gradients with bileaflet mechanical valves, limited validation of valve area calculations for mechanical valves, and the problem of differentiating "normal" from pathologic prosthetic valve regurgitation.

Importantly, the same factors that can lead to errors in evaluation of native valves also are significant limitations in evaluation of prosthetic valves. Most notably, these factors include ultrasound tissue penetration, Doppler intercept-angle assumptions, accurate measurement of 2D images, correct image orientation, and correct identification of the origin of Doppler signals.

When the echocardiographic examination is negative or yields results discordant with other clinical findings, other diagnostic procedures may be indicated. Cardiac catheterization can be performed with direct measurement of intracardiac pressures to confirm the pressure gradient across the valve and measure pulmonary artery pressures. In combination with cardiac output measurement, Gorlin formula valve area and pulmonary vascular resistance can be calculated. For some mechanical valves, catheterization may be complicated by a risk of inducing valve dysfunction if a catheter is passed retrograde across the valve. In these cases, evaluation of a mechanical aortic valve requires transseptal catheterization with measurement of left ventricular pressures by advancing the catheter across the mitral valve into the left ventricle. With a mitral valve prosthesis, transseptal catheterization is more reliable than the pulmonary wedge pressure in evaluating the left atrial to left ventricular pressure gradient. In a patient with both a mechanical aortic and mitral valve, measurement of left ventricular pressure may require direct left ventricular puncture.

Angiographic evaluation (left ventricle for mitral regurgitation, aortic root for aortic regurgitation) is helpful in evaluating prosthetic regurgitation on a semiquantitative (0 to 4+) scale or for calculating regurgitant volumes and fractions in conjunction with other quantitative cardiac output data.

Fluoroscopy of the valve is important for some valve types. For bileaflet and single-disk mechanical valves, the angle of opening can be measured from a view oriented perpendicular to the plane of the open leaflet(s). In a small number of now discontinued valve models, the occluder undergoes degeneration, resulting in a smaller size that can be detected by fluoroscopic measurements. None of the valves prone to this type of wear (and subsequent leaflet escape) are currently implanted, and there are few patients with these prostheses still in place.

Neither magnetic resonance imaging nor computed tomographic imaging has proved particularly helpful in evaluation of prosthetic valves. Newer approaches to imaging regurgitant jets with these techniques may yield useful data in the future.

CLINICAL UTILITY

Prosthetic Valve Stenosis

Echocardiography is the initial diagnostic approach to evaluation of suspected prosthetic valve stenosis. The antegrade velocity and mean gradient across the prosthetic valve, particularly in comparison with previous data in that patient, may be diagnostic. Valve area can be calculated by the continuity equation for valves in the aortic (Fig. 12–23) or pulmonic position and by the pressure half-time method for valves in the mitral or tricuspid (Fig. 12–24) position. Despite the overestimation of the average transvalvular gradient that occurs with Doppler evaluation of bileaflet mechanical valves, this approach still is helpful in assessing changes over time in an individual patient.

The differential diagnosis of an increased antegrade velocity across the valve includes a high cardiac output state or coexisting valvular re-

FIGURE 12–23. A 46-year-old man with chronic renal failure and a porcine valve replacement 8 years ago presented with presyncope. Echocardiography showed severely reduced left ventricular systolic function, a left ventricular outflow tract velocity of only 0.4 m/s *(top)*, and an aortic jet of 4 m/s *(middle)*. Continuity equation valve area was 0.5 cm². At autopsy, the porcine valve leaflets were severely calcified and stiff *(bottom)*.

gurgitation, as well as prosthetic valve stenosis. A significant prosthetic or paraprosthetic regurgitant jet can increase the antegrade volume flow rate across the valve substantially, resulting in a high velocity and a high transvalvular gradient. Valve area, however, remains relatively normal.

With careful examination techniques, the antegrade velocity across the prosthetic valve can be recorded in nearly all patients. When signal strength is suboptimal, invasive evaluation may be required. This is most likely for evaluation of a prosthetic valve in a conduit (typically right ventricle or right atrium to pulmonary artery). In this situation, the valve is difficult to image due to shadowing by the vascular graft, and it is difficult to obtain a window where the Doppler beam is parallel to flow across the prosthetic valve.

Prosthetic Valve Regurgitation

Transthoracic echocardiography is accurate for the diagnosis of prosthetic aortic valve regurgitation and for the differentiation of normal from pathologic regurgitation (Fig. 12–25). Standard methods for evaluating regurgitant severity can be used for aortic valve prostheses. Because of acoustic shadowing, the sensitivity for detection of mitral prosthetic regurgitation is lower, and it is more difficult to distinguish normal from pathologic regurgitation. Transesophageal echocardiography imaging is needed when this diagnosis is suspected on clinical grounds. Transesophageal echocardiography has a high accuracy for detection of prosthetic regurgitation and reliably distinguishes transprosthetic from paraprosthetic regurgitation.

Prosthetic Valve Endocarditis

Detection of valvular vegetations on prosthetic valves is difficult with transthoracic echocardiography due to reverberations and acoustic shadowing. Features that might increase the suspicion of prosthetic valve endocarditis on a transthoracic echocardiographic examination include Doppler evidence of valve dysfunction (either regurgitation due to incomplete closure or stenosis due to an infected pannus on the inflow surface of the valve), evidence of valve instability (i.e., "rocking" on 2D images), an unexplained increase in pulmonary artery pressures, or an interval change in chamber dimensions. Prosthetic valve endocarditis often involves the sewing ring and annulus, resulting in formation of a paravalvular abscess ("ring" abscess) rather than the typical vegetation seen with

FIGURE 12–24. A 36-year-old man with a prior tricuspid valve replacement for endocarditis presented with right-sided heart failure. The apical four-chamber view showed a severely calcified porcine tricuspid valve replacement *(above)* with an increased antegrade velocity and prolonged pressure half-time *(below)*.

native valve infection. Identification of an abscess may be limited on transthoracic echocardiography (Fig. 12–26).

Thus, given the technical and pathologic peculiarities of evaluation of suspected prosthetic valve endocarditis, transesophageal imaging is needed in the majority of these patients. Transesophageal echocardiography has a high sensitivity for detection of prosthetic valve endocarditis and/or abscess formation. As for native

valve endocarditis (see Chap. 13), cardiac abscesses may be echodense or relatively echo-free (Fig. 12–27).

Prosthetic Valve Thrombosis

In patients with embolic events presumed secondary to prosthetic valve thrombosis, even transesophageal echocardiographic results may be negative if the thrombi are small or if new thrombus has not formed since the embolic event. When thrombi are documented on transesophageal echocardiography, this finding may be important in patient management in some cases. However, an embolic event in a patient with a prosthetic valve (especially mechanical) presumably is related to the presence of a prosthetic valve even if transesophageal echocardiography is negative. Thus the potential clinical implications of the study results should be considered *before* the examination. If the treatment and subsequent management would be the same whether or not a thrombus is documented, then transesophageal echocardiogra-

phy may be unnecessary. If documentation of thrombus or exclusion of other possible abnormalities would affect patient management, then transesophageal echocardiography examination is appropriate. Of course, infected pannus due to prosthetic valve endocarditis cannot be differentiated from thrombus on 2D imaging. Careful clinical and bacteriologic correlation is

FIGURE 12–25. A 60-year-old man with a previous porcine aortic valve replacement presented with congestive heart failure. Angiography *(above)* showed severe prosthetic aortic regurgitation (the left ventricle is densely opacified with an aortic root contrast injection). Echocardiography was technically limited due to poor ultrasound tissue penetration, but the continuous-wave Doppler signal *(below)* is diagnostic for significant aortic regurgitation.

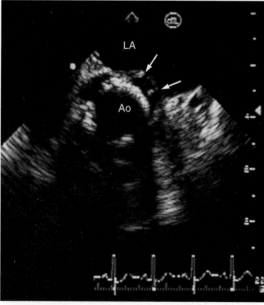

FIGURE 12–26. Prosthetic valve endocarditis of a porcine valve in the aortic position. The vegetation *(arrow)* is seen on the transthoracic parasternal long-axis view *(above)*, but the paravalvular abscess *(arrows)* was diagnosed on transesophageal imaging *(below)*.

FIGURE 12–27. Prosthetic valve endocarditis of a mitral porcine valve seen on transesophageal imaging with a large vegetation prolapsing into the left ventricle in diastole *(above)* and into the left atrium in systole *(below)*.

FIGURE 12–28. Transesophageal view of thrombus *(T)* on the left atrial side of a bileaflet mechanical valve in a 56-year-old woman who was noncompliant with Warfarin therapy.

lishing baseline Doppler findings in each patient soon after implantation serves as a reference point should prosthetic valve dysfunction be suspected in the future. Approximately 6 to 8 weeks after surgery is a reasonable time to obtain this baseline study because the patient has recovered from surgery, is returning to cardiology follow-up, and has stable hemodynamic status with a normal cardiac output. This timing of the examination also allows an initial evaluation of regression of left ventricular hypertrophy or dilation, recovery of left ventricular systolic function, changes in pulmonary artery pressures, and other long-term effects of the valve surgery.

SUGGESTED READING

General Reviews

1. Nottestad SY, Zabalgoitia M: Echocardiographic recognition and quantitation of prosthetic valve dysfunction. *In* Otto CM (ed): The Practice of Clinical Echocardiography. Philadelphia, WB Saunders, 1997, pp. 797–820.

  Advanced level review and discussion of echocardiographic evaluation of prosthetic valve dysfunction. Numerous tables summarize normal values for prosthetic valves and findings reported with abnormal valve function. Excellent photographs and echocardiographic images of each valve type. Complications reviewed include mechanical failure, thrombosis, endocarditis, patient-prosthesis mismatch, prosthetic stenosis, and regurgitation. 109 references.

needed whenever an abnormal valve-associated mass is observed (Fig. 12–28).

"Routine" Follow-up of Prosthetic Valve Function

While it is difficult to justify routine periodic echocardiographic examinations of prosthetic valve function in clinically stable patients, the importance of a baseline examination in each patient with a prosthetic valve should not be overlooked. There is wide variability in normal antegrade velocities and in the degree of "normal" regurgitation across prosthetic valves even for a given size, type, and position. Estab-

2. Vongpatanasin W, Hillis LD, Lange RA: Prosthetic heart valves. *N Engl J Med* 335:407–416, 1996.

Concise review of the clinical aspects of prosthetic valve function and dysfunction. Excellent description and chart of the normal and abnormal auscultatory findings for each valve type.

Normal Doppler Flow Patterns

3. Yoganathan AP, Heinrich RS, Fontaine AA: Fluid dynamics of prosthetic valves. *In* Otto CM (ed): The Practice of Clinical Echocardiography. Philadelphia, WB Saunders, 1997, pp. 773–796.

Review of the basic principles of fluid dynamics and the application of fluid dynamics to evaluation of prosthetic heart valves. Extensive tables summarize in vitro data for each valve type and size. Illustrations show the flow patterns for each valve type. Mathematical descriptions of fluid dynamics are included.

4. Reisner SA, Meltzer RS: Normal values of prosthetic valve Doppler echocardiographic parameters: A review. *J Am Soc Echocardiogr* 1:201–210, 1988.

Summary of normal Doppler velocities across prosthetic valves, including data from 18 studies with a total of 1105 patients. 32 references.

5. Zabalgoitia M: Echocardiographic assessment of prosthetic heart valves. *Curr Prob Cardiol* 17:269–325, 1992.

Review of echocardiographic evaluation of prosthetic valve function. 203 references.

6. Jones M, McMillan ST, Eidbo EE, et al: Evaluation of prosthetic heart valves by Doppler flow imaging. *Echocardiography* 3:513–525, 1986.

Description of laser Doppler anemometry flow characteristics of prosthetic valves in comparison with color Doppler flow patterns. Flow velocity profiles and turbulence patterns are shown for several valve types.

7. Jaffe WM, Coverdale HA, Roche AHG, et al: Doppler echocardiography in the assessment of the homograft aortic valve. *Am J Cardiol* 63:1466–1470, 1989.

Doppler echocardiographic findings in 27 patients with normal functioning aortic homograft valves and 30 patients with suspected valve dysfunction. Significant regurgitation of the aortic homograft was unlikely with an antegrade velocity <2.0 m/s.

8. Sagar KB, Wann LS, Paulsen WHJ, Romhilt DW: Doppler echocardiographic evaluation of Hancock and Bjork-Shiley prosthetic valves. *J Am Coll Cardiol* 7:681–687, 1986.

Doppler echocardiographic findings in 50 patients with clinically normal valve function and 46 patients with suspected prosthetic valve dysfunction.

9. Connolly HM, Miller FA Jr, Taylor CL, et al: Doppler hemodynamic profiles of 82 clinically and echocardiographically normal tricuspid valve prostheses. *Circulation* 88:2722–2727, 1993.

In 41 patients with clinically normal heterograft tricuspid valves, Doppler echo studies showed a mean early filling velocity of 1.3 ± 0.2 m/s, a mean gradient of 3.2 ± 1.1 mmHg, and a pressure half-time of 146 ± 39 ms. In 22%, mild prosthetic regurgitation was detected. Values were similar for ball-cage, bileaflet, and tilting-disk valve prostheses.

Validation of Doppler Echo Pressure Gradients

10. Baumgartner H, Khan S, DeRobertis M, et al: Discrepancies between Doppler and catheter gradients in aortic prosthetic valves in vitro. A manifestation of localized gradients and pressure recovery. *Circulation* 82:1467–1475, 1990.

In vitro study emphasizing the importance of pressure recovery downstream from the valve as a cause of discrepancies between Doppler and invasive pressure gradient measurements, with an overestimation of 13% ± 11% for mean gradients across the Hancock bioprosthetic valve. High localized gradients in the narrow central orifice at the valve plane of the St. Jude (bileaflet) valve were measured accurately by Doppler echo. However, this localized gradient was greater than the gradient measured 30 mm downstream from the valve.

11. Wilkins GT, Gillam LD, Kritzer GL, et al: Validation of continuous-wave Doppler echocardiographic measurements of mitral and tricuspid prosthetic valve gradients: A simultaneous Doppler-catheter study. *Circulation* 74:786–795, 1986.

Simultaneous Doppler and catheter pressure gradients were measured across prosthetic mitral valves in 12 patients, showing an excellent correlation for both porcine and mechanical valves.

12. Burstow DJ, Nishimura RA, Bailey KR, et al: Continuous wave Doppler echocardiographic measurement of prosthetic valve gradients. A simultaneous Doppler-catheter correlative study. *Circulation* 80:504–514, 1989.

Simultaneous Doppler and catheter pressure gradients were measured in 36 patients. Correlations for maximum and mean pressure gradients were excellent for both aortic and mitral prostheses and for bioprosthetic and mechanical valves.

13. Stewart SFC, Nast EP, Arabia FA, et al: Errors in pressure gradient measurement by continuous-wave Doppler ultrasound: Type, size and age effects in bioprosthetic aortic valves. *J Am Coll Cardiol* 18:769–779, 1991.

Consistent overestimation of pressure gradients across prosthetic valves as measured by Doppler echocardiography was observed in detailed in vitro studies of four types of bioprosthetic valves. Pressure recovery downstream did not account for this overestimation. Instead, this error may be related to neglect of proximal velocities in the Bernoulli equation. For example, a mean proximal velocity of 0.66 ± 0.02 m/s at a mean flow rate of 5.6 L/min would result in an error of 1.74 ± 0.10 mmHg for mean gradient and 3.48 ± 0.21 mmHg for maximum gradient. These differences are even larger at higher flow rates.

14. Baumgartner H, Khan S, DeRobertis M, et al: Effect of prosthetic aortic valve design on the Doppler-catheter gradient correlation: An in vitro study of normal St. Jude, Medtronic-Hall, Starr-Edwards and Hancock valves. *J Am Coll Cardiol* 19:324–332, 1992.

This in vitro study shows that smaller valve sizes have higher antegrade velocities and pressure gradients than larger valve sizes. The 19-mm St. Jude and Han-

cock valves can have velocities as high as 4.7 m/s with a gradient of 89 mmHg even with normal prosthetic valve function. Doppler gradients consistently overestimated catheter gradients for St. Jude and Starr-Edwards valves (differences as great as 44 mmHg were seen). Agreement was closer for Hancock and Medtronic-Hall valves.

Prosthetic Valve Area

15. Chafizadeh ER, Zoghbi WA: Doppler echocardiographic assessment of the St. Jude medical prosthetic valve in the aortic position using the continuity equation. *Circulation* 83:213–223, 1991.

    In 67 patients with recent implantation (and clinically normal valve function) of St. Jude aortic valve prostheses, continuity equation valve areas (0.73 to 4.23 cm²) correlated well with the reported actual orifice area (r = 0.83). The Doppler velocity index—the ratio of left ventricular outflow tract to aortic jet velocity—provides a useful simple index of valve function and is less dependent on valve size.

16. Baumgartner H, Khan SS, DeRobertis M, et al: Doppler assessment of prosthetic valve orifice area: An in vitro study. *Circulation* 85:2275–2283, 1992.

    Continuity equation valve areas correlated well with invasively derived Gorlin formula valve areas for St. Jude, Medtronic-Hall, and Hancock aortic valves in a pulsatile flow model. However, valve area of St. Jude valves was significantly underestimated due to the localized high velocities in the narrow central orifice. Valve areas decrease with low flow in Hancock valves consistent with incomplete opening of the leaflets at low flow rates.

17. Rothbart RM, Castriz JL, Harding LV, et al: Determination of aortic valve area by two-dimensional and Doppler echocardiography in patients with normal and stenotic bioprosthetic valves. *J Am Coll Cardiol* 15:817–824, 1990.

    In 22 patients undergoing catheterization for suspected dysfunction of bioprosthetic aortic valves, Doppler continuity equation valve areas agreed well with invasively determined Gorlin valve areas.

18. Dumesnil JG, Honos GN, Lemieux M, Beauchemin J: Validation and applications of indexed aortic prosthetic valve areas calculated by Doppler echocardiography. *J Am Coll Cardiol* 16:637–643, 1990.

    In 31 patients with a Medtronics Intact Bioprosthesis in the aortic position, both standard and simplified continuity equation valve areas correlated well with in vivo and known in vitro prosthetic valve areas (r = 0.86, SEE = 0.16 cm²).

19. Baumgartner H, Schima H, Kuhn P: Effect of prosthetic valve malfunction on the Doppler-catheter gradient relation for bileaflet aortic valve prostheses. *Circulation* 87:1320–1327, 1993.

    Malfunction of bileaflet mechanical valves was simulated in a pulsatile flow model by restricting opening of one leaflet. While Doppler and catheter gradients correlated well for each degree of prosthetic valve stenosis, the slope of the regression line progressively approached 1 with increasing stenosis. Thus, while Doppler overestimates bileaflet prosthetic valve gradients with normal valve function, the Doppler gradients are accurate when stenosis is present. The mechanism of this observation most likely is a reduction in the central orifice size. Clinically, these findings suggest that the development of stenosis of a bileaflet mechanical valve may not be reflected in increases in velocity across the prosthesis.

20. Chambers JB, Cochrane T, Black MM, Jackson G: The Gorlin formula validated against directly observed orifice area in porcine mitral bioprostheses. *J Am Coll Cardiol* 13:348–353, 1989.

    In an in vitro pulsatile flow system, measured orifice area and the modified Gorlin relation (Q/V_{max}) correlated well (r = 0.88). Maximum valve orifice area, measured by a high-speed video camera, decreased at low flow rates for all four Carpentier-Edwards prostheses.

Natural History of Doppler Echo Findings

21. Reimold SC, Yoganathan AP, Sung H-W, et al: Doppler echocardiographic study of porcine bioprosthetic heart valves in the aortic valve position in patients without evidence of cardiac dysfunction. *Am J Cardiol* 67:611–615, 1991.

    Several studies over 5 years showed a decrease in Doppler-derived effective orifice area >0.20 cm² in 10 of 16 patients. The mean decrease in effective orifice area was 0.25 ± 0.29 cm² (at 34 ± 1 month follow-up) with an increase in mean gradient from 12 ± 4 to 15 ± 7 mmHg.

Exercise Studies with Prosthetic Valves

22. Leavitt JI, Coats MH, Falk RH: Effects of exercise on transmitral gradient and pulmonary artery pressure in patients with mitral stenosis or a prosthetic mitral valve: A Doppler echocardiographic study. *J Am Coll Cardiol* 17:1520–1526, 1991.

    The feasibility of measurements of transmitral mean gradient and pulmonary artery pressure immediately after exercise was demonstrated in 12 patients with mitral stenosis and 11 patients with a normally functioning prosthetic valve (10 of 11 mechanical). Mean gradient increased from 5 ± 2 to 8 ± 3 mmHg and pulmonary artery systolic pressure from 28 ± 8 to 39 ± 16 mmHg with an increase in heart rate from 79 ± 9 to 104 ± 21 bpm with exercise in the prosthetic valve patients.

23. van den Brink RB, Verhuel HA, Visser CA, et al: Value of exercise Doppler echocardiography in patients with prosthetic or bioprosthetic cardiac valves. *Am J Cardiol* 69:367–372, 1992.

    In 61 asymptomatic patients with an aortic (n = 24) or mitral (n = 39) prosthetic valve, postexercise Doppler data could be obtained within 60 seconds in 92%. In the mitral group, heart rate increased from 80 ± 12 to 116 ± 14 bpm, mean gradient from 6 to 14 mmHg, and pulmonary artery systolic pressure from 34 to 57 mmHg. In the aortic group, heart rate increased from 74 ± 10 to 105 ± 18 bpm and mean gradient from 24 (range 12 to 50) to 39 (range 18 to 100) mmHg.

Prosthetic Valve Regurgitation

24. Baumgartner H, Khan S, DeRobertis M, et al: Color Doppler regurgitant characteristics of normal mechanical mitral valve prostheses in vitro. *Circulation* 85:323–332, 1992.

    Patterns of normal regurgitation for bileaflet and tilting-disk mechanical mitral valves in a pulsatile flow model are described. Bileaflet valves showed two converging jets from the pivot points, a small central jet, and a variable number of peripheral jets. Normal bileaflet regurgitant jets showed little signal aliasing. Tilting-disk (with a central strut and hole) valves showed a large central jet and one or two small peripheral jets. The large central jet showed aliasing extending distally into the atrium.

25. Flachskampf FA, O'Shea JP, Griffin BP, et al: Patterns of normal transvalvular regurgitation in mechanical valve prostheses. *J Am Coll Cardiol* 18:1493–1498, 1991.

    In an in vitro system, bileaflet valves showed peripheral convergent jets in a plane parallel to the two disk axes and several diverging jets in the orthogonal place. Tilting-disk (with central strut and hole) valves showed a prominent central jet with minor jets along the periphery of the disk.

26. Bargiggia GS, Tronconi L, Raisaro A, et al: Color Doppler diagnosis of mechanical prosthetic mitral regurgitation: Usefulness of the flow convergence region proximal to the regurgitant orifice. *Am Heart J* 120:1137–1142, 1990.

    On transthoracic imaging, identification of flow acceleration on the left ventricular side of the prosthesis aids in identifying the presence and location of prosthetic regurgitation. Proximal acceleration was detected in 19 of 20 (95%) of the subgroup with mechanical prosthetic mitral regurgitation, whereas a jet in the left atrium was detected in only 12 of 20 (60%) due to acoustic shadowing of the left atrium.

Transesophageal Echocardiography

27. Khandheria BK, Seward JB, Oh JK, et al: Value and limitations of transesophageal echocardiography in assessment of mitral valve prostheses. *Circulation* 83: 1956–1968, 1991.

    In reviewing the clinical experience at the Mayo Clinic, 50 patients with a prosthetic mitral valve had a transesophageal study followed by confirmatory cardiac catheterization, surgery, or both. For mechanical valves, 10 of 25 (40%) were considered abnormal on transthoracic echocardiography, while 16 of 25 (64%) had abnormalities detected on transesophageal echocardiography. Findings were concordant at surgery in 20 of 23 (87%). For bioprosthetic valves, 9 of 25 (36%) had an abnormal prosthesis on transthoracic echocardiography, while 20 of 25 (80%) had an abnormal transesophageal echocardiography examination. Transesophageal echocardiographic findings were confirmed at surgery in all cases.

28. Alton ME, Pasierski TJ, Orsinelli DA, et al: Comparison of transthoracic and transesophageal echocardiography in evaluation of 47 Starr-Edwards prosthetic valves. *J Am Coll Cardiol* 20:1503–1511, 1992.

    The high sensitivity of transesophageal echocardiography for detection of prosthetic valve vegetations, abscess formation, and thrombus is emphasized in this study of 37 patients with 47 Starr-Edwards valves. All the normal mitral valves (13) had a small degree of early systolic mitral regurgitation with a central jet directed posteriorly.

29. Karalis DG, Chandrasekaran K, Ross JJ Jr, et al: Single-plane transesophageal echocardiography for assessing function of mechanical or bioprosthetic valves in the aortic valve position. *Am J Cardiol* 69:1310–1315, 1992.

    In 89 patients, with 69 mechanical and 20 bioprosthetic aortic valves, transesophageal echocardiography was superior to transthoracic echocardiography for evaluation of prosthetic aortic regurgitation only when transthoracic echocardiographic image quality was poor. Transesophageal echocardiography was superior for detection of perivalvular abscess, subaortic perforation, valve dehiscence, and abnormal bioprosthetic valve cusps, as well as in differentiating valvular from paravalvular regurgitation.

30. Daniel WG, Mugge A, Grote J, et al: Comparison of transthoracic and transesophageal echocardiography for detection of abnormalities of prosthetic and bioprosthetic valves in the mitral and aortic positions. *Am J Cardiol* 71:210–215, 1993.

    In 126 patients with 148 prosthetic valves (35 mechanical, 113 bioprosthetic), transesophageal echocardiography had a higher sensitivity (35 of 41, 85%) than transthoracic echocardiography (13 of 41, 32%) for detection of prosthetic valve endocarditis and thrombi. Transesophageal echocardiography also had a higher sensitivity for anatomic bioprosthetic valve abnormalities (87% versus 65%).

31. Barbetseas J, Crawford ES, Sail HJ, et al: Doppler echocardiographic evaluation of pseudoaneurysms complicating composite grafts of the ascending aorta. *Circulation* 85:212–222, 1992.

    Description of the echo Doppler findings in eight patients with pseudoaneurysms of ascending aortic grafts. An echo-free space adjacent (often posterior) to the aortic graft with flow from the graft lumen into the pseudoaneurysm is seen. Identification is facilitated by transesophageal echocardiography imaging when image quality is suboptimal on a transthoracic echocardiographic approach.

32. Garcia MJ, Vandervoort P, Stewart WJ, et al: Mechanisms of hemolysis with mitral prosthetic regurgitation. Study using transesophageal echocardiography and fluid dynamic simulation. *J Am Coll Cardiol* 27: 399–406, 1996.

    In 27 patients with prosthetic regurgitation, echocardiographic factors associated with hemolysis (present in 16 patients) were examined. Hemolysis was associated with a paravalvular origin of the regurgitant jet (8/16 with hemolysis versus 2/11 without hemolysis). In addition, patterns of flow fragmentation, collision, or rapid acceleration were associated with hemolysis.

The Role of Echocardiography in Suspected or Definite Endocarditis

13

BASIC PRINCIPLES

ECHOCARDIOGRAPHIC APPROACH
Valvular Vegetations
Transthoracic Echocardiography
Transesophageal Imaging
Diagnostic Accuracy of Echocardiography for Detection of Vegetations
Functional Valvular Abnormalities Due to Endocarditis
Other Echocardiographic Findings
Diagnosis of Paravalvular Abscess and Intracardiac Fistula

LIMITATIONS/TECHNICAL CONSIDERATIONS
Active versus Healed Vegetations
Nonbacterial Thrombotic Endocarditis
Diagnosis of Vegetations with Underlying Valve Disease
Endocarditis of Prosthetic Valves

CLINICAL UTILITY
"Rule Out" Endocarditis
Cardiac Evaluation of the Patient with Endocarditis

SUGGESTED READING

Echocardiography is an essential component of the evaluation of a patient with infective endocarditis. In combination with clinical and bacteriologic data, the echocardiographic finding of a valvular vegetation allows an accurate diagnosis of endocarditis. In addition, echocardiographic assessment of the degree of valve dysfunction and detection of complications, such as a paravalvular abscess or fistula, are needed for optimal patient care.

While transthoracic echocardiography is adequate in some cases, transesophageal imaging is more sensitive and specific, both for the detection of valvular vegetations and for detection of complications. Further, demonstration of normal valve anatomy and function on transesophageal imaging reliably excludes endocarditis in patients in whom this diagnosis is suspected.

BASIC PRINCIPLES

The diagnosis of endocarditis is most secure when there is pathologic confirmation of a valvular vegetation with active infection, local tissue destruction, and/or paravalvular abscess formation. In the clinical setting, endocarditis is diagnosed based on a combination of echocar-diographic, laboratory, and physical examination findings as detailed in Table 13–1. The major criteria for the diagnosis of endocarditis are persistent bacteremia with typical organisms and echocardiographic evidence of endocardial involvement. Minor criteria include less specific bacteriologic and echocardiographic findings, factors predisposing to endocarditis (such as preexisting valve disease or intravenous drug use), vascular events (such as pulmonary or systemic emboli), immunologic phenomenon (such as glomerulonephritis), and signs of systemic infection (such as fever).

The goals of echocardiography in a patient with an infective endocarditis are:

1. To identify the presence, location, size, and number of valvular vegetations.

2. To assess functional abnormalities of the affected valve(s), especially valvular regurgitation.

3. To identify the underlying anatomy of the affected valve(s) and any coincident valvular disease.

4. To assess the impact of valvular disease on chamber dimensions and function, most importantly left ventricular size and systolic function.

329

TABLE 13–1	Duke Criteria for Definite Infective Endocarditis

Pathologic Criteria
Microorganisms: demonstrated by culture of histology in a vegetation, *or* in a vegetation that has embolized, *or* in an intracardiac abscess, *or*
  Pathologic lesions: vegetation or intracardiac abscess present, confirmed by histology showing active endocarditis

Clinical Criteria*
Major criteria
  Positive blood culture for infective endocarditis
    Typical microorganism for infective endocarditis from two separate blood cultures
      Viridans streptococci,† *Streptococcus bovis*, HACEK group, *or*
      Community-acquired *Staphylococcus aureus* or enterococci, in the absence of a primary focus, *or*
    Persistently positive blood culture, defined as recovery of a microorganism consistent with infective endocarditis from:
      (i) Blood cultures drawn more than 12 hours apart, *or*
      (ii) All of three or a majority of four or more separate blood cultures, with first and last drawn at least 1 hour apart
  Evidence of endocardial involvement
    Positive echocardiogram for infective endocarditis
      (i) Oscillating intracardiac mass, on valve or supporting structures, *or* in the path of regurgitant jets, *or* on implanted material, in the absence of an alternative anatomic explanation, *or*
      (ii) Abscess, *or*
      (iii) New partial dehiscence of prosthetic valve, *or*
    New valvular regurgitation (increase or change in preexisting murmur not sufficient)

Minor criteria
  Predisposition: predisposing heart condition *or* intravenous drug use
  Fever: ≥38.0°C (100.4°F)
  Vascular phenomena: major arterial emboli, septic pulmonary infarcts, mycotic aneurysm, intracranial hemorrhage, conjunctival hemorrhages, Janeway lesions
  Immunologic phenomena: glomerulonephritis, Osler's nodes, Roth's spots, rheumatoid factor
  Microbiologic evidence: positive blood culture but not meeting major criterion as noted previously‡ or serologic evidence of active infection with organism consistent with infective endocarditis
  Echocardiogram: consistent with infective endocarditis but not meeting major criterion as noted previously

HACEK = *Haemophilus* spp., *Actinobacillus actinomycetemcomitans*, *Cardiobacterium hominis*, *Eikenella* spp., and *Kingella kingae*.
*Two major criteria, *or* one major and three minor criteria, *or* five minor criteria.
†Including nutritional variant strains.
‡Excluding single positive cultures for coagulase-negative staphylococci and organisms that do not cause endocarditis.
From Durack DT, Lukes, AS, Bright DK: New criteria for diagnosis of infective endocarditis: Utilization of specific echocardiographic findings. Duke Endocarditis Service. *Am J Med* 96:200–209, 1994.

5. To identify other complications of endocarditis (e.g., paravalvular abscess, pericardial effusion).

6. To provide prognostic data on the anticipated clinical course, risk of systemic embolization, and potential need for surgical intervention.

In a patient with a lower likelihood of endocarditis on clinical grounds, an echocardiogram often is requested to "rule out" endocarditis. In this setting, the goals of the echocardiographic examination are:

1. Identification of any valvular vegetations.
2. Assessment of valve anatomy and function with respect to anatomic or physiologic

factors that increase the likelihood of endocarditis (e.g., bicuspid aortic valve, myxomatous mitral valve).

If an abnormality is identified, complete evaluation is directed toward the goals listed for clinical endocarditis.

ECHOCARDIOGRAPHIC APPROACH

Valvular Vegetations

Transthoracic Echocardiography

Although transesophageal echocardiography is more sensitive and specific than transthoracic echocardiography for detection of valvular vegetations, transthoracic echocardiography remains the initial procedure of choice in most cases due to the lower cost and risk of this approach.

On two-dimensional (2D) echocardiography, a valvular vegetation typically appears as an abnormal echogenic, irregular mass attached to the upstream side of the valve leaflet with a pattern of motion that is dependent on, but more chaotic than, normal valve motion. For example, an aortic valve vegetation prolapses into the left ventricular outflow tract in diastole and extends into the aortic root in systole (Fig. 13–1). The mass is attached to the left ventricular side of the valve leaflet but shows motion in excess of normal valve excursion with rapid oscillations in diastole (best appreciated on M-mode recordings). A mitral valve vegetation is attached on the atrial side of the valve, prolapses into the left atrium in systole, and moves into the left ventricle, beyond the normal range of mitral valve opening, in diastole (Fig. 13–2).

Valvular vegetations vary in size from so small as to be undetectable with current imaging techniques to greater than 3 cm in length. Vegetations may be attached at any area of the leaflet, although lesions at the coaptation line are most common. More than one valve can be involved, either by direct extension of infection or as a separate process, emphasizing the caveat that each valve requires careful examination even if a vegetation has been identified on another valve. In most cases, endocarditis occurs on a previously abnormal valve.

Multiple acoustic windows and 2D views are needed for detection of a valvular vegetation. First, since the vegetation is a discrete structure, it may be seen only in certain tomographic planes. Slow scanning between the standard image planes—for example, between the parasternal long-axis view and the right ventricular inflow view—increases the likelihood of identifying a valvular vegetation. Orthogonal views further ensure that all segments of the valve leaflets are examined. In a patient with suspected endocarditis, a complete examination is needed with scanning from parasternal, apical, subcostal, and suprasternal notch views for careful evaluation of each valve. The reported sensitivity of transthoracic echocardiography for detection of valvular vegetations ranges from less than 50% to as high as 90% (Table 13–2). To some extent, the reported sensitivity of transthoracic echocardiography increased between the advent of 2D instruments in the late 1970s and the improved image quality with advances in instrumentation in the 1980s.

Aortic Valve. Aortic valve vegetations most often are detected in parasternal long- and short-axis views. Careful angulation from medial to lateral in the long-axis plane and from inferior to superior in the short-axis plane is needed because vegetations often are eccentrically located. Image quality is optimized by use

Aortic Valve Vegetation

Diastole

Systole

FIGURE 13–1. Schematic diagram of an aortic valve vegetation attached to the ventricular side of the leaflet with prolapse into the left ventricular outflow tract in diastole. AR = aortic regurgitation.

Mitral Valve Vegetation

Diastole

Systole

FIGURE 13–2. Schematic diagram of a mitral valve vegetation attached to the atrial side of the leaflet with prolapse into the left atrium in systole. MR = mitral regurgitation.

| TABLE 13–2 | Accuracy of Echocardiographic Diagnosis of Valvular Vegetations (Selected Studies) | | | | | | |

First Author/ Year	Study Entry Criteria/Standard of Reference	No. of Valves	Percent Prosthetic	Transthoracic Echo		Transesophageal Echo	
				Sensitivity	Specificy	Sensitivity	Specificity
1. Mugge/ 1989	Definite endo-carditis *plus* surgery/autopsy	91	24%	53/91 (58%)	—	82/91 (90%)	—
2. Jaffe/1990	Definite endo-carditis *plus* surgery/autopsy	38	16%	38/44 (86%)	—	Not done	
3. Burger/ 1991	Suspected endo-carditis and clinical outcome	101	—	35/39 (90%)	61/62 (98%)	Not done	
4. Shively/ 1991	Suspected endo-carditis and clinical outcome	66	18%	7/16 (44%)	49/50 (98%)	15/16 (94%)	50/50 (100%)
5. Pedersen/ 1991	Suspected endo-carditis and clinical outcome	24	42%	5/10 (50%)	13/14 (93%)	10/10 (100%)	14/14 (100%)
6. Daniel/ 1993	Prosthetic valve with surgically confirmed endo-carditis	33	100%	12/33 (36%)	—	27/33 (82%)	—
7. Sochowski/ 1993	Suspected endo-carditis with ini-tially negative TTE study	65	32%	—	—	Negative predictive value = 56/65 (86%)	
8. Shapiro/ 1994	Suspected endo-carditis	68	—	23/34 (68%)	31/34 (91%)	33/34	31/34 (91%)

Data from Mugge et al: JACC 14:631–638, 1989; Jaffe et al: JACC 15:1227–1233, 1990; Burger et al: Angiology 42:552–560, 1991; Shiveley et al: JACC 18:391–397, 1991; Pedersen et al: Chest 100:351–356, 1991; Daniel et al: AJC 71:210–215, 1993; Sochowski and Chan: JACC 21:216–221, 1993; Shapiro et al: Chest 105:377, 1994.

of a minimum depth setting and adjustment of gain and processing parameters. An echogenic mass attached to the ventricular side of the leaflet with independent motion and prolapse into the outflow tract in diastole is diagnostic for a valvular vegetation (Fig. 13–3). Rapid os-cillating motion may be best appreciated on an M-mode recording.

Less typically, a vegetation may be attached to the aortic side of the leaflet or may show lit-tle independent motion. A definitive diagnosis may be difficult if the underlying valve anatomy is abnormal. For example, a vegetation on a calcified aortic valve may be difficult to visual-ize. In these cases, the findings of independent motion and prolapse into the left ventricle in di-astole are particularly helpful signs. Compari-son with previous echocardiograms may allow recognition of recent changes, increasing the

likelihood of valve infection, or may show no significant difference, decreasing the likelihood of an acute process.

Findings that may be mistaken for an aortic valve vegetation include beam-width artifact re-lated to either a calcified nodule, a prosthetic valve, the normal leaflet apposition zone, or the normal leaflet thickening at the central coapta-tion region (the nodule of Arantius). Occasion-ally, a linear echo representing a normal variant called a *Lambl's excrescence* is seen. These small fibroelastic protrusions from the ventric-ular side of the leaflet closure zone occur with increasing frequency with age and are present in a high percentage of patients. As image qual-ity improves, these normal structures are seen more frequently (Fig. 13–4).

Apical views of the aortic valve, both from an anteriorly angulated four-chamber view and from an apical long-axis view, may show an aortic valve vegetation. The finding of an abnormality in both parasternal and apical views decreases the likelihood of an ultrasound artifact, since the relationship of the ultrasound beam and aortic valve is entirely different from these two windows.

Two-dimensional imaging of a definite or suspected aortic valve vegetation is accompanied by evaluation of the functional abnormalities due to valve destruction, as discussed in the following sections.

Mitral Valve. Mitral valve vegetations typically are located on the atrial side of the leaflets. Diagnostic features include rapid independent motion, prolapse into the left atrium in systole, and functional evidence of valve dysfunction. Parasternal long- and short-axis views with careful scanning across the valve apparatus in both image planes allows assessment of the presence, size, and location of any vegetation (Fig. 13–5). Apical four-chamber, two-chamber, and long-axis views again are helpful both in visualizing valve and vegetation anatomy and in distinguishing a true valve mass from an ultrasound artifact.

As for the aortic valve, beam-width artifacts can be mistaken for a vegetation. A particular artifact to be aware of is the appearance of a "mass" on the atrial side of the anterior mitral leaflet in the apical four-chamber view due to beam-width artifact from a calcified or prosthetic aortic valve. Other types of mitral valve pathology may be difficult to distinguish from a valvular vegetation, including a severely myxomatous leaflet, a partial flail leaflet, or a ruptured papillary muscle (Fig. 13–6).

Again, comparison with previous studies may help differentiate an acute process from chronic underlying valve disease. With mitral

FIGURE 13–3. In a 29-year-old intravenous drug abuser with *S. aureus* endocarditis, aortic valve vegetations are seen in transthoracic parasternal long-axis *(above)* and short-axis *(below)* views. Irregularly shaped echogenic masses are attached to the ventricular side of the aortic valve leaflets with prolapse into the outflow tract in diastole (seen in the long-axis view) and extension into the aortic root in systole (seen in the short-axis view). Severe aortic regurgitation was present. The short-axis view also shows a paravalvular abscess *(three arrows)*.

FIGURE 13–4. Lambl's excrescence or beam-width artifact at the aortic closure line that might be mistaken for a valvular vegetation.

FIGURE 13-6. Abnormal valve (myxomatous) with flail leaflet *(arrow)* but no vegetation on transesophageal imaging. Angulation showed this "mass" to be a flail leaflet. The patient had no clinical evidence of endocarditis.

FIGURE 13-5. A 31-year-old woman with a history of intravenous drug abuse and *S. aureus* endocarditis has a typical-appearing mitral valve vegetation (VEG) seen in a parasternal long-axis view *(above)* and in a focused apical four-chamber view *(below)*. The mass is attached to the atrial side of the leaflets near the coaptation line with prolapse into the left atrium in systole and extension into the left ventricle in diastole.

valve endocarditis, mitral regurgitation typically, but not invariably, is present.

Tricuspid Valve. Tricuspid valve endocarditis occurs most often in intravenous drug abusers, is associated with large vegetations due to *Staphylococcus aureus* infection, and tends to have a better prognosis than left-sided valvular involvement.

The right ventricular inflow view often is diagnostic, showing a large, mobile mass of echoes attached to the atrial side of the leaflet with prolapse into the right atrium in systole (Fig. 13-7). Given the range of excursion and mobility of these vegetations, it is not surprising that septic pulmonary emboli are a frequent complication of tricuspid valve endocarditis.

The apical and subcostal four-chamber views allow further evaluation of the presence and extent of tricuspid valve infection. Assessment of tricuspid regurgitant severity and consequent right atrial and right ventricular dilation also can be performed from these windows.

Transesophageal Imaging

Transesophageal imaging clearly has a greater sensitivity for detection of vegetations. Some echocardiographers propose that transesophageal echocardiography should be performed whenever endocarditis is suspected. It is generally agreed that transesophageal echocardiography should be considered when transthoracic imaging is suboptimal or when the level of clinical suspicion is high and the presence of a valvular vegetation would affect therapy. It is noteworthy that the reported sensitivity of transthoracic echocardiography is highest from laboratories that did not have transesophageal echocardiography at the time of the study (studies 2 and 3 in Table 13-2). This supports the view that the sensitivity of the echocardiographic examination is directly related to the completeness and care with which the examination is performed. However, since transesophageal echocardiography clearly has a higher diagnostic accuracy, it should be used in appropriate clinical settings.

From the transesophageal approach, the aortic valve is examined in multiple image planes including a standard long-axis (typically at about 120° rotation) and short-axis (about 45° rotation) views. As with transthoracic imaging, careful scanning from medial to lateral in the long-axis view and from superior to inferior in the short-axis view is needed to fully evaluate valve anatomy and to achieve a high sensitivity for detection of valvular vegetations (Figs. 13–8 and 13–9). When the image plane is oblique, an aortic leaflet may be seen *en face*, mimicking an aortic valve mass. Evaluation in more than one image plane and assessment of the pattern of motion (rapid oscillating independent motion

versus motion *with* the valve) avoids this potential error. Since image quality tends to be superior from the transesophageal approach, small normal variants of valve anatomy may be appreciated and should not be interpreted as

FIGURE 13–8. Transesophageal long-axis view of the aortic valve showing valvular vegetations *(above)* and a flail aortic leaflet *(below)* with slight angulation of the image plane in a 75-year-old woman with endocarditis who died after emergency aortic valve replacement for severe acute aortic regurgitation.

FIGURE 13–7. Transthoracic imaging in a right ventricular inflow view of a 28-year-old woman with a history of intravenous drug use and *S. aureus* tricuspid valve endocarditis. In diastole *(above)*, a mobile mass is seen in the right ventricle attached to the tricuspid valve leaflet *(arrow)*. In systole *(below)* the vegetation (VEG) prolapses into the right atrium.

FIGURE 13–9. Color flow imaging in the same view as 13-8 *(bottom panel)* shows acute severe aortic regurgitation (AR) due to the flail leaflet in this patient. RPA = right pulmonary artery. (See Color Plate 14, p. 274.)

abnormalities. Image quality may be enhanced by use of a higher-frequency transducer and a smaller area of interest. Sometimes the aortic valve can be evaluated from a transgastric apical view; however, image quality may be no better than from a transthoracic approach due to the distance from the transducer to the aortic valve.

The mitral valve is well seen from a high esophageal position. Since the mitral valve plane is perpendicular to the ultrasound beam from this approach, excellent images can be obtained in multiple views by slowly rotating the multiplane transducer from 0 to 180°. Particular attention should be paid to standard four-chamber (at 0°), two-chamber (at 60°), and long-axis (at 120°) views. The degree of mitral regurgitation can be assessed with color flow imaging in these same views. Given the distance of the mitral valve from the chest wall in both parasternal and apical transthoracic views, transesophageal imaging often provides dramatically better images and important clinical data (Figs. 13–10 and 13–11).

FIGURE 13–10. Transthoracic *(above)* and transesophageal *(below)* imaging in a 61-year-old man with group B streptococcal endocarditis. The valvular vegetation *(arrow)* is seen on transthoracic imaging but is better defined on transesophageal imaging. In addition, there was evidence for a mitral annular abscess. There was no detectable mitral regurgitation. At surgery, the patient had an extensive mitral annular abscess and purulent pericarditis. PE = pericardial effusion.

FIGURE 13–11. Transesophageal echocardiography in a 34-year-old man with a history of intravenous drug use and blood cultures positive for *S. aureus*. There is a small vegetation attached to the ridge between the left atrial appendage and body of the left atrium *(top)*. There was an associated perforation of the base of the mitral valve leaflet with color flow imaging *(bottom)* showing a mitral regurgitant jet through the perforation. A successful patch repair of the mitral perforation was performed. (See Color Plate 14, p. 274.)

The tricuspid valve is seen in the transesophageal four-chamber view and from a transgastric approach. Since the tricuspid valve lies closer to the chest wall than the mitral valve, transthoracic imaging often is diagnostic, and information that would change patient therapy or management may not be obtained on transesophageal imaging (Fig. 13–12).

Diagnostic Accuracy of Echocardiography for Detection of Vegetations

While numerous studies have evaluated the sensitivity of echocardiography for diagnosis of valvular vegetation by comparing the echo findings with subsequent surgical or autopsy findings, there are fewer data on the specificity of echocardiography for valvular vegetations. This stems from two study design problems. (1) Most studies only include subjects with a definite diagnosis of endocarditis. Thus there are no subjects without the disease in the study group. (2) When surgical or autopsy inspection of the valve is the standard of reference, only patients who are sick enough to need surgery or who have died are included in the study group. Direct inspection of valves that appeared normal on echocardiography rarely is available.

A few studies (for example, studies 3 through 5 in Table 13–2) have circumvented these study design problems by including all patients with *suspected* endocarditis (some have the disease and some do not) and using clinical outcome rather than direct valve inspection as the standard of reference. All these studies demonstrate a high specificity of transthoracic (93% to 98%) and transesophageal (100%) echocardiography in excluding the diagnosis of endocarditis. Another study (study 7 in Table 13–2) found that the negative predictive value of a negative transesophageal study also is high (86%).

The specificity of echocardiography depends on distinguishing a valvular vegetation from other intracardiac masses and from ultrasound artifacts (Table 13–3). In a patient with abnormal valve leaflets (e.g., myxomatous, calcified), it may be difficult to distinguish the abnormal tissue from a valvular vegetation unless a study performed before onset of the illness is available for comparison. Mistaking ultrasound artifacts for a vegetation can be avoided by identification of the characteristic findings in more than one view. Note that not all valvular vegetations are "typical." Some may be on the downstream side of the valve or may show little independent motion. These atypical findings further decrease the sensitivity and speci-

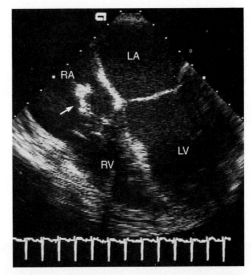

FIGURE 13–12. Transesophageal view of a tricuspid valve vegetation *(arrow)* attached to the atrial side of the septal leaflet of the tricuspid valve in a 38-year-old woman undergoing tricuspid valve repair for *S. aureus* endocarditis.

TABLE 13–3	Anatomic Abnormalities That May Mimic Infectious Endocarditis on Echocardiography

Papillary fibroma

Myxomatous mitral valve disease (especially with partial flail leaflet or ruptured chordae)

Old, "healed" vegetation

Nonbacterial thrombotic endocarditis

Systemic lupus cardiac involvement

Thrombus (especially with prosthetic valve)

Beam-width artifact from calcific valve disease or prosthesis

Aortic valve Lambl's excrescence or nodule of Arantius

ficity of echocardiography for valvular vegetations.

Endocarditis most often occurs on a previously abnormal valve or a prosthetic valve. Evaluation of the underlying valve disease is an important aspect of the ultrasound examination.

Functional Valvular Abnormalities Due to Endocarditis

Valve leaflet destruction by the infectious process plus the distortion of leaflet closure by the vegetation mass result in valvular regurgitation. Regurgitation can occur at the closure line or through a perforation in the leaflet itself. The degree of regurgitation varies from none to mild, moderate, or severe.

Assessment of valvular regurgitation in endocarditis is performed using the pulsed, color flow, and continuous-wave Doppler approaches described in Chapter 11 with careful attention to the features that distinguish acute from chronic regurgitation. Since endocarditis often affects a previously abnormal valve, acute regurgitation may be superimposed on chronic regurgitation, resulting in mixed findings on echocardiography.

FIGURE 13–13. Transthoracic parasternal long-axis *(above)* and short-axis *(below)* views in a 34-year-old man with a bicuspid aortic valve and suspected endocarditis. Definite evidence for valvular vegetations and a paravalvular abscess *(arrows)* is seen. Doppler allowed assessment of the severity of aortic regurgitation.

Valvular stenosis due to endocarditis is rare. Occasionally, a large vegetation will partially obstruct the orifice of the open valve, resulting in some degree of functional stenosis.

Note that not all patients with endocarditis have a new murmur (about 10% do not) and a few have no regurgitation detectable on Doppler examination. This is most likely to occur if the vegetation is located at the base of the leaflet, resulting in little distortion of leaflet closure. Echocardiographic recognition of the diagnosis in this subgroup is all the more important in that endocarditis often is not suspected clinically with the echocardiogram having been ordered for other reasons.

Other Echocardiographic Findings

In addition to direct assessment of valvular disease, the examination includes evaluation of cardiac chamber size and function. Acute aortic regurgitation results in only mild left ventricular dilation, but a subacute or acute course superimposed on mild to moderate chronic disease may result in significant ventricular dilation. Severe valve destruction may result in a flail aortic leaflet (see Figs. 13–8 and 13–9). Mitral regurgitation results in left atrial and left ventricular enlargement. Left ventricular systolic dysfunction may be seen either due to long-standing valvular disease or to the acute infectious process.

Pulmonary pressures may be elevated due to mitral regurgitation directly resulting in an elevated left atrial pressure or to aortic regurgitation with a high end-diastolic left ventricular pressure.

A small pericardial effusion often is seen with endocarditis. A larger effusion raises the concern of purulent pericarditis due to direct extension from a paravalvular abscess.

Diagnosis of Paravalvular Abscess and Intracardiac Fistula

Unlike abscesses elsewhere in the body, a cardiac abscess may be either echolucent or echo-dense on ultrasound examination. Typically, abscesses occur in the valve annulus adjacent to the infected leaflet tissue and are more common with aortic than with mitral valve endocarditis. For diagnosis of aortic annular abscess, findings include increased echogenicity or an echolucent area in the base of the septum or increased thickness of the posterior aortic root (Figs. 13–13 to 13–15). Involvement of the aortic annulus may extend into the contiguous anterior mitral valve leaflet with evidence of increased thickness of the leaflet tissue, a valvular

FIGURE 13–14. Transesophageal long- *(top)* and short-axis *(bottom)* views of the aortic valve in the same patient as in Figure 13–13. While the bicuspid valve, valvular vegetations, and paravalvular abscess *(arrows)* are more clearly seen, no additional diagnostic information was obtained compared with the transthoracic study. At surgery, a paravalvular abscess due to α-hemolytic *Streptococcus* was found.

FIGURE 13–15. Transesophageal echocardiographic long- *(top)* and short-axis *(bottom)* views showing a contour abnormality of the right coronary sinus of Valsalva *(arrows)* suggestive of a paravalvular abscess in a 43-year-old man with *S. aureus* endocarditis on a congenital bicuspid valve. This patient had an embolic cerebrovascular event and died of acute congestive heart failure.

vegetation, and/or leaflet perforation (Figs. 13–16 and 13–17). A sinus of Valsalva aneurysm can occur due to infection of the aortic wall and may be detected by echocardiography, before rupture occurs, as a dilated and distorted sinus. In effect, this represents an abscess that is in direct communication with the bloodstream.

Rupture of an aortic annular abscess can occur in several fashions. The region of the noncoronary cusp can rupture into the right ventricular outflow tract either in the sinus of Valsalva (an aortic to right ventricular connection) or from the left ventricular outflow tract through the septum into the right ventricle (a ventricular septal defect) (Figs. 13–18 and 13–19). An aortic to right ventricular fistula shows both systolic and diastolic left to right flow on Doppler interrogation, while a ventricular septal defect shows predominantly systolic flow. Rupture also can occur from the left ventricle into the abscess in the region of the mitral-aortic intervalvular fibrosa with flow into and out of the abscess cavity from the left ventricular outflow tract (Fig. 13–20).

The right coronary sinus region can rupture into the right ventricle or right atrium and can lead to involvement of the adjacent septal

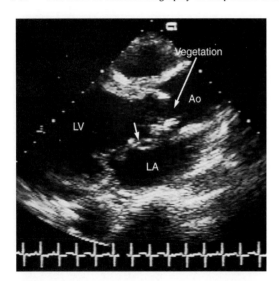

FIGURE 13–16. Aortic valve endocarditis with vegetations and extension into the base of the anterior mitral valve leaflet resulting in mitral leaflet perforation.

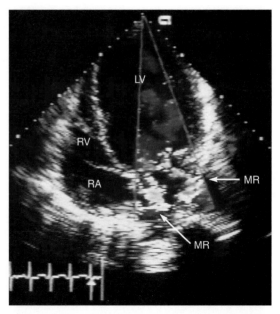

FIGURE 13–17. In the same patient as in Figure 13–16, the apical four-chamber color flow image showed two jets of mitral regurgitation—one through the leaflet perforation and one through the valve coaptation zone. (See Color Plate 14, p. 274.)

leaflet of the tricuspid valve. Again, rupture can occur either from the aorta or from the left ventricular outflow tract into the right side of the heart. Note that a small segment of ventricular septum (the atrioventricular septum) actually separates the left ventricle from the right *atrium* so that a ventriculoatrial communication can occur. The left coronary sinus of the aortic valve can rupture into the left or right atrium, or infection may extend directly into the interatrial septum.

A mitral annular abscess appears as increased thickening and echogenicity in the posterior aspect of the mitral annulus. Infection may extend into the basal segments of the ventricular myocardium or into the pericardial space. Again, identification may be difficult on echocardiographic imaging, and the diagnosis should be pursued with transesophageal echocardiography when suspected on clinical grounds. An unusual complication of mitral valve endocarditis is a persistent contour abnormality, in effect a pseudoaneurysm of the valve leaflet, which persists even after the infection is treated (Figs. 13–21 and 13–22).

Tricuspid valve endocarditis may be associated with a ring abscess, again manifested as increased thickening and echogenicity in the annulus region.

Diagnosis of paravalvular abscess by transthoracic echocardiography has a markedly lower sensitivity and specificity (Table 13–4), compared with transesophageal imaging, due to poor ultrasound tissue penetration resulting in suboptimal image quality. A high in-

dex of suspicion is needed by the echocardiographer, and subtle abnormalities that may suggest a valve abscess should not be ignored. However, even with careful imaging from several acoustic windows in multiple tomographic planes, a definite diagnosis may not be possible. Transesophageal imaging is especially important in patients with prosthetic valve endocarditis as paravalvular abscesses are common and shadowing and reverberations from the valve prosthesis compromise the examination (see Chap. 12).

The superior image quality of transesophageal echocardiography is associated with a higher sensitivity (87%) and specificity (96%) for diagnosis of paravalvular abscess. In addition to 2D findings of abnormal areas of increased echogenicity or abnormal echolucent areas adjacent to the valve, color flow imaging and conventional pulsed Doppler may allow demonstration of flow into and out of these abnormal areas consistent with an abscess that partially communicates with the bloodstream.

Usually, both transthoracic and transesophageal approaches are needed for complete evaluation of the patient with endocarditis. One advantage of transthoracic imaging is the ability to align a continuous-wave Doppler beam parallel to high-velocity flows of interest. When abnormal intracardiac communications complicate endocarditis due to abscess rupture,

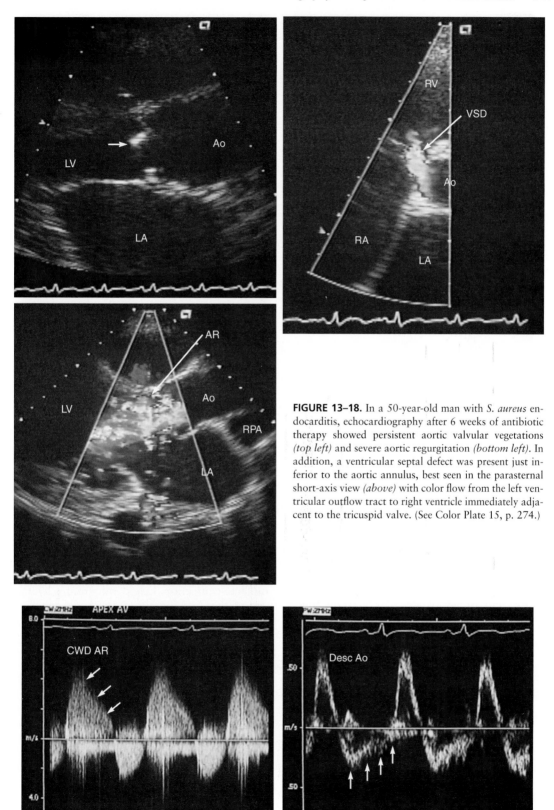

FIGURE 13–18. In a 50-year-old man with *S. aureus* endocarditis, echocardiography after 6 weeks of antibiotic therapy showed persistent aortic valvular vegetations *(top left)* and severe aortic regurgitation *(bottom left)*. In addition, a ventricular septal defect was present just inferior to the aortic annulus, best seen in the parasternal short-axis view *(above)* with color flow from the left ventricular outflow tract to right ventricle immediately adjacent to the tricuspid valve. (See Color Plate 15, p. 274.)

FIGURE 13–19. In the same patient as in Figure 13–18, evidence for acute severe aortic regurgitation is present including a dense continuous-wave Doppler signal *(left)* with a steep deceleration slope *(arrows)* and holodiastolic flow reversal in the proximal abdominal aorta *(right)*.

FIGURE 13–20. In this 26-year-old woman with a history of intravenous drug use and *S. aureus* endocarditis, transesophageal echocardiography shows an abscess of mitral-aortic intervalvular fibrosa *(top left)*. This cavity communicated with the left ventricular outflow tract with flow into the abscess in systole *(bottom left)* with diastolic regurgitation *(right)* into the left ventricle. The abscess was débrided and an aortic homograft was placed but the patient did not survive the surgical procedure. (See Color Plate 15, p. 274.)

identification of an abnormal high-velocity jet may be the first clue to the diagnosis. The transthoracic approach also allows measurement of chamber dimensions in standard views, quantitation of left ventricular systolic function, and measurement of pulmonary artery pressures.

LIMITATIONS/TECHNICAL CONSIDERATIONS
(Table 13–5)

Active versus Healed Vegetations

Sequential echocardiographic studies in a patient undergoing treatment for endocarditis may show a gradual reduction in size, decreased mobility, and increased echogenicity of the valvular vegetation. However, vegetations may either abruptly "disappear" from the heart due to embolization or may remain unchanged in size or appearance long after the acute episode. Thus a patient with active endocarditis may have no

visible vegetation if recent embolization has occurred. Conversely, a patient with prior endocarditis may have a persistent vegetation without active infection. Echocardiography, by itself, can neither exclude nor establish a diagnosis of endocarditis. Correlation of the echocardiographic findings with the patient's clinical presentation (fevers, systemic emboli, new murmur, peripheral manifestation of endocarditis) plus the results of microbiologic cultures is needed for diagnosis as detailed in Table 13–1. Obviously, echocardiography provides no information regarding the causative organism. While certain etiologic agents (fungal endocarditis, *Haemophilus influenzae*) are associated with larger vegetations, this observation is not diagnostically useful in an individual patient.

Nonbacterial Thrombotic Endocarditis

The echocardiographic appearance of nonbacterial thrombotic endocarditis, as has been described in patients with malignancy and in patients with systemic lupus erythematosus, is similar to that of infectious endocarditis. Although the vegetations of nonbacterial thrombotic endocarditis tend to be smaller, to be located near the leaflet base, and to show variable echo density and less independent motion, again, clinical and bacteriologic correlation is needed for a correct diagnosis (Fig. 13–23).

Diagnosis of Vegetations with Underlying Valve Disease

Endocarditis most often occurs on a previously abnormal valve, since the local flow disturbance increases the likelihood of bacterial deposition. When the underlying disease is anatomically straightforward, such as a bicuspid aortic valve, this poses little problem in diagnosing superimposed valvular vegetations. Often, however, the presence of an abnormal valve makes exclusion or confirmation of a valvular vegetation more difficult. For example, with calcific aortic stenosis, the irregular areas of increased echogenicity on the valve leaflets could represent a vegetation or chronic fibrocalcific changes. Findings of independent rapid motion and prolapse into the outflow tract on diastole increase the likelihood of a vegetation, but the absence of these findings does not allow a definite conclusion as to the absence of a vegetation.

Another example is myxomatous mitral valve disease where an independently mobile mass of echoes attached to the leaflet and prolapsing into the left atrium in systole could represent either a valvular vegetation or a flail leaflet segment and attached chordae. When underlying valve disease is present, the improved images obtained by the transesophageal approach may increase the certainty of diagnosis. In any case, careful integration with other clinical findings usually leads to a correct diagnosis.

Endocarditis of Prosthetic Valves

Evaluation of prosthetic valves for suspected endocarditis is problematic for two reasons. First, infection often involves the area around the sewing ring of the prosthetic valve rather than resulting in a discrete valvular vegetation.

FIGURE 13–21. Chronic mitral valve pseudoaneurysm in a 69-year-old man with a remote history of bacterial endocarditis. In the apical long-axis *(above)* and four-chamber *(below)* views a circular echolucent structure is seen at the base of the anterior mitral leaflet *(arrow)*.

FIGURE 13–22. In the same patient as Figure 13–21, color flow imaging shows two aortic regurgitant jets *(arrow)*, with one jet directed at the pseudoaneurysm of the anterior mitral valve leaflet. (See Color Plate 15, p. 274.)

First Author/ Year	Study Entry Criteria	No. of Valves	Percent Prosthetic	Transthoracic Echo		Transesophageal Echo	
				Sensitivity	Specificy	Sensitivity	Specificity
1. Daniel/ 1991	Endocarditis with surgery or autopsy	137	25%	13/46 (28%)	90/91 (99%)	40/46 (87%)	87/91 (96%)
2. Jaffe/ 1990	Endocarditis with surgery or autopsy	7		5/7 (71%)			
3. Karalis/ 1992	Endocarditis with surgery or autopsy	55	46%	13/24 (54%)		24/24 (100%)	

TABLE 13-4 Accuracy of Echocardiographic Diagnosis of Paravalvular Abscess (Selected Series)

Data from Daniel et al: NEJM 324:795–800, 1991; Jaffe et al: JACC 15:1227–1233, 1990; Karalis et al: Circ 86: 353–362, 1992.

TABLE 13-5 Limitations of Echocardiography in Evaluation of Patients with Endocarditis

1. Active versus healed vegetation
2. Nonbacterial thrombotic endocarditis (NBTE)
3. Abnormal underlying valve anatomy
4. Prosthetic valve
5. Detection of abscess
6. Need for clinical and microbiologic correlation

Second, reverberations and shadowing by the prosthesis limit the ability of echocardiography to detect abnormalities. This is a particular problem with transthoracic imaging of mitral prostheses, where the left atrial side of the valve is "masked" by the prosthesis so that neither the paravalvular infection in the mitral annulus nor the resulting valvular incompetence can be detected (see Chap. 12). Acoustic shadowing is less of a problem with aortic valve prostheses because aortic regurgitation can be evaluated from both apical and parasternal windows without "masking" by the valve prosthesis. However, since the anterior part of the valve prosthesis shadows the more posterior portions, images of the valve leaflets may be suboptimal.

With suspected prosthetic valve endocarditis, the transthoracic examination may provide clues that suggest the diagnosis even when definitive findings are not present. For example, if color flow imaging is nondiagnostic due to

FIGURE 13–23. Transesophageal echocardiography in a 49-year-old woman with the antiphospholipid antibody syndrome and multiple embolic events shows a typical mass on the mitral valve (arrows) consistent with nonbacterial thrombotic endocarditis. She was afebrile and had negative blood cultures.

shadowing and color flow artifacts, a careful continuous-wave Doppler examination may show a regurgitant signal. Care is needed in assessment of the *severity* of regurgitation in this situation, and it may be prudent to state only that regurgitation is present but quantitation is not possible. Other clues to prosthetic valve dysfunction include an increased antegrade flow velocity across the prosthesis (reflecting increased antegrade volume flow due to prosthetic regurgitation) and an elevated tricuspid regurgitant jet velocity due to pulmonary hypertension.

Whenever prosthetic valve endocarditis is suspected, transesophageal imaging should be strongly considered (Figs. 13–24 to 13–26). If the transthoracic images are diagnostic, or if the results of transesophageal imaging will not change patient management, it may not be needed. Otherwise, this technique is warranted given its higher sensitivity and specificity for detection of prosthetic valve endocarditis, paravalvular abscess, and prosthetic mitral regurgitation.

Endocarditis rarely can result in prosthetic valve stenosis due to impingement of the infected mass on leaflet opening or to an infected pannus on the upstream side of the valve. Again, visualization of the infected mass may not be possible on transthoracic imaging. Prosthetic valve stenosis is recognized by findings of an increased transvalvular pressure gradient and a decreased valve area (by pressure half-time or by continuity equation).

FIGURE 13–24. In a 24-year-old woman with an aortic homograft valve replacement for a prior episode of endocarditis, reinfection with *S. aureus* has resulted in a paravalvular abscess (or pseudoaneurysm) posterior to the homograft. The transthoracic parasternal long-axis view shows the abscess cavity *(top)* and color flow imaging shows flow from the aortic root into the abscess cavity *(bottom)*. (See Color Plate 16, p. 274.)

FIGURE 13–25. Short-axis views in the same patient as Figure 13–24 show the proximity of the abscess cavity to the left atrium *(top)* and color flow Doppler shows a fistula from the abscess cavity into the left atrium *(bottom)*. (See Color Plate 16, p. 274.)

In an individual patient, a *change* in the appearance or flow characteristics of a prosthetic valve is more diagnostic than an observation at one point in time. Review of previous studies (if available) performed when the patient clinically was well can improve the diagnostic yield of echocardiography.

CLINICAL UTILITY

"Rule Out" Endocarditis

In Figure 13–27, the posttest likelihood of endocarditis has been calculated using Bayesian analysis based on the reported sensitivities and specificities of transthoracic and transesophageal echocardiography. In the setting of a low pretest likelihood of disease—the echocardiogram ordered to "rule out" endocarditis—although the posttest likelihood of disease appears to be high, the studies these data are based on may not have included the findings of old, healed vegetations, artifacts, or abnormal (but not infected) valve tissue being mistaken for active endocarditis.

When the pretest likelihood of disease is high (>80%), even a "negative" transthoracic echocardiogram decreases the posttest likelihood of disease only modestly (still >50%). In some patients, when endocarditis is present, a repeat echocardiogram after several days may show vegetations when the initial study result was negative. A negative transesophageal echocardiogram results in a much lower posttest

likelihood of disease even when the pretest likelihood is high. Thus transesophageal echo is most useful when the clinical findings support a diagnosis of endocarditis, especially if the transthoracic study result is "negative."

Cardiac Evaluation of the Patient with Endocarditis

In a patient with endocarditis, an echocardiogram is an invaluable adjunct to clinical decision making concerning potential surgical intervention and prediction of short- and long-term prognosis. Echocardiography often allows

FIGURE 13–26. Continuous-wave Doppler in the same patient as Figures 13–24 and 13–25 shows continuous high-velocity flow in systole and diastole *(arrows)* consistent with a fistula from a high-pressure (aorta) to low-pressure (left atrium) chamber.

Diagnostic Utility of Echo for Endocarditis

FIGURE 13–27. Bayesian analysis of the posttest likelihood of endocarditis for transthoracic (TTE) and transesophageal (TEE) echocardiography, using the overall sensitivity (sens) and specificity (spec) determined from the data in Table 13–2 (TTE sens = 64%, spec = 98%; TEE sens = 90%, spec = 99%).

clear definition of which (and how many) valves are affected.

Diagnosis of acute severe valvular regurgitation or a paravalvular abscess is a clear indication for surgical treatment. Associated left ventricular dysfunction, involvement of more than one valve, and secondary pulmonary hypertension as evaluated by echocardiography are important determinants of the surgical approach and timing of intervention.

The occurrence of a systemic embolic event generally is accepted as an indication for valve replacement; however, the importance of vegetation size and appearance by echocardiography remains controversial. If patients with embolization prior to echocardiography are excluded, several studies have shown a trend toward a higher incidence of systemic embolization with a vegetation diameter greater than 1 cm (Table 13–6). However, other studies contest this conclusion. Infection with *H. influenzae* and mitral valve involvement also have been shown to predict a higher rate of systemic emboli. Recent studies have suggested that sequential transesophageal echocardiographic evaluation of patients with endocarditis can predict whether antimicrobial therapy is effective by demonstrating progressive decreases in vegetation size. However, the cost-effectiveness (and patient acceptance) of this approach is unclear.

In the current era, with aggressive and prompt surgical intervention, severe regurgitation and heart failure do *not* predict mortality, since these patients undergo early valve replacement. With antibiotic therapy and appropriate surgical intervention, risk factors for in-hospital death are prosthetic valve infection, systemic embolism, and infection with *S. aureus*. Long-term outcome in survivors is related to the residual degree of valve damage, the effects of chronic valvular regurgitation on ventricular function and pulmonary artery pressures, and the risk of recurrent episodes of endocarditis.

SUGGESTED READING

General Reviews

1. Schiller NB: Clinical decision making in patients with endocarditis: the role of echocardiography. *In* Otto CM (ed): The Practice of Clinical Echocardiography. Philadelphia, WB Saunders, 1997. pp. 389–404.

   Review of the current role of echocardiography in management of the patient with suspected or known endocarditis. In addition to a review of the literature, this chapter provides useful tips on the echocardiographic approach with clear illustrations.

Clinical Diagnosis

2. Durack DT, Lukes AS, Bright DK: New criteria for diagnosis of infective endocarditis: utilization of specific echocardiographic findings. Duke Endocarditis Service. *Am J Med* 96:200–209, 1994.

   Proposed criteria for the clinical diagnosis of endocarditis as detailed in Table 13–1 incorporate echocardiographic findings as key factor in the diagnosis. Includes validation of sensitivity and specificity of this approach compared to older diagnostic approaches. The Duke criteria are used at many medical centers.

TABLE 13–6	Size of Vegetation by Two-Dimensional Echocardiography versus Risk of Embolism				
			Embolism		
Study	**n**	**Total No. of Emboli**	**No Vegetation or < 10 mm**	**Vegetation >10 mm**	**P Value**
Lutas et al.	76	17	16% (8/50)	45% (9/26)	0.065‡
Buda et al.*	42	14	26% (8/31)	55% (6/11)	0.08‡
Wann et al.†	21	7	21% (3/14)	57% (4/7)	0.16§
Wong et al.	31	6	20% (3/15)	19% (3/16)	0.64§
Jaffe et al.	50	10	11% (2/18)	26% (8/32)	0.19§
Total	251	56	19% (24/128)	33% (30/92)	0.018‡

*Excludes patients with right-sided endocarditis.
†Vegetation size graded qualitatively on 1+ to 3+ scale; 3+ was considered >10 mm.
‡Chi-square analysis.
§Fisher exact test.
Data from Lutas et al: Am Heart J 112:107, 1986; Buda et al: Am Heart J 112:1291, 1986; Wann et al: Circulation 60:728, 1979; Wong et al: Arch Intern Med 143:1874, 1983; Jaffe et al, J Am Coll Cardiol 15: 1227, 1990.
From Jaffe WM, Morgan DE, Pearlman AS, Otto CM: Infective endocarditis, 1983–1988: Echocardiographic findings and factors influencing morbidity and mortality. *J Am Coll Cardiol* 15:1227–1233, 1990. Reprinted with permission from the American College of Cardiology.

3. Dodds GA, Sexton DJ, Durack DT, et al: Negative predictive value of the Duke criteria for infective endocarditis. *Am J Cardiol* 77:403–407, 1996.

   In 405 episodes of suspected endocarditis, 52 were classified as "rejected" endocarditis based on the Duke criteria. With clinical outcome used as the standard of reference, none of these patients subsequently developed endocarditis, although one had possible endocarditis at autopsy, indicating a negative predictive value of the Duke criteria of at least 92%.

4. Lindner JR, Case RA, Dent JM, et al: Diagnostic value of echocardiography in suspected endocarditis: an evaluation based on the pretest probability of disease. *Circulation* 93:730–736, 1996.

   This study suggests that echocardiography is not necessary in patients with a low pretest likelihood of the diagnosis. In those with an intermediate or high pretest likelihood (positive blood cultures plus new murmur or predisposing heart disease), transthoracic echocardiography should be performed first. Transesophageal echocardiography is needed primarily when the transthoracic study is technically inadequate, indicates an intermediate probability of endocarditis, or when a prosthetic valve is present.

5. Yvorchuk KJ, Chan KL: Application of transthoracic and transesophageal echocardiography in the diagnosis and management of infective endocarditis. *J Am Soc Echocardiogr* 14:294–308, 1994.

   Review article on the utility of echocardiography in patients with known or suspected endocarditis. An excellent synthesis of the literature with tables summarizing data, clear examples, and a proposed diagnostic approach. 61 references.

Transthoracic versus Transesophageal Echocardiography

6. Burger AJ, Peart B, Jabi H, Touchon RC: The role of two-dimensional echocardiography in the diagnosis of infective endocarditis. *Angiology* 42:552–560, 1991.

   In 106 patients with suspected endocarditis, vegetations were present on echocardiography in 36 patients, 35 of whom had active infective endocarditis. Of the 65 patients with no vegetation on the initial echo, only 4 patients had clinical endocarditis.

7. Shiveley BK, Gurule FT, Roldan CA, et al: Diagnostic value of transesophageal compared with transthoracic echocardiography in infective endocarditis. *J Am Coll Cardiol* 18:391–397, 1991.

   Transesophageal echocardiography was more sensitive and specific than transthoracic echocardiography for diagnosis of endocarditis. A negative transesophageal echocardiographic study resulted in a low probability of disease in patients with an intermediate pretest likelihood of disease.

8. Pedersen WR, Walker M, Olson JD, et al: Value of transesophageal echocardiography as an adjunct to transthoracic echocardiography in evaluation of native and prosthetic valve endocarditis. *Chest* 100:351–356, 1991.

   In 24 consecutive patients with possible endocarditis (10 with prosthetic valves), transesophageal echocardiography was more sensitive than transthoracic echocardiography for diagnosing vegetations or abscesses.

9. Daniel WG, Mugge A, Grote J, et al: Comparison of transthoracic and transesophageal echocardiography for detection of abnormalities of prosthetic and bioprosthetic valves in the mitral and aortic positions. *Am J Cardiol* 71:210–215, 1993.

   Detection of prosthetic valve endocarditis was enhanced by transesophageal echocardiography. Of 148 prosthetic valves, 124 were abnormal at surgery or autopsy (33 endocarditis, 8 thrombi, and 83 degeneration). Endocarditis was correctly identified in 12 of 36 (36%) by transthoracic echocardiography and 27 of 33 (82%) by transesophageal echocardiography.

10. Sochowski RA, Chan K-L: Implication of negative results on a monoplane transesophageal echocardiographic study in patients with suspected infective endocarditis. *J Am Coll Cardiol* 21:216–221, 1993.

    In 65 patients with a negative transesophageal echocardiographic study for suspected endocarditis, 56 remained free of clinical evidence of endocarditis, 4 were treated empirically, and 5 had infective endocarditis either on repeat transesophageal echocardiography study (3), at autopsy (1), or based on the subsequent clinical course (1). Factors associated with endocarditis and a negative initial transesophageal echocardiography study were gram-positive bacteremia and an aortic valve prosthesis.

11. Shapiro SM, Young E, DeGuzman, et al: Transesophageal echocardiography in diagnosis of infective endocarditis. *Chest* 105:377–382, 1994.

    In 64 patients with suspected endocarditis, transesophageal echocardiography was more sensitive (97%) than transthoracic echocardiography (68%) for detection of valvular vegetations. Based on strict clinical criteria, 30 of 64 (47%) had acute infective endocarditis. Both transthoracic and transesophageal echocardiography were highly specific (91%) for this diagnosis with false-positive echocardiographic findings in 3 patients, 2 of whom had a prior history of endocarditis. All 9 perivalvular abscesses were diagnosed by transesophageal echocardiography versus 2 of 9 on transthoracic echocardiography.

12. Lowry RW, Zoghbi WA, Baker WB, et al: Clinical impact of transesophageal echocardiography in the diagnosis and management of infective endocarditis. *Am J Cardiol* 73:1089–1091, 1994.

    In 93 consecutive patients undergoing transesophageal echocardiography for suspected endocarditis, the negative predictive value of transesophageal echocardiography was 100% for native valves and 90% for prosthetic valves. Transesophageal echocardiography resulted in a change in the subsequent diagnostic or therapeutic plan in >90% of patients.

Diagnosis of Paravalvular Abscess

13. Daniel WG, Mugge A, Martin RP, et al: Improvement in the diagnosis of abscesses associated with endocarditis by transesophageal echocardiography. *N Engl J Med* 324:795–800, 1991.

In 118 consecutive patients with endocarditis, 44 (37%) had surgical or autopsy evidence of abscess formation. Abscesses were more common with infection with Staphylococcus (52% of cases) and with aortic valve involvement. The hospital mortality rate in patients with an abscess was 23% versus 14% in the remainder of the study group. Transesophageal echocardiography was much more sensitive than transthoracic echocardiography for diagnosis of paravalvular abscess.

14. Karalis DG, Bansal RC, Huack AJ, et al: Transesophageal echocardiographic recognition of subaortic complications in aortic valve endocarditis: Clinical and surgical implications. Circulation 86:353–362, 1992.

Detailed description (with illustrations) of the patterns of paravalvular and subaortic abscess formation in patients with aortic valve endocarditis. The authors note that eccentric jets of mitral regurgitation in patients with aortic valve endocarditis raise the possibility of involvement (perforation) of the anterior mitral leaflet by the infectious process.

Risk of Embolic Events

15. Mügge A, Daniel WG, Frank G, Lichtlen PR: Echocardiography in infective endocarditis: Reassessment of prognostic implications of vegetation size determined by the transthoracic and the transesophageal approach. J Am Coll Cardiol 14:631–638, 1989.

In 105 patients with endocarditis, a vegetation size >10 mm on transthoracic or transesophageal echocardiography was predictive of embolic events (22 of 47 with vegetation ≤10 mm, P < .01). Mitral valve endocarditis also was associated with a higher likelihood of embolism. Heart failure and survival were not related to vegetation size.

16. Steckelberg JM, Murphy JG, Ballard D, et al: Emboli in infective endocarditis: The prognostic value of echocardiography. Ann Intern Med 114:635–640, 1991.

In 207 patients with endocarditis, the likelihood of first embolic events was 6.2 per 1000 patient days (95% confidence interval, 4.2 to 9.2). The risk of embolic events was related to infection with Streptococcus viridans infections but not to vegetation size. The likelihood of embolization decreased over time, falling to 1.2 per 1000 patient days after 2 weeks of therapy.

17. Sanfilippo AJ, Picard MH, Newell JB, et al: Echocardiographic assessment of patients with infectious endocarditis: Prediction of risk for complications. J Am Coll Cardiol 18:1191–1199, 1991.

In 204 patients with endocarditis, multivariate predictors of complications (persistent fever, congestive heart failure, systemic emboli, surgery, and mortality) were vegetation size, extent, and mobility. The authors propose an echo score for vegetation appearance to predict the likelihood of complications.

Long-term Outcome

18. Jaffe WM, Morgan DE, Pearlman AS, Otto CM: Infective endocarditis, 1983–1988: Echocardiographic findings and factors influencing morbidity and mortality. J Am Coll Cardiol 15:1227–1233, 1990.

In 70 patients with endocarditis, predictors of in-hospital mortality were prosthetic valve endocarditis, occurrence of a systemic embolic event, and infection with S. aureus. Abnormal (≥2+) valvular regurgitation was noted on transthoracic Doppler examination in 88% of patients.

19. Werner GS, Schulz R, Fuchs JB, et al: Infective endocarditis in the elderly in the era of transesophageal echocardiography: Clinical features and prognosis compared with younger patients. Am J Med 100: 90–97, 1996.

Compared to younger patients, elderly patients (age >70 years) with endocarditis more often have predisposing valve conditions, including calcified and prosthetic valves, which decrease the sensitivity of transthoracic imaging for detection of valvular vegetations. The sensitivity of transthoracic echocardiography was only 45% in those older than age 70 compared to 75% in those younger than age 50 years in this study.

20. Erbel R, Liu F, Ge J, et al: Identification of high-risk subgroups in infective endocarditis and the role of echocardiography. Eur Heart J 16:588–602, 1995.

High-risk subgroups with endocarditis can be identified based on clinical and echocardiographic features. Factors associated with a poor clinical outcome include increased age, delayed diagnosis, infection with S. aureus, aortic valve involvement, large vegetations, embolic events, prosthetic valves, and failed antibiotic therapy.

21. Rohmann S, Erbel R, Darius H, et al: Prediction of rapid versus prolonged healing of infective endocarditis by monitoring vegetation size. J Am Soc Echocardiogr 4:465–474, 1991.

Increasing vegetation size during antibiotic therapy was associated with a higher rate of valve replacement, embolic events, paravalvular abscess formation, and mortality in 83 patients with echocardiographic evidence of endocarditis

22. Fowler VG, Li J, Corey R, et al: Role of echocardiography in evaluation of patients with Staphylococcus aureus bacteremia: Experience in 103 patients. J Am Coll Cardiol 30:1072–1078, 1997.

In a consecutive series of patients with S. aureus bacteremia, definite endocarditis (Duke criteria) was present in only 25%. Transthoracic echocardiography had a low sensitivity (32%) but was 100% specific for detection of vegetations. Transesophageal echocardiography had a sensitivity of 100% and a specificity of 99% (one false-positive result). Death due to sepsis was significantly (P = .03) more likely in those with endocarditis (15%) compared to those with bacteremia alone (3%), even though evidence for eradication of the infection was similar in both groups.

Right-sided Endocarditis

23. Hecht SR, Berger M: Right-sided endocarditis in intravenous drug users: Prognostic features in 102 episodes. Ann Intern Med 117:560–566, 1992.

Clinical study of 132 patients with right-sided endocarditis emphasizes the high prevalence of S. aureus infection (82%), tricuspid valve involvement (96%), large vegetation size (>10 mm in 80%), and low mortality (7%) in right-sided (versus left-sided) endocarditis.

Nonbacterial Thrombotic Endocarditis

24. Roldan CA, Shively BK, Crawford MH: An echocardiographic study of valvular heart disease associated with systemic lupus erythematosus. *N Engl J Med* 335:1424–1430, 1996.

   Valvular abnormalities were seen on echocardiography in two-thirds of 69 patients with lupus. Valve thickening was most common, but vegetations were seen in 43% and significant valvular regurgitation was seen in 25%. Echocardiographic findings often changed on follow-up examination with some patients having resolution of valvular abnormalities and others having increased valve dysfunction.

25. Edoute Y, Haim N, Rinkevich D, et al: Cardiac valvular vegetations in cancer patients: A prospective echocardiographic study of 200 patients. *Am J Med* 102: 252–258, 1997.

   In 200 ambulatory patients with solid tumors, echocardiography showed valvular vegetations (most often on the aortic or mitral valve) in 19% of patients. Cardiac abnormalities were most common in patients with carcinoma of the pancreas and lung and with lymphoma. Systemic thromboembolism occurred in 11% of the total study group.

26. Lopez JA, Ross RS, Fishbein MC, Siegel RJ: Non-bacterial thrombotic endocarditis: A review. *Am Heart J* 113:773–784, 1987.

   Review of nonbacterial thrombotic endocarditis. Diagnosis often is missed antemortem but, if suspected, may be seen on echocardiography. Advocates use of heparin to prevent embolization.

27. Roldan CA, Shively BK, Lau CC, et al: Systemic lupus erythematosus valve disease by transesophageal echocardiography and the role of antiphospholipid antibodies. *J Am Coll Cardiol* 20:1127–1134, 1992.

   In 54 patients with lupus erythematosus, diffuse leaflet thickening was common (50%) in those with antiphospholipid antibody and was associated with valve regurgitation in 64% or a valve mass in 41% or with both. Even in patients with lupus erythematosus who had no antiphospholipid antibody, 47% had leaflet thickening, 25% had valve masses, and 59% had valve regurgitation. In contrast to infective endocarditis, lupus-associated valve lesions tended to occur near the leaflet bases, were heterogeneous in echo density, and showed little independent motion.

Clinical Guidelines

28. Bayer AS, Bolger AF, Taubert KA, et al: Diagnosis and management of infective endocarditis and its complications. From the Ad Hoc Writing Group of the Committee on Rheumatic Fever, Endocarditis, and Kawasaki Disease; American Heart Association. *Circulation* 98:2936–2948, 1998.

   American Heart Association scientific statement supporting use of the Duke criteria for diagnosis of infective endocarditis. The role of echocardiography is discussed in detail including a flow chart of the use of transthoracic versus transesophageal echocardiography when endocarditis is suspected. Medical and surgical therapy also are reviewed. 141 references.

Echocardiographic Evaluation of Cardiac Masses and Potential Cardiac "Source of Embolus"

14

BASIC PRINCIPLES
ECHOCARDIOGRAPHIC APPROACH
  Infectious Cardiac Masses
  Cardiac Tumors
    Nonprimary
    Primary
    Technical Considerations/Alternate Approaches
  Left Ventricular Thrombus
    Predisposing Conditions
    Identification of Left Ventricular Thrombi
    Clinical Implications
    Alternate Approaches

Left Atrial Thrombus
  Predisposing Factors
  Identification of Left Atrial Thrombi
  Prognosis/Clinical Implications
  Alternate Approaches
  Right Heart Thrombi
CARDIAC SOURCE OF EMBOLUS
  Basic Principles
  Identifiable Cardiac Sources of Emboli
  Predisposing Conditions
  Indications for Echocardiography in Patients with
    Systemic Embolic Events
SUGGESTED READING

A cardiac mass is defined as an abnormal structure within or immediately adjacent to the heart. There are three basic types of cardiac masses: tumor, thrombus, and vegetation. Abnormal mass lesions must be distinguished from the occasional unusual appearance of a normal cardiac structure, which may be mistakenly considered as an apparent "mass." Echocardiography allows dynamic evaluation of intracardiac masses with the advantage, compared with other tomographic techniques, that both the anatomic extent and the physiologic consequences of the mass can be evaluated. In addition, associated abnormalities (e.g., valvular regurgitation associated with a vegetation) and conditions that predispose to development of a mass (e.g., apical aneurysm leading to left ventricular thrombus or rheumatic mitral stenosis resulting in left atrial thrombus) can be evaluated. Disadvantages of echocardiography include suboptimal image quality in some patients, a relatively narrow field of view compared with computed tomography (CT) or magnetic resonance imaging (MRI), and the possibility of mistaking an ultrasound artifact for an anatomic mass.

BASIC PRINCIPLES

The first step in assessing a possible cardiac mass is to ensure that the echocardiographic findings represent an actual mass rather than an ultrasound artifact. As discussed in detail in Chapter 1, artifacts can be caused by electrical interference, characteristics of the ultrasound transducer/system, or various physical factors influencing image formation from the reflected ultrasound signals. These include beam-width artifact, near-field "ring-down," and multipath artifact. Appropriate transducer selection, scanning technique, and evaluation from multiple examining windows will help to distinguish artifacts from actual anatomic structures.

Besides ultrasound artifacts, several normal structures and normal variants may be mistaken for a cardiac mass (Table 14–1). In the ventricles, normal trabeculae, aberrant trabeculae or chordae (ventricular "webs" or false tendons) (Fig. 14–1), muscle bundles (such as the moderator band), or the papillary muscles may be mistaken for abnormal structures.

Valvular anatomy includes a wide range of normal variation, and the appearance of a normal (but often unrecognized) structure such as a

TABLE 14–1	Structures that May Be Mistaken for an Abnormal Cardiac Mass
Left atrium	Dilated coronary sinus (persistent left superior vena cava) Raphe between left superior pulmonary vein and left atrial appendage Atrial suture line after cardiac transplantation Beam-width artifact from calcified aortic valve, aortic valve prosthesis, or other echogenic target adjacent to the atrium Interatrial septal aneurysm
Right atrium	Crista terminalis Chiari network (Eustachian valve remnants) Lipomatous hypertrophy of the interatrial septum Trabeculation of right atrial appendage Atrial suture line after cardiac transplantation Pacer wire, Swan-Ganz catheter, or central venous line
Left ventricle	Papillary muscles Left ventricular web (aberrant chordae) Prominent apical trabeculations Prominent mitral annular calcification
Right ventricle	Moderator band Papillary muscles Swan-Ganz catheter or pacer wire
Aortic valve	Nodules of Arantius Lambl's excrescences Base of valve leaflet imaged tangentially
Mitral valve	Redundant chordae Myxomatous mitral valve tissue
Pulmonary artery	Left atrial appendage (just caudal to pulmonary artery)
Pericardium	Epicardial adipose tissue Fibrinous debris in a chronic organized pericardial effusion

FIGURE 14–1. Left ventricular aberrant trabeculation or "web" seen in an apical four-chamber view in a 35-year-old woman with a normal echo.

nodule of Arantius on the aortic valve may be considered incorrectly to represent a cardiac mass. The belly of a valve leaflet, if cut tangentially, may appear as a "mass" when it actually is a portion of the leaflet itself seen *en face*. In the atrium, normal ridges adjacent to the venous entry sites (Figs. 14–2 and 14–3), normal trabeculations (Fig. 14–4), postoperative changes (Fig. 14–5), and distortion of the free wall contour by structures adjacent to the atrium (Fig. 14–6) all may be diagnosed erroneously as a cardiac mass.

Definitive diagnosis of an intracardiac mass by echocardiography is based on:

1. Excellent image quality, which may require use of a high-frequency (5- or 7.5-MHz) short-focus transducer to evaluate the left ventricular apex from the transthoracic approach

FIGURE 14–2. Normal appearance of the crista terminalis *(arrow)* in the right atrium in a transthoracic apical four-chamber view *(left)* and in a transesophageal view *(right)* in two different patients.

FIGURE 14–3. Prominent valve at the entrance of the inferior vena cava into the right atrium seen obliquely on transesophageal imaging *(left)* might be mistaken for a cardiac mass. A more longitudinal view *(right)* shows the inferior vena cava and valve more clearly.

and the use of transesophageal imaging to evaluate posterior cardiac structures (e.g., left atrium, mitral valve).

2. Identification of the mass throughout the cardiac cycle, in the same anatomic region of the heart, from more than one acoustic window. This decreases the likelihood of an ultrasound artifact.

3. Knowledge of the normal structures, normal variants, and postoperative changes that may simulate a cardiac mass.

4. Integration of other echocardiographic findings (e.g., rheumatic mitral stenosis and left atrial enlargement in a patient with suspected left atrial thrombus) and clinical data in the final echocardiographic interpretation.

FIGURE 14–4. The normal ridge between the left atrial appendage (LAA) and left superior pulmonary vein (LSPV) may be mistaken for an abnormal mass *(left)*. Slight angulation of the image plane shows a more typical appearance *(right)*.

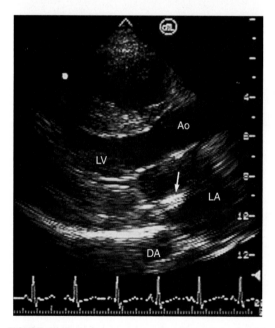

FIGURE 14–5. Prominent suture line *(arrow)* in the left atrium in a parasternal long-axis view of a patient after cardiac transplantation.

ECHOCARDIOGRAPHIC APPROACH
(Table 14–2)

Once it is clear that a cardiac mass is present, the next step is to determine whether that mass most likely is a tumor, a vegetation, or a thrombus. A definitive diagnosis generally cannot be made from the echocardiographic images alone, since the microscopic and bacteriologic characteristics of the structure cannot be determined. However, a reasonably secure diagnosis often can be made by integrating the clinical data, echocardiographic appearance, and associated echo Doppler findings.

Infectious Cardiac Masses

Infectious cardiac masses include valvular vegetations, which are seen in patients with endocarditis (bacterial or fungal). Noninfectious vegetations also occur in patients with nonbacterial thrombotic endocarditis (NBTE, or *marantic* endocarditis). Vegetations typically are irregularly shaped, attached to the upstream side of the valve leaflet (e.g., left atrial side of the mitral valve, left ventricular side of the aortic valve), and exhibit chaotic motion that differs from that of the leaflets themselves (see Figs. 13–1 and 13–2). Valvular regurgitation is a frequent but not invariable accompaniment of endocarditis. Valvular stenosis *due to* the vegetation is rare. Paravalvular abscess, which also presents as a cardiac mass, may be difficult to recognize on transthoracic imaging but can be diagnosed with a high sensitivity and specificity on transesophageal echocardiography. Infectious cardiac masses are discussed in detail in Chapter 13.

Cardiac Tumors

Nonprimary

Nonprimary cardiac tumors are about 20 times more common than primary cardiac tumors. Tumors can involve the heart by direct invasion from adjacent malignancies (lung, breast), by lymphatic spread, or by metastatic

FIGURE 14–6. Persistent left superior vena cava resulting in a dilated coronary sinus (CS) posterior to the left atrium seen in a parasternal long-axis view *(top left)*. If there is ultrasound "dropout" from the wall of the coronary sinus, the abnormal contour of the left atrium may be mistaken for a mass. In the posteriorly angulated apical four-chamber view, the dilated coronary sinus connects to the right atrium *(top right)*. Contrast injection in a left arm vein results in opacification of the coronary sinus, confirming the diagnosis *(right)*.

TABLE 14–2	Distinguishing Characteristics of Intracardiac Masses		
Characteristic	**Thrombus**	**Tumor**	**Vegetation**
Location	LA (especially when enlarged or associated with MV disease) LV (in setting of reduced systolic function or segmental wall abnormalities)	LA (myxoma) Myocardium Pericardium Valves	Usually valvular Occasionally on ventricular wall or Chiari network
Appearance	Usually discrete and somewhat spherical in shape *or* laminated against LV apex or LA wall	Various: may be circumscribed or may be irregular	Irregular shape, attached to the proximal (upstream) side of the valve with motion independent from the valve
Associated findings	Underlying etiology usually evident LV systolic dysfunction or segmental wall motion abnormalities (exception: eosinophilic heart disease) MV disease with LA enlargement	Intracardiac obstruction depending on site of tumor Clinically: fevers, systemic signs of endocarditis, positive blood cultures	Valvular regurgitation usually present

LA = Left atrium; MV = mitral valve; LV = left ventricle.

spread of distant disease (lymphoma, melanoma). In autopsy series of patients with a malignancy, cardiac involvement is present in approximately 10% of cases, although clinical recognition of cardiac involvement occurs less frequently. Melanoma has the highest rate of pericardial metastases, but since there are relatively few patients with melanoma, a cardiac tumor is more likely to represent a more prevalent malignancy, as shown in Table 14–3. Almost three-fourths of cardiac metastases are due to lung, breast, or hematologic malignancies. It is noteworthy that lymphomas associated with acquired immunodeficiency syndrome (AIDS) have frequent and extensive cardiac involvement.

Tumors can affect the heart by (1) invasion of the pericardium, epicardium, myocardium, or endocardium, (2) production of biologically active substances, or (3) toxic effects of treatment on the heart (e.g., radiation or chemotherapy).

Cardiac malignancies most often involve the pericardium and epicardium (about 75% of metastatic cardiac disease), presenting as a pericardial effusion, with or without tamponade physiology (Figs. 14–7 and 14–8). Since echocardiographic diagnosis of the *cause* of a pericardial effusion rarely is possible, the diagnosis of a pericardial effusion (and particularly tamponade) in a patient with a known malignancy should alert the clinician to the possibility of cardiac involvement. Confirmation of the diagnosis requires examination of pericardial fluid

TABLE 14–3	Origin of Metastatic Cardiac Tumors in Adults (in order of frequency)
Lung	
Lymphoma	
Breast	
Leukemia	
Stomach	
Melanoma	
Liver	
Colon	

Data from Abraham KP, Reddy V, Gattuso P: Neoplasms metastatic to the heart: Review of 3314 consecutive autopsies. *Am J Cardiovasc Pathol* 3:195–198, 1990.

and, if necessary, pericardial biopsy. The differential diagnosis of a pericardial effusion in a patient with a known malignancy includes radiation pericarditis and idiopathic pericarditis (which is common in patients with cancer), as well as metastatic disease. The prognosis of a patient with a malignant pericardial effusion is extremely poor, with a predicted 1-year survival less than 50%. Repeat echocardiographic evaluation of these patients often is needed after the initial diagnosis for assessment of therapeutic interventions and follow-up for recurrent effusion.

Myocardial involvement by metastatic dis-

FIGURE 14–7. Metastatic tumor to the heart with an irregular epicardial mass invading the myocardium at the right ventricular apex and an associated pericardial effusion.

FIGURE 14–8. Metastatic lymphoma has filled the pericardial space resulting in compression of the heart and tamponade physiology in the absence of free pericardial fluid.

FIGURE 14–9. Renal cell carcinoma extending up the inferior vena cava (IVC) is seen on a subcostal view *(above)* and in an apical four-chamber view *(below)* protruding into the right atrium and across the tricuspid valve into the right ventricle. This tumor was resected *en bloc* at the time of surgery.

ease is less common than pericardial involvement, but does occur, particularly with lymphoma or melanoma. Intramyocardial masses can project into or compress cardiac chambers, resulting in hemodynamic compromise. Endocardial involvement is rarely seen.

A specific type of cardiac involvement by tumor that should be recognized by the echocardiographer is extension of *renal cell carcinoma* up the inferior vena cava (Fig. 14–9). A "finger-like" projection of tumor may protrude into the right atrium from the inferior vena cava, and the tumor can be followed retrograde (from a subcostal approach) back to the kidney. Collaboration with the abdominal ultrasound laboratory is needed for full delineation of the tumor extent. Identification is important, since curative en bloc resection may be possible. *Uterine tumors* occasionally present in this fashion as well.

Tumors also can affect the cardiac structures indirectly, as is seen in *carcinoid heart disease* (Fig. 14–10). Metastatic carcinoid tissue in the liver produces biologically active substances, including serotonin, which cause abnormalities of the right-sided cardiac valves and endocardium. Typical changes include thickening, retraction, and increased rigidity of the tricuspid and pulmonic valve leaflets, resulting in valvular regurgitation or, less often, valvular stenosis. Left-sided valvular involvement is rarely seen, possibly due to a lower concentration of the active molecules after passage through the lungs. While metastatic carcinoid disease is rare, the echocardiographic findings

are pathognomonic and may lead to the diagnosis in a patient in whom it was not considered previously. Although only a third of patients with carcinoid tumors have cardiac involvement, half the deaths in carcinoid patients are due to heart failure resulting from severe tricuspid regurgitation.

FIGURE 14–10. Carcinoid heart disease with thickening and shortening of the tricuspid leaflets *(arrows)* seen in a right ventricular inflow view *(left)*. Mild stenosis and severe regurgitation of the tricuspid valve were present as seen on color flow imaging in the right ventricular inflow view *(right)*. (See Color Plate 16, p. 274.)

TABLE 14–4	Primary Cardiac Tumors in Adults	
Benign		
Myxoma	27%	
Lipoma	10%	
Papillary fibroelastoma	10%	
Hemangioma	3%	
Mesothelioma of the AV node	1%	
Malignant		
Angiosarcoma	9%	
Rhabdomyosarcoma	5%	
Mesothelioma	4%	
Fibrosarcoma	3%	
Malignant lymphoma	2%	
Extraskeletal osteosarcoma	1%	
Cysts		
Pericardial	18%	
Bronchogenic	2%	

AV = Atrioventricular.
Data from McAllister HA, Fenoglio JJ: Tumors of the cardiovascular system. *In Atlas of Tumor Pathology.* fascicle 15, second series. Armed Forces Institute of Pathology, 1978.

FIGURE 14–11. Left atrial myxoma arising from a thin stalk attached to the fossa ovalis of the interatrial septum seen in a transesophageal view.

Primary (Table 14–4)

As for tumors elsewhere in the body, the distinction between benign and malignant primary cardiac tumors is based on pathologic examination of tissue and its tendency to invade adjacent tissue or metastasize to distant sites. Although 75% of primary cardiac tumors are benign, a pathologically benign cardiac tumor can have "malignant" hemodynamic consequences if it obstructs the normal pattern of blood flow. Thus the echocardiographic examination includes definition of both the anatomic extent of a cardiac tumor and its physiologic consequences.

Benign Primary Cardiac Tumors. *Myxomas* account for 27% of primary cardiac tumors.

Cardiac myxomas most often are single, arising from the fossa ovalis of the interatrial septum and protruding into the left atrium (in about 75% of cases) (Fig. 14–11). Other sites of origin include the right atrium (18%), the left ventricle (4%), and the right ventricle (4%). More than one site can occur in an individual patient (5% of cases).

The clinical presentation of a cardiac myxoma can include constitutional symptoms (fever, malaise), clinically evident embolic events, and symptoms of mitral valve obstruction. A myxoma also may be an unexpected finding on a study requested for other clinical indications.

A left atrial myxoma may nearly fill the left atrial chamber (Fig. 14–12), with prolapse of the tumor mass across the mitral annulus into the left ventricle in diastole (accounting for the tumor "plop" on auscultation). The mass often has an irregular shape characterized by protruding "fronds" of tissue or a "grape cluster" appearance. The echogenicity of the mass may be nonhomogeneous, and sometimes areas of calcification are noted.

The degree to which the tumor causes functional obstruction to left ventricular diastolic filling can be evaluated qualitatively by color flow imaging and quantitatively by the pressure half-time method (Fig. 14–13). Careful echocardiographic evaluation from multiple views, often including transesophageal, is needed in planning the surgical approach. Important goals of the echo examination are to identify the site of tumor attachment, to ensure that the tumor does not involve the valve leaflets themselves, and to exclude the possibility of multiple masses. Postoperatively, complete excision should be documented by echocardiography. Sequential long-term follow-up may be indicated, since recurrent myxomas have been reported, particularly with a familial form of this disease, with multiple myxomas, or with a less than full-thickness excision.

The echocardiographic approach to myxomas arising in other locations is similar to that described for left atrial myxomas, except that the two-dimensional (2D) views and Doppler examination should be tailored toward evaluating the specific region of tumor involvement in that patient. Again, it should be emphasized

FIGURE 14–12. Large left atrial myxoma (M) in an 84-year-old woman with prolapse across the mitral annulus in diastole *(above)* in an apical four-chamber view. Doppler left ventricular filling *(below)* shows normal filling at valve opening *(arrow)* followed by obstruction as the myxoma obstructs the mitral orifice.

FIGURE 14–13. Color flow imaging also shows the partial obstruction to left ventricular diastolic filling due to the atrial myxoma (M) in the same patient as Figure 14–12. (See Color Plate 16, p. 274.)

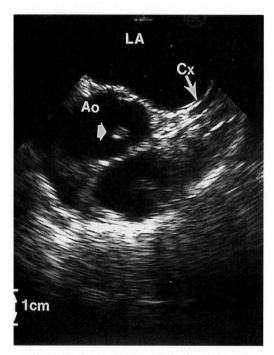

FIGURE 14–14. Small papillary fibroelastoma attached to the left coronary cusp of the aortic valve (with independent motion) as seen on transesophageal imaging *(arrow)*. This mass was not seen on transthoracic imaging. In this patient with increased thrombogenicity, this benign valve tumor had associated thrombus which resulted in embolic events (Cx = circumflex coronary artery). (From Huth M, Gordon D, Verner ED, Otto CM: Aortic valvular fibroma as a source of systemic emboli in POEMS syndrome. *J Am Soc Echocardiogr* 4:401, 1991. Used with permission.)

FIGURE 14–15. Lipomatous hypertrophy *(arrows)* of the interatrial septum seen on transesophageal imaging with typical sparing of the thin fossa ovalis.

that the diagnosis of a myxoma, based on the clinical features, anatomic location, and echocardiographic appearance of the tumor, is only presumptive until confirmed histologically. A "typical" myxoma may turn out to be a metastatic malignancy or a primary cardiac malignancy on pathologic examination. Hence the echocardiographic examination should be as complete as possible to exclude tissue invasion by the tumor, multiple sites of involvement, or atypical features.

A *papillary fibroelastoma* is a benign cardiac tumor that arises on valvular tissue, thus mimicking the appearance of a valvular vegetation. A papillary fibroelastoma appears as a small mass attached to the mitral or (less often) aortic valve with motion independent from the normal valve structures (Fig. 14–14). Unlike a vegetation, fibroelastomas are more often found on the downstream side of the valve (left ventricular side of mitral valve, aortic side of aortic valve). The histologic appearance is very similar to the smaller Lambl's excrescences,

which can be seen on normal valves in the elderly. Usually a papillary fibroelastoma is of no clinical significance, but may cause consternation on the part of the physicians caring for the patient and lead to further diagnostic tests with their associated costs and complications. Occasional cases of superimposed thrombus formation resulting in systemic embolic events have been described.

Other benign cardiac tumors seen in adults include hemangiomas, and mesotheliomas of the atrioventricular node.

Lipomatous hypertrophy of the interatrial septum presents as a cardiac mass that may be mistaken for a tumor. Lipomatous hypertrophy typically involves the superior and inferior fatty portions of the atrial septum, sparing the fossa ovalis region (Fig. 14–15). However, symmetric ellipsoid-shaped enlargements of the interatrial septum also have been described. If the etiology of atrial septal hypertrophy is unclear on echocardiography, CT scanning may establish the diagnosis of lipomatous hypertrophy by showing the characteristic radiographic density of adipose tissue.

Malignant Primary Cardiac Tumors. Malignant primary cardiac tumors are rare. In adults, angiosarcomas, rhabdomyosarcomas (Fig. 14–16), mesotheliomas, and fibrosarcomas are seen (see Table 14–3). The clinical presentation is variable, ranging from an "incidental" finding on echocardiography or nonspecific systemic symptoms (fever, malaise, fatigue) to signs and symptoms of cardiac tamponade. Since metastatic disease is far more likely than a primary cardiac origin, thorough evaluation must include a search for potential primary sites. Ultimately, the diagnosis depends on examination of tissue from the cardiac mass.

The echocardiographic examination focuses on the anatomic location and extent of the tumor involvement, the physiologic consequences of the tumor (e.g., valve regurgitation, chamber obliteration, obstruction), and associated findings (pericardial effusion, evidence of tamponade physiology). Along with other imaging techniques, the echocardiographic examination may help guide therapy by determining whether the tumor is resectable or whether palliative cardiac procedures are likely to be beneficial. Specific attention also is directed toward possible involvement of the valves, coronary arteries, or conducting system.

FIGURE 14–16. Large, recurrent left atrial rhabdomyosarcoma attached to the ridge between the left atrial appendage and left superior pulmonary vein. Note that this malignant tumor appears similar on echocardiography to a benign myxoma.

Technical Considerations/Alternate Approaches

Although echocardiography has definite advantages for evaluating cardiac tumors, it has significant disadvantages as well. These include (1) poor acoustic access, resulting in suboptimal image quality, which limits the confidence with which tumor location and extent can be defined or results in a missed diagnosis (transesophageal imaging may obviate this limitation in some patients), (2) the need for a careful and meticulous examination to detect and fully evaluate the cardiac tumor (as for other applications, echocardiography is operator dependent, and a significant learning curve for obtaining optimal data can be observed), and (3) the limited "field of view" inherent in echocardiography (i.e., structures adjacent to the heart in the mediastinum and lung are difficult to evaluate). Other tomographic imaging techniques, specifically CT and MRI, have the advantage of a wide field of view so that the relationship between cardiac and extracardiac tumor involvement can be evaluated. Often judicious use of both echocardiographic techniques (to assess cardiac involvement in detail and to evaluate the physiologic consequences of the tumor mass) and CT or MRI (to assess potential extracardiac involvement) may be needed in an individual patient for optimal clinical decision making. Both CT and MRI may provide data on the tissue characteristics of the abnormal mass, which currently cannot be obtained with echocardiography (Fig. 14–17).

Left Ventricular Thrombus

Predisposing Conditions

Thrombus formation in the left ventricle tends to occur in regions of blood stasis or low-

FIGURE 14–17. *Left,* MRI scan in a patient with angiosarcoma shows a large nonhomogeneous right atrial mass. *Right,* CT scan at the level of the pulmonary artery and ascending aorta in a different patient (who also had an angiosarcoma) shows extensive intrapericardial tumor involvement. These cases illustrate the advantage of the wide field of view of MRI and CT techniques compared with the narrow field of view of echocardiography.

velocity blood flow. The most familiar example of blood flow stasis in the left ventricle is a ventricular aneurysm, in which low-velocity swirling blood flow patterns are seen. Stasis also may occur with less severe segmental wall motion abnormalities (e.g., apical akinesis) and with diffuse left ventricular dysfunction (e.g., dilated cardiomyopathy). Left ventricular thrombus formation is extremely rare in the absence of an akinetic or dyskinetic apex or diffuse left ventricular dysfunction. Thrombus formation also often accompanies a left ventricular pseudoaneurysm. In this case, the thrombus lines an area of left ventricular rupture that has been contained by the pericardium (see Fig. 7–28).

Even when a definite left ventricular thrombus is not seen on an echocardiographic examination, the likelihood of thrombus formation remains high in patients with left ventricular aneurysm, apical akinesis, or diffuse left ventricular systolic dysfunction with an ejection fraction less than 20%. Doppler analysis of apical flow patterns has been suggested to help identify which of these patients are at highest risk of thrombus formation. Evidence of apical flow stasis or of continuous swirling of flow around the apex is thought to identify patients at particular risk for apical thrombus.

Identification of Left Ventricular Thrombi

The sensitivity of echocardiography for detecting left ventricular thrombi is extremely operator-dependent (Table 14–5). A careful and thorough examination requires not only standard views but also angulated apical views and the use of higher-frequency short-focus transducers to improve near-field resolution. It is advantageous to use a 5- or 7.5-MHz transducer from the standard apical four-chamber window and also to move the transducer slightly laterally while angulating it medially to obtain an apical short-axis view. Scanning across the apex in several views usually allows distinction of apical thrombi from prominent apical trabeculations or false tendons, which are bright linear structures that attach to mural trabeculae. Thrombus is often (though not always) somewhat more echogenic than the underlying myocardium, and has a contour distinct from the endocardial border.

The diagnosis of left ventricular thrombus is most secure when an echogenic mass is seen with a convex surface that is not a "ring-down" artifact, is clearly distinct from the endocardium, and is located in a region of abnormal wall motion (Fig. 14–18). The diagnosis of laminated thrombus is more problematic unless a clear demarcation between the thrombus and the underlying myocardium is seen, but it can be suspected when the apex appears "rounded" and akinetic with apparent excessively thick apical myocardium (Fig. 14–19).

Clinical Implications

In some cases, apical images are suboptimal despite careful examination technique. In this situation, definite exclusion of apical thrombus may not be possible. Even so, clinical management (e.g., chronic anticoagulation) may depend more on assessment of overall left ventricular function or the presence of an apical aneurysm than on the presence or absence of an echocardiographically documented thrombus.

The presence of a left ventricular thrombus on echocardiographic examination is a strong predictor of subsequent embolic events, particularly when the thrombus protrudes into the ventricular cavity or shows independent mobility. Sessile, nonprotruding thrombi may have lower embolic potential.

Alternate Approaches

Transthoracic echocardiography is the clinical procedure of choice for identification of left ventricular thrombi. Transesophageal imaging rarely is helpful and may be less sensitive, as the apex may not be visualized in standard image planes and since the left ventricular apex is at

FIGURE 14–18. Protruding thrombus *(arrows)* in an akinetic apex in a 53-year-old man with a dilated cardiomyopathy seen in an apical four-chamber view.

FIGURE 14–19. Apical thrombus "obliterating" the left ventricular apex in a 53-year-old woman with an old anterior myocardial infarction.

considerable distance from the transducer, thereby limiting resolution of structural detail. Left ventricular contrast angiography and radionuclide ventriculography both have a low sensitivity and specificity for diagnosing left ventricular thrombus. In the research setting, indium 114–labeled platelets with gamma-camera imaging have shown a high specificity, but this approach is not available for routine clinical use.

Left Atrial Thrombus

Predisposing Factors

Left atrial thrombi tend to form when there is stasis of blood flow in the left atrium. In general, low-velocity flow in the left atrium is associated with atrial enlargement, mitral valve disease, and atrial fibrillation. The highest incidence of left atrial thrombus is in patients with rheumatic mitral stenosis and atrial fibrillation. However, in the presence of mitral stenosis or poor left ventricular function, even patients in sinus rhythm and those with only modest left atrial enlargement can have left atrial thrombi.

Left atrial thrombi are less common in patients with mitral regurgitation, presumably because the high-velocity regurgitant jet mechanically disrupts the area of blood stasis within the left atrium.

Identification of Left Atrial Thrombi

Visualization of left atrial thrombi using transthoracic echocardiography is limited by two factors:

1. The left atrium is in the far field of the image from both parasternal and apical windows,

TABLE 14–5	Sensitivity and Specificity of Diagnostic Tests for Intracardiac Thrombus Formation		
		Sensitivity	Specificity
LA thrombus			
Echo-TTE[a]		59–63%	95–99%
Echo-TEE[b]		100%	100%
Radionuclide angiography		67%	54%
CT[c]		100%	91%
Angiography[c]		70%	88%
LV thrombus			
Echo-TTE[d]		92–95%	86–88%
Radionuclide angiography[e]		77%	88%
MRI[f]		93%	85%
Indium-111 platelet scintigraphy[g]		71%	100%

[a]Shrestha et al: Am J Cardiol 48:954–960, 1981; Chiang et al: J Ultrasound Med 6:525–529, 1987; Bansal et al: Am J Cardiol 64:243–246, 1989.
[b]Aschenberg et al: JACC 7, 163–166, 1986; Olson et al: JASE 5:52–56, 1992.
[c]Tomoda et al: Am Heart J 100: 306, 1980.
[d]Visser et al: Chest 83:228–232, 1983; Stratton et al: Circulation 66:156–165, 1982.
[e]Stratton et al: Am J Cardiol 48:565–572, 1981.
[f]Sechtem et al: Am J Cardiol 64:1195–1199, 1989.
[g]Stratton et al: Am J Cardiol 47:874–881, 1981; Seabold et al: JACC 9:1057–1066, 1987.
LA = left atrium; LV = left ventricle; MRI = magnetic resonance imaging; TEE = transesophageal echocardiography; TTE = transthoracic echocardiography.

FIGURE 14–20. Transthoracic parasternal short-axis view of the left atrial appendage (LAA).

FIGURE 14–21. Transthoracic apical two-chamber view showing a definite thrombus (T) in the left atrial appendage in a 51-year-old man with dilated cardiomyopathy.

thus limiting resolution of left atrial structures and possible thrombi.

2. A large percentage of left atrial thrombi are found in the left atrial appendage, which is difficult to image from the transthoracic approach.

In some patients, the left atrial appendage can be visualized from a parasternal approach (Fig. 14–20), starting in the short-axis view at the aortic valve level and angulating the transducer inferiorly and laterally to demonstrate the triangular appendage just inferior to the pulmonary artery. From the apical two-chamber view, the left atrial appendage may be visualized by slight superior angulation of the transducer. If a discrete echogenic mass is seen in the left atrium of a patient with mitral stenosis and atrial fibrillation, the specificity of this finding for left atrial thrombi is very high (Fig. 14–21). Of course, the differential diagnosis includes tumor, but this possibility is much less likely in this setting. Nonetheless, the sensitivity of transthoracic echocardiography for detection of left atrial thrombus remains modest at best. If *no* left atrial thrombus is seen in a patient in whom the diagnosis is suspected, a transthoracic echo study certainly does *not* exclude this possibility.

Transesophageal imaging has a much greater sensitivity and a high negative predictive value for the diagnosis of left atrial thrombi. Hence transesophageal evaluation should be considered when the presence or absence of left atrial thrombus is important for patient management. From the transesophageal approach, the left

atrium lies close to the transducer, and usually it can be visualized clearly with a 5- or 7.5-MHz transducer in at least two orthogonal views. Optimally, the left atrial appendage is evaluated by centering the appendage in the image plane at the 0° transducer position, using a small field of view and a high-frequency transducer. Then the image plane is slowly rotated through 180°, keeping the atrial appendage centered in the image, to evaluate for possible thrombus. In addition, the body of the left atrium and atrial septal region are evaluated using rotational scanning from 0 to 180° from a high esophageal position (Fig. 14–22).

Stasis of blood flow may be seen on transesophageal imaging as "spontaneous" echo contrast, that is, echogenic reflections from the low-velocity blood flow appearing as white swirls on the 2D echocardiographic image (Fig. 14–23). While the appearance of "spontaneous" contrast depends on technical factors such as transducer frequency and instrument gain, as well as the pattern of blood flow, it clearly is associated with an increased risk of left atrial thrombus formation. An increased risk of embolic complications that appears to be independent of associated atrial thrombus also has been reported. Doppler recordings of the pattern of blood flow in the left atrial appendage also may be helpful in identifying patients at highest risk of thrombus formation (Fig. 14–24).

Prognosis/Clinical Implications

The importance of a left atrial thrombus depends on the clinical setting. In a patient with new atrial fibrillation and an embolic stroke, the most likely cause of the stroke is a left atrial thrombus whether or not one is actually imaged, and thus the demonstration of a left atrial thrombus would be unlikely to change clinical management. In contrast, in a patient with rheumatic mitral stenosis, the presence of a left atrial thrombus is a contraindication to mitral balloon commissurotomy.

Alternate Approaches

While few direct comparisons of echocardiography versus CT or MRI have been performed, these imaging modalities have been reported to have a high sensitivity for detection of left atrial thrombus.

Right Heart Thrombi

Formation of thrombi in the right side of the heart is rare, although it has been reported in cases of severe right ventricular dilation and systolic dysfunction. A more likely source of thrombi seen within the right side of the heart is venous thrombi that have embolized and be-

FIGURE 14–22. Thrombus in the left atrial appendage seen on transesophageal imaging in a 42-year-old man with severe rheumatic mitral stenosis.

FIGURE 14–23. "Spontaneous" contrast with a swirling motion in real time is seen in the body of the enlarged left atrium in a patient with atrial fibrillation and mitral stenosis.

FIGURE 14–24. Left atrial appendage blood flow pattern recorded on transesophageal echocardiography in sinus rhythm *(top)*, atrial fibrillation *(middle)*, and atrial flutter *(bottom)*. Notice that both the P wave in sinus rhythm and the flutter waves are associated with a flow velocity out of the atrial appendage are >40 cm/s. In contrast, only very low flow velocities are seen in atrial fibrillation leading to stasis of blood in the atrial appendage. (AF = atrial fibrillation, NSR = normal sinus rhythm.)

come entrapped in the tricuspid valve apparatus or right ventricular trabeculations during passage from the peripheral veins toward the pulmonary artery. Thrombi also can form on indwelling catheters or pacer wires. While thrombi in the right side of the heart can sometimes be demonstrated by meticulous transthoracic imaging (Figs. 14–25 and 14–26), transesophageal echo is better able to resolve the presence, extent, and attachment of right-sided heart thrombi.

When mobile echogenic targets are seen within the right heart chambers, it is important to distinguish thrombi from eustachian valve remnants, microbubbles, or reverberation artifacts. Eustachian valve remnants, which are persistent portions of the embryologic valves of the sinus venosus, are typically mobile, thin linear structures attached at the junction of the inferior or superior cavae and the right atrial cavity. They may be extensive and can cross the atrium, attaching to the fossa ovalis. They do not extend antegrade to cross the tricuspid valve in diastole, however. Microbubbles, which are encapsulated gas bubbles that can be seen in patients with indwelling venous access, appear as discrete echogenic targets that are usually located in different parts of the heart during successive cycles.

CARDIAC SOURCE OF EMBOLUS

Basic Principles

In a patient with a suspected cardiac origin of a systemic embolic event, echocardiographic evaluation is directed toward one or all of the following:

1. Identification of an abnormal intracardiac mass (e.g., left ventricular thrombus, left atrial tumor, valvular vegetation), *or*
2. Identification of an abnormality that may predispose the patient to development of intracardiac thrombi (e.g., left ventricular aneurysm, mitral stenosis, atrial flow stasis), *or*
3. Identification of a cardiac abnormality that may serve as a potential source for systemic embolism (patent foramen ovale, atrial septal aneurysm, atheromatous aortic debris).

Note that echocardiographic evaluation *after* an index embolic event may fail to demonstrate a cardiac thrombus even if it was the etiology of the clinical event, since now the thrombus has embolized and is no longer in the heart. Recurrent intracardiac thrombus formation may not yet have occurred.

FIGURE 14–25. Extracardiac localized thrombus after coronary artery surgery is seen indenting the right atrium in a four-chamber view.

FIGURE 14–26. Right atrial thrombus *(arrows)* in a patient with a dilated cardiomyopathy.

Identifiable Cardiac Sources of Emboli

In patients with an echocardiographically demonstrated abnormal intracardiac mass in the aftermath of a recent systemic embolic event, the likelihood is very high that a portion of the mass embolized, thereby causing the clinical event. Cardiac masses known to be associated with clinical systemic embolic events include valvular vegetations, left ventricular and atrial thrombi, and cardiac tumors (especially left atrial myxomas). Other potential pathways for systemic embolization (patent foramen ovale) and possible cardiac sources (atrial septal aneurysm, aortic atherosclerosis) are discussed in the following section. In patients with suspected systemic embolic events, a definite cardiac source is documented by transthoracic echocardiography in approximately 10% to 15% of sequential cases. To some extent, the low prevalence of a definite source may relate to imaging *after* the event (when the mass is no longer in the heart). On the other hand, in many patients the source of embolus may have been noncardiac (e.g., atheromas with or without superimposed thrombus in the carotid arteries or ascending aorta), or the intracardiac thrombi may have embolized soon after formation. In this latter group, it is especially important to search for conditions that predispose to intracardiac thrombus formation, even though an intracardiac thrombus is not identified at the time of the examination.

Predisposing Conditions

Apical aneurysms have a high incidence of associated thrombus formation. Other segmental wall motion abnormalities and diffuse left ventricular systolic dysfunction also predispose to left ventricular thrombus formation. A left ventricular *pseudoaneurysm* is almost invariably accompanied by thrombus lining the pseudoaneurysm cavity.

Rheumatic mitral stenosis is associated with left atrial thrombus formation. *Atrial fibrillation,* even when it occurs without coexisting mitral valve disease, is strongly associated with systemic embolic events, presumably due to left atrial thrombi. In a patient with a systemic embolic event and either paroxysmal or sustained atrial fibrillation, left atrial thrombus formation is so likely that even if transesophageal echocardiography fails to demonstrate a left atrial clot, it still may be appropriate to treat the patient with systemic anticoagulants to prevent recurrent atrial thrombus formation.

Intracardiac thrombi may occur in patients with *congenital heart disease,* particularly those with atrial dilation or ventricular dysfunction. Patients with a large atrial septal defect are at risk for "paradoxical" systemic embolization of peripheral venous thrombi. Thrombi can pass from the right to the left atrium even when the shunt is predominantly left to right, owing to streaming of flow or transient shifts in the right-to-left atrial pressure gradient. While patients with Eisenmenger's complex and a large ventricular septal defect are at risk of systemic embolization from peripheral venous thrombus formation, such paradoxical embolization is unlikely when the ventricular septal defect is small and there is a large pressure difference between the left and right ventricles.

Prosthetic valves are another potential source of embolic events; the incidence of clinical events is higher with mechanical compared with tissue valves. Demonstration of small thrombi on prosthetic valves is difficult even with transesophageal imaging, owing to shadowing and reverberations from the prosthetic leaflets and sewing ring. Hence the diagnosis often is presumptive when there is evidence of suboptimal anticoagulation at the time of the event or when other causes for the clinical event have been excluded even if the level of anticoagulation appears to have been adequate. In these patients, the primary goals of the echocardiographic examination are to assess prosthetic valve function (since significant thrombus may result in stenosis and/or regurgitation) and to exclude other intracardiac sources of thrombus formation (e.g., associated left ventricular systolic dysfunction).

The advent of transesophageal echocardiography has made it possible to image atrial structures in more detail and has led to the recognition of other anatomic variants and disease processes that may be associated with systemic embolic events: (1) patent foramen ovale, (2) interatrial septal aneurysm, (3) a swirling pattern of blood flow in the left atrium in the absence of an exogenous "contrast" agent (thought to represent flow stasis and often called *spontaneous contrast*), and (4) atherosclerotic debris in the aorta.

A *patent foramen ovale* is present in 25% to 35% of unselected patients at autopsy. During fetal development, incomplete closure of the interatrial septum shunts oxygenated placental blood from the right to left atrium and then to the brain. This potential interatrial communication fuses within the first few days after birth in most individuals. If the flap valve covering the fossa ovalis remains unfused, there usually is no passage of blood across the interatrial septum. The "flap" is functionally closed because left atrial pressure normally exceeds right atrial pressure. However, if right atrial pressure transiently exceeds left atrial pressure (as during a cough or the Valsalva maneuver), or if right atrial pressure chronically exceeds left atrial pressure (e.g., after pulmonary embolization or with chronic lung disease), there can be right-to-left passage of blood (or thrombi) across the interatrial septum.

Echocardiographic demonstration of a patent

FIGURE 14–28. Another example of a patent foramen ovale seen on transesophageal echocardiography in a short-axis image plane. Careful adjustment of transducer position and angulation often in needed to demonstrate the defect.

FIGURE 14–27. Atrial septal aneurysm *(top)* with a patent foramen ovale *(bottom)* demonstrated on transesophageal echocardiography in a four-chamber view after injection of agitated saline solution in peripheral vein. Small microbubbles *(arrow)* are seen traversing the defect from the opacified right into the unopacified left atrium.

foramen ovale is possible with color flow Doppler imaging from a transesophageal approach in only about 5% to 10% of patients, with a lesser number detected by transthoracic color Doppler imaging. Detection of a patent foramen is enhanced by intravenous injection of echo contrast material (such as agitated saline solution) providing opacification of the right-sided heart structures. Passage of contrast across the interatrial septum is seen as bright echo contrast in the left atrium within one to three beats of its appearance in the right atrium

(Figs. 14–27 and 14–28). It is important to use a view in which the contrast effect does not obscure identification of microbubbles in the left side of the heart. Often the site of origin of the contrast in the left atrium can be identified on frame-by-frame analysis. Using echo contrast, a patent foramen is detectable at rest in about 5% of the general population. When maneuvers to transiently increase right atrial pressure are performed simultaneously with contrast injection, the prevalence of detectable patent foramen ovale by contrast transesophageal echocardiography increases to approximately 25%—similar to the incidence at autopsy.

Accurate detection of a patent foramen ovale is more likely on transesophageal imaging due to improved image quality. However, contrast injections still are needed to detect all cases. Passage of very small microbubbles through the pulmonary capillaries can occur; these typically appear in the left atrium via the pulmonary veins late after the appearance of contrast material in the right atrium. The examiner should evaluate whether contrast material in the left atrium detected on transesophageal imaging passed across the interatrial septum or reflects transpulmonary passage. Meticulous evaluation using multiplane transesophageal echocardiography often is helpful.

In young patients (<45 years of age) with transient ischemic attacks or cerebrovascular events, a higher incidence of patent foramen ovale is found than in the general population, suggesting that passage of thrombi across the atrial septum may be a significant cause of systemic embolic events in these patients. This diagnosis is most secure in a patient with a patent foramen ovale when a peripheral venous source of thrombi is also identified.

An *interatrial septal aneurysm* is defined as a transient bulging of the fossa ovalis region of the interatrial septum (total excursion from the septal plane) greater than 15 mm in the absence of chronically elevated left or right atrial pressure (Fig. 14–29). Septal aneurysms are associated with a high likelihood (up to 90%) of associated fenestration. Until recently, the diagnosis rarely was made from transthoracic echo imaging due to suboptimal image quality, and this finding was thought to be of little clinical significance. The excellent views of the interatrial septum on transesophageal echocardiography have resulted in an increasing recognition of this anatomic variant. Several investigators have suggested a possible relationship between the presence of an atrial septal aneurysm and an increased risk of systemic embolic events.

"Spontaneous" contrast is seen in the left atrium when there is stasis of blood flow. It is seen more often on transesophageal than transthoracic imaging due to the higher transducer frequency and the closer proximity of the left atrium when interrogated from the esophagus but can be seen on transthoracic imaging in some patients. Spontaneous contrast is associated with left atrial enlargement and left atrial

FIGURE 14–29. Incidental finding of an atrial septal aneurysm (ASA) in an elderly patient seen in a transthoracic apical four-chamber view.

thrombus formation, and it may be a marker for a "prethrombotic" state when definite atrial thrombi are not seen. In extreme cases of spontaneous contrast in mitral stenosis patients, the jet of diastolic blood flow across the stenotic mitral orifice can be seen on 2D imaging due to the contrast effect.

Spontaneous contrast can be seen in the left ventricle when there is stasis of blood flow, such as in the region of an apical aneurysm. Spontaneous contrast also is observed frequently in patients with mechanical prosthetic valves. Here the mechanism of spontaneous contrast formation may be different, relating to the mechanical impact of the valve occluder during closure and resulting in microcavitation or liberation of gas from solution. Of course, patients with mitral prosthetic valves also may have stasis of blood flow in the left atrium if long-standing disease has resulted in left atrial enlargement and atrial fibrillation.

Indications for Echocardiography in Patients with Systemic Embolic Events

Current understanding of potential cardiac etiologies for systemic embolism is incomplete, and there is considerable controversy as to the indications for transthoracic and transesophageal echocardiography in patients with suspected systemic embolic events. Transthoracic echocardiography rarely demonstrates abnormalities in patients without clinical evidence of heart disease, and most authorities do not recommend transthoracic echo evaluation unless there is clinically apparent heart disease. The proper role of transesophageal echo is more controversial. At one extreme, some clinicians advocate echocardiography in nearly all patients on the principle that even if a cardiac abnormality is unlikely, the risk of echocardiography is so low that evaluation still is warranted. At the other extreme, some clinicians argue that echocardiography is indicated only if there is definite evidence for cardiac disease by history or physical examination.

Current guidelines recommend echocardiography in patients with neurologic or other vascular occlusive events if (1) there is abrupt occlusion of a major peripheral or visceral artery in patients of any age, (2) in younger patients (<45 years of age) with a cerebrovascular embolic event, (3) in older patients with a neurologic event without other evidence of cerebrovascular disease, and (4) in patients in whom the clinical therapeutic decision would be altered based on the echocardiographic results. The use of echocardiography in patients with cerebrovascular disease of questionable significance or with other evident causes for the cerebrovascular event remains controversial. If transthoracic studies are unrevealing, transesophageal imaging should be performed, given its higher sensitivity for diagnosis of a patent foramen ovale, left atrial thrombus, interatrial septal aneurysm, valvular vegetation, and small intracardiac tumors.

In older patients, the yield of echocardiographic imaging is highest in those without evidence for an extracardiac source (e.g., those without carotid disease) and with evidence (or risk factors) for underlying cardiac disease. The possibility that atheromas of the ascending aorta may lead to embolic events also should be considered in this age group (see Chap. 15).

Currently accepted definite indications for echocardiography in patients with suspected cerebral embolism include clinical evidence of heart disease or age younger than 45 years. Opinion is divided on the appropriateness of echocardiography in patients older than age 45 with suspected cerebral embolism but no clinical evidence of heart disease. Most cardiologists agree that echocardiography is not indicated in patients with known noncardiac causes of cerebral embolism.

SUGGESTED READING

General Reviews

1. Waller BF (ed): Pathology of the Heart and Great Vessels. New York, Churchill-Livingstone, 1988.

   Multiauthor textbook of cardiac pathology in the current era emphasizing surgical findings. Chapters are included on prosthetic valve dysfunction, endomyocardial biopsy, and diseases of the great vessels, as well as valvular heart disease and cardiac tumors.

2. Becker AE, Anderson RH: Cardiac Pathology: An Integrated Text and Colour Atlas. New York, Raven Press, 1982.

   An atlas of cardiac pathology with excellent illustrations and concise descriptions.

3. Reeder GS, Khandheria BK, Seward JB, Tajik AJ: Transesophageal echocardiography and cardiac masses. *Mayo Clin Proc* 66:1101–1109, 1991.

   Descriptive article of the Mayo Clinic's experience with transesophageal echo for detection of cardiac masses over a 2-year period (83 masses were identified). Several illustrative 2D echocardiograms.

Cardiac Tumors

4. Salcedo EE, Cohen GI, White RD, Davison MB: Cardiac tumors: Diagnosis and management. *Curr Prob Cardiol* 17:75–137, 1992.

   Review of the clinical aspects of diagnosis and management of cardiac tumors. 174 references.

5. Hancock EW: Neoplastic pericardial disease. *Clin Cardiol* 8:673–682, 1990.

   Review article focusing on the presentation and management of malignant pericardial disease. 43 references.

6. Abraham KP, Reddy V, Gattuso P: Neoplasms metastatic to the heart: Review of 3314 consecutive autopsies. *Am J Cardiovasc Pathol* 3:195–198, 1990.

   Autopsy study (n = 3314) with malignant disease in 24% (n = 806) and cardiac involvement in 12% of these cases (n = 95). Analysis of frequency of primary tumors. Used as the source of data for Table 14–4.

7. Klatt EC, Heitz DR: Cardiac metastases. *Cancer* 65:1456–1459, 1990.

   A large autopsy series of patients with a malignancy (n = 1029) with a rate of cardiac involvement of 11%. In this study the lung was the most common primary tumor site (36%). More than 75% of metastatic cardiac disease involved the epicardium, and 34% of such patients had a pericardial effusion.

8. Klarich KW, Enriquez-Sarano M, Gura GM, et al: Papillary fibroelastoma: Echocardiographic characteristics for diagnosis and pathologic correlation. *J Am Coll Cardiol* 30:784–790, 1997.

   At the Mayo Clinic, 54 patients with papillary fibroelastomas seen on echocardiography were identified over a 15-year period. Pathologic confirmation of the diagnosis was available in 17 patients. On echocardiography, papillary fibroelastomas typically were small (about 1 cm in diameter on average), pedunculated, mobile masses attached to valves (60%) or other endocardial surfaces (40%). Clinically, valve dysfunction was rare and most patients were asymptomatic. Overall, 12 of 54 (22%) patients had either a history of or a subsequent embolic neurologic event.

Left Ventricular Thrombi

9. Stratton JR, Lighty GW Jr, Pearlman AS, Ritchie JL: Detection of left ventricular thrombus by two-dimensional echocardiography: Sensitivity, specificity, and causes of uncertainty. *Circulation* 66:156–165, 1982.

   In 78 patients with surgical, autopsy, or indium-111 platelet imaging evidence of left ventricular thrombus, the 2D transthoracic echo result was positive or equivocal in 21 of the 22 patients with a thrombus (sensitivity 95%) and was negative in 48 of 56 without a thrombus (specificity 86%). A definitely positive echo study had a positive predictive accuracy of 86%, while an equivocal study had a positive predictive value of only 29%.

10. Ezekowitz MD, Wilson DA, Smith EO, et al: Comparison of indium-111 platelet scintigraphy and two-dimensional echocardiography in the diagnosis of left ventricular thrombi. *N Engl J Med* 306:1509–1513, 1982.

    In 53 patients with autopsy or surgical proof of left ventricular thrombus, 2D echo had a sensitivity of 77% and specificity of 93%, while indium–111 platelet scintigraphy had a sensitivity of 71% and a specificity of 100%.

11. Stratton JR, Ritchie JL, Hammermeister KE, et al: Detection of left ventricular thrombi with radionuclide angiography. *Am J Cardiol* 48:565–572, 1981.

Radionuclide angiography had a sensitivity of 77% (10 of 13) and a specificity of 88% (23 of 22) for detection of left ventricular thrombi. In a subset of these patients (n = 13), 2D echo had a sensitivity and specificity of 100% for detection of left ventricular thrombus.

12. Delemarre BJ, Visser CA, Bot H, Dunning AJ: Prediction of apical thrombus formation in acute myocardial infarction based on left ventricular spatial flow pattern. *J Am Coll Cardiol* 15:355–360, 1990.

    Data are presented supporting the hypothesis that abnormal left ventricular apical flow patterns can be used to predict the risk of thrombus formation. A normal apical flow pattern is characterized by simultaneous onset of flow at the mitral valve and apex with a discontinuous (diastolic toward and systolic away from the transducer) Doppler signal along the lateral wall and septum in the apical four-chamber view. Accompanying editorial.

13. Visser CA, Kan G, Meltzer RS, et al: Embolic potential of left ventricular thrombus after myocardial infarction: A two-dimensional echocardiographic study of 119 patients. *J Am Coll Cardiol* 5:1276–1280, 1985.

    In 119 patients with acute myocardial infarction (98 anterior), systemic embolization occurred in 26 patients (22%). Embolization was more likely with protrusion or free mobility of the thrombus.

Left Atrial Thrombi

14. Shrestha NK, Moreno FL, Narciso FV, et al: Two-dimensional echocardiographic detection of intra-atrial masses. *Am J Cardiol* 48:954–960, 1981.

    One of the few studies comparing detection of left atrial thrombi by transthoracic echo with surgical results. Of the 51 patients with left atrial thrombus at surgery, lesions in 30 were detected by 2D echo (sensitivity 59%). Of the 242 patients without thrombus at surgery, in 239 the 2D echo did not show a thrombus (3 false-positive results, specificity 99%).

15. Herzog CA, Bass D, Kane M, Asinger R: Two-dimensional echocardiographic imaging of left atrial appendage thrombi. *J Am Coll Cardiol* 3:1340–1344, 1984.

    Description of visualization of the left atrial appendage on transthoracic imaging in the parasternal short-axis view by slight superiomedial angulation of the transducer.

Management of Atrial Fibrillation

16. Manning WJ, Chafizadeh ER: Echocardiographic aspects of atrial fibrillation and flutter. *In* Otto CM (ed): The Practice of Clinical Echocardiography. Philadelphia, WB Saunders, 1997, pp. 649–664.

    Review of the literature on left atrial thrombus formation and the risk of embolic events with cardioversion. An approach to the use of echocardiography in management of patients with atrial fibrillation of unknown duration is proposed. 97 references.

17. Manning WJ, Silberman DI, Gordon SPF, et al: Cardioversion from atrial fibrillation without prolonged anticoagulation with the use of transesophageal echocardiography to exclude the presence of atrial thrombi. *N Engl J Med* 328:750–755, 1993.

    Transesophageal echocardiography was performed in 119 patients with atrial fibrillation longer than 2 days in duration, who were not receiving long-term anticoagulant therapy and had no contraindications to the transesophageal procedure. Left atrial thrombi were identified in 12 (13%) patients. In the 78 patients without detectable atrial thrombi and successful conversion to sinus rhythm, none had an embolic event. Most of these patients received short-term heparin therapy before cardioversion and warfarin for 1 month after cardioversion.

18. Grimm RA, Stewart WJ, Black IW, et al: Should all patients undergo transesophageal echocardiography before electrical cardioversion of atrial flutter? *J Am Coll Cardiol* 23:533–541, 1994.

    Review article proposing that transesophageal echocardiography can be used to allow early cardioversion if atrial thrombus is absent (although anticoagulation at the time of cardioversion and for 4 weeks after cardioversion is recommended in all patients). In patents with thrombus identified on transesophageal echocardiography, cardioversion is delayed to avoid risk of embolization. 71 references.

19. Zabalgiotia M, Halperin JL, Pearce LA, et al: Transesophageal echocardiographic correlates of clinical risk of thromboembolism in nonvalvular atrial fibrillation. *J Am Coll Cardiol* 31:1622–1666, 1998.

    Clinical factors associated with increased risk of thromboembolism in nonvalvular atrial fibrillation included women older than 75 years, hypertension, congestive heart failure, and a history of prior thromboembolism. Features on transesophageal echocardiography associated with an increased thromboembolic risk included appendage thrombi, dense spontaneous echo contrast in the left atrium, an appendage peak flow velocity ≤20 cm/s, and complex aortic plaque.

Cardiac Source of Embolus

20. Redberg RF: Echocardiographic evaluation of the patient with an embolic event. *In* Otto CM (ed): The Practice of Clinical Echocardiography. Philadelphia, WB Saunders, 1997, pp. 629–648.

    Review and discussion of the association of various echocardiographic findings and the risk of systemic embolic events. Topics include left atrial thrombus, spontaneous echo contrast, Chiari's network, mitral valve strands, intracardiac tumors, papillary fibroelastomas, thoracic aortic debris, atrial septal aneurysm, and patent foramen ovale. 144 references.

21. Meltzer RS, Visser CA, Fuster V: Intracardiac thrombi and systemic embolization. *Ann Intern Med* 104:689–698, 1986.

    Review of the utility of transthoracic echocardiography in evaluation of intracardiac thrombi. 96 references.

22. Pearson AC, Labovitz AJ, Tatineni S, Gomez CR: Superiority of transesophageal echocardiography in detecting cardiac source of embolism in patients with cerebral ischemia of uncertain etiology. *J Am Coll Cardiol* 17:66–72, 1991.

    In 79 patients with unexplained cerebrovascular events, transthoracic echocardiography detected a potential cardiac source of embolus in only 15% com-

pared with 57% by transesophageal echocardiography. Abnormalities detected included atrial septal aneurysms with a patent foramen ovale (9), left atrial thrombus or tumor (6), and left atrial "spontaneous" contrast (13).

23. DeRook FA, Comess KA, Albers GW, Popp RL: Transesophageal echocardiography in the evaluation of stroke. *Ann Intern Med* 117:922–931, 1992.

    Review of the utility of transesophageal echo in evaluation of patients with cerebrovascular events possibly due to cardiogenic emboli. 66 references.

24. Black IW, Hopkins AP, Lee LCL, Walsh WF: Left atrial spontaneous echo contrast: A clinical and echocardiographic analysis. *J Am Coll Cardiol* 18:398–404, 1991.

    Spontaneous left atrial contrast was found in 75 of 400 patients (19%) undergoing transesophageal echocardiography. Atrial fibrillation or mitral stenosis was present in 71 (95%) of the patients with "spontaneous" contrast. In the 60 patients with nonvalvular atrial fibrillation, the only independent predictors of left atrial thrombus or systemic embolism were spontaneous left atrial contrast and age.

25. Fatkin D, Kelly RP, Feneley MP: Relations between left atrial appendage blood flow velocity, spontaneous echocardiography contrast and thromboembolic risk in vivo. *J Am Coll Cardiol* 23:961–969, 1994.

    In 140 patients with atrial fibrillation, left atrial spontaneous contrast was present in 78 (56%) patients and left atrial thrombus was present in 15 (11%) patients. On multivariate analysis, spontaneous echo contrast was the only significant predictor for the presence of thrombus. Left atrial appendage velocity was negatively associated with the degree of spontaneous contrast, and an appendage velocity <35 cm/s was associated with a 30 times higher risk of spontaneous contrast.

26. Pearson AC, Nagelhout D, Castello R, et al: Atrial septal aneurysm and stroke: A transesophageal echocardiographic study. *J Am Coll Cardiol* 18:1223–1229, 1991.

    In 410 patients undergoing transesophageal echocardiography, an atrial septal aneurysm (defined as a base width ≥1.5 cm with ≥1.1 cm total excursion) was found in 32 (8%) patients. Atrial septal aneurysm was diagnosed more frequently in patients with stroke (15% versus 4%; P < .05).

27. Fatkin D, Kelly RP, Feneley MP: Relations between left atrial appendage blood flow velocity, spontaneous echocardiographic contrast and thromboembolic risk in vivo. *J Am Coll Cardiol* 23:961–969, 1994.

    In 140 patients with atrial fibrillation, left atrial spontaneous contrast was seen in 56% on transesophageal echocardiography. Increasing grades of spontaneous contrast were associated with decreasing atrial appendage blood flow velocities. On multivariate analysis, spontaneous contrast was the cardiac factor most strongly associated with left atrial thrombus (identified in 11% of patients) and a history of embolic events (36% of patients).

28. Schneider B, Hofmann T, Justen MH, Meinertz T: Chiari's network: Normal anatomic variant or risk factor for arterial embolic events? *J Am Coll Cardiol* 26:203–210, 1995.

    A Chiari network was present on 29 of 1436 (2%) of consecutive transesophageal echocardiographic studies. The presence of a Chiari network was associated with a patent foramen ovale in 83%, evidence for right-to-left shunting in 55%, and atrial septal aneurysm in 24% of patients.

29. Roldan CA, Shively BK, Crawford MH: Valve excrescences: Prevalence, evolution and risk for cardioembolism. *J Am Coll Cardiol* 30:1308–1314, 1997.

    Valve excrescences (thin, elongated, mobile structures attached near the leaflet closure line) are seen in about 40% of normal individuals on transesophageal echocardiography and do not appear to be associated with an increased risk of thromboembolism.

Aortic Atheroma

30. Karalis DG, Chandrasekaran K, Victor MF, et al: Recognition and embolic potential of intraaortic atherosclerotic debris. *J Am Coll Cardiol* 17:73–78, 1991.

    In 556 patients undergoing transesophageal echocardiography, intraaortic atherosclerotic debris was identified in 7%. The incidence of embolism was higher with pedunculated and mobile versus layered and immobile debris (8 of 11 versus 3 of 25; P < .002).

31. Katz ES, Tunick PA, Rusinek H, et al: Protruding aortic atheromas predict stroke in elderly patients undergoing cardiopulmonary bypass: Experience with intraoperative transesophageal echocardiography. *J Am Coll Cardiol* 20:70–77, 1992.

    Protruding atheromas were identified in 23 of 130 (18%) of patients undergoing transesophageal echocardiography. Strokes occurred in 3 of 12 patients with mobile atheroma versus 2 of 118 without a mobile atheroma (P = .001).

32. Tunick PA, Rosenzweig BP, Katz ES, et al: High risk for vascular events in patients with protruding aortic atheromas: A prospective study. *J Am Coll Cardiol* 23:1085–1090, 1994.

    Of 521 consecutive patients undergoing transesophageal echocardiography, 42 had protruding atheromas and no other potential source of emboli. Compared with 42 age- and gender-matched control subjects, multivariate analysis identified protruding atheromas as the only independent predictor of subsequent vascular events (odds ratio 4.3; 95% confidence intervals 1.2 to 15).

33. Vaduganathan P, Ewton A, Nagueh SF, Weilbaecher DG, et al: Pathologic correlates of aortic plaques, thrombi and mobile "aortic debris" imaged in vivo with transesophageal echocardiography. *J Am Coll Cardiol* 30:357–363, 1997.

    The echocardiographic appearance of aortic plaques was compared with histologic examination in 31 patients undergoing aortic aneurysm or dissection repair. Agreement between histologic and echocardiographic grading of lesion severity was high (73%); the major limitation of ultrasound was its inability to detect superficial ulcerations. Transesophageal echocardiography had a sensitivity of 91% and specificity of 90% for detection of thrombus associated with the atheroma.

Clinical Echocardiography for Diseases of the Great Vessels

15

BASIC PRINCIPLES
ECHOCARDIOGRAPHIC APPROACH
    Transthoracic Imaging of the Aorta
        2D and Doppler Echo
        Limitations of Transthoracic Imaging of the Aorta
    Transesophageal Imaging
        2D Echo
        Doppler Flows
CLINICAL UTILITY
    Chronic Aortic Dilation
    Aortic Dissection
        Transthoracic Imaging
        Transesophageal Imaging
        Alternate Approaches
    Sinus of Valsalva Aneurysm

Preoperative and Postoperative Evaluation of Aortic
    Disease
    Preoperative Evaluation
    Residual Dissection Flaps
    Aortic Graft Pseudoaneurysms
    Atherosclerotic Aortic Disease
    Aortic Atherosclerosis as a Potential Source of
        Embolus
    Aortic Atherosclerosis as a Marker for Coronary
        Artery Disease
    Pulmonary Artery Abnormalities

LIMITATIONS/TECHNICAL CONSIDERATIONS/ALTERNATE
APPROACHES

SUGGESTED READING

Echocardiographic evaluation of the aortic root and main pulmonary artery is a routine part of the standard echocardiographic examination. In addition, further evaluation of the ascending aorta, arch, and descending aorta can be performed when disease is suspected clinically. Transthoracic images often are suboptimal due to overlying or adjacent air-filled structures, so transesophageal imaging has greatly enhanced the diagnostic utility of echocardiography for diseases of the aorta.

BASIC PRINCIPLES

The most common abnormality of the aorta is *dilation,* or an increase in diameter greater than expected for age and body size. Dilation of the ascending aorta occurs in a wide variety of diseases. Most cases of ascending aortic dilation are due to hypertension, atherosclerosis, cystic medical necrosis, or are poststenotic in etiology. In addition, aortic root dilation is seen in collagen vascular and inflammatory disorders such as Marfan's syndrome, rheumatoid arthritis, systemic lupus erythematosus, and Reiter's syndrome. With poststenotic dilation or with dilation due to hypertension or athero-

sclerosis, the contours of the sinuses of Valsalva and the normal narrowing at the sinotubular junction typically are preserved. In contrast, Marfan's syndrome is characterized by effacement of the sinotubular junction and enlargement of the sinuses of Valsalva, as well as dilation of the ascending aorta, resulting in a "water balloon" appearance of the aortic root (Fig. 15–1).

When aortic dilation is severe, the term *aneurysm* is used. Aneurysms can involve one or more segments of the aorta (ascending, arch, descending) and may be tubular or saccular in configuration. Aortic aneurysms most often are due to cystic medial necrosis, Marfan's syndrome, hypertension, atherosclerosis, or collagen-vascular or inflammatory diseases. Aneurysms also may be seen in tertiary syphilis (with a characteristic pattern of calcification), aortic arteritis (such as Takayasu's arteritis), and as a result of blunt or penetrating chest trauma. Aortic aneurysms are prone to rupture, so prophylactic repair often is recommended.

An *aortic dissection* is a life-threatening situation in which an intimal tear in the aortic wall allows passage of blood into a "false" channel between the intima and the media (Fig. 15–2).

FIGURE 15–1. Schematic diagram of the typical 2D echo findings in Marfan's syndrome as seen in a long-axis view. The aortic root is markedly dilated with effacement of the sinotubular junction. Aortic annular dilation results in inadequate aortic leaflet apposition with a central jet of aortic regurgitation (AR) and consequent left ventricular enlargement (LVE). Often the anterior mitral leaflet (AMVL) is long and redundant.

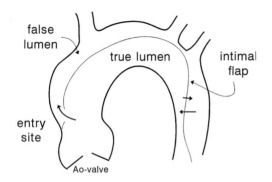

FIGURE 15–2. Schematic diagram of an aortic dissection showing an entry site above the sinotubular junction into a false lumen. In real time, the intimal flap shows rapid undulating motion, independent of the cardiac cycle. As indicated by the *arrows* across the intimal flap in the descending aorta, multiple flow communications between the true and false lumens may be seen with color flow imaging.

This false channel may be localized or may propagate downstream, often in a spiral fashion, due to the pressure of blood flow in the channel. The false lumen may (1) expand, compressing the true aortic lumen (which supplies major branch vessels), (2) propagate down major branch vessels, (3) thrombose, or (4) rupture. An accurate, rapid diagnosis of the presence or absence of aortic dissection and the site of the entry tear is crucial in management of patients with suspected dissection. Aortic dissection is associated with aortic valve disease, with a risk of aortic dissection of approximately five times normal in individuals with a congenital bicuspid or unicuspid aortic valve. Dissection

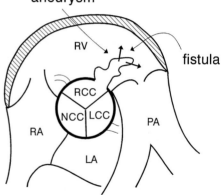

FIGURE 15–3. Schematic diagram of a congenital sinus of Valsalva aneurysm. A long "wind sock"–like membranous outpouching of the right coronary cusp (RCC) protrudes into the right ventricular (RV) outflow tract. If there are fenestrations in the aneurysm, an aortic-to-right ventricular fistula is seen. Note that an aneurysm of the left coronary cusp (LCC) would protrude into the left atrium (LA), whereas an aneurysm of the right coronary cusp (RCC) would protrude into the right atrium (RA).

also is more likely in patients with a preexisting aneurysm, although dissection can occur in the absence of dilation in patients with Marfan's syndrome. The most prevalent risk factor for aortic dissection is chronic hypertension.

Sinus of Valsalva aneurysms (Fig. 15–3) may be congenital or may be due to infection, Marfan's syndrome, or previous surgical procedures. A sinus of Valsalva aneurysm protrudes into adjacent chambers and may be associated with a fistula. Specifically, an aneurysm of the right coronary sinus protrudes into the right ventricular outflow tract, the left coronary sinus into the left atrium, and the noncoronary sinus into the right atrium.

Atherosclerosis of the aorta may lead to dilation, aneurysm, or dissection. In addition, the presence of atheroma may be important as a marker for coexisting coronary artery disease and as a potential source of embolic cerebrovascular events.

ECHOCARDIOGRAPHIC APPROACH

Transthoracic Imaging of the Aorta
(Fig. 15–4)

2D and Doppler Echo

On transthoracic imaging, the *aortic root* is well seen in parasternal long- and short-axis views. Depending on ultrasound penetration, images of additional segments of the ascending aorta may be obtained by moving the transducer cephalad one or more interspaces. Image quality is enhanced by positioning the patient in a steep left lateral decubitus position, bringing the aorta in contact with the anterior chest wall (Figs. 15–5 and 15–6). Doppler interrogation of the ascending aorta from the parasternal approach is limited to qualitative evaluation of the flow pattern in the proximal root and assessment of aortic regurgitation severity (if present) given the nonparallel intercept angle from this position. The aortic root also may be imaged from the apical approach in an anteriorly angulated four-chamber view and in an apical long-axis view. While two-dimensional (2D) image quality may be limited at the depth of the ascending aorta from the apical approach, this view does allow a parallel intercept angle between the Doppler beam and the direction of blood flow. In some individuals, images of the ascending aorta can be obtained from the subcostal approach.

The *aortic arch* is imaged from a suprasternal notch or supraclavicular approach with the patient in a supine position with the neck extended. Both longitudinal (Fig. 15–7) and transverse (Fig. 15–8) views of the arch are obtainable in nearly all individuals. Usually only a short segment of the ascending aorta is visible from the suprasternal notch window, but this is variable between patients. Also note that the

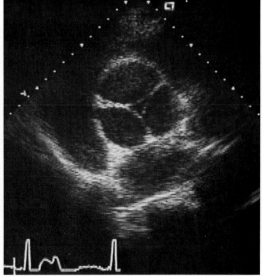

FIGURE 15–5. Parasternal long-axis view in a patient with Marfan's syndrome showing a dilated root with effacement of the sinotubular junction and a dissection flap in the descending thoracic aorta seen posterior to the left atrium *(arrow) (top)*. In short axis the stretched trileaflet valve shows a small central regurgitant orifice *(bottom)*.

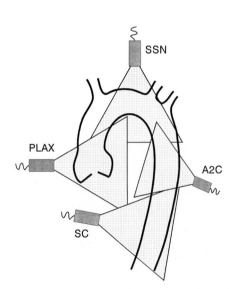

FIGURE 15–4. The use of several acoustic windows for complete evaluation of the aorta from a transcutaneous approach is shown. From a parasternal long-axis (PLAX) window, the root and a segment of the ascending aorta are seen. From the suprasternal notch (SSN) window, the arch and proximal descending thoracic aorta are seen; from a posteriorly angulated apical two-chamber (A2C) approach, the midsegment of the descending thoracic aorta is seen; and from a subcostal (SC) approach, the distal thoracic and proximal abdominal aortae are seen. In some individuals, the segment of ascending aorta between the standard PLAX and SSN views can be imaged from a high parasternal position. However, in other patients, this segment of the aorta is "missed" on transthoracic imaging.

FIGURE 15–6. A long-axis view of the ascending aorta and arch obtained from a right suprasternal notch window in the patient with Marfan's syndrome shown in Figure 15–5 shows that the aortic dilation extends only to the proximal segment of the arch.

descending aorta appears to taper due to an oblique image plane with respect to its curvature (i.e., the descending aorta is only partially in the image plane).

Pulsed or continuous-wave Doppler record-ings of descending aortic flow from the suprasternal notch show systolic flow away from the transducer at a velocity of about 1 m/s. Normally, there is (1) brief, low-velocity, early diastolic flow reversal, (2) low-velocity antegrade flow in mid-diastole, and (3) low-velocity flow reversal at end-diastole. The use of low wall filter settings is needed to appreciate this normal flow pattern (Fig. 15–9).

Even though 2D imaging of the ascending aorta is suboptimal from the suprasternal approach, high-quality Doppler flow signals may be obtained because the Doppler beam is aligned parallel to flow. Antegrade flow toward the transducer in systole is seen, the reciprocal of the ascending aortic flow signal recorded from the apex.

The *descending thoracic aorta* is seen in cross section posterior to the left atrium in the parasternal long-axis view. A longitudinal section of this segment of the descending aorta may be obtained by clockwise rotation and lateral angulation of the transducer. From the suprasternal notch approach, a small portion of the descending thoracic aorta is seen. From the apical two-chamber view, a longitudinal section of a segment of the descending aorta is seen by lateral angulation and clockwise rotation of the transducer (Fig. 15–10). Doppler interrogation of descending thoracic aortic flow is most easily performed from the suprasternal notch long-axis view. Flow abnormalities may be related to

FIGURE 15–7. Suprasternal notch view in the long-axis of the aorta in a normal individual *(left)*. With slight lateral rotation and angulation, the left pulmonary artery (LPA) can be visualized *(right)*.

aortic disease (e.g., coarctation), shunts (e.g., patent ductus arteriosus), or aortic valve disease (e.g., regurgitation).

From the subcostal approach, the *distal thoracic* and *proximal abdominal aorta* is seen as it traverses the diaphragm. From this approach, the angle between the transducer and the aorta allows Doppler interrogation of antegrade flow (Fig. 15–11).

Thus, by combining images from multiple acoustic windows, visualization of much of the aortic root, ascending aorta, arch, and descending thoracic aorta is possible using transthoracic echocardiography.

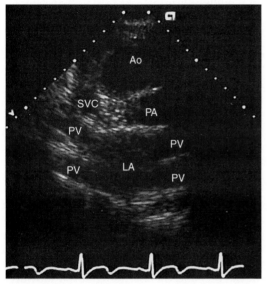

FIGURE 15–8. Short-axis suprasternal notch view in a normal individual showing the aortic arch (Ao), pulmonary artery (PA), superior vena cava (SVC), left atrium (LA), and four pulmonary veins (PV).

FIGURE 15–10. Posteriorly angulated apical two-chamber view showing the descending thoracic aorta (DA) along its long axis in the patient with Marfan's syndrome.

FIGURE 15–9. Normal pulsed Doppler recording of flow in the descending thoracic aorta from a suprasternal notch long-axis view. Antegrade flow in systole has a maximum velocity of 1.4 m/s with a normal systolic ejection curve. In diastole, there is brief early diastolic flow reversal, followed by low-velocity antegrade flow in middiastole and absence of flow (or low-velocity reversal) in end-diastole.

FIGURE 15–11. Subcostal view of the distal thoracic and proximal abdominal aorta. Although a nonparallel intercept angle from this window limits the quantitative velocity data, velocity recordings are helpful for evaluation of blood flow patterns.

In patients with a left pleural effusion, images of the aorta can be obtained by imaging through the fluid from the left posterior chest (paraspinal) with the patient in a right lateral decubitus position (Fig. 15–12).

Limitations of Transthoracic Imaging of the Aorta

The major limitations of the transthoracic approach to ultrasound evaluation of the aorta are acoustic access and image quality. In many individuals, acoustic access is suboptimal or minimal from one or more of the windows needed for full evaluation of the aorta, leaving

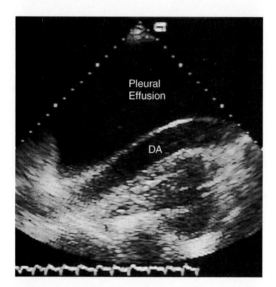

FIGURE 15–12. Descending thoracic aorta (DA) recorded through a large left pleural effusion with the patient lying on his left side and transducer positioned on the left posterior chest wall.

"gaps" in the echocardiographic examination. Even when acoustic access is adequate, image quality often is poor due to beam width at the depth of the aorta—particularly the descending thoracic aorta from apical and parasternal windows. Beam-width artifact, noise, and poor lateral resolution make differentiation of intraluminal defects from artifacts difficult. Because of these limitations, there has been increasing enthusiasm for transesophageal echocardiography in patients with suspected aortic disease.

Transesophageal Imaging

2D Echo

The aortic valve, *aortic root,* and ascending aorta are seen in an oblique image plane with the transducer at 0° rotation from a high esophageal probe position. A short-axis view at the aortic valve level is obtained by rotating the image plane to about 45°, with a short-axis view of the proximal few centimeters of the ascending aorta obtained by slight withdrawal of the probe in the esophagus. In the short-axis plane, evaluation of more distal segments of the ascending aorta is obscured by the position of the air-filled trachea between the esophagus (and transducer) and the ascending aorta. However, by rotating the image plane to about 120°, a long-axis view of the aortic valve, sinus of Valsalva, and ascending aorta can be obtained in most patients (Fig. 15–13). Further cephalad segments of the ascending aorta may be seen by slowly moving the transducer to a higher esophageal position.

The *aortic arch* is best imaged from a high esophageal position. Starting with a short-axis view of the descending thoracic aorta, the probe

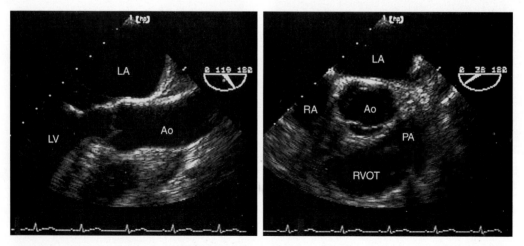

FIGURE 15–13. Normal ascending aorta seen on transesophageal imaging in long-axis *(left)* and short-axis *(right)* views using a multiplane probe to align the image plane appropriately relative to the aortic long axis.

FIGURE 15–14. On transesophageal imaging, a 2D view *(left)* of the descending thoracic aorta shows a dissection flap *(arrow)*, with flow between the true (TL) and false lumens (FL) seen on color flow imaging *(right)*. (See Color Plate 17, p. 386.)

FIGURE 15–15. Transesophageal imaging in another patient with an aortic dissection shows prominent spontaneous contrast in the false lumen (FL) due to low flow.

is withdrawn to the level of the arch and then the entire probe is turned toward the patient's right and angulated inferiorly to obtain a long-axis view of the arch. In some patients, images of the aortic arch may be suboptimal due to the positions of the trachea and bronchi. In many cases, transthoracic suprasternal notch views of the arch provide superior image quality.

The *descending thoracic* and *proximal abdominal aorta* are well seen by the transesophageal approach. The descending thoracic aorta lies immediately lateral and slightly posterior to the esophagus so that posterior rotation of the probe provides excellent images in either a cross-sectional (transverse plane at 0°) or long-axis (at 90° to 120°) view (Figs. 15–14 and 15–15). Slight turning of the transesophageal probe is needed at different levels as the aorta curves relative to the esophagus. From a transgastric position, the proximal abdominal aorta is seen posterior to the stomach. Many examiners prefer to examine the length of the aorta in sequential cross-sectional views as the probe is slowly withdrawn from the stomach and esophagus, with imaging of the aortic arch just prior to probe removal. Any areas of abnormality are then examined in both long- and short-axis views.

Doppler Flows

Color flow imaging of the aorta shows the normal antegrade flow pattern in the ascending aorta and arch. For the descending aorta, the ultrasound beam is nearly perpendicular to the direction of blood flow. In addition, normal flow shows a hemicylindrical swirling pattern so that normal flow appears red in one half and blue in the other half of a cross-sectional view of descending aorta. Given the constraints of the probe position, alignment of the Doppler beam parallel to aortic flow is difficult from a transesophageal approach. It may be possible to obtain ascending aortic flow from a transgastric "apical" view, but underestimation of flow velocity due to a nonparallel intercept angle should be considered. Quantitative evaluation of aortic flow velocity from other transgastric or transesophageal views rarely is feasible. Aortic flow signals preferably are recorded from a transthoracic approach.

CLINICAL UTILITY

Chronic Aortic Dilation

Aortic dilation often is first recognized on the chest radiograph (Fig. 15–16) or on an echocardiographic examination requested for other reasons. In specific clinical settings, such as Marfan's syndrome, aortic dilation is an expected consequence of a systemic disease. In these cases, echocardiography is requested to assess the presence and degree of aortic abnormality.

Measurements of aortic diameter on echocardiography are accurate and reproducible when care is taken to obtain a true short-axis dimension (nonoblique), gain settings are appropriate, and standard measurement conventions (leading edge to leading edge) are used. In patients with aortic dilation, it is important to measure aortic diameter at several locations and to specify the measurement sites. Typical measurements include (1) the aortic annulus (the site used for left ventricular outflow tract diameter measurement), (2) the aortic leaflet tip level (the standard position of an M-mode of the aortic valve), (3) the sinotubular junction, (4) the ascending aorta, (5) the aortic arch, and (6) the descending thoracic aorta (Fig. 15–17). While all these measurements are not needed in every patient, quantitative evaluation of the extent and severity of aortic dilation is extremely useful in follow-up and management of pa-

tients with chronic, progressive aortic dilation. With discrete aneurysms, maximum diameter and length also are measured.

Sequential transthoracic studies of the degree of aortic dilation are used to follow patients with Marfan's syndrome. Prophylactic aortic root and valve replacement may be recommended when the degree of ascending aortic dilation reaches a critical range (some authorities suggest a value between 50 and 60 mm maximum diameter). For other etiologies of aortic dilation, sequential studies also may be used to assess whether the dilation is progressive or stable over time. Transesophageal evaluation of chronic aortic dilation is reserved for patients with inadequate transthoracic images.

Aortic Dissection

Transthoracic Imaging

Evaluation of the Aorta. A transthoracic echocardiographic examination for aortic dissection includes evaluation of the ascending aorta from the standard and high parasternal windows, the aortic arch from the suprasternal notch window, the descending aorta from parasternal and apical windows, and the proximal abdominal aorta from a subcostal approach. When a left pleural effusion is present, the descending thoracic aorta can be imaged through the effusion with the transducer positioned on the left posterior chest wall.

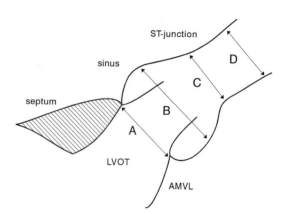

FIGURE 15–17. Schematic diagram of the aortic root and ascending aorta showing the possible measurement sites for "aortic" diameter. Left ventricular outflow tract (LVOT) diameter *(A)* is used for transaortic stroke volume calculations in the continuity equation. The aortic leaflet tips *(B)* in systole define the usual site for M-mode measurements and usually indicate maximum diameter of the sinuses of Valsalva. The sinotubular (ST) junction typically is the narrowest segment of the ascending aorta *(C)*, with variable degrees of dilation in the ascending aorta itself *(D)*. The site of measurement should be specified in the echocardiographic report.

FIGURE 15–16. Chest radiography showing a dilated ascending aorta and wide mediastinum, raising the diagnostic possibility of aortic dissection (same patient as in Figure 15–18).

The echocardiographic diagnosis of aortic dissection is most secure when a linear, mobile echogenic structure is seen within a dilated aortic lumen (Figs. 15–18 and 15–19). When a definite, undulating intimal flap is seen, the specificity of transthoracic echocardiography for diagnosis of dissection is high (Table 15–1). However, beam-width artifact and reverberations can be mistaken for intraluminal structures by an inexperienced observer, resulting in a specificity of less than 100%, particularly when the images are not "classic" or image quality is suboptimal.

Conversely, the sensitivity of transthoracic echocardiography for aortic dissection is quite low (i.e., the inability to demonstrate an internal flap does not reliably exclude the diagnosis). This low sensitivity is due to poor image quality, particularly of the segment of ascending aorta between the sinotubular junction and the aortic arch, and the poor far-field resolution of the descending thoracic aorta from the transthoracic approach.

Complications of Aortic Dissection (Table 15–2). Indirect signs of aortic dissection on transthoracic imaging include aortic root dilation, the presence of aortic regurgitation, or evidence of complications of aortic dissection (Fig. 15–20). While the presence of these abnormalities does not confirm the diagnosis (since there are many other etiologies for these findings), their presence or absence may weight the clinical evidence toward or away from a diagnosis of dissection. Complications of aortic dissection can be recognized on echocardiography and have important clinical implications both for diagnosis and therapy. Aortic regurgitation is nearly always present. Chronic regurgitation is due to aortic root dilation and/or associated anatomic valve abnormalities. Acute regurgitation (often superimposed on chronic) is due to further root dilation or to inadequate leaflet support due to retrograde extension of the dissection. In extreme cases, a flail aortic leaflet is seen.

Coronary artery ostial occlusion can occur as a result of the dissection flap separating the coronary artery from normal blood flow or by compression of the vessel. The resultant wall motion abnormalities—inferior for right coro-

FIGURE 15–18. A 36-year-old man with known aortic valve disease presented with severe chest pain. Echocardiography shows a unicuspid stenotic aortic valve in the parasternal short-axis view in systole with the orifice indicated by the dots.

FIGURE 15–19. In a long-axis view, a dilated aorta with a dissection flap *(arrow)* is seen in the same patient as Figure 15–18. *(left).* Moving the transducer cephalad two interspaces provides better separation of the dissection flap *(arrow)* from a reverberation artifact *(right)* (RPA = right pulmonary artery).

TABLE 15–1	Diagnosis of Aortic Dissection				
First Author/ Year	**N**	**Approach**	**Sensitivity**	**Specificity**	**Standard of Reference**
Victor/1981	42	TTE	80% (12/15)	96% (26/27)	Angiography
Erbel/1987	21	TTE	29% (6/21)	All had dissection	Surgery or angiography
		TEE	100% (21/21)		
Hashimoto/ 1989	22	TTE	71% (15/21)	All had dissection	Angiography (17), surgery (12)
		TEE	100% (22/22)		
		CT	100% (8/8)		
Ballal/1991	61	TEE	97% (33/34)	100% (27/27)	Angiography, surgery, or autopsy
		CT	67% (16/24)	100% (7/7)	
Nienaber/1992	53	TTE	83% (26/31)	63% (14/22)	Surgery, autopsy, or angiography
		TEE	100% (31/31)	66% (15/22)	
		MRI	100% (31/31)	100% (22/22)	
Nienaber/1993	110	TTE	59% (37/62)	83% (39/48)	Surgery (62), autopsy (7), angiography (64)
		TEE	98% (43/44)	98% (25/26)	
		MRI	98% (58/59)	87% (27/31)	
		CT	94% (45/48)	83% (38/46)	

TTE = Transthoracic echocardiography; TEE = transesophageal echocardiography; CT = computed tomography; MRI = magnetic resonance imaging.

Data from Victor et al: Am J Cardiol 48:1155–1159, 1981; Erbel et al: Br Heart J 58:45–51, 1987; Hashimoto et al: JACC 14:1253–1262, 1989; Ballal et al: Circ 84:1903–1914, 1991; Neinaber et al: Circ 85:434–447, 1992; Neinaber et al: NEJM 328:1–9, 1993.

TABLE 15–2	Complications of Thoracic Aortic Dissection

I. Aortic valve regurgitation
  A. Due to aortic root dilation
  B. Due to leaflet flail
II. Coronary artery occlusion due to dissection at the orifice
  A. Ventricular fibrillation
  B. Acute myocardial infarction
III. Distal vessel obstruction or occlusion
  A. Carotid (stroke)
  B. Subclavian (upper limb ischemia)
IV. Aortic rupture
  A. Into the pericardium
    1. Pericardial effusion
    2. Pericardial tamponade
  B. Into the mediastinum
  C. Into the pleural space
    1. Pleural effusion
    2. Exsanguination

nary obstruction, anterolateral for left main obstruction—are easily recognized on echocardiography. The diagnostic difficulty in this situation is recognizing that the wall motion abnormalities are a secondary event due to aortic dissection rather than the primary event (e.g., acute myocardial infarction due to coronary thrombosis).

Distal vessel obstructions rarely will be recognized during the cardiac ultrasound examination. However, the possibility of aortic dissection should be considered in patients with distal vessel obstructions referred for echocardiography to "rule out" a cardiac source of embolus. The correct diagnosis of distal vessel obstruction due to a dissection flap (rather than an embolus) may be made by the astute echocardiographer.

Aortic dissections can rupture in one of several ways. *External* rupture into the mediastinum or pleural space often results in exsanguination with acute hemodynamic collapse. If the rupture *thromboses*, the patient may exhibit a mediastinal hematoma and/or pleural effusion (more often left than right). Alternatively, the dissection can rupture at the aortic annulus into the pericardial space. Again, uncontrolled rupture leads to an acute pericardial effusion with tamponade and rapid hemodynamic collapse. However, a partial rupture or a leak may result in a smaller pericardial effusion. Obviously, the presence of any amount of pericardial fluid in a patient with an aortic dissection is an alarming sign and should prompt rapid intervention.

Echocardiographic Differential Diagnosis. In most cases where transthoracic echocardiography is requested to "rule out" aortic dissection, the differential diagnosis is broad, with aortic dissection being one of many (and often the least likely) possible diagnoses. Thus, if the echocardiographic appearance of the aorta is normal, echocardiographic examination for other possible etiologies of chest pain is needed, including coronary artery disease (e.g., wall motion abnormalities), valvular disease (e.g., aortic stenosis), pulmonary embolus, and pericarditis.

When the clinical suspicion of aortic dissection is low to intermediate, a normal aorta on echocardiography further decreases the posttest likelihood of disease, so other diagnoses might be pursued. However, when the clinical suspicion is moderate to high, a "negative" transthoracic echocardiogram does *not* substantially decrease the posttest likelihood of disease, so prompt further evaluation is needed. In fact, when the clinical suspicion is high, many clinicians would argue that transthoracic echocardiography is inappropriate; either transesophageal echocardiography, magnetic resonance imaging, computed tomography, or angiographic evaluation should be performed promptly.

Transesophageal Imaging

Transesophageal images of the aorta are far superior to transthoracic images in most patients because of (1) the shorter distance between the transducer and aorta, (2) the use of a higher frequency transducer, and (3) better ultrasound tissue penetration (higher signal-to-noise ratio). The descending thoracic aorta can be examined in its entirety from the diaphragm to the arch in both long- and short-axis planes.

A dissection flap appears as a linear, bright echogenic structure in the aortic lumen with erratic motion compared with normal systolic pulsations (Figs. 15–21 and 15–22). Color flow imaging may show blood flow in both true (bounded by endothelium) and false (bounded by media) lumens. Both the entry site into the false lumen and other communications between the two channels are seen as high-velocity turbulent flow jets on color flow imaging. The false lumen may be thrombosed, which is more difficult to appreciate than a false lumen with blood flow. In some cases, hematoma in the wall of the aorta is seen rather than an initial flap, reflecting an impending dissection or rupture of a thrombosed false lumen. This area of hematoma appears as an echogenic mass adjacent to the aortic lumen and bounded by the bright adventitial echo signal (Figs. 15–23 and 15–24).

The proximal segment of the aortic root is seen on transesophageal imaging in the short-axis plane at the aortic valve level. However, evaluation of the ascending aorta depends on use of a long-axis view. Evaluation of the ascending aorta is particularly important because the decision between emergency surgical intervention and medical therapy hinges on whether the dissection originates in (or involves) the ascending aorta. Note that even a localized dissection flap in the ascending aorta carries a grim prognosis and warrants surgical treatment. Again, color flow imaging may further define the entry site and demonstrate flow in true and false lumens.

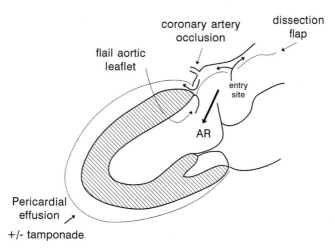

FIGURE 15–20. Potential complications of dissection of the ascending aorta are shown schematically. If the dissection proceeds retrograde (as well as antegrade) from the entry site, the false lumen can cause (1) occlusion in the coronary artery ostium with resultant myocardial infarction, (2) loss of support of an aortic leaflet with consequent severe aortic regurgitation (AR), or (3) rupture into the pericardium, which may result in tamponade physiology.

FIGURE 15–21. Transesophageal long-axis *(above)* and short-axis *(below)* views of an aortic dissection localized to the sinus of Valsalva in a 37-year-old woman with renal failure, hypertension, and acute chest pain. The flap is indicated by the *arrow.*

FIGURE 15–22. Transesophageal echocardiography showing a typical ascending aortic dissection in a long-axis view *(top)*. Color flow imaging shows flow in both the true and false lumen *(bottom)*. (See Color Plate 17, p. 386.)

The sensitivity of transesophageal echocardiography for the diagnosis of aortic dissection is high (>97%; see Table 15–1). Although specificity also is high, it is less than 100% due to misinterpretation of ultrasound artifacts, such as reverberations, beam-width artifacts, and oblique imaging planes. Careful evaluation from multiple views with adjustment of instrument settings helps avoid these false-positive diagnoses.

Alternate Approaches (Table 15–3)

Several centers have suggested that transesophageal echocardiography is the procedure of choice for evaluation of acute aortic dissections given its high sensitivity/specificity plus the ability to perform the study quickly at the patient's bedside. Alternate techniques for evaluation of possible acute aortic dissection include contrast aortic root angiography, chest computed tomography, and magnetic resonance imaging (Figs.15–25 to 15–27).

The choice of a particular procedure in an individual patient depends not only on availability of these tests but also on the differential diagnosis in the individual patient. Contrast angiography may be most appropriate when acute myocardial infarction is a likely diagnosis, since evaluation (and treatment) of coronary artery obstruction can be performed quickly if dissection is not present. Wide-angle tomographic imaging procedures (computed tomography, magnetic resonance imaging) may be most helpful in cases where the differential diagnosis includes mediastinal tumor. Echocardiography has the advantage of allowing evaluation of aortic valve anatomy and function, overall and regional left ventricular systolic function, and the presence and significance of a pericardial effusion.

Alternatively, the choice of imaging procedures may be driven by the specific additional

FIGURE 15–23. In a transesophageal short-axis view of the descending thoracic aorta (DA) a "thick" or double-walled appearance is seen *(left)* suggestive of an intramural hematoma. In a long-axis view, the atherosclerotic plaque *(small arrows)* is "lifted" off the posterior aortic wall *(large arrow)*. This patient was treated medically and has done well.

FIGURE 15–24. Potential false-positive echocardiographic findings with transesophageal imaging in two patients with no clinical evidence of aortic disease. On the *left,* lymphoma is seen surrounding the descending thoracic aorta. On the *right,* prominent paraaortic adipose tissue is seen.

TABLE 15–3	Diagnostic Imaging Procedures in Aortic Disease	
Procedure	**Advantages**	**Disadvantages**
Transthoracic echocardiography	Portable, rapid Inexpensive Evaluation of LV function Evaluation of aortic valve function Evaluation of pericardial effusion	Moderate sensitivity/specificity due to poor acoustic access and suboptimal image resolution
Transesophageal echocardiography	High sensitivity/specificity Portable, rapid Evaluation of LV function Evaluation of aortic valve function Evaluation of pericardial effusion Can assess proximal coronary arteries	Some risks (especially if esophageal disease is present) Cannot evaluate distal coronary arteries
Chest computed tomography	High sensitivity/specificity Wide field of view	Site of intimal tear not well defined Not portable Ionizing radiation Little data on LV, aortic valve Cannot evaluate coronary involvement
Magnetic resonance imaging	High sensitivity/specificity Wide field of view Evaluation of pericardial effusion	High cost, not portable, limited availability Limited evaluation of valvular and ventricular function Cannot evaluate coronary involvement
Contrast aortography	High sensitivity/specificity Branch vessel anatomy Evaluation of AR Can assess and intervene for coronary artery disease	Expensive, invasive Ionizing radiation Limited availability Not portable No evaluation for pericardial effusion

LV = Left ventricle; PE = pericardial effusion; AR = aortic regurgitation.

information needed in an individual patient. Examples include distal vessel anatomy (angiography), adjacent mediastinal disease (computed tomography or magnetic resonance imaging), or valvular function (echocardiography).

Sinus of Valsalva Aneurysm

A sinus of Valsalva aneurysm can be congenital or due to an acute infectious or inflammatory process. Echocardiographically, a dilated and distorted sinus of Valsalva is seen both in long- and short-axis views at the aortic valve level either from a transesophageal or transthoracic approach. A congenital aneurysm often is complex in shape with a "wind sock" appearance of a mass of irregular, mobile echos protruding from the aortic sinus into adjacent cardiac structures (Fig. 15–28). If the aneurysm is not fenestrated, Doppler flow examination is unremarkable. More commonly, multiple fenestrations are present, with high-velocity turbulent flow from the high-pressure aorta to the low-pressure adjacent chambers detectable by continuous-wave, pulsed wave, and color flow Doppler techniques. Note that infection of a previously competent congenital sinus of Valsalva aneurysm may result in flow across a necrotic area of infection.

Acquired sinus of Valsalva aneurysms tend to be less irregular in shape. The dilation of the sinuses that occurs in Marfan's syndrome symmetrically involves all three sinuses with a rounded, smooth pattern of root dilation. Because of persistent sinus of Valsalva dilation in patients with Marfan's syndrome, ascending aorta root replacements are performed with a composite valve and graft (with reimplantation of the coronaries) to avoid sinus dilation and rupture with separate root and valve replacements. A sinus of Valsalva aneurysm due to endocarditis tends to result in a more spherical, but still irregular-appearing dilation of the sinus (Fig. 15–29). Again, the aneurysm protrudes and may rupture into adjacent cardiac structures depending on which sinus is involved.

Color Plate 17

FIGURE 15–14. For legend, see page 379.

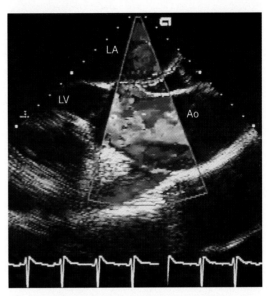

FIGURE 15–22. For legend, see page 384.

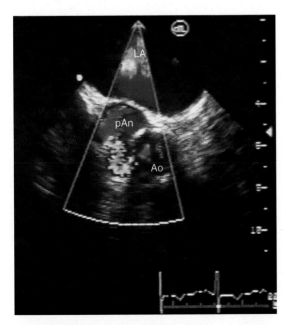

FIGURE 15–31. For legend, see page 389.

FIGURE 16–4. For legend, see page 401.

Color Plate 18

FIGURE 16–5. For legend, see page 404.

FIGURE 16–7. For legend, see page 406.

FIGURE 16–11. For legend, see page 408.

FIGURE 16–12. For legend, see page 409.

Color Plate 19

FIGURE 16–13. For legend, see page 410.

FIGURE 16–14. For legend, see page 411.

FIGURE 16–16. For legend, see page 412.

FIGURE 16–21. For legend, see page 416.

FIGURE 16–22. For legend, see page 417.

Color Plate 20

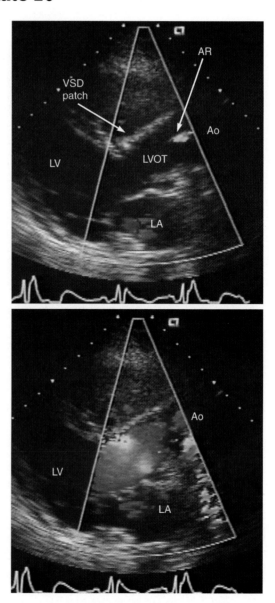

FIGURE 16–24. For legend, see page 418.

FIGURE 16–27. For legend, see page 422.

FIGURE 16–28. For legend, see page 423.

Preoperative and Postoperative Evaluation of Aortic Disease

Preoperative Evaluation

In some cases, the suspicion of aortic dissection is so high that transesophageal echocardiographic examination may be performed initially

FIGURE 15–25. Subtraction contrast angiogram shows an aortic dissection extending from the aortic valve level to the proximal descending thoracic aorta. The true lumen is more densely opacified than the false lumen.

in the operating room with the patient anesthetized and undergoing preparation for surgery. In these cases, the echocardiographer aims to rapidly confirm or exclude the suspected diagnosis. If a dissection is present, evaluation of the entry site and extent of dissection is helpful in planning the surgical approach. Recognition of complications such as aortic regurgitation, coronary ostial occlusion, or pericardial effusion also may affect acute patient management.

Residual Dissection Flaps

Transesophageal echocardiography may be used intraoperatively to assess for residual dissection following surgical repair. A residual dissection flap, with flow in both true and false lumens, persists in most patients (possibly as many as 70% to 80%) following emergency surgery for acute dissection. The usual operative procedure is to close the entry site by replacing a segment of the involved aorta with a prosthetic graft. At the distal graft anastomosis, the flap may persist. Often this persistence is intentional since some branch vessels may be supplied by the false lumen and other vessels by the true lumen. Thus the finding of a dissection flap in the aortic arch or descending aorta of a patient with a prior ascending aortic dissection and graft repair may represent stable residual disease or a second acute process. These conditions are differentiated by comparison with previous imaging studies (when available) and careful clinical evaluation. Some investigators have suggested that persistence of an intimal flap and flow in the false lumen are poor prognostic signs.

In patients with ascending aortic grafts, echocardiographic follow-up is warranted to assess for late complications. In patients with a

FIGURE 15–26. On chest computed tomography, a clear dissection flap *(arrow)* is seen in the aortic arch *(left)*. In a second patient, an atypical dissection is seen with displacement of intimal calcification *(arrow)* by an intramural thrombus in the descending thoracic aorta *(right)*.

valved conduit, a baseline study is indicated postoperatively to allow comparison with future studies in terms of prosthetic valve function (see Chap. 12). The prosthetic aortic graft itself appears as an echodense, cylindrical structure with a uniform diameter (Fig. 15–30). Although most surgeons now resect the native diseased aorta, in the past, the native aorta often was "wrapped around" the prosthetic graft resulting in irregular areas of thickening anterior and posterior to the graft on echocardiography. Even with resection of the native aortic segment, postoperative periaortic scar tissue may be prominent. The coronary arteries retain

FIGURE 15–27. In a 61-year-old man with cystic medial necrosis and prior ascending aortic dissection and graft placement, a magnetic resonance imaging scan in the coronal plane shows persistent dilation and a chronic dissection flap (arrow) in the aortic arch.

their normal insertions if a segment of the native aorta has been preserved. In these cases, careful examination for dilation of the remaining aortic tissue and the sinuses of Valsalva is needed. When the graft extends to the aortic valve level, the right and left coronary ostia are reimplanted into the graft along with a small "button" of native aortic tissue. Dilation or loss of structural integrity of this aortic tissue or dehiscence of the coronary reimplantation suture line results in myocardial infarction due to disruption of coronary blood flow. In addition, this complication can lead to aortic rupture or pseudoaneurysm formation.

Aortic Graft Pseudoaneurysms

A pseudoaneurysm, escape of blood from the graft lumen into an area contained by surrounding scar tissue or the native aorta, can occur at the proximal or the distal graft anastomoses to the aorta or at the coronary reimplantation sites. Rarer instances of rupture of the graft material itself have been reported. A pseudoaneurysm appears as an echolucent area adjacent to the aortic graft (Fig. 15–31). Flow into this region can be demonstrated with color flow imaging, although a transesophageal study often is necessary for adequate image quality. The pseudoaneurysm may rupture into the mediastinum or pleural spaces (both of which are likely to be fatal) or back across the aortic annulus into the left ventricle. This pseudoaortic regurgitation consists of flow from the pseudoaneurysm into the left ventricle

FIGURE 15–28. Congenital sinus of Valsalva aneurysm of the right coronary cusp (arrows) protruding into the right ventricular outflow tract on a transesophageal short-axis view.

FIGURE 15–29. Acquired sinus of Valsalva aneurysm (arrow) after aortic valve replacement in an apical long-axis view protruding into the left atrium.

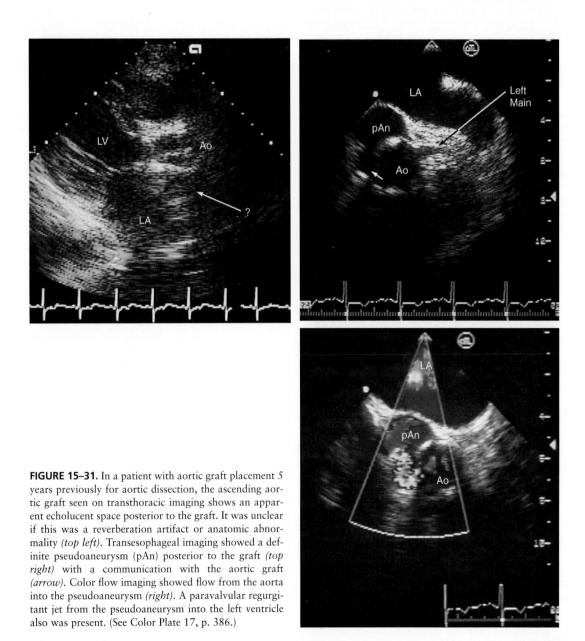

FIGURE 15–30. Composite ascending aortic graft and valve replacement postoperatively in a patient with Marfan's syndrome.

FIGURE 15–31. In a patient with aortic graft placement 5 years previously for aortic dissection, the ascending aortic graft seen on transthoracic imaging shows an apparent echolucent space posterior to the graft. It was unclear if this was a reverberation artifact or anatomic abnormality *(top left)*. Transesophageal imaging showed a definite pseudoaneurysm (pAn) posterior to the graft *(top right)* with a communication with the aortic graft *(arrow)*. Color flow imaging showed flow from the aorta into the pseudoaneurysm *(right)*. A paravalvular regurgitant jet from the pseudoaneurysm into the left ventricle also was present. (See Color Plate 17, p. 386.)

in diastole, with flow from the left ventricle into the pseudoaneurysm in systole. The characteristics of this flow signal on pulsed and continuous-wave Doppler are similar to those of transvalvular aortic regurgitation. Color flow imaging shows the flow around, rather than through, the prosthetic aortic valve.

Atherosclerotic Aortic Disease

Aortic Atherosclerosis as a Potential Source of Embolus

The excellent-quality images of the aorta obtained by transesophageal echocardiography have led to the observation of extensive atherosclerotic plaque in many individuals, with mobile thrombus attached to the atheroma in some cases. These observations have generated the hypothesis that atherosclerosis of the ascending aorta and arch may serve as a nidus for embolic material, resulting in cerebrovascular events. (See Suggested Readings 30 to 33 in Chapter 14.) These areas of atherosclerosis rarely are seen on transthoracic imaging due to poor image quality related to acoustic access, the depth of the aorta from the transthoracic approach, and the use of a lower frequency transducer. Echocardiographic evaluation of the extent and severity of atheroma correlates well with histologic examination, and transesophageal echocardiography is both sensitive and specific for detection of atheroma-related thrombus formation.

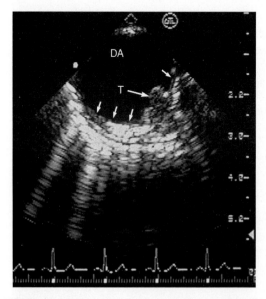

FIGURE 15–32. Transesophageal short-axis view of the descending thoracic aorta (DA) showing a large atherosclerotic plaque *(small arrows)* with attached thrombus (T), which showed independent motion in real time.

Aortic Atherosclerosis as a Marker for Coronary Artery Disease

The presence of detectable atherosclerotic plaques in the descending aorta on transesophageal echocardiography (Fig. 15–32) indicates the presence of atherosclerosis and thus is a marker of coronary artery disease with a sensitivity of 90%. Conversely, the absence of detectable atherosclerosis in the descending thoracic aorta suggests that significant coronary artery disease is not present with a specificity of 90%.

Pulmonary Artery Abnormalities

Most abnormalities of the pulmonary artery are congenital, including poststenotic dilation, branch pulmonary artery stenosis, and an abnormal position of the pulmonary artery, as in transposition of the great vessels. However, the pulmonary artery may be involved by systemic diseases that affect the aorta, such as Takayasu's arteritis. Pulmonary artery dissection is rare but has been reported in patients with chronic pulmonary hypertension.

The finding of a dilated pulmonary artery raises the possibility of right-sided volume overload (e.g., atrial septal defect) or pressure overload (e.g., pulmonary hypertension). Occasionally, a patient is seen with a dilated main pulmonary artery and no other cardiac abnormalities (idiopathic dilation of the pulmonary artery).

The pulmonary artery can be visualized on transthoracic echocardiography in a parasternal short-axis view at the aortic valve level or in a right ventricular outflow view. In adults, it may be difficult to visualize the anterior pulmonary artery wall due to overlying lung tissue. In younger patients, the pulmonary artery can be visualized from the anteriorly angulated apical four-chamber view by further anterior angulation. The subcostal short-axis view allows an alternate approach to visualize the pulmonary artery in most patients. From the suprasternal notch window, the right pulmonary artery is seen in cross section in the long-axis view of the aortic arch (see Fig. 15–7) and in its long axis in the orthogonal view (see Fig. 15–8). The left pulmonary artery can be imaged by slight lateral angulation and posterior rotation from the standard long-axis suprasternal notch view.

Transesophageal images of the pulmonary artery can be obtained in a 0° image plane by slowly withdrawing the probe to an esophageal level superior to the left atrium. This view shows the long axis of the pulmonary artery

FIGURE 15–33. Transesophageal view of the pulmonary artery from a high esophageal position in the 0° image plane orientation. This view cannot be obtained in all patients due to interposition of the air-filled bronchus.

and its bifurcation, but may not be obtained in all patients due to interposition of the air-filled bronchus (Fig. 15-33). The pulmonary artery also can be imaged in the 90° plane (analogous to the transthoracic right ventricular outflow view) by turning the transducer to the patient's right from the left ventricular long-axis view. However, image quality may be suboptimal due to the distance of the pulmonary artery from the transducer in this view.

Alternate approaches to evaluation of the pulmonary artery include computed tomographic or magnetic resonance image scanning and contrast angiography.

LIMITATIONS/TECHNICAL CONSIDERATIONS/ALTERNATE APPROACHES

The major limitations of echocardiographic evaluation of diseases of the great vessels are acoustic access and image quality. From the transthoracic approach, images of each segment of the aorta can be obtained, but image quality depends on the body habitus of the patient, the skill of the sonographer, and careful attention to the technical details of image acquisition. Interpretation of the images obtained must consider the likelihood of false-positive findings from beam-width artifacts, reverberations, and oblique image planes, as well as false-negative findings due to limited acoustic access and poor resolution.

Transesophageal imaging obviates many of these limitations by providing optimal acoustic access and excellent resolution. However, reverberations, beam-width artifacts, and oblique image planes still can result in apparent intraluminal "abnormalities," particularly in the ascending aorta, that in fact represent ultrasound artifacts. Use of a biplane or multiplane probe is essential, since the ascending aorta is visualized only at its base using the transverse image plane (single-plane probe). Even with a multiplane probe, a few centimeters of the ascending aorta at its junction with the arch may not be adequately visualized due to the interposed air-filled bronchial tree. Images of the ascending aorta are of particular importance in suspected aortic dissection because the entry site (ascending or descending aorta), rather than the simple presence or absence of disease, determines therapy.

Alternate approaches provide excellent quality images of the aorta with sensitivities and specificities for diagnosis of aortic dissection at least comparable with those of transesophageal echocardiography. Chest computed tomography can be used to evaluate aortic disease with the advantages of a wide field of view, high accuracy, and wide availability. Disadvantages include the use of ionizing radiation and the nonportable nature of the study. Chest computed tomography may identify associated pericardial effusion but is of limited value in evaluation of left ventricular or aortic valve function.

Magnetic resonance imaging of the aorta has the advantages of high resolution, high diagnostic accuracy, wide field of view, and the ability to orient the images along the long axis of the aorta. Like chest computed tomography, magnetic resonance imaging equipment is not portable. In addition, it is not as widely available, is expensive, and provides limited data on ventricular and valvular function in routine clinical use. However, both chest computed tomography and magnetic resonance imaging can provide data on branch vessel involvement, information that rarely is obtainable by echocardiography.

Contrast aortography allows accurate diagnosis of aortic disease, including aortic dissection, and may be the initial diagnostic procedure if the possibility of coronary artery disease is high on the differential diagnosis. Aortography allows evaluation of the degree of aortic regurgitation, involvement of branch vessels, and (by separate contrast injection) left ventricular systolic function. Cardiac catheterization, with contrast aortography, is the only diagnostic procedure that provides detailed coronary anatomy and allows rapid intervention should coronary artery obstruction be present. Disadvantages of contrast aortography are that it is not portable, uses ionizing radiation, is invasive, and is expensive.

Again, the choice of imaging procedures in a patient with suspected aortic disease depends largely in the differential diagnosis, the specific data needed in that patient, and procedure availability.

SUGGESTED READING

Aortic Dissection

1. Bolger AF: Aortic dissection: value and limitations of echocardiography. *In* Otto CM (ed): The Practice of Clinical Echocardiography. Philadelphia, WB Saunders, 1997, pp. 547–564.

   Review of the pathophysiologic and clinical presentation of aortic dissection and the role of echocardiography both for the initial diagnosis, management at the time of surgery and long-term follow-up. 112 references.

2. Roberts WC: Aortic dissection: Anatomy, consequences, and causes. *Am Heart J* 101:195–215, 1981.

   Excellent review of the pathology and anatomy of aortic dissection with clear diagrams and photographs. Emphasizes complications and etiology.

3. DeSanctis RW, Doroghazi RM, Austen WG, Buckley MJ: Aortic dissection. *N Engl J Med* 317:1060–1067, 1987.

   Review of pathogenesis, predisposing factors, clinical findings, diagnosis, and treatment of aortic dissection.

4. Roberts CS, Roberts WC: Dissection of the aorta associated with congenital malformation of the aortic valve. *J Am Coll Cardiol* 17:712–716, 1991.

   Of 186 patients with aortic dissection, 7.5% had a bicuspid aortic valve and 1.1% had a unicuspid aortic valve. The dissection entry site was in the ascending aorta in 100% of (16 of 16) patients with an abnormal aortic valve but only 68% of those with a trileaflet aortic valve. A congenitally abnormal aortic valve is approximately five times more common in patients with (compared with patients without) aortic dissection.

5. Hahn RT, Roman MJ, Mogtader AH, Devereux RB: Association of aortic dilation with regurgitant, stenotic and functionally normal bicuspid aortic valves. *J Am Coll Cardiol* 19:283–288, 1992.

   In 83 adults with a bicuspid aortic valve, ascending aortic dilation was present in 50% of those with a functionally normal valve (n = 19) and in 63% of those with aortic regurgitation or aortic stenosis, with mean aortic diameters of 3.6 ± 0.7 and 3.8 ± 0.7 cm, respectively, compared with 2.9 ± 0.7 cm in control subjects.

6. Goldstein SA, Mintz GS, Lindsay J Jr: Aorta: Comprehensive evaluation by echocardiography and transesophageal echocardiography. *J Am Soc Echocardiogr* 6:634–659, 1993.

   Review of the use of transthoracic and transesophageal echocardiography for evaluation of diseases of the aorta. 104 references.

7. Kotler MN: Is transesophageal echocardiography the new standard for diagnosing dissecting aortic aneurysms? *J Am Coll Cardiol* 14:1263–1265, 1989.

   Editorial on transesophageal echocardiography for diagnosis of aortic dissection reviews previous studies of transthoracic echocardiography in which sensitivity ranged from 79% to 100% with a specificity of 90%. Emphasizes that transesophageal echocardiography allows evaluation of entrance sites, differentiation of true from false lumen, evaluation of aortic regurgitation, and detection of pericardial effusion in addition to identification of the intimal flap.

8. Cigarroa JE, Isselbacher EM, DeSanctis RW, Eagle KA: Diagnostic imaging in the evaluation of suspected aortic dissection. Old standards and new directions. *N Engl J Med* 328:35–43, 1993.

   Excellent review, with examples, of diagnostic imaging procedures for aortic dissection, including aortography, computed tomographic scanning, magnetic resonance imaging, and echocardiography. Discusses the choice of imaging procedure in patients with suspected aortic dissection.

9. Victor MF, Mintz GS, Kotler MN, et al: Two-dimensional echocardiographic diagnosis of aortic dissection. *Am J Cardiol* 48:1155–1159, 1981.

   Transthoracic echocardiographic study of patients with suspected aortic dissection.

10. Erbel R, Borner N, Steller D, et al: Detection of aortic dissection by transesophageal echocardiography. *Br Heart J* 58:45–51, 1987.

    Evaluation of transthoracic and transesophageal echocardiography in 21 patients, all of whom had aortic dissection.

11. Hashimoto S, Kumada T, Osakada G, et al: Assessment of transesophageal Doppler echography in dissecting aortic aneurysm. *J Am Coll Cardiol* 14:1253–1262, 1989.

    Use of transesophageal echocardiography in aortic dissection emphasizing identification of sites of entry and detection of thrombus in the false channel.

12. Ballal RS, Nanda NC, Gatewood R, et al: Usefulness of transesophageal echocardiography in assessment of aortic dissection. *Circulation* 84:1903–1914, 1991.

    Besides diagnosis of dissection, transesophageal echocardiography correctly identified the type of dissection in all 29 patients. Complications detected by transesophageal echocardiography included involvement of the coronary arteries, communications between the true and false lumens, presence of thrombus in the false lumen, and localized rupture with pseudoaneurysm formation.

13. Nienaber CA, Spielmann RP, von Kodolitsch Y, et al: Diagnosis of thoracic aortic dissection. Magnetic resonance imaging versus transesophageal echocardiography. *Circulation* 85:434–447, 1992.

    Comparison of magnetic resonance imaging and transesophageal echocardiography in suspected aortic dissection. False-positive results on transesophageal echocardiography were related to reverberations, extensive plaque formation, and previous periaortic trauma. Magnetic resonance imaging was helpful in resolving these false-positive echocardiographic findings.

14. Nienaber CA, von Kodolitsch Y, Nicolas V, et al: The diagnosis of thoracic aortic dissection by noninvasive imaging procedures. *N Engl J Med* 328:1–9, 1993.

Further extension of the authors' study (Suggested Reading 13), including computed tomography, magnetic resonance imaging, transthoracic echocardiography, and transesophageal echocardiography diagnosis of aortic dissection. Again, the specificity of transesophageal echocardiography was lowest (86%) for the ascending aorta due to echo reverberation and atherosclerotic plaque. Magnetic resonance imaging and transesophageal echocardiography had the highest overall predictive value, and neither computed tomography nor aortography provided further significant information in the patients in this series. The authors advocate that transthoracic echocardiography should be followed by either magnetic resonance imaging or transesophageal echocardiography to provide a definitive diagnosis before surgical intervention.

15. Chan K-L: Usefulness of transesophageal echocardiography in the diagnosis of conditions mimicking aortic dissection. *Am Heart J* 122:495–504, 1991.

In 22 patients with suspected (but absent) aortic dissection, ischemic disease was present in 5. Of the remaining 17, transesophageal echocardiography demonstrated aortic disease in 16 patients with dilation in 10 (63%), atheromas in 7 (41%) (5 also had dilation), an extrinsic aortic mass in 2, a posttraumatic clot in the descending aorta in 1, and an anastomotic leak at a coronary reimplantation site in 1 patient. Thus transesophageal echocardiography provided valuable clinical data, even when aortic dissection was excluded.

16. Mohr-Kahaly S, Erbel R, Rennollet H, et al: Ambulatory follow-up of aortic dissection by transesophageal two-dimensional and color-coded Doppler echocardiography. *Circulation* 80:24–33, 1989.

Persistent dissection flaps were observed in 5 of 7 (71%) patients with aortic dissection treated surgically and 9 of 11 (82%) treated medically. Flow in the false lumen was present in 14 patients, and multiple persistent communications between the true and false lumens were detected frequently.

17. Erbel R, Oelert H, Meyer J, et al for the European Cooperative Study Group on Echocardiography: Effect of medical and surgical therapy on aortic dissection evaluated by transesophageal echocardiography: Implications for prognosis and therapy. *Circulation* 87: 1604–1615, 1993.

Of 168 patients treated for acute aortic dissection, a persistent patent false lumen was seen at follow-up in 93% (28 of 30) after surgery for ascending aortic dissection that extended into the descending aorta but in only 11% (2 of 18) with dissection confined to the ascending aorta. The authors propose that thrombus formation in the false lumen is a good prognostic sign, which is associated with a lower rate of complications and reoperation.

Aortic Pseudoaneurysms

18. Zoghbi WA: Echocardiographic recognition of unusual complications after surgery on the great vessels and cardiac valves. *In* Otto CM (ed): The Practice of Clinical Echocardiography. Philadelphia, WB Saunders, 1997, pp. 821–836.

Review and discussion of complications after aortic surgery including pseudoaneurysms of composite aortic grafts and complications after total root replacement. Excellent illustrations of the surgical techniques and echocardiographic findings.

19. Barbetseas J, Crawford ES, Sail HJ, et al: Doppler echocardiographic evaluation of pseudoaneurysms complicating composite grafts of the ascending aorta. *Circulation* 85:212–222, 1992.

Description of the echocardiographic appearance of pseudoaneurysm formation after ascending aortic graft surgery in eight cases. Periannular and coronary artery dehiscences were detected by echocardiography using both 2D imaging (transthoracic or transesophageal or both) and Doppler flow studies.

Marfan's Syndrome

20. Pyeritz RE, McKusick VA: The Marfan syndrome: Diagnosis and management. *N Engl J Med* 300:772–777, 1979.

Concise review article on the clinical manifestations of Marfan's syndrome. Nearly all patients with Marfan's syndrome have (or develop) aortic root dilation as seen on echocardiography. Annual echocardiographic examination is advocated.

21. Roman MJ, Devereux RB, Kramer-Fox R, O'Loughin J: Two-dimensional echocardiographic aortic root dimensions in normal children and adults. *Am J Cardiol* 64:507–512, 1989.

Aortic root dimensions can be normalized for the expected value for age and body size as:

Children *(<18 years)*	*Predicted sinus dimension =* *1.02 ± (0.98 BSA)*
Adults *(age 18–40 years)*	*Predicted sinus dimension =* *0.97 ± (1.12 BSA)*
Adults *(>40 years)*	*Predicted sinus dimension =* *1.92 ± (0.74 BSA)*

Where BSA = body surface area in m^2.

22. Simpson IA, de Belder MA, Treasure T, et al: Cardiovascular manifestations of Marfan's syndrome: Improved evaluation by transesophageal echocardiography. *Br Heart J* 69:104–108, 1993.

Transesophageal echocardiography studies in 11 patients with Marfan's syndrome, suspected aortic dissection, and inadequate transthoracic echocardiography images revealed evidence for dissection in 6 subjects with surgical confirmation in all 6 cases.

23. Shores J, Berger KR, Murphy EA, Pyeritz RE: Progression of aortic dilatation and the benefit of long-term beta-adrenergic blockade in Marfan's syndrome. *N Engl J Med* 330:1335–1341, 1994.

Echocardiography was used to follow the rate of aortic root dilation in 70 patients with Marfan's syndrome in a randomized trial of beta-blockade therapy. Maximal measured aortic root diameter was divided by the predicted diameter for the patient age, height, and weight. This "aortic ratio" was comparable both between patients and in the same patient during growth of the body. The rate of progression, measured as the slope of the aortic ratio regression line, was significantly lower in the treatment group compared with control subjects ($P < .001$).

24. Legget ME, Unger TA, O'Sullivan CK, et al: Aortic root complications in Marfan's syndrome: Identification of a lower risk group. *Heart* 75:389–395, 1996.

Echocardiography was used to follow disease progression in 89 patients with Marfan's syndrome. To compare aortic root dimensions as patients aged, the normalized root ratio was used as a measure of disease progression. A ratio of actual to predicted root dimension ≥1.3 predicted an increased likelihood of ascending aortic dissection. An increase in the root ratio ≥5% also predicted a poor clinical outcome.

Aortic Atheroma

25. Fazio GP, Redberg RF, Winslow T, Schiller NB: Transesophageal echocardiographically detected atherosclerotic aortic plaque is a marker for coronary artery disease. *J Am Coll Cardiol* 21:144–150, 1993.

In 61 patients (31 females) with previous coronary angiography, transesophageal echocardiography showed atherosclerotic plaque in the descending thoracic aorta in 37 of 41 (sensitivity 90%) with documented coronary artery disease (>50% left main or >70% left anterior descending artery, right coronary artery, or circumflex). Of the 20 patients without significant coronary disease, 18 (specificity 90%) had no evidence for atherosclerosis in the descending aorta on transesophageal echocardiography.

Traumatic Aortic Rupture

26. Smith MD, Cassidy JM, Souther S, et al: Transesophageal echocardiography in the diagnosis of traumatic rupture of the aorta. *N Engl J Med* 332:356–362, 1995.

Transesophageal echocardiography was attempted in 101 patients with possible aortic trauma and was successful in 93 patients. Aortic rupture was diagnosed on transesophageal images in 11 (12%) studies with confirmation by aortography, surgery, or autopsy showing a sensitivity of 100% and a specificity of 98% (1 false-positive result). The typical appearance of aortic trauma on transesophageal echocardiography is a mobile 2- to 3-cm intraluminal flap or mass just distal to the junction of the aortic arch and descending thoracic aorta.

27. Vignon P, Gueret P, Vedrinne JM, et al: Role of transesophageal echocardiography in the diagnosis and management of traumatic aortic disruption. *Circulation* 92:2959–2968, 1995.

In 32 consecutive trauma patients with suspected traumatic disruption of the aorta, two distinct echocardiographic patterns were seen: subadventitial traumatic disruption in 10 patients and traumatic intimal flaps in 3 patients. The remaining 18 patients had a normal echo and angiogram. Transesophageal echocardiography had a sensitivity of 91% and a specificity of 100% for diagnosis of subadventitial traumatic disruption compared to confirmation by aortography, surgery, or autopsy. Disruption can be recognized on transesophageal echocardiography by the presence of a thick flap (the disrupted aortic wall) that traverses the lumen at the level of the aortic isthmus, an irregular appearance to aortic wall due to pseudoaneurysm formation, and similar flow patterns on both sides of the disrupted aortic wall.

Aortic Intramural Hemorrhage

28. Mohr-Kahaly S, Erbel R, Kearney P, et al: Aortic intramural hemorrhage visualized by transesophageal echocardiography: Findings and prognostic implications. *J Am Coll Cardiol* 23:658–664, 1994.

Localized intramural hemorrhage results in a layered appearance of the aorta on transesophageal imaging. This variant of aortic dissection was seen in 15 of 114 patients. The length of the intramural hematoma ranged from 3 to 20 cm with a thickness of 0.7 to 3 cm. At 11-month follow-up, the mortality rate was 53% (8 of 15)—5 (33%) patients had classic aortic dissection, 4 (27%) had aortic rupture, and 5 (33%) became asymptomatic with medical therapy.

29. Keren A, Kim CB, Hu BS, et al: Accuracy of biplane and multiplane transesophageal echocardiography in diagnosis of typical acute aortic dissection and intramural hematoma. *J Am Coll Cardiol* 28:627–636, 1996.

In a consecutive series of 112 patients undergoing transesophageal echocardiography for suspected aortic dissection, echocardiographic findings were compared to findings at surgery or autopsy. The sensitivity of transesophageal echocardiography for the presence of aortic dissection was 98% with a specificity of 95%. The sensitivity of transesophageal echocardiography for detection of intramural hematoma was 90% with a specificity of 99%. Echocardiography also was highly accurate for detection of associated aortic regurgitation and pericardial tamponade.

Echocardiographic Evaluation of the Adult With Congenital Heart Disease

16

ECHOCARDIOGRAPHIC APPROACH
Congenital Stenotic Lesions
Congenital Regurgitant Lesions
Abnormal Intracardiac Communications (Shunts)
Abnormal Chamber and Great Vessel Connections

CONGENITAL DEFECTS SEEN IN ADULTS WITH OR WITHOUT PRIOR CARDIAC SURGERY
Congenital Aortic Valve Abnormalities
Congenital Obstructions to Right Ventricular
    Outflow
Congenital Abnormalities of the Aorta
    Aortic Coarctation
    Marfan's Syndrome
    Sinus of Valsalva Aneurysm
Coronary Arteriovenous Fistula
Congenital Regurgitant Lesions
    Ebstein's Anomaly of the Tricuspid Valve
    Myxomatous Mitral Valve Disease
Atrial Septal Defects
    Anatomy
    Two-Dimensional Imaging
    Doppler Examination
    Contrast Echo
    After Atrial Septal Defect Repair

Ventricular Septal Defects
    Anatomy
    Two-Dimensional Echocardiographic Findings
    Doppler Findings
Patent Ductus Arteriosus
Ventricular Inversion
"Incidental" Congenital Anomalies
Other Congenital Cardiac Diseases Presenting in
    Adults

ADULT CONGENITAL HEART DISEASE WITH PRIOR SURGICAL PROCEDURES
Classification of Types of Procedures
Tetralogy of Fallot
Transposition of the Great Arteries
Tricuspid Atresia
Truncus Arteriosus

LIMITATIONS OF ECHOCARDIOGRAPHY/ALTERNATE APPROACHES
Calculations of Shunt Ratios
Imaging
Intracardiac Hemodynamics
Integrating the Diagnostic Approach

SUGGESTED READING

There are two basic categories of congenital heart disease in adults:

1. The initial clinical presentation of previously undiagnosed and untreated congenital defects.

2. Survival into adulthood of patients with known congenital heart disease and previous surgical procedures.

In adult patients with no prior diagnosis of heart disease, a congenital defect often is not considered as a potential cause of symptoms, and thus the initial diagnosis may be made at the echocardiographic examination. In these patients, the diagnostic challenge is to recognize and correctly evaluate the congenital abnormality. In patients with known congenital disease and prior surgical procedures, the diagnostic challenge for the echocardiographer is to identify the postoperative anatomy and assess the physiologic consequences of residual defects in each patient. With "corrective" surgery, as well as with "palliative" procedures, many patients have significant residual or progressive abnormalities.

Both these challenges can be met by a logical and methodical approach to the echocardiographic examination with application of the basic principles of two-dimensional (2D) imaging and Doppler ultrasound described throughout this text. Unusual imaging planes and careful integration of imaging and Doppler data may be needed for complete assessment of congenital heart disease. In addition, the physician and sonographer must have a thorough understanding of the three-dimensional (3D) anatomic relationships for each type of congenital defect.

Obviously, a comprehensive discussion of the echocardiographic findings in adult congenital heart disease is beyond the scope of this text. Instead, an overview of the echocardiographic approach to these patients and examples of the more common abnormalities will be presented. The reader is referred to the specialized references listed at the end of the chapter for more detailed information.

ECHOCARDIOGRAPHIC APPROACH (Table 16–1)

Congenital Stenotic Lesions

Congenital stenotic lesions are common, including obstruction to right or left ventricular outflow (either subvalvular, valvular, or supravalvular), obstruction to left ventricular inflow (congenital mitral stenosis, cor triatriatum), and narrowings in the great vessels (aortic coarctation, branch pulmonary artery stenosis).

The anatomy of a congenital stenotic lesion is specific for each condition (as discussed below), although, in adult patients, 2D images of the stenotic region may be suboptimal. The physiology and fluid dynamics of congenital stenosis are identical to those seen in acquired disease. There is laminar, normal-velocity flow upstream and a flow disturbance downstream from the narrowing. In the narrowed region itself, a high-velocity laminar jet of flow is present, with velocity (V, in m/s) related to the pressure difference (ΔP, in mmHg) across the narrowing as stated in the simplified Bernoulli equation:

$$\Delta P = 4V^2$$

When a parallel intercept angle can be obtained between the jet and the ultrasound beam, quantitative data on stenosis severity and intracardiac hemodynamics can be derived. For example, if the maximum velocity across a subpulmonic stenosis is 4.5 m/s, then the maximum right ventricular to pulmonary artery systolic pressure difference is approximately 80 mmHg. Quantitative evaluation of stenosis severity for a congenitally stenotic lesion includes calculation of maximum and mean pressure gradients as for acquired valve stenosis. Similarly, when possible, valve area calculations are performed using either the continuity equation (aortic valve) or the pressure half-time method (mitral valve).

Several significant differences between congenital and acquired stenosis should be noted. First, congenital stenosis of ventricular outflow, for both right and left ventricles, may involve the subvalvular or supravalvular region rather than (or in addition to) stenosis of the valve itself. Careful evaluation with conventional pulsed Doppler or color flow imaging to identify the poststenotic flow disturbance is helpful in determining the exact site of obstruction. Second, when serial stenoses are present, quantitation of the contribution of each level of obstruction to the overall degree of stenosis can be difficult using Doppler echo methods. Third, the proximal flow pattern in congenital stenosis often is characterized by a greater increase in velocity due to anatomic tapering of the proximal flow region (e.g., in aortic coarctation or in the congenitally stenotic pulmonic valve). In these situations, accurate pressure gradient calculations should include the proximal velocity (V_{prox}) as well as the jet velocity (V_{jet}) in the Bernoulli equation:

$$\Delta P = 4(V^2_{jet} - V^2_{prox})$$

Otherwise, evaluation of congenital stenosis is similar to evaluation of acquired stenosis in adults, and the methods described in detail in Chapter 10 can be applied in this patient group.

Congenital Regurgitant Lesions

Careful 2D imaging of a congenitally regurgitant valve may reveal the specific mechanism of regurgitation in that patient. For the atrioventricular valves, particular attention is focused on the number and position of papillary muscles; the chordal attachments (especially aberrant ones); leaflet size, shape, thickness, redundancy, and motion; and annulus size and shape. Malformations can include myxomatous changes of the leaflets, abnormal leaflet position (Ebstein's anomaly), and abnormal chordal attachments (atrioventricular canal defect). The

TABLE 16–1	Categories of Congenital Heart Disease

Congenital Stenotic Lesions
Subvalvular
Valvular
Supravalvular
Peripheral great vessels

Congenital Regurgitant Lesions

Abnormal Intracardiac Communications
Atrial septal defect
Ventricular septal defect
Patent ductus arteriosus

Abnormal Chamber and Great Vessel Connections

semilunar valves may be regurgitant due to great vessel dilation or a leaflet fenestration.

The physiology of congenital regurgitation is no different from that of acquired regurgitation. There is a flow disturbance in the chamber receiving the regurgitant flow with progressive dilation (and eventual dysfunction) of the volume-overloaded cardiac chambers. Evaluation of congenital regurgitation is similar to evaluation of acquired regurgitation, as detailed in Chapter 11.

Abnormal Intracardiac Communications (Shunts)

An abnormal intracardiac communication is characterized by blood flow across the defect, with the direction, timing, and volume of flow determined by the size of the orifice, the pressure gradient across the defect, and the relative resistance to flow of the vascular beds on each side of the defect. If left-sided heart pressures exceed right-sided pressures (pulmonary vascular resistance is low), left-to-right flow across the defect predominates. Small degrees of right-to-left shunting may be present briefly during the cardiac cycle, since right-sided pressures may transiently exceed left-sided pressures.

With conventional pulsed Doppler ultrasound or with color flow imaging, a flow disturbance is found downstream from the defect: on the right side of the interventricular septum for a ventricular septal defect, in the right atrium for an atrial septal defect, and in the pulmonary artery for a patent ductus arteriosus.

Analogous to a stenotic or regurgitant orifice, the velocity of blood flow through the shunt orifice is related to the pressure gradient across the defect, as stated in the Bernoulli equation. Thus a small ventricular septal defect results in a high-velocity systolic flow signal (about 5 m/s), since left ventricular systolic pressure greatly exceeds right ventricular systolic pressure (by about 100 mmHg). Conversely, flow across an atrial septal defect typically is low in velocity because only a modest left atrial to right atrial pressure difference is present.

A left-to-right intracardiac shunt imposes a chronic volume overload on the receiving chamber(s) with consequent dilation of the affected chamber(s). With an atrial septal defect, both right atrial and right ventricular dilation, along with paradoxical septal motion, are seen. With a patent ductus arteriosus, the volume overload is imposed on the left atrium and left ventricle. Although it might seem that a ventricular septal defect would cause right ventric-

ular volume overload, in fact, right ventricular size usually is normal since the left ventricle effectively ejects the shunt flow across the defect directly into the pulmonary artery in systole. Instead, left atrial and left ventricular dilation are seen, since these chambers receive the increased pulmonary blood flow as it returns to the left side of the heart via the pulmonary veins.

The volume of blood flow (Q) across an intracardiac shunt—the ratio of pulmonary to systemic blood flow (Q_p:Q_s)—can be determined by Doppler echo measurements of stroke volume at two intracardiac sites (Fig. 16–1). In the case of an atrial septal defect, transpulmonic volume flow (Q_p) is calculated from pulmonary artery (PA) cross-sectional area (CSA) and velocity-time integral (VTI), while systemic volume flow (Q_s) is calculated from measurements of left ventricular outflow tract (LVOT) cross-sectional area and velocity-time integral:

Shunt ratio

$$Q_p = CSA_{PA} \times VTI_{PA}$$

$$Q_s = CSA_{LVOT} \times VTI_{LVOT}$$

$$\text{so that } Q_p{:}Q_s = \frac{CSA_{PA} \times VTI_{PA}}{CSA_{LVOT} \times VTI_{LVOT}}$$

This approach is accurate when 2D images are of adequate quality for precise diameter measurements (for calculation of a circular cross-sectional area) and when Doppler velocity data are recorded at a parallel intercept angle to flow. Potential errors in estimation of the Q_p:Q_s ratio may arise as for any Doppler echo stroke volume measurement (see Chap. 5).

With significant left-to-right shunting, pulmonary pressures become elevated, and irreversible pulmonary hypertension may develop over time. When pulmonary vascular resistance equals or exceeds systemic vascular resistance, the direction of shunt flow reverses, resulting in decreased systemic oxygen saturation and cyanosis. Irreversible pulmonary hypertension with equalization of pulmonary and systemic pressures due to an intracardiac shunt is known as *Eisenmenger's physiology*. This phenomenon can occur in infancy, particularly with a large ventricular septal defect, but also can occur later in life when the pulmonary-to-systemic shunt ratio chronically exceeds 2:1.

Abnormal Chamber and Great Vessel Connections

Echocardiographic diagnosis is more difficult when there are abnormal connections between the atrium and the ventricles and/or be-

FIGURE 16–1. Schematic diagram of Doppler echo shunt ratio calculation. Pulmonary flow (Q_p) is calculated from transpulmonic stroke volume calculation using pulmonary artery (PA) diameter measured at the site of the Doppler sample position and the velocity-time integral (VTI) of pulmonary artery flow. A circular cross-sectional area (CSA) is assumed. Similarly, systemic flow (Q_s) is calculated from left ventricular outflow tract (LVOT) diameter and the velocity-time integral of left ventricular outflow tract.

tween the ventricles and great vessels. In adults, poor acoustic access may further compromise the examination. However, with a systematic approach, a correct anatomic evaluation usually is possible.

Since the position of the heart in the chest may be abnormal, the echocardiographer cannot rely on the intrathoracic position of the chambers for correct identification of cardiac anatomy. In *dextrocardia* the heart is located in the right hemithorax with the apex in the right midclavicular line. With *situs inversus,* there is right-to-left reversal of thoracic and abdominal viscera. *Dextroversion* is a rightward shift in the cardiac apex without mirror-image inversion.

The first step in a systemic examination of complex congenital heart disease is determination of *atrial situs.* The inferior vena cava nearly always drains into the right atrium, allowing correct identification of this chamber by imaging the inferior vena cava from a subcostal approach and following it into the right atrium. Thus the subcostal window often is a useful starting point for examination of a patient with complex congenital heart disease. The left atrium, then, is the "other" atrial chamber, since although the pulmonary veins normally drain into the left atrium, this is not always the case (e.g., partial or total anomalous pulmonary venous return).

The *anatomic right and left ventricles* (Table 16–2) can be distinguished from each other by several features. The anatomic right ventricle

TABLE 16–2	Echocardiographic Features Distinguishing the Anatomic Right Ventricle from the Left Ventricle

Feature	Right Ventricle	Left Ventricle
Atrioventricular valve	Trileaflet	Bicuspid—unless cleft anterior mitral leaflet present
Annulus location	More apical	More basal
Trabeculation	Prominent	Less prominent
Moderator band	Present	Absent
Infundibulum	Present	Absent—fibrous continuity between anterior mitral valve leaflet and great vessel

has more prominent trabeculation than the left ventricle and has a moderator band. The infundibular region is seen only in the right ventricle, so fibrous continuity of the anterior mitral valve leaflet and the aortic valve occurs only with a normally related left ventricle and aortic root. When the anatomic right ventricle connects to the aortic root, a band of myocardium is seen between the base of the atrioventricular valve leaflet and the great vessel. The atrioventricular valves develop with the appropriate anatomic ventricle, so identification of the mitral valve is another feature that differentiates the left from the right ventricle. Caution is needed if a cleft anterior mitral valve leaflet is present because it may superficially resemble the tricuspid valve. In addition to the number of atrioventricular valve leaflets, the relative positions of the atrioventricular valve annuli are helpful, since the tricuspid valve annulus lies slightly closer to the apex than the mitral valve annulus. Note that ventricular size, shape, and/or wall thickness do not distinguish the two ventricles, since congenital lesions can result in dilation and hypertrophy of either chamber.

After identifying the atrium and ventricles, attention is directed toward the *great vessels*. The aortic root is best identified by following the vessel downstream to image the arch and head and neck vessels. Origins of the coronary arteries also may be seen, but anomalous origin of the coronary arteries from the pulmonary artery must be considered. The pulmonary artery is identified by its bifurcation into right and left branches. The position of the great vessels within the thorax and relative to each other often are altered in congenital disease. Normally, the pulmonary artery lies anterior and slightly medial to the aortic root at its origin and then courses posteriorly and laterally, with the right pulmonary artery lying posterior to the

ascending aorta. The aortic annulus normally lies posterior to the right ventricular outflow tract, with the aortic root extending medially and anteriorly before turning posterolaterally to form the aortic arch. The normal relationship of the aortic and pulmonic valve planes is approximately perpendicular to each other, with the pulmonary valve slightly more superior within the chest than the aortic valve. With transpositions of the great vessels, these relationships are altered so that the semilunar valves lie in the same tomographic plane, and the aorta and pulmonary artery lie parallel to each other instead of in their normal "crisscross" positions (Fig. 16–2). If the aorta is located anterior and to the left, L (for *levo*) *transposition* is present. An anterior and medial (rightward) aorta is termed D (for *dextro*) *transposition*.

Most patients with abnormal connections between the cardiac chambers and great vessels have associated abnormalities that require echocardiographic evaluation. These include intracardiac shunts, stenotic and regurgitant lesions, pulmonary hypertension, and ventricular dysfunction. The echocardiographic examination in these patients is facilitated by the following (Table 16–3):

1. Knowledge of the clinical history, including prior surgical procedures and diagnostic tests.

2. Formulation of specific clinical questions to be answered by the echocardiographic examination.

FIGURE 16–2. Transposed great arteries seen on a transesophageal view with an anterior aorta and a smaller posterior pulmonary artery with a bicuspid valve in a 42-year-old with congenital transposition of the great arteries, pulmonic stenosis, and a ventricular septal defect.

TABLE 16–3	Approach to Echocardiographic Examination in Adults with Complex Congenital Heart Disease

Before the Examination

Review the clinical history

Obtain details of any prior surgical procedures

Review results of prior diagnostic tests

Formulate specific questions

Sequence of Examination

Identify cardiac chambers, great vessels, and their connections

Identify associated defects, and evaluate the physiology of each lesion
  Regurgitation and/or stenosis
  Shunts
  Pulmonary hypertension
  Ventricular dysfunction

After the Examination

Integrate echo and Doppler findings with clinical data

Summarize findings

Identify which clinical questions remain unanswered, and suggest appropriate subsequent diagnostic tests

During the examination, the physician and sonographer work together in:

1. Identifying the cardiac chambers, great vessels, and their connections.

2. Identifying associated defects, and evaluating the physiologic consequences of each defect with appropriate Doppler modalities.

3. Identifying which clinical questions remain unanswered at the end of examination, and proposing appropriate alternate diagnostic tests that can provide answers to these questions.

CONGENITAL DEFECTS SEEN IN ADULTS WITH OR WITHOUT PRIOR CARDIAC SURGERY (Table 16–4)

Congenital Aortic Valve Abnormalities

Although a congenital bicuspid aortic valve is the most common type of congenital heart disease (reported to occur in 1% to 2% of the general population), the bicuspid valve often is functionally normal until about age 50 to 60 years, when superimposed fibrocalcific changes lead to aortic valve stenosis. Significant regurgitation of a congenital bicuspid valve occurs somewhat less commonly but presents in young adulthood with a diastolic murmur and symptoms of exercise intolerance.

The presentation of significant left ventricular outflow obstruction in a young adult should prompt consideration of abnormalities other than a bicuspid valve—specifically a unicuspid aortic valve, a subaortic membrane, or hypertrophic cardiomyopathy. A unicuspid aortic valve will appear as a thickened, deformed valve with systolic bowing of the valve on 2D imaging. A high parasternal short-axis view may show the eccentric unicuspid opening in systole, even allowing 2D planimetry of the valve orifice (see Fig. 15–18). Doppler echocardiography can be used to determine the transvalvular gradient and valve area as for any type of aortic valve stenosis. Restenosis of the aortic valve in patients who previously underwent surgical valvotomy in childhood or adolescence is common. Restenosis occurs in up to 40% of patients a mean of 13 years after open surgical valvotomy.

Congenital subaortic obstruction can range anatomically from a muscular ridge to a thin membrane (Fig. 16–3). Although typically located 1 to 1.5 cm apically from the aortic valve plane, the membrane may be located immediately adjacent to the aortic valve. In either case, a subaortic membrane can be difficult to visualize in adults due to poor acoustic access. The possibility of a subaortic membrane should be considered when high-velocity flow is recorded in the left ventricular outflow tract, but the aortic valve leaflets appear normal. Transesophageal echocardiography may allow direct imaging of the subaortic membrane, especially if multiple image planes are used to identify this thin structure. Conventional pulsed Doppler, high-pulse-repetition-frequency Doppler, and color flow imaging can be extremely helpful from either transthoracic or transesophageal approaches in demonstrating that, in contrast to valvular aortic stenosis, the increase in antegrade velocity and poststenotic flow disturbance occur on the *left ventricular* side of the aortic valve, indicating that subaortic obstruction is present (Fig. 16–4). Coexisting aortic regurgitation may be present due to chronic exposure of the aortic valve leaflets to the high-velocity subaortic flow, resulting in a "jet lesion" on the aortic valve, or (rarely) due to fibrous attachments from the subaortic membrane to the aortic valve leaflets.

FIGURE 16–3. Parasternal long-axis 2D view *(above)* and M-mode *(below)* in a patient with a subaortic membrane *(arrow)*. Note the early systolic notch on the aortic valve M-mode *(arrow)*.

Congenital Obstructions to Right Ventricular Outflow

Right ventricular outflow obstruction may be subvalvular (in the muscular outflow tract), valvular, or supravalvular (either in the main pulmonary artery or its major branches). Pulmonic stenosis can occur as an isolated anomaly but more often is part of a complex of abnormalities for example, tetralogy of Fallot or is associated with other abnormalities—for example, ventricular inversion.

The level of outflow obstruction can be determined using pulsed Doppler and color flow to identify the anatomic site at which the flow velocity increases and the poststenotic flow disturbance appears. The obstruction itself may be visualized on 2D echocardiography as a muscular subpulmonic ridge; as deformed, doming pulmonic valve leaflets; or as a narrowing in the pulmonary artery. If significant obstruction is

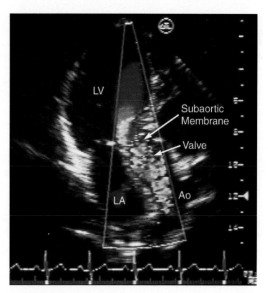

FIGURE 16–4. Color Doppler in an apical long-axis view in the same patient as in Figure 16–3 showing that the flow disturbance occurs proximal to the aortic valve *(arrow)*. (See Color Plate 17, p. 386.)

present, compensatory right ventricular hypertrophy typically is seen.

The degree of obstruction can be measured by Doppler ultrasound using the Bernoulli equation (Fig. 16–5) with the proviso that only an estimate of the total obstruction may be possible if serial stenoses are present. Note that in the presence of pulmonic stenosis, the tricuspid regurgitant jet velocity remains an accurate reflection of the right ventricular to right atrial systolic pressure difference but no longer indicates pulmonary artery systolic pressure. Instead, pulmonary artery systolic pressure can be estimated by (1) calculation of the right ventricular systolic pressure by adding the right ventricular to right atrial gradient ($\Delta P_{\text{RV-RA}}$ calculated from the tricuspid regurgitant jet) to an estimate of right atrial pressure (P_{RA}) and then (2) subtracting the right ventricular to pulmonary artery gradient ($\Delta P_{\text{RV-PA}}$) calculated from the pulmonic stenosis jet:

$$\text{Estimated pulmonary artery systolic}$$
$$\text{pressure} = (\Delta P_{\text{RV-RA}} + P_{\text{RA}}) - \Delta P_{\text{RV-PA}}$$

The end-diastolic velocity in the pulmonic regurgitation jet also may give useful data on pulmonary artery pressures because it reflects the diastolic pressure difference between the pulmonary artery and the right ventricle (high in patients with pulmonary hypertension, low in patients with pulmonic stenosis and normal pulmonary artery diastolic pressures).

TABLE 16–4	Common Unoperated Congenital Heart Disease Seen in Adults	
Congenital Defect	**2D Echo Findings**	**Doppler Findings**
Bicuspid aortic valve	Bicuspid valve identified in systole (raphe seen in diastole).	Mild stenosis and/or regurgitation.
Unicuspid aortic valve	Abnormal, deformed aortic valve with systolic doming; sometimes the unicuspid orifice can be imaged.	Aortic stenosis (may be severe) and/or aortic regurgitation.
Subaortic membrane	Membrane from anterior MV leaflet to ventricular septum; TEE may be needed for visualization.	High-velocity signal just proximal to aortic valve; AR due to nonsupport of aortic annulus or to a "jet lesion."
Pulmonic stenosis	Thickened pulmonic valve leaflets with systolic doming, increased a wave on pulmonic M-mode.	Mild pulmonic stenosis (more severe stenosis is recognized and treated in childhood).
Aortic coarctation	Coarctation may not be easy to visualize since descending thoracic aorta goes out of the image plane from SSN; associated with bicuspid aortic valve; highly pulsatile aortic root and akinetic abdominal aorta.	High-velocity systolic flow in descending thoracic aorta with extension of flow into diastole with severe obstruction; nonparallel intercept angle limits quantitation of severity in unoperated patients.
Marfan's syndrome	Dilated aortic root with loss of the sinotubular junction; elongated, redundant anterior MV leaflet; dilation of ascending aorta, arch, and descending aorta may be present.	AR
Sinus of Valsalva aneurysm	Dilated, thin sinus with "wind sock" type of projection into adjacent cardiac structures depending on sinus involved.	May have fistula from aorta into RA, LA, RV, or LV depending on cusp involved.
Coronary AV fistula	May not be able to visualize fistula, but coronary sinus may be dilated; proximal coronary artery may be dilated.	Disturbed flow in coronary sinus or in abnormal epicardial echolucent structures.
Epstein's anomaly	Septal tricuspid valve leaflet is adherent to RV wall, appearing "apically displaced"; apparent RA enlargement (part of anatomic RV is physiologically part of RA); associated with WPW and with right-to-left atrial shunt.	Tricuspid regurgitation.
Myxomatous mitral valve disease	Thick, redundant, prolapsing mitral valve leaflets; LV and LA enlargement depending on severity of MR; tricuspid and aortic valves also may be affected; can be seen in syndrome of polyvalvular dysplasia.	MR
Atrial septal defects	Right ventricular and right atrial volume overload with RVE, RAE, and paradoxical ventricular septal motion. *Secundum ASD:* Absence of interatrial septum in fossa ovalis region best seen on subcostal or parasternal four-chamber view.	$Q_p:Q_s$ can be calculated from Doppler stroke volume measurements in LVOT (or Ao) versus PA. Color flow imaging of left-to-right flow across interatrial septum; IV echo contrast shows some right-to-left shunting.

Ao = aorta, AR = aortic regurgitation, ASD = atrial septal defect, AV = atrioventricular, CW = continuous-wave, IAS = interatrial septum, IV = intravenous, LA = left atrium, LVOT = left ventricular outflow tract, LV = left ventricle, MR = mitral regurgitation, MV = mitral valve, PA = pulmonary artery, Q = volume flow rate, Q_p = pulmonic volume flow rate, Q_s = systemic volume flow rate, RA = right atrium, RAE = right atrial enlargement, RV = right ventricle, RVE = right ventricular enlargement, RVOT = right ventricular outflow tract, SSN = suprasternal notch, SVC = superior vena cava, TEE = transesophageal echocardiography, VSD = ventricular septal defect, WPW = Wolff-Parkinson-White (pre-excitation) syndrome.

TABLE 16–4	Common Unoperated Congenital Heart Disease Seen in Adults *Continued*	
Congenital Defect	**2D Echo Findings**	**Doppler Findings**
Atrial septal defects *Continued*	*Primum ASD:* Defect in IAS adjacent to central fibrous body; associated with AV valve abnormalities (cleft anterior MV leaflet).	Color flow imaging of left-to-right flow across interatrial septum; may have associated mitral regurgitation.
	Sinus venosus ASD: Defect at SVC-RA junction (may be associated with anomalous PVR); TEE helpful for imaging defect; suspect when $Q_p{:}Q_s$ is elevated without clear evidence of secundum or primum ASD.	TEE to visualize site of defect and left-to-right flow with color imaging.
Partial anomalous pulmonary venous return	RVE, RAE, and paradoxical septal motion reflecting right-sided volume overload (may be associated with ASD).	Suspect when $Q_p{:}Q_s > 1$ with no evidence for flow across interatrial septum.
Ventricular septal defects	*Small VSD:* Membranous, muscular, or outflow defects may be difficult to image; membranous defects may be partially or completely closed (ventricular septal aneurysm) by the septal leaflet of the tricuspid valve.	High-velocity jet from left to right in systole with pulsed or CW Doppler; color flow imaging shows flow disturbance on right ventricular side of the defect; normal PA pressures.
	Eisenmenger VSD: Large defect, often membranous or subaortic, with equal size and wall thickness of LV and RV.	Low-velocity bidirectional flow across the ventricular defect; severe pulmonary hypertension.
Patent ductus arteriosus	Mild LV and LA enlargement; duct itself rarely visualized in adults.	Diastolic flow reversal in the pulmonary artery (typically along the anterior PA wall); diastolic flow reversal in the descending thoracic aorta.
Ventricular inversion (corrected transposition)	RV-LV reversal; pattern of blood flow is physiologic: RA to LV to PA; LA to RV to Ao. Associated defects are common, including pulmonic stenosis, VSD, heart block, and Ebstein's type anomaly of the inverted tricuspid valve with systemic AV valve regurgitation.	Normal physiology in absence of associated defects; Doppler findings of pulmonic stenosis, VSD, AV valve regurgitation when present.
Persistent left SVC	Dilated coronary sinus; absence of innominate vein on SSN view; small right SVC.	Contrast injection from left arm opacifies coronary sinus first, then right atrium.
Hypertrophic cardiomyopathy	Asymmetrically hypertrophied LV with several patterns of involvement; 2D and M-mode signs of dynamic LVOT obstruction.	Dynamic LVOT obstruction; mitral regurgitation; diastolic LV dysfunction.
Tetralogy of Fallot	Large, overriding aorta, VSD, subvalvular or valvular pulmonic stenosis.	High-velocity flow in RVOT and/or across pulmonic valve; bidirectional flow across VSD.

Congenital Abnormalities of the Aorta

Aortic Coarctation

A congenital narrowing in the proximal descending thoracic aorta most often is located just upstream from the entry site of the ductus arteriosus. Less often, postductal coarctation is seen. The coarctation may be relatively discrete, with involvement of only a short segment of the aorta, or may be a long, tubular narrowing. Imaging of the coarctation site is difficult from transthoracic or suprasternal notch windows in adults. From the suprasternal notch approach, the descending thoracic aorta has a tapering appearance, even in normal individuals, due to the oblique tomographic view of the descending aorta obtained as the descending aorta leaves the image plane. Adults with prior

FIGURE 16–5. 2D parasternal long-axis view *(top left)* of the same patent as in Figure 16–2 showing the transposed great vessels. Color flow imaging *(bottom left)* shows an eccentric jet with proximal acceleration across the stenotic bicuspid pulmonic valve. Note the proximal isovelocity surface area. Continuous-wave Doppler from a high right parasternal position *(top right)* shows a maximum velocity of 5.6 m/s consistent with a maximum pulmonic stenosis (PS) pressure gradient of 125 mmHg. (See Color Plate 18, p. 386.)

surgical repair of a coarctation may present with restenosis, depending on the specific surgical procedure used and the patient's age at the time of repair. For both operated and unoperated coarctations, transesophageal imaging with a long-axis view of the descending aorta may be helpful.

Doppler examination shows an increased velocity across the coarctation and, if the obstruction is severe, persistent antegrade flow into diastole (Fig. 16–6). If elevated, the proximal velocity should be included in the Bernoulli equation for pressure gradient estimation. The jet direction in an unoperated coarctation may be very eccentric, so it rarely is possible to achieve a parallel alignment between the ultra-

sound beam and jet direction, leading to underestimation of the severity of obstruction. In restenosis of a previously operated coarctation, the jet orientation tends to be more symmetrical, and a parallel intercept angle with correct estimation of the pressure gradient is more likely. In either case, other clinical methods for assessing severity of the coarctation are available (e.g., upper versus lower extremity blood pressure).

Marfan's Syndrome

Marfan's syndrome is inherited in an autosomal dominant pattern with variable penetrance. It is characterized by a specific, but variable, gene defect coding for fibrillin, a com-

Aortic Coarctation

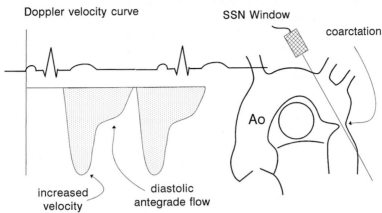

FIGURE 16–6. Aortic coarctation. From a suprasternal notch (SSN) window, continuous-wave Doppler of the coarctation shows an increased velocity in systole with persistent antegrade flow into diastole. Imaging of the coarctation often is suboptimal in adults.

ponent of microfibrils (a key structure in elastic fibers), resulting in musculoskeletal, ocular, and cardiovascular manifestations.

Cardiovascular abnormalities of Marfan's syndrome include dilation, aneurysm formation, and rupture of peripheral arteries, an abnormally redundant anterior mitral valve leaflet, and most important, dilation and dissection of the aortic root. Echocardiography may be helpful in confirming or excluding a diagnosis of Marfan's syndrome in patients with a suspected diagnosis. Examination also is indicated to screen first-degree relatives of an affected individual.

Characteristic echocardiographic findings include dilation of the aortic annulus, aortic root, sinuses of Valsalva, and ascending aorta with loss of a clearly defined sinotubular junction (see Figs. 15–1, 15–5, and 15–6). Aortic annular dilation results in aortic regurgitation and consequent left ventricular volume overload. Aortic dissection occurs frequently and can occur even when aortic dilation is not severe. With an aortic root diameter of more than 50 to 55 mm, the risk of spontaneous rupture is high, so many clinicians recommend periodic echocardiographic examination with prophylactic aortic root replacement with a valved aortic conduit when ascending aortic diameter exceeds this limit (see Fig. 15–30).

Sinus of Valsalva Aneurysm

A congenital aneurysm of the aortic sinuses of Valsalva appears as a thin, dilated area that projects into adjacent cardiac structures, often with a fistulous communication depending on which sinus is involved. On 2D imaging, a con-

genital aneurysm often has a "wind sock" appearance with a long, convoluted, mobile sac of tissue extending from the aortic sinus into adjacent cardiac structures (see Fig. 15–3). This appearance contrasts with the more symmetrical dilation seen in aneurysms due to endocarditis. An aneurysm of the noncoronary sinus projects into the right atrium, the left coronary cusp into the left atrium, and the right coronary cusp into the right ventricular outflow tract. If a fistula is present, pulsed and color Doppler flow imaging demonstrate a left-to-right shunt with a flow disturbance in the receiving chamber. Continuous-wave Doppler shows a high-velocity systolic and diastolic flow signal.

Coronary Arteriovenous Fistula

A coronary arteriovenous fistula is a rare congenital anomaly that may present in young adults as a continuous murmur. Abnormal communication from a coronary artery to the coronary sinus or right atrium has been described. A coronary arteriovenous fistula is recognized echocardiographically as an abnormal area of dilation with diastolic or continuous flow plus a flow disturbance at the site of entry into the cardiac chamber (Fig. 16–7).

Other coronary artery abnormalities may be diagnosed on echocardiography, particularly when transthoracic or transesophageal images are of high quality, allowing identification of the proximal coronary arteries, such as the origin of the circumflex coronary artery from the right sinus of Valsalva, the origin of the right coronary artery from the left sinus of Valsalva, or the origin of the left main coronary from the

right sinus of Valsalva. An anomalous coronary artery arising from the pulmonary artery rarely is diagnosed initially in adulthood because the resulting myocardial ischemia leads to significant clinical manifestations at a younger age.

Congenital Regurgitant Lesions

Ebstein's Anomaly of the Tricuspid Valve

Ebstein's anomaly is characterized by adherence of the basal segments of one (most often the septal) or more of the leaflets of the tricuspid valve to the right ventricular endocardium, resulting in the appearance of apical displacement of the tricuspid valve attachment (Fig.

16–8). In Ebstein's anomaly, the distance from the apex to the tricuspid versus mitral annulus exceeds the normal 10-mm difference. In severe cases, the tricuspid valve may be displaced nearly to the right ventricular apex. In addition, the tricuspid valve leaflets are thickened and malformed. Functionally, tricuspid regurgitation nearly always is present and may be severe. Typically, there is no antegrade obstruction to right ventricular diastolic filling (Fig. 16–9).

Owing to the apical displacement of the tricuspid leaflet insertion, a portion of the anatomic right ventricle physiologically serves as part of the right atrium. This "atrialized" ventricle adds to the appearance of right atrial en-

FIGURE 16–7. Coronary arteriovenous fistula from the left main coronary artery to the right atrium in a 20-year-old woman with a continuous murmur on auscultation. Transthoracic echocardiography showed an abnormal flow pattern in the right atrium. Transesophageal imaging showed a dilated left main coronary artery *(above, left)* with a tortuous channel *(above, right)* leading to an entrance in the right atrium *(below, left)*. Color flow imaging shows disturbed systolic and diastolic flow in the fistula *(below, right)*. (See Color Plate 18, p. 386.)

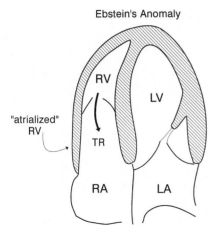

Ebstein's Anomaly

FIGURE 16–8. Schematic diagram of Ebstein's anomaly showing apical displacement of the tricuspid valve, and "atrialization" of the base of the right ventricle. Tricuspid regurgitation with right ventricular and right atrial enlargement typically is present.

FIGURE 16–9. Apical four-chamber view of a 52-year-old man with Ebstein's anomaly showing the apically displaced tricuspid valve *(arrow)*, compared to the tricuspid annulus *(open arrows)*, and right ventricular and right atrial enlargement. Color flow imaging showed severe tricuspid regurgitation.

largement, which is augmented by chronic atrial volume overload from tricuspid regurgitation. Ebstein's anomaly may be seen as an isolated anatomic defect or may be associated with an aberrant atrioventricular conduction bypass tract (Wolff-Parkinson-White syndrome), an atrial septal defect, or other congenital anomalies (e.g., ventricular inversion). Ebstein's

anomaly of the anatomic tricuspid valve in a patient with ventricular inversion results in systemic atrioventricular valve regurgitation and chronic volume overload of the systemic ventricle.

Myxomatous Mitral Valve Disease

Like a bicuspid aortic valve, myxomatous mitral valve disease may be silent clinically until late in life, when progressive leaflet changes result in significant mitral regurgitation and symptom onset. The thickened, redundant mitral valve leaflets of myxomatous disease may result in slowly increasing severity of chronic mitral regurgitation with progressive volume overload of the left ventricle and atrium. Alternatively, chordal rupture can result in acute mitral regurgitation with abrupt symptom onset. Myxomatous involvement of tricuspid and, less often, aortic valves also may be present. Myxomatous mitral valve disease is discussed in detail in Chapter 11.

Atrial Septal Defects

Anatomy

There are three basic anatomic types of atrial septal defect (Fig. 16–10). The most common is a *secundum* defect, in which the central section of the atrial septum (the fossa ovalis) is absent due to failure of the secundum atrial septum to cover the foramen secundum during development.

A *primum* atrial septal defect is absence of the section of the interatrial septum adjacent to the central fibrous body. Developmentally, there is abnormal formation of the septum primum with failure of closure of the foramen primum. Primum defects often are associated with abnormalities of the atrioventricular valves, especially a cleft anterior mitral leaflet. A cleft anterior leaflet can be visualized in parasternal short-axis and long-axis views, demonstrating the cleft and differing motion of the medial and lateral segments of the anterior leaflet (Fig. 16–11). In the long-axis view, lateral to medial angulation of the image plane shows the differing patterns of leaflet motion. The cleft mitral valve may be competent if adequate apposition of the edges of the cleft occurs in systole or may result in mitral regurgitation if closure is functionally inadequate. In a more severe developmental abnormality—atrioventricular canal defect—the entire central fibrous body is absent, resulting in a primum atrial septal defect, a ventricular septal defect, and abnormalities of the atrioventricular valves.

FIGURE 16–10. Schematic of primum, secundum, and sinus venosus atrial septal defects (ASDs). A secundum atrial septal defect is seen in the midsection of the atrial septum with prominent left-to-right flow on color imaging *(stippled area)*. Paradoxical septal motion and right ventricular and right atrial enlargement are present when the shunt is significant. A primum atrial septal defect is located near the atrioventricular connection and may be associated with abnormalities of the atrioventricular valves. A sinus venosus atrial septal defect is located at the base. Imaging may be difficult on transthoracic views but sometimes can be demonstrated from a subcostal approach.

FIGURE 16–11. Cleft anterior mitral valve leaflet seen in a parasternal short-axis view *(above)*. Discontinuity of the anterior leaflet is seen *(arrow)*. On color flow imaging in a long-axis view *(below)*, an eccentric regurgitant jet with proximal acceleration is present. (See Color Plate 18, p. 386.)

The third type of atrial septal defect is the *sinus venosus* defect. This abnormal communication between right and left atrium is located near the junction of either the superior or inferior vena cava and the right atrium. Developmentally, it is related to abnormal fusion between the embryologic sinus venosus and the atrium. A sinus venosus defect may be associated with partial anomalous pulmonary venous return. Partial anomalous pulmonary venous return also may be seen as an isolated defect and may not present until adulthood. The anomalous veins can drain directly into the right atrium or into the superior or inferior vena cava.

Two-Dimensional Imaging

Two-dimensional imaging of an atrial septal defect is most reliable from a subcostal approach so that the ultrasound beam is perpendicular to the plane of the interatrial septum. From apical or parasternal windows, apparent loss of signal from the atrial septum may be due to a parallel alignment between the ultrasound beam and the structures of interest (i.e., no ultrasound is reflected back to the transducer).

Secundum atrial septal defects are seen in the central portion of the atrial septum (Fig.

16–12), and primum defects (Fig. 16–13) are seen adjacent to the annuli of the atrioventricular valves. Imaging of a sinus venosus defect may not be possible on a transthoracic study. However, because the defect is located in the superior and posterior aspects of the interatrial septum, a subcostal approach can visualize the defect in some patients. Transthoracic 2D echocardiography from a subcostal approach has a sensitivity of 89% for detection of a secundum atrial septal defect and 100% for a primum defect but only 44% for a sinus venosus defect. Sinus venosus defects are well visualized from the transesophageal approach (Figs. 16–14 to 16–16).

If an atrial septal defect is associated with a significant left-to-right shunt (Fig. 16–17), right atrial enlargement, right ventricular enlargement, and paradoxical septal motion consistent with right-sided volume overload (Fig. 16–18) are uniformly present. In fact, evidence for right-sided heart volume overload often is the first abnormality noted during the echocardiographic examination. When evidence for right-sided heart volume overload is present in the absence of a visualized atrial septal defect or other definable cause for volume overload (e.g., tricuspid regurgitation), transesophageal imaging should be performed to evaluate for the possibility of a sinus venosus defect or partial anomalous pulmonary venous return.

Doppler Examination

Color flow imaging often allows reliable identification of the atrial septal defect flow based on the spatial distribution of the flow disturbance from the left to right atrium. However, multiple tomographic image planes are needed for correct identification of the origin of the flow signal. In some cases, the diastolic/systolic low-velocity flow signal across the atrial septal defect can be difficult to distinguish from other venous flow signals in the right atrium. Care must be taken to avoid mistaking superior vena cava flow into the right atrium, which often streams along the interatrial septum, for atrial septal defect flow. This appearance can be particularly misleading in high-volume flow states, such as pregnancy. Occasionally, a tricuspid regurgitant jet directed along the interatrial septum results in a confusing flow pattern, as well.

The subcostal window is optimal for color imaging of flow across the atrial septal defect, since the direction of flow is parallel to the ultrasound beam. Color flow imaging from other windows (including parasternal and apical) also is helpful, since it is the location and timing of the flow disturbance—rather than the absolute velocity of flow—that are diagnostic of the defect in the atrial septum. Color flow imaging shows a broad flowstream from left to right atrium in both diastole and systole with a more prominent diastolic component. With large shunts, the flow across the atrial septum extends across the open tricuspid valve into the right ventricle in diastole. Proximal flow acceleration on the left atrial side of the septum usually is evident.

Transesophageal echocardiography is helpful for further definition of the site and size of an atrial septal defect if transthoracic images are suboptimal. In addition, transesophageal imaging usually is needed when a sinus venosus defect or partial anomalous pulmonary venous return is suspected. Using a biplane or multiplane approach, 2D and color flow imaging will identify the abnormal defect and flow communication in the superior aspect of the posterior portion of the interatrial septum. Small secundum defects also are most likely to be detected from a transesophageal approach.

The severity of left-to-right shunting across the atrial septal defect can be measured as described above (Fig. 16–19).

FIGURE 16–12. Secundum atrial septal defect demonstrates a large color flow area across the central region of the atrial septum (in an apical four-chamber view) into an enlarged right atrium and ventricle. (See Color Plate 18, p. 386.)

FIGURE 16–13. Ostium primum atrial septal defect *(above)* in a 25-year-old woman with trisomy 21 and a complete atrioventricular canal defect seen in a subcostal four-chamber view *(top).* Note the intact superior aspect of the atrial septum and the large atrial septal defect *(between arrows).* There are two separate atrioventricular valves with mild regurgitation of both valves *(middle).* Schematic of an atrioventricular canal defect in a four-chamber view *(bottom).* (See Color Plate 19, p. 386.)

Contrast Echo

In a patient with a primum or secundum atrial septal defect, peripheral venous injection of echo contrast material shows passage of microbubbles across the interatrial septum, even when the shunt is predominantly left to right in direction. The explanation for this observation is that right atrial pressure transiently and briefly exceeds left atrial pressure, allowing passage of a small volume of blood from right to left. This small volume can be visualized when contrast echoes from the right atrium appear in the left atrium. Dense contrast in the right atrium also allows visualization of a "negative" contrast jet across the atrial septal defect; that is, the blood flow from the left atrium into the right atrium will appear as an area with no echo contrast.

Contrast echo studies are rarely needed for diagnosis of an atrial septal defect when typical 2D echo, Doppler, and color flow imaging findings are present. The principle of using echo contrast to identify very small degrees of right-to-left shunting can be used to detect a patent foramen ovale as a potential etiology for a systemic embolic event (see Chap. 14).

After Atrial Septal Defect Repair

With a prior atrial septal defect repair, there may be mild residual right ventricular and right atrial dilatation. More than mild persistent dilation should prompt a search for a residual defect or a leak around the patch repair.

Ventricular Septal Defects

Anatomy

There are four anatomically different types of ventricular septal defects (Fig. 16–20). The most common type is a membranous defect located in the region of the membranous septum immediately inferomedial to the aortic valve and lateral to the septal leaflet of the tricuspid valve. Small membranous ventricular septal defects may close spontaneously during childhood by approximation of the tricuspid valve septal leaflet across the defect. A completely closed defect may be undetectable in adulthood, or a residual anatomic abnormality—a ventricular septal aneurysm—may be visualized at the closure site without evidence of blood flow from the left to the right ventricle. Incom-plete closure leads to a persistent, albeit smaller, ventricular septal defect, which may be difficult to distinguish from septal aneurysm on 2D imaging. However, color flow and continuous-wave Doppler show typical evidence for an abnormal flow communication between the left and right ventricle even when the defect is small.

Muscular ventricular septal defects occur at any location in the muscular portion of the septum and may be multiple. When small, imaging the defect may not be possible with a tomographic imaging technique (such as echocardiography) even when multiple image planes are examined. Again, Doppler data are diagnostic in this situation.

Inlet ventricular septal defects are the result of failure of complete formation of the central

FIGURE 16–14. Transesophageal echocardiographic demonstration of an atrial septal defect in a 53-year-old woman. In a standard four-chamber view, the septum appears intact *(top left)*. However, with slight anterior angulation, a defect is seen adjacent to the aortic root *(top right)* with color flow showing left-to-right flow across the defect *(right)*. (See Color Plate 19, p. 386.)

fibrous body. This defect is located inferior to the aortic valve plane, adjacent to the mitral and tricuspid valve annuli. Inlet defects often are associated with other anomalies of the central fibrous body such as a primum atrial septal defect, atrioventricular valve abnormalities, or a complete atrioventricular canal defect.

Supracristal ventricular septal defects are located in the right ventricular outflow portion of the septum (above the crista ventricularis), lateral and just inferior to the aortic valve. These defects are rarely initially diagnosed in adulthood.

Two-Dimensional Echocardiographic Findings

As noted, while large defects may easily be imaged with 2D echocardiography, small defects may be very difficult to demonstrate. Membranous defects are imaged best in a parasternal long-axis view angulated slightly medially (Fig. 16–21). In the short-axis view just below the aortic valve level, the defect is seen in a 10-o'clock position inferior to the right coronary cusp of the aortic valve and adjacent to the septal leaflet of the tricuspid valve. In this view, a supracristal defect is located at the 2-o'clock position, inferior to the left coronary leaflet of the aortic valve and adjacent to the pulmonic valve. A supracristal defect is imaged in the long-axis plane by lateral angulation of the transducer from the standard long-axis view. Muscular ventricular septal defects may be seen in sequential basal-to-apical short-axis views of the left ventricle or in the apical

four-chamber view. Inlet defects are best imaged in the apical four-chamber view or from the parasternal window in a short-axis view at the mitral valve level.

With a ventricular septal defect and a left-to-right shunt, dilation of the left ventricle and left atrium is seen due to volume overload of these chambers. Right ventricular size usually is normal, since the systolic flow across the defect is ejected directly into the pulmonary artery. Left ventricular systolic function typically is preserved because the shunt flow is ejected into the low-impedance pulmonary vascular bed. With large shunts, pulmonary vascular hypertension

FIGURE 16–16. In the same patient as in Figure 16–15, the region of the atrial septum just inferior to the superior vena cava is absent *(above)*, and color flow demonstrates left-to-right flow across this defect *(below)*. (See Color Plate 19, p. 386.)

FIGURE 16–15. Sinus venosus atrial septal defect in a 74-year-old man. Although the transesophageal four-chamber view shows marked volume overload of the right side of the heart, the atrial septum appears intact in this view.

FIGURE 16–18. Paradoxical septal motion (note anterior motion in systole) and right ventricular enlargement on M-mode in a 21-year-old women with an atrial septal defect.

FIGURE 16–17. Right ventricular enlargement due to a secundum atrial septal defect in a 65-year-old woman with new-onset atrial fibrillation seen in a parasternal short-axis view in diastole *(above)* and in systole *(below)*.

supervenes, resulting in Eisenmenger's physiology with right ventricular hypertrophy and dilation (Fig. 16–22).

Doppler Findings

Pulsed or color Doppler flow imaging shows a flow disturbance on the right side of the ventricular septum (with a left-to-right shunt). The presence and location of this flow disturbance are diagnostic even in the absence of a demonstrable defect on 2D imaging. The flow disturbance is detectable in the defect itself with proximal acceleration on the left side of the septum, immediately adjacent to the defect. Conventional pulsed Doppler ultrasound has a sensitivity of 90% and a specificity of 98% for detection of a ventricular septal defect. The sensitivity of color flow imaging probably is even greater.

Continuous-wave Doppler ultrasound shows a high-velocity left-to-right signal, with the shape of the velocity curve similar to that of mitral regurgitation, as determined by the instantaneous left ventricular to right ventricular pressure differences. In diastole, left-to-right shunting persists at a lower velocity (proportional to the diastolic left ventricular to right ventricular pressure differences) with the shape of the time-velocity curve similar to that of mitral stenosis. Brief reversal of flow may be, but is not always, present during isovolumic relaxation and contraction phases. Both the diastolic flow and brief reversals during the isovolumic periods are low velocity and thus may not be appreciated except at low high-pass filter settings on the Doppler spectral recording. Because this reversal of flow may not occur, intravenous injection of echo contrast material is less sensitive for detection of an intracardiac shunt at the ventricular level than at the atrial level.

Calculation of a pulmonic to systemic shunt ratio rarely is needed in adults with ventricular septal defects because either (1) the defect is small with a small volume of left-to-right shunt or (2) a large defect with a significant shunt in childhood now has resulted in Eisenmenger's physiology with equalization of right and left ventricular pressures. If calculation of a shunt ratio is needed, systemic flow can be calculated in the aorta, and pulmonary flow can be calculated either in the pulmonary artery (if not disturbed by the septal defect flow) or across the mitral valve (pulmonary venous return).

Patent Ductus Arteriosus

A patent ductus arteriosus often is difficult to image in adults because of limited acoustic access. However, the chronic volume overload of the left atrium and left ventricle is manifested as dilation of these chambers. Left-to-right flow through the ductus can be detected with either conventional pulsed or color Doppler flow imaging using both parasternal short-axis and right ventricular outflow views of the pulmonary artery (Figs. 16–23 and 16–24). Dia-

stolic ductal flow in the pulmonary artery, typically seen along the lateral wall of this vessel, has a sensitivity of 96% and specificity of 100% for diagnosis of a patent ductus arteriosus. Recording of flow in the descending aorta, from a suprasternal notch approach, shows holodiastolic flow reversal due to antegrade flow into the ductus in diastole. This finding must be distinguished from diastolic flow reversal due to aortic regurgitation, since the two conditions may coexist in adult patients.

Ventricular Inversion

Congenitally corrected transposition of the great arteries (TGA) is more clearly designated "ventricular inversion," since the anatomic

FIGURE 16–19. In a 23-year-old man with an atrial septum defect (shown in Fig. 16–12), systemic flow (Q_s) is calculated from the left ventricular outflow tract diameter (2 cm) and Doppler flow curve (VTI 17.3 cm) *(left)*, while pulmonary blood flow is calculated from the pulmonary artery diameter (2.8 cm) and Doppler flow curve (VTI 25.1 cm) *(right)*. In this example, Q_s is 54 ml, Q_v is 154, with a $Q_p:Q_s$ of 2.9:1.

FIGURE 16–20. Schematic of types of ventricular septal defects (VSDs). A membranous VSD is seen in a medially angulated parasternal long-axis view, immediately adjacent to the aortic valve. A supracristal VSD is seen well in a short-axis view just below the aortic valve with flow from the left ventricular outflow tract (LVOT) into the outflow region of the right ventricle. A muscular VSD can be located anywhere in the muscular portion of the ventricular septum and may be multiple. An inlet VSD is seen in the apical four-chamber view and may be associated with an atrioventricular canal defect.

right ventricle serves as the systemic ventricle, and the anatomic left ventricle serves as the venous ventricle. Physiologically, the pathway of venous and systemic blood flow is normal in uncomplicated ventricular inversion (Fig. 16–25). Systemic venous blood returns to the right atrium, crosses the mitral valve into an anatomic left ventricle, and then is ejected into the pulmonary artery. Pulmonary venous return to the left atrium crosses the tricuspid valve into an anatomic right ventricle and then is ejected into the aorta. In the absence of associated defects, the diagnosis may be made "incidentally" in adulthood (Fig 16–26). However, associated defects are common, including ventricular septal defects, pulmonic stenosis, complete heart block, and Ebstein's anomaly of the "inverted" tricuspid valve. Dilation, and eventual systolic dysfunction, of the systemic ventricle is common, although it is unclear whether this is due to the anatomy of the right ventricle being less suited to performing as the systemic ventricle, to inadequate coronary blood flow via the right coronary artery, or to associated systemic atrioventricular valve regurgitation.

On echocardiographic examination, ventricular inversion is recognized by identifying the anatomic ventricles in a side-by-side orientation (see Table 16–2) and demonstrating the pathway of blood flow. Associated defects have 2D echo and Doppler findings as described for each abnormality. In addition, the position of the great vessels is abnormal, with the two semilunar valves lying in the same image plane—best seen in parasternal short-axis views—and with the great vessels parallel to each other—best seen in parasternal long-axis views. Typically, the aortic annulus is anterior and to the left of the pulmonic valve. Ventricular inversion also is associated with dextroversion (apex points toward the right), which makes the echocardiographic examination technically more difficult because the cardiac structures lie directly behind the sternum, limiting acoustic access.

"Incidental" Congenital Anomalies

A few congenital anomalies have no known adverse clinical effects but are important in that, if not recognized, they can be mistaken for pathologic conditions and prompt other (possibly harmful) diagnostic tests. A *persistent left superior vena cava* is seen in a small percentage (0.3% to 0.5%) of otherwise normal individuals and in a higher percentage (3% to 10%) of patients with other congenital heart abnormalities. Since this vein drains into the coronary sinus, dilation of the coronary sinus is seen on parasternal long- and short-axis views and on an apical four-chamber view angulated posteriorly (see Fig. 14–6). This latter view nicely illustrates the entry of the dilated coronary sinus into the right atrium. The diagnosis can be confirmed (if questions remain) by injection of echo contrast material into the left arm, which will first opacify the coronary sinus and then the right atrium. Injection of echo contrast material into the right arm will opacify only the right atrium. The dilated coronary sinus can protrude into the left atrium, particularly on the parasternal long-axis view, sometimes being mistaken for a left atrial mass.

Idiopathic dilation of the pulmonary artery is another uncommon benign abnormality. The diagnosis is made when the pulmonary artery is enlarged but there is no evidence of pulmonic stenosis (which might result in poststenotic dilation) or other congenital abnormalities.

A *Chiari network* is a prominent inferior vena cava valve with fibrous extensions to the crista terminalis and/or coronary sinus valve seen in 2% of patients undergoing transesophageal echocardiography. These fibrous connections are fenestrated and lax, forming a "network" which shows rapid chaotic motion during the cardiac cycle. On 2D imaging, the appearance of small, echogenic targets moving rapidly in the right atrium suggests this diagnosis. Although the Chiari network itself is be-

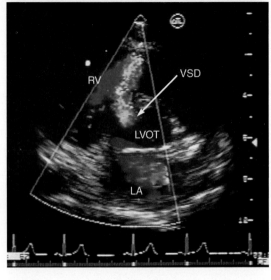

FIGURE 16–21. Small membranous ventricular septal defect with associated ventricular septal aneurysm *(arrow)* seen in a medially angulated parasternal long-axis view *(top left)* in a 21-year-old man. In short axis, a deformity *(arrows)* just inferior to the right coronary sinus of Valsalva is seen *(top right)*. Color flow demonstrates left-to-right flow across this defect *(right)*. (See Color Plate 19, p. 386.)

FIGURE 16–22. Large ventricular septal defect *(between arrows)* in a 32-year-old woman with Eisenmenger's physiology seen on a transesophageal four-chamber view *(top left)*. Severe right ventricular hypertrophy is present, and color flow *(bottom left)* shows bidirectional flow across the defect due to equalization of right and left ventricular pressures. Continuous-wave Doppler *(right)* of the tricuspid regurgitant jet shows a maximum velocity of 4.6 m/s, confirming that right ventricular pressure is equal to systemic pressure. (See Color Plate 19, p. 386.)

FIGURE 16–23. Schematic of a patent ductus arteriosus. Flow *(stippled area* and *arrow)* from the descending aorta into the pulmonary artery often streams along the lateral wall of the pulmonary artery on color flow imaging. Pulsed or continuous-wave Doppler shows holodiastolic flow reversal in the pulmonary artery. Systolic flow typically is abnormal as well, since aortic pressure exceeds pulmonary artery pressure throughout the cardiac cycle (giving rise to a continuous murmur on auscultation).

FIGURE 16–24. Patent ductus arteriosus (PDA) in a 22-year-old asymptomatic man. The parasternal short-axis view shows the pulmonary artery and descending aorta (DA) *(top left)*. Color flow *(bottom left)* and pulsed Doppler *(right)* images show characteristic diastolic flow reversal extending into systole *(arrows)* and disturbed systolic flow in the pulmonary artery. (See Color Plate 20, p. 386.)

nign, there is a high likelihood of an associated atrial septal aneurysm or patent foramen ovale.

A *left ventricular web* or *chord* is a bright linear band which traverses the ventricular chamber but is attached to the endocardium at both ends. It appears to represent an "aberrant" mitral valve chordae or a prominent trabeculation of the ventricle. Occasionally, this benign structure is mistaken for the edge of an apical thrombus.

Other Congenital Cardiac Diseases Presenting in Adults

In addition to conditions considered under the category of congenital heart disease, other cardiac diseases in adults are congenital (or genetic) in origin but usually present in adult-

hood. For example, hypertrophic cardiomyopathy and Marfan's syndrome are inherited disorders (see Chap. 8 and 15). Other types of cardiomyopathy may show a familial pattern, suggesting a genetic component. As our knowledge of molecular cardiology expands, other "acquired" diseases may be found to be genetic in origin.

ADULT CONGENITAL HEART DISEASE WITH PRIOR SURGICAL PROCEDURES (Table 16–5)

Classification of Types of Procedures

Numerous palliative and corrective surgical treatments for congenital heart disease have been developed since the first closure of a patent ductus arteriosus in 1938. These procedures can be grouped in several categories, as indicated in Table 16–5. The approximate years during which each procedure was performed are shown to indicate which are likely to be encountered in a patient of a given age and to provide a historical explanation of why a patient may have had a particular procedure.

In conditions with low pulmonary blood flow, such as tetralogy of Fallot, transposition of the great arteries, pulmonary atresia, or tricuspid atresia, an intracardiac shunt is created to increase pulmonary blood flow. Shunts may be made from a systemic artery to a pulmonary artery (Blalock-Taussig, Potts, Waterston), from a systemic vein to the pulmonary artery (Glenn), or at the atrial level (Blalock-Hanlon or balloon atrial septostomy). In some cases these shunts are removed ("taken down") at the time of subsequent corrective surgery. Complications of surgical shunts include (1) inadequate pulmonary blood flow due to kinking or closure of the shunt, (2) excessive pulmonary blood flow resulting in pulmonary hypertension, and (3) thrombus formation.

Procedures to close congenital intracardiac shunts—atrial septal defects, ventricular septal defects, patient ductus arteriosus—are conceptually straightforward and may be performed by suturing the edges of the defect (primary closure) or by using a pericardial or synthetic patch. The most common long-term complication of a shunt closure is a residual shunt.

Pulmonary banding is a palliative procedure that creates functional pulmonary stenosis to reduce pulmonary blood flow and "protect" the pulmonary vasculature from irreversible pulmonary hypertension. It is performed in patients with a large left-to-right shunt if definitive repair is not possible or must be delayed. If the degree of banding is not adequate, pulmonary hypertension still may ensue. Distal migration of the band can result in unequal right versus left pulmonary artery obstruction.

Atrial baffle procedures for transposition of the great arteries are designed to redirect intraatrial flow so that systemic venous return goes to the pulmonary artery (via the anatomic mitral valve and left ventricle) and pulmonary venous return goes to the aorta (via the anatomic tricuspid valve and right ventricle). The 3D anatomy of these baffles is complex and may be difficult to demonstrate on a transthoracic study due to poor ultrasound penetration at that depth. A transesophageal approach improves image quality, but an experienced examiner and multiple tomographic

Ventricular Inversion

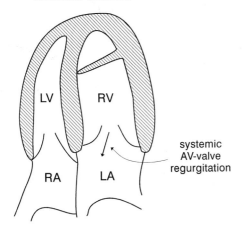

FIGURE 16–25. Schematic of ventricular inversion. With ventricular inversion (or "corrected" transposition of the great arteries), systemic venous blood returns to the right atrium, passes across the mitral valve into an anatomic left ventricle, and exits the left ventricle into the pulmonary artery. Pulmonary venous return into the left atrium is directed across the tricuspid valve into an anatomic right ventricle (with moderate band) and from there into the aorta. Common associated abnormalities are an Ebstein's-type malformation of the tricuspid valve resulting in systemic atrioventricular valve regurgitation, pulmonic stenosis, a ventricular septal defect, and complete heart block.

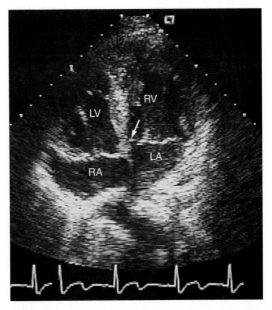

FIGURE 16–26. Apical four-chamber view in a patient with ventricular inversion in the standard display format in a 22-year-old man. The anatomic right ventricle (RV) is on the patient's left and serves as the systemic ventricle. Note the slightly more apical insertion of the tricuspid valve leaflets *(arrow)*.

TABLE 16–5	Common Operations for Congenital Heart Disease Seen in Surviving Adults			
Type	**Procedure**	**Description**	**Defects Treated**	**Years**
Shunts	Blalock-Taussig	Anastomosis of subclavian artery to PA (with or without modification)	Reduced pulmonary blood flow (TOF, TGA, pulmonary atresia, tricuspid atresia)	1945–present
		Conduit (subclavian remains intact)		
	Blalock-Hanlon	Surgical atrial septostomy (largely replaced by percutaneous blade-and-balloon septostomy)	TGA (early palliation), mitral atresia, complex congenital heart disease	1950–early 1980s (occasionally still performed)
	Rashkind balloon	Percutaneous atrial	TGA	1966–present
	Potts	Descending aorta to left PA	Alternate to Blalock	1946–mid-1960s
	Waterston	Ascending aorta to right PA	Alternate to Blalock	1962–present
	Glenn	SVC to divided right PA (bidirectional = SVC to right PA without isolation from left PA)	Tricuspid atresia, pulmonic atresia, constitutes a portion of a hemi-Fontan	1959–present (1985–present)
Closures	Atrial septal defect	Primary or patch closure	ASD with $Q_p{:}Q_s \geq 2{:}1$	1954–present
	Ventricular septal defect	Primary or patch closure	Isolated VSD or with other anomalies (TOF)	1955–present
	Patent ductus arteriosus	Ligation ± division of PDA (transcatheter technique 1981)	PDA	1938–present
	Endocardial cushion defect repair	Closure of ASD and VSD, repair of atrioventricular valve abnormalities (e.g., cleft mitral leaflet)		
PA banding		PA band to decrease PA flow and pressure	Large left-to-right shunts	1952–present
Atrial baffles	Mustard	Dacron or pericardial baffle directs systemic venous return to PA via LV, pulmonary venous return to aorta via RV	TGA (replaced by arterial switch procedures at many centers)	1964–present
	Senning	RA free wall and interatrial septal tissue used for similar baffle	TGA (replaced by arterial switch procedures at many centers)	1959–1964, 1980–present
Relief of stenosis	Aortic coarctation repair	Various procedures including end-to-end anastomosis, patch enlargement, Gore-Tex graft; balloon dilation for recoarctation	Aortic coarctation	1944–present Balloon dilation 1983–present
	Pulmonic valvotomy	Brock trans-RV approach; direct surgical repair; Balloon dilation	TOF, pulmonic stenosis	1948–1960s
	Aortic valvotomy	Direct surgical valvotomy or percutaneous balloon dilation	Congenital aortic stenosis	1960s–present
	Mitral repair	Open commissurotomy	Congenital mitral stenosis	1982–present
	Konno procedure	LVOT enlargement by creation of a VSD which is then patched, plus aortic valve replacement	LV outflow obstruction not amenable to valvotomy	1976–present

ASD = atrial septal defect, LVOT = left ventricular outflow tract, LV = left ventricle, PA = pulmonary artery, PDA = patent ductus arteriosus, Q_p = pulmonic volume flow rate, Q_s = systemic volume flow rate, RA = right atrium, RV = right ventricle, SVC = superior vena cava, TGA = transposition of the great arteries, TOF = tetralogy of Fallot, VSD = ventricular septal defect.

TABLE 16-5	Common Operations for Congenital Heart Disease Seen in Surviving Adults *Continued*		
Type	**Procedure**	**Description**	**Defects Treated**	**Years**
Great vessel switch	Jatene procedure	Switch of aortic root and PA trunk, coronaries transposed to neoaorta	TGA	1976 (Brazil) 1988–present
	Fontan procedure	Conduit from RA to PA with prosthetic conduit (± valve)	TGA, double-inlet ventricle with pulmonic stenosis, tricuspid atresia	1971–present
Conduits	Rastelli procedure	Valved conduit from RV to transected PA. LV to aorta via VSD and intraventricular patch	TGA + VSD + subvalvular pulmonic stenosis, truncus arteriosus, double-outlet RV	1968–present
	Damus-Kaye Stansel	Supravalvular anastomosis of aorta and PA (functions as aortopulmonary window) to relieve subvalvular stenosis	Irreparable subaortic obstruction with a double-inlet ventricle	1975–present
	Norwood procedure	Ascending aorta enlarged with pulmonary trunk; Fontan from RV to PA (two-stage procedure)	Aortic valve atresia, hypoplastic left heart	1983–present

planes are needed to fully assess the interatrial baffle. Late complications of this procedure include baffle obstruction, baffle leaks, systolic dysfunction of the systemic (anatomic right) ventricle, and arrhythmias. More recently, the great vessel switch procedure have been used to treat patients with transposition. Complications of this procedure are related to reimplantation of the coronary arteries and supravalvular great vessel obstruction at the anastomotic sites.

Procedures to relieve congenital stenotic lesions include aortic coarctation repair; pulmonic, aortic, or mitral valvotomy either with direct surgical inspection or with a percutaneous balloon; and the Konno procedure to relieve left ventricular outflow obstruction. A residual gradient may be present after these procedures, and valvular regurgitation may be induced.

More complex intracardiac repairs that use conduits (with or without valves) include (1) the Fontan procedure (right atrial to pulmonary artery), (2) the Rastelli procedure, (3) the Damus-Kaye-Stansel procedure, and (4) the Norwood procedure, as indicated in Table 16–5. Many patients with a prior Rastelli or Fontan procedure are now being seen as young adults (Figs. 16–27 and 16–28). Complications of the Rastelli procedure include subaortic obstruction in the left ventricular to aortic baffle, obstruction of the right-sided conduit, and residual ventricular septal defects. Evaluation of patients with a Fontan procedure

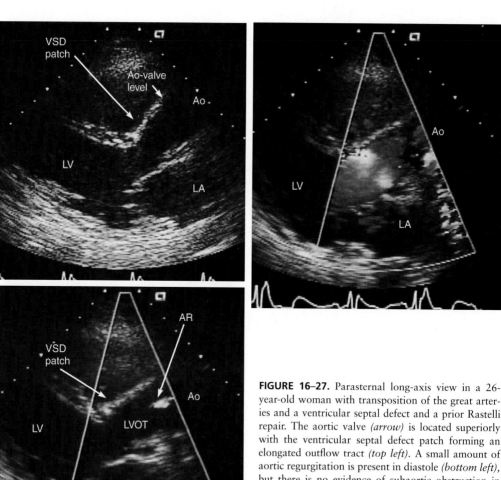

FIGURE 16–27. Parasternal long-axis view in a 26-year-old woman with transposition of the great arteries and a ventricular septal defect and a prior Rastelli repair. The aortic valve *(arrow)* is located superiorly with the ventricular septal defect patch forming an elongated outflow tract *(top left)*. A small amount of aortic regurgitation is present in diastole *(bottom left)*, but there is no evidence of subaortic obstruction in systole *(right)*. (See Color Plate 20, p. 386.)

FIGURE 16–28. In a 33-year-old asymptomatic woman with transposition of the great arteries and a prior Rastelli repair, transesophageal imaging shows severe calcification of the prosthetic valve *(arrow)* in the right ventricular to pulmonary artery conduit with a stenotic jet seen on color flow imaging *(top)* with a velocity of 4.2 m/s by continuous-wave Doppler recording *(bottom)*. (See Color Plate 20, p. 386.)

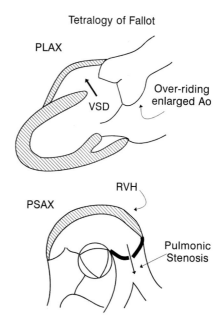

FIGURE 16–29. Schematic of tetralogy of Fallot. Tetralogy of Fallot is characterized by a large ventricular septal defect with an enlarged aorta that spans (or overrides) the defect, pulmonic stenosis (which may be subpulmonic or valvular), and compensatory right ventricular hypertrophy (RVH).

is complicated by the numerous variations of the surgical approach, which often require transesophageal imaging for visualization. Late complications of the Fontan procedure include baffle obstruction, interatrial shunts, and thrombus formation.

When patients with prior surgical procedures for congenital heart disease present for echocardiographic evaluation, more detailed references on congenital heart disease can be helpful in planning, performing, and interpreting the echocardiographic examination. Echocardiographers dealing with these patients should consult these sources (see Suggested Readings 1 to 8).

Tetralogy of Fallot

The three primary characteristics of tetralogy of Fallot are a membranous ventricular septal defect, a large aorta that is positioned across the ventricular septal defect ("overriding"), and right ventricular outflow obstruction that may be sub-, supra-, or valvular in location (Fig. 16–29). The fourth feature of this tetralogy is right ventricular hypertrophy secondary to outflow obstruction.

Adults with an untreated tetralogy of Fallot are rarely seen due to the high mortality of this condition without surgical intervention. In adults with a repaired tetralogy of Fallot, the ventricular septal defect patch is evident, the aortic root is enlarged, and some degree of residual right ventricular outflow obstruction may be present (Fig. 16–30).

Transposition of the Great Arteries

Adults with surgical treatment of TGA present for echocardiographic evaluation either for routine follow-up in the asymptomatic patient or for recurrent cardiac symptoms. Adults with a prior interatrial baffle procedure are most often seen given the more recent introduction of the arterial switch procedure (Fig. 16–31). Echocardiographic evaluation includes identification of the transposed great arteries, correct identification of the two ventricles, evaluation of the blood flow pathway, and evaluation of the intraatrial baffle with transthoracic and transesophageal echocardiography.

Tricuspid Atresia

Evaluation of the adult patient with tricuspid atresia includes assessment of the prior surgical procedures to increase pulmonary blood flow. A complete surgical history is very helpful in directing the echocardiographic examination since the exact location of the conduit and the use of a valved versus nonvalved conduit vary from patient to patient. Systemic arterial or venous shunts to the pulmonary artery may be difficult to demonstrate if image quality is suboptimal, in which case other tomographic imaging procedures or angiography may be needed. If a Fontan conduit or anastomosis

from the right atrium to pulmonary artery is present, it usually can be visualized anteromedially and superiorly to the right atrium (Fig. 16–32).

Transposition of the Great Arteries

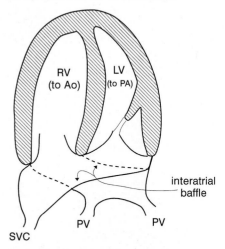

FIGURE 16–31. Schematic of interatrial baffle repair for transposition of the great arteries which directs systemic venous return to the anatomic left ventricle (and then to the pulmonary artery) and pulmonary venous return to the anatomic right ventricle (and then aorta). With this repair, the anatomic right ventricle serves as the systemic ventricle. Adequate visualization of the interatrial baffle usually requires transesophageal imaging in adults.

FIGURE 16–30. A 23-year-old woman with repaired tetralogy of Fallot. The overriding aorta and ventricular septal defect patch are seen in the parasternal long-axis view *(top)*. This patient has mild residual pulmonic stenosis (jet velocity 2.3 m/s) after a patch enlargement of the right ventricular outflow tract *(bottom)*.

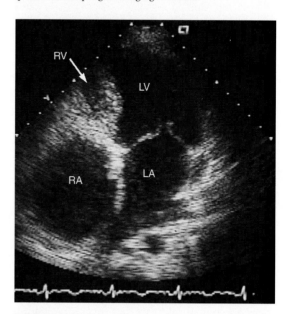

FIGURE 16–32. Tricuspid atresia in a 24-year-old woman with a previous Fontan conduit from the right atrium to pulmonary artery. The large right atrium, absent tricuspid valve, and small residual right ventricular chamber (connected to the left ventricle via a ventricular septal defect) are seen.

Truncus Arteriosus

A surgically treated patient with truncus arteriosus will have variable 2D echocardiographic findings depending on the anatomic type of truncus present and the specific repair performed. Again, obtaining a complete surgical history before performing the study is very helpful. The echocardiographic examination then is directed toward the specific clinical question, after demonstrating the basic anatomy and pathway of blood flow in the patient.

LIMITATIONS OF ECHOCARDIOGRAPHY/ ALTERNATE APPROACHES

Calculations of Shunt Ratios

Accurate calculation of shunt ratios by Doppler echocardiography depends on accurate stroke volume determinations at two intracardiac sites. Each of these stroke volume determinations can be affected by several factors, as discussed in Chapter 5. Specifically, both the mean spatial flow velocity and the cross-sectional area of flow must be measured correctly. Flow at each site is assumed to be laminar with a flat flow velocity profile. Furthermore, accuracy depends on a parallel intercept angle between the direction of blood flow and the ultrasound beam. The cross-sectional area of flow typically is assumed to be circular and is calculated from a 2D echo diameter measurement. Small errors in diameter measurement (which is squared in calculating a circular area) translate into large errors in stroke volume determinations. In adult patients, imaging of the diameter of the pulmonary artery often is difficult and thus is the major source of error in Doppler-derived shunt ratios.

Alternate methods for calculation of pulmonary to systemic shunt ratios include (1) cardiac catheterization with measurement of intracardiac oxygen saturations and total body oxygen consumption, and (2) first-pass radionuclide estimation from the early recirculation pattern of the time-activity curve.

Imaging (Table 16–6)

Two-dimensional transthoracic echocardiographic imaging in adult patients with congenital heart disease may be limited by poor acoustic access. Even when image quality is acceptable, evaluation of posterior structures may be limited by lateral resolution at the depth of interest. This can be problematic, particularly in the evaluation of posterior conduits, interatrial baffle repair procedures, sinus venosus atrial septal defects, or anomalous pulmonary venous return. Transesophageal echocardiography offers improved image quality, especially of posterior structures, and is a useful adjunct to transthoracic imaging in this patient population.

Evaluation of extracardiac anatomy also is difficult. This limits evaluation of the pulmonary artery branches, systemic arterial or venous shunts to the pulmonary artery, and abnormalities of the ascending aorta and aortic arch. Other tomographic imaging techniques are especially helpful in assessing the position of the cardiac structures in the chest and in evaluating mediastinal abnormalities not accessible by ultrasound. Both chest computed tomography and magnetic resonance imaging can be used, with the advantage of a wide field of view for both techniques. With magnetic resonance imaging, the data can be reformatted, in an orientation based on the long axis of the left ventricle, into standard long- and short-axis views, facilitating identification of abnormal structures.

Other limitations of echocardiography are due to the use of a tomographic approach. For example, coronary anatomy cannot be assessed adequately with tomographic techniques. Angiography, with injection of dye into the coronary arteries, followed by cine- or digital radiographic recording is needed. Another example of potential shortcomings of echocardiography is that multiple ventricular septal defects may be missed unless careful evaluation in numerous tomographic planes is performed. A silhouette technique, such as ventriculography from an angle where the septum forms one of the borders of the ventricular chamber, has a higher reliability for this diagnosis. Limitations of angiography include the risks of contrast dye injection and its cost and invasive nature. Recent improvements in 3D echocardiographic displays may soon provide a clinically useful approach to evaluation of complex congenital heart disease.

Intracardiac Hemodynamics

While the definitive method for assessment of intracardiac hemodynamics remains cardiac catheterization with direct pressure measurement, much indirect information on intracardiac hemodynamics can be derived from the continuous-wave Doppler signal. Pulmonary artery pressure can be approximated by evaluation of pulmonic regurgitation and/or the tricuspid regurgitant jet. Maximum and mean pressure gradients across stenotic valves can be measured accurately with Doppler techniques.

TABLE 16–6	Alternate Diagnostic Imaging Procedures in Congenital Heart Disease	
Diagnostic Test	**Strengths**	**Weaknesses**
Echocardiography (transthoracic, including Doppler)	Detailed 2D anatomy allowing identification of anatomic chambers, valves, and great vessels; blood flow pathway; structural abnormalities Assessment of stenotic and regurgitant lesions by Doppler Detection of intracardiac shunts Assessment of ventricular size and systolic function $Q_p:Q_s$ calculations Estimate of PA pressure Noninvasive, no discomfort	Poor acoustic access limits image quality in some individuals Definition of posterior structures is suboptimal $Q_p:Q_s$ calculation depends on accurate diameter measurements No direct measures of intracardiac pressures Cannot accurately calculate pulmonary vascular resistance
Transesophageal echocardiography	Excellent image quality, especially of posterior structures Detailed Doppler evaluation of pulmonary veins, interatrial septum atrioventricular valves is possible	Anterior cardiac structures now in far field of ultrasound image Apex may not be visualized Oblique image planes limit quantitative measurements of chamber size Some risk of procedure, plus discomfort to patient
Radionuclide ventriculography	Nongeometric accurate EF determination Detection and quantitation of intracardiac shunts using first-pass time-activity curve	EF less accurate with irregular rhythms (e.g., atrial fibrillation) With abnormal position of the ventricle, it may be difficult to "isolate" LV for accurate EF calculations Limited anatomic data No evaluation of valve function
Computed tomography	Detailed anatomic images if gated to cardiac cycle Excellent for posterior structures, extracardiac vascular abnormalities, and exact position of cardiac structures in the chest	Limited image quality if not "gated" to cardiac cycle May need intravenous contrast injection Radiation exposure Little physiologic data
MRI	Detailed anatomic images on gated cardiac cycle Excellent for posterior structures, extracardiac vascular abnormalities, and position related to chest wall Blood has intrinsic "contrast" using different MRI sequences Images can be realigned to cardiac major and minor axes Cine-MRI images allow assessment of ventricular function	Tomographic sections at different times in the cardiac cycle Still images provide little data on dynamic cardiac function Research on assessment of valve dysfunction with MRI is in progress Expensive, not portable
Cardiac catheterization	Direct measurement of intracardiac pressures Allows calculation of pulmonary vascular resistance Detection and quantitation of intracardiac shunts Assessment of ventricular size and systolic function Only method that adequately assesses coronary anatomy	Invasive (risks and discomfort) Expensive Requires contrast injection for visualization of structures

EF = ejection fraction, LV = left ventricle, MRI = magnetic resonance imaging, PA = pulmonary artery, Q_p = pulmonic volume flow rate, Q_s = systemic volume flow rate.

Inferences about the chronicity of regurgitation and the presence or absence of v waves can be made from the shape of the regurgitant velocity curve. Estimates of left ventricular end-diastolic pressure may be possible based on aortic regurgitant velocity at end-diastole, the pattern of left ventricular diastolic filling, or pulmonary venous flow patterns. However, invasive pressure measurements still are often needed for appropriate clinical decision making in adults with congenital heart disease. In particular, evaluation of pulmonary vascular resistance, which requires invasive data, is a key factor in patient management.

Integrating the Diagnostic Approach

Whichever diagnostic imaging procedure is performed first in an individual patient—be it echocardiography, catheterization, or a magnetic resonance imaging scan—the next step should be to consider the data acquired in terms of both the anatomic and physiologic diagnoses and the certainty that these diagnoses are correct. Then, the remaining important clinical questions should be formulated and the most appropriate study to answer those questions performed next. When this approach is used, the echocardiogram may be the initial test to assess cardiac anatomy and physiology or may be performed only to answer a specific clinical question.

SUGGESTED READING

1. Snider AR: General echocardiographic approach to the adult with suspected congenital heart disease. *In* Otto CM (ed): The Practice of Clinical Echocardiography. Philadelphia, WB Saunders, 1997, pp. 665–696.
   A detailed discussion of the echocardiographic approach to segmental analysis of the heart and a review of the echocardiographic features of frequently encountered complex congenital cardiac defects.

2. King ME: Echocardiographic evaluation of the adult with unoperated congenital heart disease. *In* Otto CM (ed): The Practice of Clinical Echocardiography. Philadelphia, WB Saunders, 1997, pp. 697–728.
   Advanced discussion of the echocardiographic evaluation of adults with congenital valvular abnormalities, obstructive outflow lesions, septal defects and shunt lesions, coronary fistulas, and complex congenital heart disease. Includes 31 illustrations and 135 references.

3. Child JS: Echocardiographic evaluation of the adult with postoperative congenital heart disease. *In* Otto CM (ed): The Practice of Clinical Echocardiography. Philadelphia, WB Saunders, 1997, pp. 729–752.
   Review of echocardiographic findings in adults with previous surgical procedures for congenital heart disease with an emphasis on expected findings and common complications. Topics include general postoperative issues, palliative procedures, corrective procedures for simple lesions (e.g., septal defects) and repair of complex malformations. More than 120 references.

4. Sahn DJ, Anderson F: Two-Dimensional Anatomy of the Heart. New York, John Wiley & Sons, 1982.
   Useful reference with comprehensive schematic drawings and echocardiographic images for each type of congenital heart disease.

5. Snider AR, Serwer GA, Ritter SB: Echocardiography in Pediatric Heart Disease (ed 2). St. Louis, Mosby, 1997.
   Detailed text with illustrations on the echocardiographic approach to congenital heart disease. Useful reference.

6. Roberts WC: Adult Congenital Heart Disease. Philadelphia, FA Davis, 1987.
   Textbook with chapters by experts in each area with excellent discussions of functional assessment and clinical syndromes seen in adults with congenital heart disease.

7. Perloff JK, Child JS: Congenital Heart Disease in Adults (ed 2). Philadelphia, WB Saunders, 1998.
   Comprehensive textbook detailed the survival patterns, medical and surgical therapy, and long-term residua and sequelae after surgical or percutaneous intervention.

8. Emmanouilides GC, Riemenschneider TA, Allen HA, Gutgesell HP (eds): Moss and Adams, Heart Disease in Infants, Children and Adolescents (Including the Fetus and Young Adult) (ed 5). Baltimore, Williams & Wilkins, 1995.
   Comprehensive detailed textbook of pediatric cardiology. Useful reference for descriptions of congenital abnormalities, clinical presentation and management, and surgical procedures.

9. McNamara DG: The adult with congenital heart disease. *Curr Probl Cardiol* 14:63–114, 1989.
   Excellent review with emphasis on problems unique to the adult with congenital heart disease, categories of cardiovascular dysfunction, and descriptions (with clear illustrations) of operations for palliative or definitive repair of congenital heart disease. 126 references.

10. Relier MD, McDonald RW, Gerlis LM, Thornburg KL: Cardiac embryology: Basic review and clinical correlations. *J Am Soc Echocardiogr* 4:519–531, 1991.
    Brief review of cardiac embryology with correlation with clinical syndromes of congenital heart disease.

11. Hagler DJ, Edwards WD, Seward JB, Tajik AJ: Standardized nomenclature of the ventricular septum and ventricular septal defects, with applications for two-dimensional echocardiography. *Mayo Clin Proc* 60: 741–752, 1985.
    Detailed description with illustrations of ventricular septal abnormalities and nomenclature.

12. Hausmann D, Daniel WG, Mugge A, et al: Value of transesophageal color Doppler echocardiography for detection of different types of atrial septal defect in adults. *J Am Soc Echocardiogr* 5:481–488, 1992.

In 121 adults with an atrial septal defect, all 6 ostium primum defects were diagnosed on transthoracic imaging (sensitivity 100%). Of the 97 secundum defects, 95% (54 of 57) of those >5 mm in diameter and 20% (8 of 40) of those <5 mm in diameter were detected on transthoracic imaging. All were detected on transesophageal study. A sinus venosus defect was diagnosed in only 9% (1 of 11) on transthoracic and 100% (11 of 11) on transesophageal imaging. Partial anomalous venous return was missed in all 12 cases on transthoracic imaging and correctly identified in 83% (10 of 12) on transesophageal study.

13. Moller JH, Anderson RC: 1000 consecutive children with a cardiac malformation with 26- to 37-year follow-up. *Am J Cardiol* 70:661–667, 1992.

    In 997 children with congenital heart disease diagnosed 30 to 40 years ago, 712 are alive, with 632 (89%) being asymptomatic without plans for further treatment.

14. Perloff JK (Conference Chairman): 22nd Bethesda Conference. Congenital heart disease after childhood: An expanding patient population. *J Am Coll Cardiol* 18:311–342, 1991.

    Series of articles describing the outcome, diagnosis, and management of adults with congenital heart disease.

15. O'Fallon WM, Weldman WH (eds): Long-term follow-up of congenital aortic stenosis, pulmonary stenosis, and ventricular septal defect: Report from the Second Joint Study on the Natural History of Congenital Heart Defects (NHS-2). *Circulation* 87(suppl 2):I1–I126, 1993.

    Reports of several long-term outcome studies of patients with congenital heart disease.

16. Lundstrom U, Bull C, Wyse RKH, Somerville J: The natural and "unnatural" history of congenitally corrected transposition. *Am J Cardiol* 65:1222–1229, 1990.

    In 111 patients with congenitally corrected transposition, only 9% had no associated anatomic abnormalities. The most common associated anomalies were a ventricular septal defect in 81%, pulmonary stenosis in 72% (valvular or subvalvular), tricuspid valve abnormalities in 33% (usually Ebstein's anomaly), atrial septal defect in 11%, and a double outlet right ventricle in 11%. The median age of survival was 20 years (range 1 to 58 years) with 46% having undergone intracardiac repair procedures.

17. Horvath KA, Burke RP, Collins JJ, Cohn LH: Surgical treatment of adult atrial septal defect: Early and long-term results. *J Am Coll Cardiol* 20:1156–1159, 1992.

    Surgical repair of secundum or sinus venosus atrial septal defects was performed in 166 adults (mean age 44 years with 35% ≥50 years old) with an operative mortality of only 1.2% and a 10-year survival rate of 94%. These results emphasize the importance of the echocardiographic recognition of atrial septal defects in adults without a previous diagnosis of congenital heart disease.

18. Driscoll DJ, Offord KP, Feldt RH et al: Five- to fifteen-year follow-up after Fontan operation. *Circulation* 85:469–496, 1992.

    The 10-year survival after the Fontan operation in 352 patients (mean age at surgery 11 years, range 1 to 42 years) was 60% with reoperations necessary in 29% of the study group. The primary congenital lesion was tricuspid atresia in 36%, and an univentricular heart in 64%. Detailed outcome measures in these patients including recurrent hospitalization, exercise capacity, arrhythmias, and functional class are reported.

19. Murphy JG, Gersh BJ, Mair DD, et al: Long-term outcome in patients undergoing surgical repair of tetralogy of Fallot. *N Engl J Med* 329:593–599, 1993.

    The 30-year actuarial survival rate for patients with a repaired tetralogy of Fallot was 90% of the expected survival rate with excellent functional status after surgery. Predictors of a poor outcome were older age (>12 years old) at surgical repair, a previous Waterston or Potts shunt procedure, and a higher postoperative ratio of right-to-left ventricular systolic pressure.

20. Hopkins WE, Waggoner AD: Right and left ventricular area and function determined by two-dimensional echocardiography in adults with the Eisenmenger syndrome from a variety of congenial anomalies. *Am J Cardiol* 72:90–94, 1993.

    Of 24 adults (age 19 to 45 years) with Eisenmenger's physiology, the 15 patients with a nonrestrictive ventricular septal defect had similar right and left ventricular sizes and preserved right ventricular systolic function. The nine patients without a ventricular septal defect (Eisenmenger's physiology due to patent ductus arteriosus or atrial septal defect), had severe right ventricular dilation and systolic dysfunction. These discordance patterns of ventricular response to differing shunt locations are reflected in the echocardiographic findings in adults with Eisenmenger's syndrome.

21. Celermajer DS, Bull C, Till JA, et al: Ebstein's anomaly: Presentation and outcome from fetus to adult. *J Am Coll Cardiol* 23:170–176, 1994.

    Of 220 cases of Ebstein's anomaly diagnosed over a 33-year period at 5 London hospitals, 23 (10%) initially presented in adulthood. Symptoms at presentation in these 23 patients were arrhythmias (44%), heart failure (26%), an incidental murmur (13%), or other (17%). Associated defects were uncommon (only 8%) in the adult patients. The severity of Ebstein's anomaly was graded using the four-chamber view at end-diastole to calculate the ratio of the area of the right atrium plus atrialized right ventricle compared with the functional right ventricle plus left heart. This severity scale, which ranged from a ratio <0.5 (mild) to ≥1.5 (severe), was a significant predictor of death. Other predictors included fetal presentation and right ventricular outflow tract obstruction.

Index

Note: Page numbers in *italics* refer to illustrations; page numbers followed by t refer to tables.

A

Abscess, paravalvular, 338–342, *338, 339, 342,* 344t, 353
Acceleration times, for left ventricular systolic function, 117, *117*
Accuracy, of test, 79–80, *80, 81*
Acoustic shadowing, in two-dimensional echocardiography, 12, *12,* 12t
Acoustic window, 30
Afterload, in ventricular systolic function, 101, 102, *102*
A-mode echocardiography, 9, *10*
Amplitude, of ultrasound wave, 3, *3*
Amyl nitrate inhalation, in hypertrophic cardiomyopathy evaluation, 194
Amyloidosis, left ventricular diastolic dysfunction in, 148–149
Aneurysm, left ventricular, after myocardial infarction, 175–177, *176*
  of aorta, 373
  of sinus of Valsalva, 374, *374,* 386, *388,* 402t, 405
  septal, interatrial, 368–369, *369*
  vs. pseudoaneurysm, 221, *221*
Angina, transthoracic echocardiography in, 86t
Angiography, contrast, for left ventricular systolic function, 118–119, *119*
  for right ventricular systolic function, 122
  in aortic dissection, *387*
  in myocardial infarction, 172, *173*
  in myocardial ischemia, 169
Angiosarcoma, atrial, 361, *361*
Annular dilation, aortic valve regurgitation and, 278
  tricuspid valve regurgitation and, 293
Aorta, 373–392
  abdominal, proximal, echocardiography of, 377, *377, 379, 379*
  aneurysm of, 373
  ascending, flow velocities of, 51t
    flow velocity of, 50t
    on transthoracic echocardiography, 34t
  atherosclerosis of, 374
  coarctation of, 402t, 403–404, *405*
    repair of, 420t
  contrast aortography of, 391
  descending, flow velocities of, on transthoracic Doppler echocardiography, 54
    holodiastolic flow reversal in, 282, *284*

Aorta *(Continued)*
  diameter of, 35t
    measurement of, 380, *380*
  dilation of, 373, *374,* 380, *380*
  dissection of, 373–374, *374, 379,* 380–386
    angiography of, *387*
    aortic regurgitation and, 278
    complications of, 381–382, 382t, *383*
    computed tomography of, *387*
    differential diagnosis of, 382–383
    false-positive echocardiography in, 383, *385*
    flap in, 383, *384*
    hematoma in, 383, *385*
    magnetic resonance imaging of, *387*
    residual flaps in, 387–389, *388*
    rupture of, 382
    transesophageal echocardiography of, 383–386, *384, 385*
    transthoracic echocardiography of, 88t, 380–383, *381,* 382t, *383*
  echocardiography of, 374–380
    aortic dilation on, 380
    aortic dissection on, 380–386, *381,* 382t, *383–385,* 386t
    aortic graft pseudoaneurysm on, 389, *389*
    atherosclerotic disease on, 390, *390*
    2D, 374–379, *375–379*
    Doppler, 376–377, *377,* 379–380
    limitations of, 391
    pleural effusion and, 377, *378*
    postoperative, 387–389, *388*
    preoperative, 387
    sinus of Valsalva aneurysm on, 386, *388*
    transesophageal, 378–380, *378, 379*
    transthoracic, 44, *45,* 374–378, *375–378*
  graft repair of, echocardiography of, 388–389, *388, 389*
  magnetic resonance imaging of, 391
  position of, 399
  thoracic, descending, echocardiography of, 377, *377, 378, 379, 379*
    flow velocities of, 51t
    on transthoracic echocardiography, 34t, 36–37, 43, 44, *45*
    distal, echocardiography of, 377, *377*
  transposition of, 399, *399,* 423–424, *424*
Aortic annular abscess, 338–339, *338, 339*
  rupture of, 339, *341*

Aortic arch, echocardiography of, 375–376, *376*, 378–379, *379*
  on transthoracic echocardiography, 34t, 44, *45*
Aortic leaflet coaptation point, on transthoracic M-mode recording, 46
Aortic regurgitant jet, velocity of, for left ventricular end-diastolic pressure estimate, 149
Aortic regurgitation, in aortic dissection, 381
Aortic root, abnormalities of, aortic regurgitation and, 278
  dilation of, in hypertensive heart disease, 202
    transthoracic echocardiography in, 87t
  motion of, in mitral valve regurgitation, 288, *289*
  on transthoracic echocardiography, 33, 43
Aortic stenosis, 232–238
  aortic jet velocity in, 242–243, 242t, *243*, 245, *245*, 247, *247*
  aortic regurgitation and, 244
  aortic valve index in, 239
  bicuspid, 233, *233, 234*
  calcific, 232–233, *233*
  case studies of, 248–249, *248, 249*
  congenital, 234
  continuity equation valve area in, 237–239, 240t, 241, *241*, 245
  diagnosis of, 89
  differential diagnosis of, 234–236, *235*, 235t
  echocardiography in, 86t, 232–241, *234–236*, 237t, *238, 239*, 240t, *241*
    aortic jet on, 242–243, 242t, *243*
    case studies of, 248–249, *248, 249*
    in asymptomatic disease, 246–247, *246, 247*
    in symptomatic disease, 244–246, *245*
    left ventricular outflow tract diameter on, 243
    left ventricular outflow tract velocity on, 243–244
    technical considerations in, 241–244, 242t
    with left ventricular systolic dysfunction, 247
    with systolic murmur, 247–248
  endocarditis and, 343
  fluid dynamics of, 230, *230, 231*
  gender differences in, 244
  left ventricular hypertrophy in, 244
  left ventricular outflow tract diameter in, 237, *239*, 243
  left ventricular response to, 244
  left ventricular systolic dysfunction, 244
  mitral regurgitation and, 244
  mitral stenosis and, 244
  outflow tract diameter in, 243
  outflow tract velocity in, 243–244
  pressure gradients in, 236–237, *236*, 237t, *238, 239*
  progression of, 246–247, *246, 247*
  proximal flow pattern in, 232
  rheumatic, 233–234, *233*
  stroke work loss in, 240–241
  valve resistance in, 240
  velocity ratio in, 239–240
  vs. hypertrophic cardiomyopathy, *235*
  vs. subaortic membrane, *235*
Aortic valve, bicuspid, 400, 402t
  congenital abnormalities of, 400, *403*
  flail leaflet of, *325*, 338
  on transesophageal Doppler echocardiography, 71–72, *73*
  on transesophageal echocardiography, 70–72, 72t, *73*
  on transthoracic echocardiography, 33–34, 34t, *36*, 39–40, *40*, 43
  on transthoracic M-mode echocardiography, 46, *46*
  schematic diagram of, *36, 39*
  unicuspid, 400, 402t
  vegetations on, *325*, 331–333, *333*
Aortic valve index, in aortic stenosis, 239–240
Aortic valve regurgitation, 178, 277–285
  aortic dissection and, 278
  aortic root abnormalities and, 278
  aortic stenosis and, 244
  echocardiography in, 277–278, 277t, *278*
    clinical utility of, 283–285
    2D/M-mode, 279, *279*, 279t
    for follow-up care, 285
    postoperative, 284–285
  endocarditis and, 278, *325*, 341
  etiology of, 278t
  in Marfan syndrome, 278
  left ventricular response to, 272, *272*, 279–280, *280*, 280t
  mitral stenosis and, 257
  reverse doming in, 279
  severity of, 280–283, 281t
    color M-mode Doppler for, 271, *271*
    continous-wave Doppler for, 280, 282, *283*
    Doppler flow mapping for, 280, *282, 283*
    holodiastolic flow reversal and, 282, *284*
    regurgitant volume and, 283
    stroke volume and, 273–274, *274*
  with prosthetic valve, 315–318, *318*, 322, *324*
Aortic valve replacement, 310t. See also *Prosthetic valve(s)*.
  antegrade velocity across, 311, *311*
  bileaflet, *306*
  bioprosthetic, 307–308, *307*
  case study of, 248, *248*
  dynamic subaortic obstruction after, 195
  echocardiography after, 284–285, 319–321
  echocardiography before, 244–246, *245*, 245t
  endocarditis and, *324, 325*
  homograft, *306*
  valve areas in, 312–314, *313*, 314t
Aortic valvotomy, 420t
Aortography, of aorta, 391
Apical window, transthoracic echocardiography, 42–44
  four-chamber view of, 42–43, *42, 43*
  long-axis view of, 44, *44*
  two-chamber view of, 43–44, *43*
Area-length method, for left systolic volume calculations, 108
Arrhythmias, screening echocardiography in, 89
Arteriovenous fistula, 402t, 405–406, *406*

Atherosclerosis, aortic, 390, *390*
Atrial baffle procedures, 419, 420t, 422
Atrial fibrillation, Doppler echocardiography of, 365, *365*
  embolus and, 367
  left ventricular filling and, 143, *143*
Atrial pressures, ventricular diastolic function and, 135–136, *135*
Atrial septal defects, 402t–403t, 407–410
  anatomy of, 407–408, *408*
  closure of, 420t
  contrast echocardiography of, 410
  Doppler echocardiography of, 409, *414*
  left-to-right shunt and, 409, *413, 414*
  paradoxical septal motion and, 123
  primum, 407, *408*, 410
  repair of, 410
  secundum, 407, *408*
  sinus venosus, 408, *408, 412*
  two-dimensional echocardiography of, 408–409, *409–413*
Atrial situs, 398
Atrium, left, dimensions of, 35t
  filling curves of, ventricular diastolic function and, *135*, 136
  filling velocities of, 50t
    on transthoracic Doppler echocardiography, 54
  flow velocities of, 50t, 51t
    on color Doppler transthoracic echocardiography, 56
    on transesophageal echocardiography, 75–76, 75t, *76*
    on transthoracic echocardiography, 34t, 36, 43
    on transthoracic M-mode recording, 46, *46*
  right, filling curves of, ventricular diastolic function and, 135–136, *135*
  filling velocities of, 50t
    on transthoracic Doppler echocardiography, 54
  flow velocities of, 50t, 51t
    on color Doppler transthoracic echocardiography, 57
  interior of, *38*
    on transesophageal echocardiography, 75t, 77, *77*
    on transthoracic echocardiography, 34t, 37–38, *37, 38*, 43
Attenuation, *3*, 4

B

Background noise, in color flow Doppler echocardiography, 24, 24t
Bayesian analysis, 81, *81*
Beam width artifact, in Doppler echocardiography, 22t, 23, *23*
  in two-dimensional echocardiography, 12t, 13–14, *13*
Bernoulli equation, 49, 230–231
Biplane apical volume formula, for left systolic volume calculations, 108

Biplane ellipsoid formula, for left systolic volume calculations, *107*, 108
Blood flow, antegrade, normal, 50–54, 50t, 51t, *52, 53*
  disturbed, 48, *48*
  Doppler evaluation of. See *Doppler echocardiography*.
  flow-velocity profile of, 48–49, *49*
  laminar, 48, *48*
Bullet formula, for left systolic volume calculations, 108
Burst length, in Doppler color flow imaging, 20–22, *21*

C

Carcinoid tumor, metastatic, 357, *358*
  tricuspid valve regurgitation and, 293
Cardiac catheterization, in congenital heart disease, 425, 426t, 427
  in pericardial constriction, 226
  in pulmonary heart disease, 208
Cardiac cycle, 101, *101*
  pressure-volume loop of, 101, *102*
Cardiac mass, 351–366. See also *Cardiac tumor*.
  echocardiography of, 351–353, *352–355*, 352t
    infection on, 354
      left atrial thrombus on, 363–365, *364, 365*
      left ventricular thrombus on, 361–363, 362t, *363*
      right heart thrombus on, 365–366, *366*
      thrombus on, 355t
      tumor on, 353–354, *356–360*, 356–361, 356t, 358t
  in embolism, 366–370, *368, 369*
  vs. normal structures, 351–352, *352–355*, 352t
Cardiac output, 103
  exercise effect on, 103
  thermodilution measurement of, 118
Cardiac transplantation, 203–205
  coronary artery disease after, 205
  echocardiographic evaluation of, 203–205
    abnormal findings on, 204–205
    atrial suture line on, 204, *204*
    normal findings on, 204, *204*
    technical considerations in, 205
  left ventricular systolic dysfunction after, 203
  rejection of, 205
  right ventricular systolic dysfunction after, 203
Cardiac tumor, 353–354, 355t, 356–361
  benign, 357–360, *358–360*, 359t
  malignant, 360–361, *360, 361*
  nonprimary, 353–354, *356–357*, 356–358, 356t
  primary, 357–361, *358–360*, 358t
  transthoracic echocardiography in, 88t
Cardiomegaly, diagnosis of, 83, *84*
  differential diagnosis of, 85t
Cardiomyopathy, 183–200
  dilated, 184–188, 184t
    B-bump (AC-shoulder) in, 186, *186*
    echocardiography in, 87t, *178*, 184–186, *185–187*, 185t

Cardiomyopathy *(Continued)*
    clinical utility of, *187,* 187–188, 187t
    Doppler, 185–186, *186, 187*
    in intensive care unit, 188, *188*
    limitations of, 186–187
    repeat studies in, 188
    technical considerations in, 186–187
  in Chagas' disease, 186–187
  left ventricular diastolic function in, 148, 186,
    187
  left ventricular systolic function in, 177t
  left ventricular thrombus in, 186, *186*
  mitral valve regurgitation in, 178
  thrombus in, 186, *186, 363, 364*
  transthoracic echocardiography in, 87t
  hypertrophic, 184t, 188–196
    anatomic features of, 188–189, *189*
    congenital, 403t
    dynamic outflow obstruction in, 189–190, *190,*
      192–194, *192, 193, 195*
      provocation of, 194
    echocardiography in, 87t, 191–194, *191–193*
      clinical utility of, 195
      Doppler, 192–194, *193*
      intraoperative, 195
      limitations of, 194–195
      preoperative, 195
      technical considerations in, 194–195
    hypertensive, 203
    left ventricular diastolic function in, 148, 190,
      191–192
    mitral regurgitation in, 189–190, *190,* 194, 286
    patterns of, 188–189, *189,* 191, *191*
    transthoracic echocardiography in, 87t
    vs. aortic stenosis, *235*
    vs. septal knuckle, 191
  restrictive, 87t, 184t, *196,* 196–200
    cardiac catheterization in, 200
    echocardiography in, 196–199, *197–199*
      clinical utility of, 199–200
      Doppler, 197, *197,* 199
      limitations of, 199
      technical considerations in, 199
    etiology of, 196, 196t
    left ventricular diastolic function in, 197–199,
      198, 199
    right atrial filling in, 199
    transthoracic echocardiography in, 87t
    vs. constrictive pericarditis, 200
    vs. pericardial constriction, 225–226, 225t
    vs. pericardial tamponade, 225–226, 225t
Cavitation, ultrasound creation of, 26
Chagas' disease, dilated cardiomyopathy in,
    186–187
Chest pain, diagnosis of, 83–84, 84t
Chiari network, 416, 418
Chordae, on transthoracic echocardiography, 40–41
Chordal disruption, mitral valve regurgitation in,
    286
Chordal elongation, mitral valve regurgitation in,
    286
Circumferential stress (σ_c), 110

Clinical decision analysis, 79–83
  Bayesian analysis in, 81, *81*
  clinical outcomes and, 82–83, *82*
  cost-effectiveness in, 82
  data integration in, 81, *81*
  test accuracy in, 79–80, *80, 81*
  test utility in, 83
  threshold approach to, 81–82, *81*
Clinical outcomes, 82–83, *82*
Compliance, ventricular, 134, *135*
  left ventricular filling and, 144
Computed tomography, in aortic dissection, *387*
  in congenital heart disease, 426t
  in pericardial constriction, 226, *226*
  of aorta, 391
Conduit, valved, 305. See also *Prosthetic valve(s).*
  2D/M-mode echocardiography of, 308
Congenital heart disease, 395–427, 396t
  cardiac catheterization in, 425, 426t, 427
  echocardiography of, 396–400, 400t, 402t–403t
    aortic coarctation on, 403–404, *405*
    aortic valve abnormalities on, 400, 402t, *403*
    atrial septal defects on, 407–410, *408–414*
    chamber abnormalities on, 397–399, 398t
    Chiari network on, 416, 418
    coronary arteriovenous fistula on, 405–406,
      406
    Ebstein's anomaly on, 406–407, *407*
    great vessel abnormalities on, 399–400, *399,*
      400t
    in Marfan's syndrome, 402t, 404–405
    left ventricular web on, 418
    limitations of, 425, 426t
    myxomatous mitral valve disease on, 407
    patent ductus arteriosus on, 414, *417, 418*
    persistent left superior vena cava on, 415–416
    pulmonary artery dilation on, 416
    regurgitant lesions on, 396–397, 406–407, *407*
    right ventricular outflow obstruction on, 401,
      405
    shunt ratio calculations and, 425
    shunts on, 397, *398*
    sinus of Valsalva aneurysm on, 405
    stenotic lesions on, 396
    surgical procedures on, 418–425, 420t–421t,
      422–424
    tetralogy of Fallot on, 423, *423,* 424
    transposition of great arteries on, 423–424, *424*
    tricuspid atresia on, 424, *424*
    truncus arteriosus on, 425
    ventricular inversion on, 414–415, *419*
    ventricular septal defects on, 411–414,
      415–417
  embolus and, 367
  surgical procedures on, 418–425, 420t–421t,
    422–424
  transthoracic echocardiography in, 88t
Continuity equation valve area, in aortic stenosis,
    237–239, 240t, *241,* 245
  in mitral stenosis, 253, 255
Contractility, in ventricular systolic function, 101
Contrast echocardiography, 92–93, *92,* 92t, *93*

Cor pulmonale, 205, 208. See also *Pulmonary heart disease.*
Coronary artery (arteries), anatomy of, segmental wall motion and, 154–156, *154–156*
    direct echocardiographic imaging of, 166–167, *167*
    intravascular imaging of, 167, *167*
    left, anatomy of, 154, *154*
        Doppler recording from, 166, *167*
        transesophageal imaging of, 166, *167*
    left-dominant, 154
    occlusion of, in aortic dissection, 381–382
    right, anatomy of, 154, *154, 155*
        transthoracic imaging of, 166, *167*
    right-dominant, 154
Coronary artery disease, 153–178. See also *Myocardial infarction; Myocardial ischemia.*
    after cardiac transplantation, 205
    aortic atherosclerosis and, 390, *390*
    global left ventricular systolic function in, 159
    of circumflex artery, 156
    of left anterior descending artery, 156
    of posterior descending artery disease, 156
    regional left ventricular systolic function in, 159–160, 159t
    stress echocardiography in, 91
    transthoracic echocardiography in, 86t–87t
Coronary sinus, on transesophageal echocardiography, 77, *77*
    on transthoracic echocardiography, 34t, 36, 38
Crista terminalis, on transthoracic echocardiography, 38, *353*
Cubed formula, for left systolic volume calculations, 107

D

Damus-Kaye-Stansel procedure, 421t, 422
Decibels, 3, *3*
Dextrocardia, 398
Dextroversion, 398
Diastasis, 133, *133*
Diastole, definition of, 123–133, *133*
    phases of, 132–133, *133*
Digoxin, in aortic valve regurgitation, 285
Dip-plateau sign, in pericardial constriction, 222, *223*
Dobutamine stress echocardiography, complications of, 161–162
    endpoints for, 161
    in myocardial ischemia, 160t, 161–163, *163*
    in myocardial viability assessment, 163
    interpretation of, 162–163, *163, 164*
Doppler echocardiography, 15–25
    antegrade blood flow on, 50–54, 50t, *52, 53*
    artifacts with, 22–25, *22–25,* 22t, 24t
    beam alignment in, 16
    beam width artifact with, 22t, 23, *23*
    color flow, 20–22, *20–22,* 21t
        artifacts with, 23–25, 24t
        atrial inflow patterns on, 56–57

Doppler echocardiography *(Continued)*
    background noise with, 24, 24t
    color scale for, 57
    electronic interference during, 24–25, 24t
    frame rate for, 21, *21,* 21t, 57
    gain for, 57
    ghosting with, 23, 24t
    intercept angle effects in, 24, *24,* 24t, 55, *55*
    normal patterns on, 54–57, *55, 56*
    physiologic valvular regurgitation on, 57
    power output for, 57
    shadowing with, 23, 24t
    signal aliasing in, 24, 24t, *25,* 55
    variance patterns with, 56
    velocity range for, 57
    ventricular inflow patterns on, 56, *56*
    ventricular outflow patterns on, 56
    continuous-wave, 17
        artifacts with, 22–23, *22–24,* 22t
    descending aorta flow on, 51t, 54
    Doppler equation for, 15–16, *15, 16*
    flow disturbance on, 49–50
    instrument controls for, 17
    left atrial filling on, 51t, 54
    left ventricular inflow on, 51t, 53–54, *53*
    left ventricular outflow on, 51–53, 51t, *52*
    mirror-image artifact with, 22t, 23, *24*
    pulsed, 17–20, *18–20*
        artifacts with, 22–23, *22–24,* 22t
        high-pulse-repetition frequency in, 19–20, *20*
        range ambiguity in, 19–20, *20*
        sample volume of, 18
        signal aliasing in, *18,* 19, *19*
    range ambiguity artifact with, 22t, 23
    right atrial filling on, 51t, 54
    right ventricular inflow on, 51t, 54
    right ventricular outflow on, 51t, *53*
    signal aliasing with, 22, 22t
    spectral analysis of, 16–17, *16*
    stress, in myocardial ischemia, 166
    transit time effect with, 22t, 23
    velocity underestimation with, 22, 22t
    velocity-pressure relationship on, 49
    volume flow on, 49
Doppler equation, 15–16, *15, 16*
Doppler shift, 15, *15*

E

Ebstein's anomaly, 406–407, *407*
    tricuspid valve regurgitation and, 293
Echocardiography, 1–27
    A-mode, 9, *10*
    basic format for, 96–97
    bioeffects of, 26
    2D, 10–14. See also *Two-dimensional echocardiography.*
    3D, 14–15
    Doppler, 15–25. See also *Doppler echocardiography.*
    education for, 97
    examination technique for, 25–26

Echocardiography *(Continued)*
  focus for, 97
  indications for, 79–98. See also *Clinical decision
      analysis.*
  interpretation of, 97–98
  M-mode, 9–10, *10*
  protocol for, 96–97
  recording devices for, 25–26
  safety during, 26–27
  training guidelines for, 97
  transesophageal, 59–77. See also
      Transesophageal echocardiography.
  transthoracic, 29–57. See also *Transthoracic
      echocardiography.*
Eisenmenger's physiology, 397
Ejection fraction, 103
Electrocardiography, exercise, in myocardial
      ischemia, 166
Electronic processing artifact, in two-dimensional
      echocardiography, 12t, 14
Embolism, differential diagnosis of, 85t
  endocarditis and, 347, 347t
  pulmonary, 208. See also *Pulmonary heart
      disease.*
Embolus, aortic atherosclerosis and, 390, *390*
  cardiac source of, 366–370
    echocardiography guidelines for, 369–370
    predisposing conditions for, 367–369, *368, 369*
    interatrial septal aneurysm and, 368–369, *369*
    patent foramen ovale and, 367–368, *368*
Endocardial cushion defect, 420t
Endocardial motion, on transthoracic
      echocardiography, 41
Endocarditis, 329–347
  aortic regurgitation and, 278
  criteria for, 329–330, 330t
  echocardiography in, 330–342
    accuracy of, 337, 337t
    clinical utility of, 346–347, *346,* 347t
    functional abnormalities on, 337–338
    goals of, 329–330
    leaflet perforation on, 339, *340*
    nonbacterial disease on, 342–343, *344,* 353
    paravalvular abscess on, 338–342, *338, 339,
        342,* 344t
    prosthetic valve disease on, 343–346, *345, 346*
    rupture on, 339, *341*
    sequential, 342
    transesophageal, 334–337, *335–337*
    transthoracic, 330–334, 332t, *333–335*
    valve disease on, 343
    vegetations on, 330–337, *331,* 332t, *333–337,*
        337t, 353, 355t
  embolism and, 347, 347t
  mitral valve regurgitation and, 286
  of prosthetic valve, 306, 322–323, *324, 325,*
      343–346, *345, 346*
  pericardial effusion with, 338
  pulmonary pressures and, 338
  tricuspid valve regurgitation and, 293
  valvular regurgitation with, *325,* 338, *338*
  ventricular response to, 338

End-systolic pressure-volume relationship (E_{max}),
      101, *102*
E-point septal separation, 104
Epstein's anomaly, 402t
Esophageal position, transesophageal
      echocardiography, 61t, 62–68
    four-chamber plane in, 62–63, *62–64*
    long-axis left ventricular plane in, 64–66,
        65, 66
    short-axis plane in, 67–68, *67*
    two-chamber plane in, 63, *64, 65*
Eustachian valve remnants, 365–366
Examination, technique of, 25–26
Exercise, cardiac output and, 103
  ventricular systolic function and, 103
Exercise electrocardiography, in myocardial
      ischemia, 166
Exercise stress echocardiography. See also *Stress
      echocardiography.*
  in myocardial ischemia, 160–161, 160t, *161,
      162*

F

False-negative test result, 80, *80*
False-positive test result, 80, *80*
Fast Fourier transform, 16, *16*
Fibroelastoma, papillary, 359–360, *360*
Flow-velocity profile, 48–49, *49*
Fontan procedure, 421t, 422
Frame rate, for color flow Doppler
      echocardiography, 21, *21,* 21t, 57
Frank-Starling curve, 101, *102*
Frequency, of sound wave, 2
Frequency bandwidth, of transducer, 5

G

Geriatric patient, echocardiography findings
      in, 34t
Ghosting, in color flow Doppler echocardiography,
      23, 24t

H

Heart failure, definition of, 196
  diagnosis of, 83, *83,* 84t
  differential diagnosis of, 187t. See also specific
      disorders.
Hemisphere cylinder formula, for left systolic
      volume calculations, *107,* 108
Hypertension. See *Hypertensive heart disease;
      Pulmonary hypertension.*
Hypertensive heart disease, 200–203, *201*
  echocardiography in, 200–202, 200t, *201*
    clinical utility of, 202–203
    limitations of, 202
    technical considerations in, 202
    left ventricular diastolic dysfunction in, 203
    left ventricular systolic dysfunction in, 203
    treatment of, 202–203

I

Impedance, acoustic, 3–4
Infarction. See *Myocardial infarction.*
Infective endocarditis. See *Endocarditis.*
Inferior vena cava, dimensions of, 35t
   on transthoracic echocardiography, 38, 44
   plethora of, in pericardial tamponade, 220
Intensity, measurement of, 26–27
Interatrial septum, aneurysm of, 368–369, *369*
   lipomatous hypertrophy of, 360, *360*
Intercept angle, in color flow Doppler
   echocardiography, 24, *24*, 24t
Intracardiac shunt, 397
Ischemia. See *Myocardial ischemia.*

J

Jantene procedure, 421t

K

Konno procedure, 420t

L

Lambl's excrescence, 40, 332, *333*
Laminar flow, *48*, 48
Left atrial compliance, in mitral valve regurgitation, 288
Left atrial filling, Doppler evaluation of, 145–147, *145, 146,* 146t
   normal pattern on, 145–146, *146*
   physiologic factors in, 146–147, 146t
   technical factors in, 145–146, *146*
  for ventricular diastolic function, 136
  respiration and, 136
Left atrial pressure, for ventricular diastolic
   function, 136
Left atrial thrombus, 355t, 363–365
  clinical implications of, 365
  echocardiography of, 76, 88t, 363–365, *364, 365*
  mitral stenosis and, 255–256, *256*
  predisposing factors for, 363
Left bundle branch block, ventricular septal motion
   with, 123, *123*
Left ventricular aneurysm, after myocardial
   infarction, 175–177, *176*
Left ventricular compliance, left ventricular filling
   and, 144
Left ventricular diastolic filling, Doppler evaluation
   of, 137–144, 137t, *138, 139,* 140t
   atrial fibrillation and, 143, *143*
   data recording for, *139,* 139–140, 139t
   left ventricular compliance and, 144
   left ventricular relaxation and, 144, *144*
   left ventricular systolic function and, 143
   mitral regurgitation and, 142, *143*
   normal rates on, 139t
   normal variations on, 140–142, *140–142,* 142t
   physiologic factors in, 142–143, *143*
   preload and, 142, *143*

Left ventricular diastolic filling *(Continued)*
   quantitative measurements with, 137–138, *138, 139*
   technical factors in, 139–140, 140t
  for left ventricular end-diastolic pressure
   estimate, 149–150
  in cardiomyopathy, 148–149
  in ischemic cardiac disease, 149
  in left ventricular hypertrophy, 148
  in myocardial ischemia, 166
  in pericardial constriction, 149, 224–225
  in pericardial tamponade, 149, 219–220, *220*
  in restrictive cardiomyopathy, 197–198, *198,* 198–199, *198, 199*
Left ventricular diastolic function, 136–144. See
   also *Left ventricular diastolic filling.*
  2D echocardiography of, 136–137
  in hypertensive heart disease, 200t, 202, 203
  in hypertrophic cardiomyopathy, 190, 191–192
  in mitral stenosis, 257
  M-mode echocardiography of, 136–137
  pseudonormalization of, 144
Left ventricular dilation, in mitral valve
   regurgitation, 288
Left ventricular end-diastolic pressure, noninvasive
   estimates of, 149–150
Left ventricular hypertrophy, in aortic stenosis, 244
  left ventricular diastolic dysfunction in, 148
Left ventricular mass, 104, 108–110, *110*
Left ventricular relative wall thickness, 104
Left ventricular relaxation, 134, *134*
  left ventricular filling and, 144
Left ventricular segmental wall motion, coronary
   artery anatomy and, 154–156, *154–156*
  echocardiographic evaluation of, 155–156, *155, 156*
   descriptive reporting of, 156, *156*
   transesophageal imaging in, 157–158
   transthoracic imaging in, 156–157, *157, 158*
   wall motion score index in, 159–160, 159t
Left ventricular stroke volume, 103
  Doppler evaluation of, 114–117, *114,* 114t, *115, 116*
Left ventricular systolic function, contrast
   angiography of, 118, *119*
  2D echocardiography of, 104–111
   accuracy of, 112
   cardiac motion during, 112
   endocardial definition on, 111–112, 111t
   geometric assumptions of, 107–108, *108,* 112
   image quality in, 111
   left ventricular mass on, 108–110, *110*
   left ventricular wall stress on, 110, *110*
   limitations of, 111–112
   mitral annulus motion on, 110
   optimization of, 111, 111t
   qualitative evaluation on, 104–105
   quantitative evaluation on, 105–110, 105t–106t, *107, 109*
   reproducibility of, 112
   respiratory motion during, 112
   technical factors in, 111–112, 111t

Left ventricular systolic function *(Continued)*
  ventricular shape changes on, 110–111
  volume measurements on, 105–110,
    105t–106t, *107, 109*
  3D echocardiography of, 112–113, 113t
  Doppler evaluation of, 114–120, 119t
    acceleration times on, 117, *117*
    dP/dt on, 117–118, *118*
    limitations of, 118, 118t
    stroke volume calculation on, 114–117, *114,*
      114t, *115, 116*
      cross-sectional area measurements for, 114,
        114t
      flow profile and, 114
      sites for, 115–117, *115, 116*
      technical factors in, 114–115
    in aortic regurgitation, 178, 279–280, 280t
    in aortic stenosis, 244, 247
    in chronic valvular disease, 177t
    in dilated cardiomyopathy, 177t, *178*
    in end-stage ischemic disease, 177–178, 177t, *178*
    in hypertensive heart disease, 200t, 202, 203
    left ventricular filling and, 143
    M-mode echocardiography of, 103–104
      aortic root motion on, 104
      E-point septal separation on, 104
      left ventricular mass on, 104
      left ventricular volume on, 104
      left ventricular wall stress on, 104
    pulmonary artery pressure and, 178
    radionuclide ventriculography of, 118, *120*
    thermodilution evaluation of, 118
    thrombi and, 178
Left ventricular thrombus, 355t, 361–363
  after myocardial infarction, 177
  clinical implications of, 362–363
  echocardiography of, 362, 362t, *363*
  in dilated cardiomyopathy, 186, *186*
  predisposing conditions for, 361–362
  transthoracic echocardiography in, 88t
Left ventricular volume, in pericardial tamponade,
    219, *220*
  on 2D echocardiography, 105–110, 105t–106t,
    107, 109
  on M-mode echocardiography, 104
Left ventricular volume overload, ventricular septal
    motion with, 123, *123*
Left ventricular wall stress, on 2D
    echocardiography, 110, *110*
  on M-mode echocardiography, 104
Left ventricular web, 418
Lipomatous hypertrophy, 360, *360*
Lymphoma, cardiac metastases from, *357*

M

Magnetic resonance imaging, in aortic dissection,
    387
  in congenital heart disease, 426t
  of aorta, 391
Marfan's syndrome, 402t, 404–405
  aortic dilation in, 373, *374, 375,* 386

Marfan's syndrome *(Continued)*
  aortic regurgitation in, 278
  descending thoracic aorta in, 377, *377*
  mitral valve regurgitation in, 286
  postoperative echocardiography in, 388–389,
    388
Mechanical index, 27
Melanoma, cardiac metastasis from, 353
Meridional stress (σ_m), 104, 110, *110*
Microbubbles, with venous catheters, 366
Mirror-image artifact, in Doppler echocardiography,
    22t, 23, *24*
Mitral annulus, abscess of, 340, *343*
  calcification of, 250
    in hypertensive heart disease, 202
    mitral regurgitation and, 285–286, *286*
  dimensions of, 35t
  motion of, for left ventricular systolic function,
    110–111
  on transthoracic echocardiography, 42
Mitral commissurotomy, percutaneous,
    echocardiography in, 257–258, *258,* 258t
Mitral regurgitant jet, *dP/dt* measurements of,
    117–118, *118*
Mitral regurgitation, 285–293
  age-related degenerative changes and, 286
  aortic root motion in, 288, *289*
  aortic stenosis and, 244
  chordal disruption and, 286
  chordal elongation and, 286
  echocardiography in, 285–287, *286, 287,* 288t
    aortic root motion on, 288, *289*
    clinical utility of, 291–292
    for follow-up care, 292
    postoperative, 293, *294, 295*
    preoperative, 293
  endocarditis, 286
  etiology of, 285, 285t
  hypertrophic cardiomyopathy and, 286
  in dilated cardiomyopathy, 178
  in endocarditis, *340*
  in hypertrophic cardiomyopathy, 189–190, *190,*
    194
  in Marfan's syndrome, 286
  in myxomatous disease, 292, *294*
  left atrial response to, 288
  left ventricular dysfunction and, 287
  left ventricular filling and, 142, *143*
  left ventricular response to, 270, 271–272, *271,*
    272, 288
  mitral annular calcification and, 285–286, *286*
  mitral stenosis and, 257
  myxomatous disease and, 286, *287*
  myxomatous disease in, 277–278, *278*
  on color Doppler transthoracic
    echocardiography, 57
  on transesophageal Doppler echocardiography,
    72, *74*
  papillary muscle disorders and, 287
  post-infarction, echocardiography of, 173, *174*
  pulmonary artery pressure in, 288
  rheumatic, 286

Mitral regurgitation *(Continued)*
  severity of, 288–290
    color M-mode Doppler for, 271, *271*
    continuous-wave Doppler for, 290, 290t, *291*
    Doppler flow mapping for, 288–289, *289*, *290*
    pulmonary vein flow reversal and, 290
    stroke volume and, 290, *291*
    upstream flow reversal and, 272, *273*
  v wave in, 290, *291*
  with prosthetic valve, 315–318, *316, 317*
Mitral stenosis, 249–261
  aortic regurgitation and, 257
  aortic stenosis and, 244
  calcific, 250
  case studies of, 259–261, *259, 260*
  continuity equation mitral valve area in, 253, 255
  2D echo valve area in, 251, *252*
  differential diagnosis of, 250–251, 251t
  echocardiography in, 86t, 249–255, *250–252*, 253t
    case studies of, 259–261, *259, 260*
    clinical utility of, 257–259, 257t, *258*, 258t
    in percutaneous commissurotomy patient, 257–258, *258*, 258t
    in pregnant patient, 258–259
    mitral valve area on, 251–254, *252*, 253t
    pressure gradients on, 251, *251*
    technical considerations in, 254–255, 254t, *255*
  left atrial enlargement and, 255–256
  left atrial thrombi and, 255–256, *256*
  left ventricular response to, 257
  mitral regurgitation and, 257
  mitral valve area in, 251–254, *252*, 253t, 254t
  pressure gradients in, 251, *251*, 254–255, *255*
  pressure half-time valve area in, 251–253, *252*, 253t, 254–255
  proximal flow pattern in, 232, *232*
  proximal isovelocity surface area in, 253–254, 255
  pulmonary hypertension and, 256–257, *256*
  rheumatic, 249–250, *250*
    case studies of, 259–261, *259, 261*
  thrombus in, 364, *364, 365*
  tricuspid regurgitant jet in, 256–257, *256*
  tricuspid stenosis and, 257
  ventricular septal motion with, 123, *123*
Mitral valve, flail leaflet of, *333, 334*
  leaflet perforation of, in endocarditis, 338–339, *340*
  movements of, 46–47, *47*
  myxomatous disease of, 277–278, *278, 286, 287, 292, 294*, 402t, 407
    endocarditis and, 343
  on transesophageal Doppler echocardiography, 72, *73, 74*
  on transesophageal echocardiography, 72, 72t, *73*
  on transthoracic echocardiography, 34, 34t, 36, *37*, 40–41, *40, 42*
  on transthoracic M-mode recording, 46–47, *47*
  schematic diagram of, *37*
  vegetations on, 333–334, *334, 336, 336*
Mitral valve area, in mitral stenosis, 251–254, *252*, 253t

Mitral valve prolapse, 287, *287*
  echocardiography in, 292, 292t, *294*
Mitral valve replacement, 310t. See also *Prosthetic valve(s)*.
  bileaflet, 304–305, *304, 305*
  clicks of, 308, *309*
  echocardiography in, 293, *294, 295*, 319–321
  left ventricular flow patterns and, *303*
  pulmonary artery pressure after, 319
  valve areas in, 314–315, 314t, *315*
M-mode echocardiography, 9–10, *10*
Momentum, of regurgitant jet, 275
Murmur, diastolic, differential diagnosis of, 85t
  systolic, differential diagnosis of, 85t
    in aortic stenosis, 247–248
Myocardial infarction, 158–159, *159*, 169–177. See also *Myocardial ischemia*.
  angiography in, 172, *173*
  complications of, echocardiography in, 173–177, *174–176*
  diagnostic criteria for, 172
  diastolic function in, 172
  echocardiography in, 170–172, *170–172*
    after interventional therapy, 173
    clinical utility of, 172–173
    in emergency room, 172–173
    limitations of, 172
    postinfarction, 173–177, *174–176*
  in circumflex artery, 171
  in left anterior descending artery, 170–171, *170, 171*
  in posterior descending artery, 171, *172*
  left ventricular aneurysm after, 175–177, *176*
  left ventricular thrombi after, 177
  mitral regurgitation after, 173, *174*
  pericardial effusion after, 175
  pseudoaneurysm after, 174–175, *176*, 220–221, *221*
  radionuclide imaging in, 172
  right ventricular infarction after, 175
  stress echocardiography after, 169
  transthoracic echocardiography in, 86t
  ventricular rupture after, 174–175, *175, 176*
  ventricular septal defect after, 173–174, *174, 175*
Myocardial ischemia, 160–169. See also *Myocardial infarction*.
  angiography in, 169
  differential diagnosis of, 177–178, 177t, *178*
  Doppler stress echocardiography in, 166
  exercise echocardiography in, 160–161, *161, 162, 164*, 165t
  exercise electrocardiography in, 166
  left ventricular diastolic function in, 149, 166
  left ventricular systolic function in, 177–178, 177t, *178*
  positron emission tomography in, 169
  pulmonary artery pressure in, 178
  radionuclide perfusion imaging in, 168–169, *168*
  stress echocardiography in, 160–164, 160t, *161–164*
    accuracy of, 169
    clinical utility of, 169

Myocardial ischemia *(Continued)*
diagnostic accuracy of, 164, 165t
dipyridamole, 163–164
dobutamine, 160t, 161–163, *163, 164*
diagnostic accuracy of, 164, 165t
Doppler, 166
exercise, 160–161, 160t, *161, 162*
diagnostic accuracy of, 164, 165t
image quality with, 164
interpretation of, 166
limitations of, 164–166
prognosis and, 169
respiratory interference in, 164–165
technical aspects of, 164–166
vs. coronary angiography, 169
tricuspid valve regurgitation in, 178
vs. dilated cardiomyopathy, 177t, *178*
Myocardium, hibernating, 170
dobutamine stress echocardiography of, 163
stunned, 170
dobutamine stress echocardiography of, 163
Myxoma, 357–359, *358, 359*

N

Nifedipine, in aortic valve regurgitation, 285
Nodules of Arantius, 40
Norwood procedure, 421t, 422
Nyquist limit, 19

P

Palpitations, evaluation of, 84t
Papillary muscle, abnormal orientation of, mitral
valve regurgitation and, 287
on transthoracic echocardiography, 41, *41,* 42
rupture of, mitral valve regurgitation and, 287
post-infarction, echocardiography of, 173, *174*
Parasternal window, transthoracic
echocardiography, 33–34, 36–42
long-axis view of, *32,* 33–34, 36–37, *36, 37*
right ventricular inflow and outflow views of,
37–38, *37–39*
short-axis views of, 39–42, *39–41*
Paravalvular abscess, 338–342, *338, 339, 342,*
344t, 353
Partial anomalous pulmonary venous return, 403t
Patent ductus arteriosus, 403t, 414, *417, 418*
closure of, 420t
Patent foramen ovale, embolus and, 367–368, *368*
Patient position, 26
Pericardial constriction, 222–226, *222*
cardiac catheterization in, 226
computed tomography in, 226, *226*
echocardiography in, 87t, 222–224, 223t
clinical utility of, 226
2D/M-mode, 222–224, *223, 224*
Doppler, 224–225, *224*
limitations of, 226
left ventricular diastolic dysfunction in, 149
pressure tracing in, 222, *223*
square-root sign in, 222, *223*

Pericardial constriction *(Continued)*
ventricular septal motion with, 123, *123*
vs. pericardial tamponade, 222, *222, 223,*
225–226, 225t
vs. restrictive cardiomyopathy, 200, 225–226,
225t
Pericardial effusion, 214t, 215–222
after myocardial infarction, 175
diffuse, 216–217, *216, 217*
echocardiography in, 216–218, *216, 217,* 221
fibrinous stranding with, 217, *217*
loculated, 217, *217*
pressure increase with, 215–216, *216*
pulsus paradoxus in, 216, *216*
size of, 217
vs. pleural fluid, 217–218, *218*
with metastatic cardiac tumor, 356, *356*
Pericardial rub, 214
Pericardial tamponade, echocardiography in, 87t,
218–220, *218–220,* 218t, 221
clinical utility of, 221–222
limitations of, 220–221
etiology of, 220
inferior vena cava plethora in, 220
left ventricular diastolic dysfunction in, 149
respiration-related changes in, 219–220, *220*
right atrial systolic collapse in, 218, *219*
right ventricular diastolic collapse in, 218–219,
219
ventricular diastolic filling changes in, 219–220,
220
ventricular volume changes in, 219, *220*
vs. pericardial constriction, 222, *222, 223,*
225–226, 225t
vs. restrictive cardiomyopathy, 225–226, 225t
Pericardiocentesis, echocardiography-guided,
221–222
Pericarditis, 214–215, 214t, *215.* See also
Pericardial effusion.
constrictive. See *Pericardial constriction.*
differential diagnosis of, 214, 214t
echocardiography in, 214–215, *215*
Pericardium, anatomy of, 213, *214*
inflammation of, 214–215, 214t, *215.* See also
Pericardial effusion.
thickening of, 215, *215*
Piezoelectric crystal, of transducer, 5, *5*
Pleural fluid, vs. pericardial effusion, 217–218,
218
Positron emission tomography, in myocardial
ischemia, 169
Power per area, 26–27
Preejection period, in left ventricular systolic
function, 117
Pregnancy, aortic stenosis in, 247–248
mitral stenosis in, 258–259
pulmonary congestion in, 258–259
Preload, in ventricular systolic function, 101, *102*
left ventricular filling pattern and, 142, *143*
Pressure half-time valve area, in mitral stenosis,
251–253, *252,* 253t, 254–255, *255*
Pressure-volume loop, of cardiac cycle, 101, *102*
Prevalence, disease, 80

Prosthetic valve(s), 301–325
  angiography of, 321
  auscultation of, 308
  bileaflet, 304–305, *304, 305, 306*
    pressure gradients across, 311–312, *312*
  bioprosthetic, 301–304, 302t, *303,* 303t
    degeneration of, 305
    2D/M-mode echocardiography of, 306–308,
      306, 307
    regurgitation with, 306
  2D/M-mode echocardiography of, 306–308, *306,
    307*
  Doppler echocardiography of, 308–318, *309,*
    310t, *311–313,* 314t, *315–319*
    antigrade velocities on, 308–309, 310t, 319
    normal regurgitation on, 309, 311
    pressure gradients on, 308–309, 310t,
      311–312, *312,* 312t
    regurgitation on, 315–318, *316–319,* 322, *324*
    stenosis on, 311–315, *311–313,* 312t, 314t,
      315, 321–322, *322*
    valve area on, 312–315, *313,* 314t, *315*
    valve clicks on, 308, *309*
  dysfunction of, 305–306
    tissue degeneration in, 305
  echocardiography of, 306–321
    clinical utility of, 321–322, *322*
    for follow-up care, 325
    limitations of, 321
    transesophageal, 320–321
    transthoracic, 319–320
  embolus and, 367
  endocarditis with, 306, 322–323, *324, 325,*
    343–346, *345, 346*
  fluoroscopy of, 321
  follow-up care for, 325
  homograft, 302t, 304
  left ventricular response to, 318–319
  mechanical, *302,* 302t, 304–305, *304, 305*
    antigrade flow profiles of, 304–305
    2D/M-mode echocardiography of, 308
    failure of, 305
    normal regurgitation with, 305, *305*
    regurgitation with, 306
  pulmonary artery pressure and, 319
  regurgitation with, 309, 311, 315–318, *316–319,*
    322, *324*
  spontaneous contrast with, 319
  stenosis of, endocarditis and, 345
  thrombosis with, 323–325, *325*
  types of, 301–305, 302t
Proximal isovelocity surface area, 232
  in mitral stenosis, 253–254, *255*
  in valvular regurgitation, 266, *266,* 273–275,
    274
Pseudoaneurysm, after myocardial infarction,
    174–175, *176,* 220–221, *221*
  of aortic graft, 388, *389*
  vs. true aneurysm, 221, *221*
Pseudonormalization, of left ventricular diastolic
    function, 144
Pulmonary artery, abnormalities of, 390–391, *391*
  dimensions of, 35t

Pulmonary artery *(Continued)*
  echocardiography of, 390–391, *391*
  flow velocity of, 50t
  idiopathic dilation of, 416
  position of, 399
  right, on transthoracic echocardiography, 36
Pulmonary artery banding, 420t
Pulmonary artery pressure, 123–129
  Doppler evaluation of, 124t
    isovolumic relaxation time on, 124t, 127
    limitations of, 127–129, *128*
    overestimation on, 127
    pulmonary artery velocity curve on, 124t,
      126–127, *127*
    right atrial pressure on, 124t, 125–126, *126,* 126t
    tricuspid regurgitant jet measurement on,
      123–126, 124t, *125, 128*
    underestimation on, 127
  in left ventricular systolic dysfunction, 178
  in mitral valve regurgitation, 288
  pulmonary artery catheter measurement of, 128–129
Pulmonary artery systolic pressure, in congenital
    right ventricular outflow obstruction, 403
Pulmonary artery wedge pressure, 134
Pulmonary banding, 419
Pulmonary embolism, 208. See also *Pulmonary
    heart disease.*
Pulmonary heart disease, 205–208
  acute, 205
  cardiac catheterization in, 208
  chronic, 205
  Doppler echocardiography in, 206, *206*
  echocardiography in, 205–207, *206–208*
    clinical utility of, 208
    limitations of, 207
    technical considerations in, 207–208
  pulmonary pressures in, 205–206, *206*
  radionuclide imaging in, 208
  right ventricular pressure overload in, 206–207,
    207, 208
  secondary tricuspid regurgitation in, 207
  ventilation-perfusion scan in, 208
Pulmonary hypertension, mitral stenosis and,
    256–257, *256*
  transthoracic echocardiography in, 87t, 88t
  tricuspid valve regurgitation and, 293
Pulmonary pressures, in pulmonary heart disease,
    205–206, *206*
Pulmonary vein, flow reversal in, in mitral valve
    regurgitation, 290
Pulmonary venous inflow, for left ventricular end-
    diastolic pressure estimate, 149
Pulmonic regurgitant jet, velocity of, 125
Pulmonic regurgitation, 297, *297*
  on color Doppler transthoracic
    echocardiography, 57
Pulmonic stenosis, 261, *261,* 402t
Pulmonic valve, movement of, 47–48, *48*
  on transesophageal Doppler echocardiography,
    72, 74
  on transesophageal echocardiography, 72t
  on transthoracic echocardiography, 34t, 38
  on transthoracic M-mode recording, 47–48, *48*

Pulmonic valvotomy, 420t
Pulse repetition frequency, of pulsed Doppler
    echocardiography, 17–18, *18*
Pulsus paradoxus, in pericardial effusion, 216, *216*

R

Radionuclide imaging, in myocardial infarction, 172
    in myocardial ischemia, 168–169, *168*
    in pulmonary heart disease, 208
Radionuclide ventriculography, for left ventricular
    systolic function, 118–119, *120*
    in congenital heart disease, 426t
Range ambiguity, in Doppler echocardiography,
    22t, 23
    in two-dimensional echocardiography, 12t, 14
Rastelli procedure, 421t, 422, *422, 423*
Recording devices, 25
Reflection, 3–4, *3*
Refraction, *3,* 4
Refraction artifact, in two-dimensional
    echocardiography, 12t, 14, *14*
Regurgitation, valvular. See *Valvular regurgitation.*
Renal cell carcinoma, cardiac metastases from, 357,
    357
Resolution, 7–9, 8t, *9*
    axial, 7–8, 8t, *9*
    elevational, 8t, *9*
    lateral, 8t, *9*
Respiration, left atrial filling and, 136
    left ventricular systolic function and, 112
    right atrial filling and, 147
    ventricular diastolic function and, 136
Reverberation artifact, in two-dimensional
    echocardiography, 12–13, 12t, *13*
Reynolds number, 48
Rhabdomyosarcoma, atrial, 360–361, *361*
Rheumatic disease, aortic stenosis in, 233–234, *233*
    mitral stenosis in, 249–250, *250*
    tricuspid regurgitation and, 293
    tricuspid stenosis in, 257, *260, 261, 261*
Right atrial dilation, in tricuspid valve
    regurgitation, 294–295
Right atrial filling, Doppler evaluation of, 147–148,
    147
Right atrial pressure, 124t, 125–126, 126, *126,*
    126t
    for ventricular diastolic function, 135–136, *135*
Right atrial thrombus, 365–366, *366*
Right ventricular diastolic filling, Doppler
    evaluation of, 144–145, *144*
    in pericardial constriction, 224–225
    in pericardial tamponade, 219–220, *220*
Right ventricular diastolic function, 144–145
    Doppler evaluation of, 144–145, *144*
Right ventricular dilation, 120–121
    in tricuspid valve regurgitation, 294–295
    ventricular septal motion with, 122
Right ventricular hypertrophy, 121–122
    ventricular septal motion with, 122
Right ventricular infarction, after myocardial
    infarction, 175

Right ventricular isovolumic relaxation time, 127
Right ventricular outflow obstruction, congenital,
    402–403, *404*
Right ventricular pressure overload, in pulmonary
    heart disease, 206–207, *207, 208*
Right ventricular stroke volume, Doppler
    evaluation of, 116–117, *116*
Right ventricular systolic function, 120–129
    2D echocardiography of, 120–122, *121*
    M-mode echocardiography of, 120–122
    interventricular septal motion on, 122–123,
        122, 123
    pulmonary artery pressure and, 123–129. See
        also *Pulmonary artery pressure.*
Right ventricular volume, in pericardial tamponade,
    219, *220*
Right ventricular volume overload, ventricular
    septal motion with, 122–123, 123, *123*

S

Safety, 26–27
Sample volume, of pulsed Doppler echocardiogra-
    phy, 18
Scattering, *3,* 4
Sector scanning, 6
Sensitivity, test, 79, 80
Septal knuckle, 191
Septum, interatrial, aneurysm of, 368–369, *369*
    on transesophageal echocardiography, 76
    on transthoracic echocardiography, 34t, 38, 43
    interventricular. See also *Ventricular septal
        defects.*
    motion of, M-mode echocardiography of,
        122–123, *122, 123*
    on transthoracic echocardiography, 37, 41, 44,
        45
Shadowing, in color flow Doppler
    echocardiography, 23, 24t
Shunt, congenital, 397, *398*
    surgical, 419, 420t
Shunt ratio, 397, *398,* 425
Signal aliasing, in color flow Doppler
    echocardiography, 24, 24t, *25, 55*
    in pulsed Doppler echocardiography, *18, 19, 19,*
        22, 22t
Simpson's rule, for left systolic volume calculations,
    108
Single plane ellipsoid formula, for left systolic
    volume calculations, 107, *107*
Sinus of Valsalva, aneurysm of, 374, *374,* 386, *388,*
    402t, 405
Situs inversus, 398
Sound waves, 1–3, *2, 3*
Spatial peak pulse average, 27
Spatial peak temporal average intensity, 27
Specificity, of test, 79, 80
Spectral analysis, of Doppler echocardiography,
    16–17, *16*
Spontaneous contrast, prosthetic valves and, 319
    thrombus and, 369
Square-root sign, in pericardial constriction, 222, *223*

Stenosis. See *Valvular stenosis.*
Stiffness, ventricular, 134
Stress echocardiography, *91*
    in myocardial ischemia, 160–164, 160t, *161–164*
    indications for, 91–92, 91t
Stroke volume, in aortic valve regurgitation, 283
    in mitral valve regurgitation, 290, *291*
    in valvular regurgitation, 267, *267,* 272–273, *274*
Stroke work loss, in aortic stenosis, 240–241
Subaortic membrane, 400, 402t, *403*
    vs. aortic stenosis, *235*
Subcostal window, for transthoracic echocardiography, 44, *45*
Superior vena cava, left, persistent, *355,* 403t, 415–416
Suprasternal notch window, for transthoracic echocardiography, 44–45, *46*
Surgery, monitoring echocardiography in, 89–90
Systole, definition of, 101, *101*

T

Temperature, ultrasound-related increase in, 26
Testing zone, in clinical decision analysis, 81–82, *81*
Tetralogy of Fallot, 403t, 423, *423, 424*
Thermodilution cardiac output, 118
Three-dimensional echocardiography, 14–15
    indications for, *94, 95, 95*
Thrombus, left atrial, 355t, 363–365
    clinical implications of, 365
    echocardiography of, 363–365, *364, 365*
    on transesophageal echocardiography, 76
    predisposing factors for, 363
    transthoracic echocardiography in, 88t
    left ventricular, 355t, 361–363
    clinical implications of, 362–363
    echocardiography of, 362, 362t, *363*
    predisposing conditions for, 361–362
    transthoracic echocardiography in, 88t
    prosthetic valve and, 323–325, *325*
    right heart, 365–366, *366*
Tissue harmonic imaging, in two-dimensional echocardiography, 10, *11*
Tissue thermal index, 27
Transaortic pressure gradient, in aortic stenosis, 236–237, *236,* 237t, *238*
Transducer(s), 5–9, *5*
    axial resolution and, 7–8, 8t, *9*
    beam geometry of, 6–7, *6–8*
    elevational resolution and, 8t, *9*
    frequency of, 5
    grating lobes of, 7, *8*
    image resolution with, 7–9, 8t, *9*
    lateral resolution and, 8t, *9*
    piezoelectric crystal of, 5, *5*
    side lobes of, 7, *8*
    types of, 5–6, 6t
Transesophageal echocardiography, 59–77, 93–94, *94,* 94t
    esophageal position for, 61t, 62–68
        four-chamber plane in, 62–63, *62–64*

Transesophageal echocardiography *(Continued)*
        long-axis left ventricular plane in, 64–66, *65, 66*
        short-axis plane in, 67–68, *67*
        two-chamber plane in, 63, *64, 65*
    protocol for, 60
    risks of, 60, 60t
    technique for, 60–62, 61t
    transducer motions for, 61–62
    transgastric apical position for, 61t, 69, *70*
        four-chamber plane in, 69, *70*
        long-axis plane in, 69
    transgastric standard position for, 61t, 68–69
        short-axis plane in, 68–69, *68, 69*
        two-chamber plane in, 69, *69*
Transgastric apical position, transesophageal echocardiography, 61t, 69, *70*
    four-chamber plane in, 69, *70*
    long-axis plane in, 69
Transgastric standard position, transesophageal echocardiography, 61t, 68–69
    short-axis plane in, 68–69, *68, 69*
    two-chamber plane in, 69, *69*
Transit time effect, in Doppler echocardiography, 22t, 23
Transmitral pressure gradient, in mitral stenosis, 251, *251,* 254–255, *255*
Transmitral stroke volume, 116, *116*
Transplantation. See *Cardiac transplantation.*
Transposition of great vessels, 399, *399,* 423–424, *424*
Transthoracic echocardiography, 29–57
    anatomic terminology for, 33t
    apical window for, 42–44
        five-chamber view of, 43
        four-chamber view of, 42–43, *42, 43*
        long-axis view of, 44, *44*
        two-chamber view of, 43–44, *43*
    baseline, 89t, 90–91
    clinical prioritization for, 90t
    Doppler, 49–57. See also *Doppler echocardiography.*
    image interpretation in, 32–33, 33t
    image orientation for, 30–31
    image planes for, 30, *31*
    image quality in, 31–32
    indications for, 83–91
        by anatomic diagnosis, 85–85, 86t–88t
        by clinical setting, 85, 89–91, 89t
        by clinical signs and symptoms, 83–84, *83, 84,* 84t, 85t
        prioritization of, 90t
    M-mode, 46–48, *46–48*
    monitoring, 89–90, 89t
    nomenclature for, 30, 30t, *31, 32*
    parasternal window for, 33–34, 36–42
        long-axis view of, *32,* 33–34, 36–37, *36, 37*
        right ventricular inflow and outflow views of, 37–38, *37–39*
        short-axis views of, 39–42, *39–41*
    postintervention, 89t, 90
    preintervention, 89t, 90
    principles of, 29–33, 30t, *31, 32,* 33t

Transthoracic echocardiography *(Continued)*
  screening, 85, 89, 89t
  subcostal window for, 44, *45*
  suprasternal notch window for, 44–45, *46*
  transducer position for, 30, *32*. See also *specific windows.*
Tricuspid annulus, on transthoracic echocardiography, 42
Tricuspid regurgitant jet, in mitral stenosis, 256–257, *256*
  velocity of, 123–126, 124t, *125, 126,* 128
    vs. regurgitant volume, 128
Tricuspid regurgitation, 293–297
  carcinoid heart disease and, 293
  Ebstein's anomaly and, 293
  echocardiography in, 294–296, *295, 296*
    clinical utility of, 296–297
  endocarditis and, 293
  etiology of, 293
  in myocardial ischemia, 178
  in pulmonary heart disease, 207
  on color Doppler transthoracic echocardiography, 57
  on transesophageal Doppler echocardiography, 74, *75*
  pulmonary hypertension and, 293
  rheumatic, 293
  right atrial dilation in, 294–295
  right ventricular dilation in, 294–295
  severity of, 295–296, *295, 296*
    upstream flow reversal and, 272, *273*
Tricuspid stenosis, *260, 261, 261*
  mitral stenosis and, 257
  rheumatic, 257
Tricuspid valve, atresia of, 424, *424*
  Ebstein's anomaly of, 406–407, *407*
  on transesophageal Doppler echocardiography, 74, *75*
  on transesophageal echocardiography, 72t
  on transthoracic echocardiography, 34t, 37–38, *37, 38*
  on transthoracic M-mode recording, 48
  vegetations on, *325, 334, 335, 337, 337*
Tricuspid valve replacement. See also *Prosthetic valve(s).*
  endocarditis and, *323*
Truncus arteriosus, 425
Tumor. See *Cardiac tumor.*
Turbulence, 48
Two-dimensional echocardiography, 10–14
  acoustic shadowing with, 12, *12,* 12t
  beam width artifact with, 12t, *13,* 13–14
  depth control for, 11
  electronic processing artifacts with, 12t, 14
  gain control for, 11
  gray scale (dynamic range) control for, 11
  image generation by, 10, *11*
  image production by, 10, *11*
  imaging artifacts with, 11–14, *12–14,* 12t
  instrument setting for, 11
  instrument settings for, 11
  power output control for, 11

Two-dimensional echocardiography *(Continued)*
  range ambiguity with, 12t, 14
  refraction artifact with, 12t, 14, *14*
  reverberations with, 12–13, 12t, *13*
  suboptimal image quality with, 12, 12t
  time-gain compensation control for, 11
  tissue harmonic imaging in, 10, *11*

U

Ultrasound. See also *Echocardiography.*
  bioeffects of, 26
  intravascular, 95
  principles of, 1–4, *2, 3*
  safety of, 26–27
Ultrasound wave, 1–3, *2, 3*
  attenuation of, *3,* 4
  reflection of, 3–4, *3*
  refraction of, *3,* 4
  scattering of, *3,* 4
  tissue interaction of, 3–4, *3*

V

Valve resistance, in aortic stenosis, 240
Valvular regurgitation, 265–297. See also *specific types.*
  congenital, 396–397
  detection of, 267–268, *268*
  Doppler detection of, 267–268
  etiology of, 266, 275
  fluid dynamics of, 266–267, *266,* 266t
  forward stroke volume in, 267, *267*
  in endocarditis, *325, 338, 338*
  in normal individuals, 268–269
  left ventricular size and, 275–276
  left ventricular systolic function in, 177t, 178
  physiologic, 268, *268*
  proximal isovelocity surface area in, 266, *266,* 273–275, *274*
  regurgitant jet momentum in, 275
  regurgitant stroke volume in, 267, *267*
  severity of, 269–275, 269t, 276–277, 277t
    color M-mode Doppler for, 270–271, *271,* 276, 277t
    continuous-wave Doppler for, 271–272, *272,* 276, 277t
    Doppler flow mapping for, 269–271, *270, 271*
    jet momentum and, 275
    proximal isovelocity surface area and, 273–275, *274*
    stroke volume and, 272–273, *274,* 276–277, 277t
    upstream flow reversal and, 272, *273*
  stroke volume in, 267, *267,* 272–275, *274*
  systolic function and, 276
  transthoracic echocardiography in, 86t
  volume overload in, 267, *267*
  with prosthetic valve, 315–318, *316–318,* 322, *324*
Valvular stenosis, 229–261. See also *specific types.*
  distal flow disturbance of, 231
  fluid dynamics of, 230–232, *230–232*

Valvular stenosis *(Continued)*
  high-velocity jet of, 230, *230, 231*
  pressure gradient of, 230–231
  proximal flow patterns of, 231–232, *232*
  stroke volume in, 232
Vegetations, 330–337, *331,* 332t, *333–337,* 337t, 353, 355t
Velocity ratio, in aortic stenosis, 239–240
Velocity underestimation, in Doppler echocardiography, 22, 22t
Velocity-pressure relationship, in Doppler echocardiography, 49
Venous catheters, microbubbles with, 366
Ventilation-perfusion scan, in pulmonary heart disease, 208
Ventricle, 398–399, 398t
  left, 398–399, 398t. See also at *Left ventricular.*
    dimensions of, 35t, 110–111
    ejection fraction of, 103
    end-diastolic volume of, 103
    end-systolic volume of, 103
    fractional shortening of, 104
    geometry of, 102–103
    inflow velocities of, 50t, 51t
      on color Doppler transthoracic echocardiography, 56, *56*
      on transthoracic Doppler echocardiography, 53–54, *53*
    mass of, 104, 108–110, *110*
    on transesophageal echocardiography, 70–72, *73, 75,* 75t, *76*
    on transthoracic echocardiography, 34t, 41, 42, 44, *45*
    on transthoracic M-mode echocardiography, 47, *48*
    outflow velocities of, 50t, 51t
      on color Doppler transthoracic echocardiography, 56
      on transthoracic Doppler echocardiography, 51–53, *52,* 54–55, *55*
    relative wall thickness of, 104
    rupture of, after myocardial infarction, 174–175, *175, 176*
  right, 398–399, 398t. See also at *Right ventricular.*
    atrialized, 293
    dilation of, 120–121
    dimensions of, 35t
    inflow velocities of, 50t, 51t
      on color Doppler transthoracic echocardiography, 56
      on transthoracic Doppler echocardiography, 54
    interior of, *39*
Ventricle *(Continued)*
    on transesophageal Doppler echocardiography, 72, 74, *74, 75*
    on transesophageal echocardiography, 75t, 77
    on transthoracic echocardiography, 34t, 37–38, *37, 38,* 42
    outflow velocities of, 50t, 51t
      on color Doppler transthoracic echocardiography, *56*
      on transthoracic Doppler echocardiography, 53
    shape of, 120
Ventricular compliance, 134, *135*
  left ventricular filling and, 144
Ventricular diastolic filling (volume) curves, 134–135
Ventricular diastolic function, 133–136. See also *Left ventricular diastolic function; Right ventricular diastolic function.*
  atrial pressures and, 135–136, *136*
  dysfunction of, 136
  respiration and, 136
  ventricular compliance and, 134, *135*
  ventricular diastolic filling curves and, 134–135
  ventricular diastolic pressures and, 134
  ventricular relaxation and, 134, *134*
Ventricular end-diastolic pressure, 134
Ventricular hypertrophy, in hypertensive heart disease, 200, 200t, *201*
Ventricular inversion, 403t, 414–415, *419*
Ventricular septal defects, 397, 403t, 411–414, *415*
  after myocardial infarction, 173–174, *174, 175*
  anatomy of, 411–412, *415*
  closure of, 420t
  Doppler echocardiography of, 413–414
  left-to-right shunt and, 412–413, *417*
  two-dimensional echocardiography of, 412–413, *416, 417*
Ventricular systolic function. See also *Left ventricular systolic function; Right ventricular systolic function.*
  exercise effect on, 103
  physiology of, 101–102, *102*
Ventriculography, radionuclide, for left ventricular systolic function, 118–119, *120*
  in congenital heart disease, 426t
Video recording devices, 25
Volume flow, in Doppler echocardiography, 49

W

Wavelength, 2–3, *2*